Biomedical Computing for Breast Cancer Detection and Diagnosis

Wellington Pinheiro dos Santos
Universidade Federal de Pernambuco, Brazil

Washington Wagner Azevedo da Silva
Universidade Federal de Pernambuco, Brazil

Maira Araujo de Santana
Universidade Federal de Pernambuco, Brazil

IGI Global
PUBLISHER of TIMELY KNOWLEDGE

A volume in the Advances in Bioinformatics and Biomedical Engineering (ABBE) Book Series

Published in the United States of America by
IGI Global
Medical Information Science Reference (an imprint of IGI Global)
701 E. Chocolate Avenue
Hershey PA, USA 17033
Tel: 717-533-8845
Fax: 717-533-8661
E-mail: cust@igi-global.com
Web site: http://www.igi-global.com

Library of Congress Cataloging-in-Publication Data

Names: Santos, Wellington Pinheiro dos, editor. | Silva, Washington Wagner Azevedo da, 1979- editor. | Santana, Maira Araujo de, 1995- editor.
Title: Biomedical computing for breast cancer detection and diagnosis / Wellington Pinheiro dos Santos, Washington Wagner Azevedo da Silva, and Maira Araujo de Santana, editors.
Description: Hershey, PA : Medical Information Science Reference, [2020] | Includes bibliographical references and index. | Summary: "This book presents a review of the physiology and anatomy of the breast; the dynamics of breast cancer; principles of pattern recognition, artificial neural networks, and computer graphics; and the breast imaging techniques and computational methods to support and optimize the diagnosis"-- Provided by publisher.
Identifiers: LCCN 2019056381 (print) | LCCN 2019056382 (ebook) | ISBN 9781799834564 (hardcover) | ISBN 9781799834571 (ebook)
Subjects: MESH: Breast Neoplasms--diagnosis | Diagnosis, Computer-Assisted
Classification: LCC RC280.B8 (print) | LCC RC280.B8 (ebook) | NLM WP 870 | DDC 616.99/449075--dc23
LC record available at https://lccn.loc.gov/2019056381
LC ebook record available at https://lccn.loc.gov/2019056382

This book is published in the IGI Global book series Advances in Bioinformatics and Biomedical Engineering (ABBE) (ISSN: 2327-7033; eISSN: 2327-7041)

British Cataloguing in Publication Data
A Cataloguing in Publication record for this book is available from the British Library.

Advances in Bioinformatics and Biomedical Engineering (ABBE) Book Series

Ahmad Taher Azar
Prince Sultan University, Riyadh, Kingdom of Saudi Arabi
and Benha University, Egypt

ISSN:2327-7033
EISSN:2327-7041

Mission

The fields of biology and medicine are constantly changing as research evolves and novel engineering applications and methods of data analysis are developed. Continued research in the areas of bioinformatics and biomedical engineering is essential to continuing to advance the available knowledge and tools available to medical and healthcare professionals.

The **Advances in Bioinformatics and Biomedical Engineering (ABBE) Book Series** publishes research on all areas of bioinformatics and bioengineering including the development and testing of new computational methods, the management and analysis of biological data, and the implementation of novel engineering applications in all areas of medicine and biology. Through showcasing the latest in bioinformatics and biomedical engineering research, ABBE aims to be an essential resource for healthcare and medical professionals.

Coverage

- Genomics
- Finite Elements
- Biomedical Sensors
- Tissue Engineering
- Dental Engineering
- Robotics and Medicine
- Algorithms
- Structural Biology
- Prosthetic Limbs
- Rehabilitation Engineering

IGI Global is currently accepting manuscripts for publication within this series. To submit a proposal for a volume in this series, please contact our Acquisition Editors at Acquisitions@igi-global.com or visit: http://www.igi-global.com/publish/.

The Advances in Bioinformatics and Biomedical Engineering (ABBE) Book Series (ISSN 2327-7033) is published by IGI Global, 701 E. Chocolate Avenue, Hershey, PA 17033-1240, USA, www.igi-global.com. This series is composed of titles available for purchase individually; each title is edited to be contextually exclusive from any other title within the series. For pricing and ordering information please visit http://www.igi-global.com/book-series/advances-bioinformatics-biomedical-engineering/73671. Postmaster: Send all address changes to above address.

Titles in this Series

For a list of additional titles in this series, please visit: http://www.igi-global.com/book-series/advances-bioinformatics-biomedical-engineering/73671

Deep Neural Networks for Multimodal Imaging and Biomedical Applications
Annamalai Suresh (Anna University, India) R. Udendhran (Bharathidasan University, India) and S. Vimal (Anna University, ndia)
Medical Information Science Reference • © 2020 • 300pp • H/C (ISBN: 9781799835912) • US $275.00

Biomedical and Clinical Engineering for Healthcare Advancement
N. Sriraam (Ramaiah Institute of Technology, India)
Medical Information Science Reference • © 2020 • 275pp • H/C (ISBN: 9781799803263) • US $285.00

Attractors and Higher Dimensions in Population and Molecular Biology Emerging Research and Opportunities
Gennadiy Vladimirovich Zhizhin (Russian Academy of Natural Sciences, Russia)
Engineering Science Reference • © 2019 • 232pp • H/C (ISBN: 9781522596516) • US $165.00

Computational Models for Biomedical Reasoning and Problem Solving
Chung-Hao Chen (Old Dominion University, USA) and Sen-Ching Samson Cheung (University of Kentucky, USA)
Medical Information Science Reference • © 2019 • 353pp • H/C (ISBN: 9781522574675) • US $275.00

Medical Data Security for Bioengineers
Butta Singh (Guru Nanak Dev University, India) Barjinder Singh Saini (Dr. B. R. Ambedkar National Institute of Technology, India) Dilbag Singh (Dr. B. R. Ambedkar National Institute of Technology, India) and Anukul Pandey (Dumka Engineering College, India)
Medical Information Science Reference • © 2019 • 340pp • H/C (ISBN: 9781522579526) • US $365.00

Examining the Causal Relationship Between Genes, Epigenetics, and Human Health
Oscar J. Wambuguh (California State University – East Bay, USA)
Medical Information Science Reference • © 2019 • 603pp • H/C (ISBN: 9781522580669) • US $295.00

Expert System Techniques in Biomedical Science Practice
Prasant Kumar Pattnaik (KIIT University (Deemed), India) Aleena Swetapadma (KIIT University, India) and Jay Sarraf (KIIT University, India)
Medical Information Science Reference • © 2018 • 280pp • H/C (ISBN: 9781522551492) • US $205.00

IGI Global
PUBLISHER of TIMELY KNOWLEDGE

701 East Chocolate Avenue, Hershey, PA 17033, USA
Tel: 717-533-8845 x100 • Fax: 717-533-8661
E-Mail: cust@igi-global.com • www.igi-global.com

Editorial Advisory Board

Table of Contents

Detailed Table of Contents

This chapter explores several steps of the thermal breast exams analysis process in detecting breast abnormality and evaluating the response of pre-surgical treatment. Topics concerning the process of acquiring, storing, and preprocessing these exams, including a novel segmentation proposal that uses collective intelligence techniques, will be discussed. In addition, various approaches to calculating statistical and geometric descriptors from thermal breast examinations are also considered of this chapter. These descriptors can be used at different stages of the analysis process of these exams. In this sense, two experiments will be presented. The first one explores the use of genetic algorithms in the feature selection process. The second conducts a preliminary study that intends to analyze some descriptors, already used in other works, in the process of evaluating preoperative treatment response. This evaluation is of fundamental importance since the response is directly associated with the prognosis of the disease.

Breast cancer, which is the second-most common and leading cause of cancer death among women, has witnessed growing interest in the two last decades. Fortunately, its early detection is the most effective way to detect and diagnose breast cancer. Although mammography is the gold standard for screening, its difficult interpretation leads to an increase in missed cancers and misinterpreted non-cancerous lesion rates. Therefore, computer-aided diagnosis (CAD) systems can be a great helpful tool for assisting radiologists in mammogram interpretation. Nonetheless, these systems are limited by their black-box outputs, which decreases the radiologists' confidence. To circumvent this limit, content-based mammogram retrieval (CBMR) is used as an alternative to traditional CAD systems. Herein, authors systematically review the state-of-the-art on mammography-based breast cancer CAD methods, while focusing on recent advances in CBMR methods. In order to have a complete review, mammography imaging principles and its correlation with breast anatomy are also discussed.

the designation of breast cancer is sensitivity limitation. To overcome this limitation, complementary imaging examinations are used that historically include screening, ultrasound, MRI, etc.

Applications that have already been developed on using infrared (IR) imaging are proposed for a better understanding of breast cancer analysis. The first part of this chapter presents the use of interval data to classify breast abnormalities. Authors have been adapting machine learning techniques to work with interval variables that can handle the intrinsic variation of data. The second part evaluates segmentation techniques applied to breast IR images. Many authors use automatic image segmentation techniques that must consider the natural anatomical variation between people. Manual segmentation techniques can be used to minimize the problem of anatomical variations. The main purpose of such techniques is to seek to avoid the errors due to the natural asymmetry of the human body. A process that uses ellipsoidal elements to represent each breast has been chosen. The manual technique is more precise and can correct possible failures presented in the automatic method. Validation of each segmentation type was also included by using Jaccard, DICE, False Positive, and False Negative methods.

In this chapter, computational tools that have been designed to analyze and classify infrared (IR) images will be presented. The function of such tools is to interconnect in a user-friendly way the algorithms that are used to map temperatures and to classify some breast pathologies. One of these performs texture mapping using IR breast images to relate temperatures measured to the points over the substitute tridimensional geometry mesh. Another computer-aided diagnosis (CAD) tool was adapted so that it could be used to evaluate individual patients. This methodology will be used when the computational framework approach for classification is described. Finally, graphical interfaces and their functionalities will be presented and explained. Some case studies will be presented in order to verify whether or not the computational classification framework is effective.

In this chapter, procedures for and applications of using infrared (IR) imaging that have been developed will be presented and proposed means by which a better detailed understanding of breast cancer can be reached. It will be shown how such applications can be used as a basis for enhancing the use of breast thermographic imaging as a user-friendly and inexpensive tool for the early detection of breast cancer. The authors intend to show that IR imaging can also be used to validate temperature profiles that have been calculated and to classify breast abnormalities as set out in previous chapters. IR images can also be used to estimate thermophysical properties of the breast, and discussion of how this is done is included. The IR images were acquired at the Outpatients Clinic of Mastology of the Hospital das Clínicas of the Federal University of Pernambuco (HC/UFPE). The research project was registered in the Brazilian Health Ministry (CEP/CCS/UFPE nº 279/05) after being approved by the Ethics Committee of UFPE.

In this chapter, deep learning-based approaches, namely deep feature extraction, fine-tuning of pre-trained convolutional neural networks (CNN), and end-to-end training of a developed CNN model, are used to classify the malignant and normal breast X-ray images. For deep feature extraction, pre-trained deep CNN models such as ResNet18, ResNet50, ResNet101, VGG16, and VGG19 are used. For classification of the deep features, the support vector machines (SVM) classifier is used with various kernel functions namely linear, quadratic, cubic, and Gaussian, respectively. The aforementioned pre-trained deep CNN models are also used in fine-tuning procedure. A new CNN model is also proposed in end-to-end training fashion. The classification accuracy is used as performance measurements. The experimental works show that the deep learning has potential in detection of the breast cancer from the X-ray images. The deep features that are extracted from the ResNet50 model and SVM classifier with linear kernel function produced 94.7% accuracy score which the highest among all obtained.

Foreword

A good research book on recent advances on Biomedical image processing techniques for Breast Cancer Detection and Diagnosis has been long overdue. This book, *Biomedical Computing for Breast Cancer Detection and Diagnosis* by Professor Wellington Pinheiro dos Santos, amply fills the void. The primary difficulty lies in addressing a very diverse set of topics and also in the different backgrounds of the potential readership. This book dealt with both. This book aims to disseminate timely to the scientific community the recent developments in Biomedical image processing techniques spanning from theoretical frameworks, algorithmic developments, to a variety of applications. The book covers advance in Breast cancer detection methods, especially those developed recently, offering academic researchers and practitioners a comprehensive update about the new development in this field. The book provides a forum for researchers to exchange their ideas, and to foster a better understanding of the state of the art of the subject. I envisage that the publication of this book will motivate new ideas and more cutting edge research activities in this area.

The book is organized into seventeen chapters. The chapters ranging from recent developments in theories, algorithms, and extensions of Breast cancer detection processes to classification of breast abnormalities and breast thermography processes. The book also focuses on low cost hardware implementation of impedance tomography to development of novel intelligence techniques for breast lesions. Finally, the book also covers current trends and future directions of breast cancer detection and classification systems.

I find this edited volume to be an excellent resource for undergraduate, postgraduate as well as other researchers working in various Biomedical image processing methods, especially on Breast cancer image processing research. I recommend it fully to everyone interested in Biomedical Image Processing research.

Ganesh R. Naik
MARCS Institute for Brain, Behaviour, and Development, Western Sydney University, Australia
March 2020

Preface

BIOMEDICAL COMPUTING, EARLY CANCER DIAGNOSIS, AND THE CHAMBER OF SECRETS

"Harry couldn't explain, even to himself, why he didn't just throw Riddle's diary away. The fact was that even though he knew the diary was blank, he kept absentmindedly picking it up and turning the pages, as though it were a story he wanted to finish. And while Harry was sure he had never heard the name T. M. Riddle before, it still seemed to mean something to him, almost as though Riddle was a friend he'd had when he was very small, and had half forgotten. But this was absurd. He'd never had friends before Hogwarts, Dudley had made sure of that.

Nevertheless, Harry was determined to find out more about Riddle, so next day at break, he headed for the trophy room to examine Riddle's special award, accompanied by an interested Hermione and a thoroughly unconvinced Ron, who told them he'd seen enough of the trophy room to last him a lifetime."

("The very secret diary", chapter of "Harry Potter and the Chamber of Secrets", 1998, by J. K. Rowling)

We are convinced diagnosis can be a deep investigative process, complex by nature. When we face the complexity of diagnosing difficult diseases, specially the several forms of cancer, we are frequently challenged to use not only the considerably large set of available technologies but, like Harry Potter facing the deep secrets of Tom Riddle's diary in J. K. Rowling's book, *Harry Potter and the Chamber of Secrets*, intuition, courage and direct action. Regarding the available technologies, the diagnostic processes have becoming much more multidisciplinary, demanding the use of an eclectic set of technological methodologies and tools, specially from the Fourth Revolution. Biosensors, Artificial Intelligence, Internet of Things, and 3D Printing have becoming common terms in health research.

From the several fields of Biomedical Engineering, Biomedical Computing has suffering the most accelerated development due to the advent of the Fourth Revolution. The intense progress of Artificial Intelligence and Internet of Things has been pushing the field forward with a plethora of contributions in Computer Science for the comprehension of several disease dynamics, bioinformatics and early diagnosis. Biomedical Computing is a rich field, combining the diagnostic and investigative aspects of Biology and Medicine and the discipline of Biomedical Engineering with the power and problem-solving capabilities of modern Computer Science. Computer tools are used to accelerate research learning, simulate patient behavior and visualize complex biological models. Several tools have been developed to promote early diagnosis and treatment, specially for complex diseases like neurodegenerative diseases and all forms of cancer.

Despite the good prognosis when diagnosed early, breast cancer is one of the most fatal forms of cancer for women. Breast cancer can target all women, regardless of social class. The availability of effective methods for the detection and classification of breast lesions can determine mortality. Imaging diagnosis is still one of the most efficient ways to detect early breast changes, among the techniques most used is mammography. However, there are other techniques that have emerged as alternatives or even complementary tests in the early detection of breast lesions, e.g. breast thermography and electrical impedance tomography. Artificial Intelligence can be used to optimize image diagnosis, increasing the reliability of the reports and supporting professionals who do not have enough knowledge or experience to make good diagnoses. In this book we propose to present a review of the physiology and anatomy of the breast; the dynamics of breast cancer; principles of pattern recognition, artificial neural networks and computer graphics; and the breast imaging techniques and computational methods to support and optimize the diagnosis.

Cancer in all its forms has become one of the biggest public health issues of the twentieth century. This phenomenon has been happening worldwide, regardless of the levels of social and economic development of the different nations. Of all types of cancer, breast cancer is the most dangerous for older and middle-aged women, also being the most common form of cancer among female population (Groot et al., 2006).

Breast cancer is among the five most common cancers worldwide. This disease has been proliferating in both developed and underdeveloped and developing countries. Its incidence rate is increasing with the average life expectancy of the population, and with the adoption of new forms of consumption (Groot et al., 2006; Shrivastava et al., 2017).

Nowadays, there are some preventive strategies for breast cancer, such as stimulating visual inspection and touching of the breasts. However, they are not efficient enough to impact breast cancer mortality rate, since the disease is still being late diagnosed in many cases (Groot et al., 2006). For this reason, there is a need to invest in tools for a deeper understanding of the disease, its risk factors, and strategies for early identification and efficient treatment. The existence and availability of these tools in healthcare systems is important, since they may contribute to increase the chances of cure and the treatment options, decreasing mortality rates. Some of these strategies are presented in this book.

This book is intended for academics, graduate and postgraduate students in Medicine, Biomedicine, Biomedical Engineering, Computer Science, and whom interested in Biomedical Computing and breast cancer diagnosis applications.

The first chapter, which is called "Prototype of a Low-Cost Impedance Tomography Based on the Open-Hardware Paradigm", Ribeiro et al. present the main procedures to create a prototype of a data acquisition system based on Electrical Impedance Tomography (EIT). This device plays an important role in the development of a complete and portable EIT equipment to be used, among other things, in the acquisition of breast images.

In the chapter "Using Extreme Learning Machines and the Backprojection Algorithm as an Alternative to Reconstruct Electrical Impedance Tomography Images", Gomes et al. propose an innovative method for image reconstruction applied to create EIT images. Their hybrid method is based on extreme learning machines and backprojection and showed promising results to be applied in breast imaging.

The chapter "Classification of Breast Lesions in Frontal Thermographic Images Using a Diagnosis Aid Intelligent System", from Santana et al., used different configuration of Extreme Learning Machines to provide breast lesion differentiation. They also chose to use the moments of Haralick and Zernike to describe the images. Using some configuration, they achieved accuracies up to 95%.

In "Feature Selection Based on Dialectical Optimization Algorithm for Breast Lesion Classification in Thermographic Images", Pereira et al. propose a features selection method using Dialectical Optimization Method (ODM) combined to a KNN classifier. This innovative approach reduced in more than 40% the amount of features used to represent thermographic images.

In "Computer Techniques for Detection of Breast Cancer and Follow up Neoadjuvant Treatment: Using Infrared Examinations", Araujo et al. propose the use of infrared technique to measure the evolution of the clinical condition of a patient, who was already diagnosed with breast cancer and is now in the neoadjuvant treatment phase. The authors believe that geometry related features and statistical features play an important role in describing those images, in order to provide useful information to the system.

Baâzaoui and Barhoumi, in "Breast Cancer Diagnosis with Mammography: Recent Advances on CBMR-Based CAD System", point out a broad overview regarding to CBMR-based CAD systems applied to breast cancer diagnosis. They review some important concepts about breast cancer screening. The authors also discuss how some of the most recent technologies may improve diagnosis accuracy.

In the chapter "The Evolution of New Trends in Breast Thermography", Araújo et al. introduce the theoretical foundations of Infrared Radiation Theory and the principles of the infrared imaging technique.

In "Thermography in Biomedicine: History and Breakthrough", written by Nola and Kolarić, talks about the main historical progresses in thermography development and their relation to thermography breakthrough in some of most interested area of biomedicine, especially breast cancer detection.

The chapter "Imaging Techniques for Breast Cancer Diagnosis", written by Saha, Vaishnav and Jha, brings a discussion regarding to the role of imaging techniques in breast cancer screening. They provide a broad overview about the history of imaging in cancer management, such as point out some new perspectives for the early future in this field of study.

In "Applications of the Use of Infrared Breast Images: Segmentation and Classification of Breast Abnormalities", Araújo et al. provide some statistical based tools to perform segmentation and classification of abnormalities in breast infrared images.

In "Developing and Using Computational Frameworks to Conduct Numerical Analysis and Calculate Temperature Profiles and to Classify Breast Abnormalities", Queiroz et al. present computational tools to assess and classify infrared images. The authors designed these tools in order to implement them in a user-friendly framework to map temperatures and classify some breast pathologies.

In "Applications of the Use of Infrared Breast Images: Numerical Calculations of Temperature Profile and Estimates of Thermophysical Properties", by Bezerra et al., presents procedures for and applications of using infrared imaging. The authors show how these applications can be used as a basis for enhancing the use of breast thermographic imaging as a user-friendly and inexpensive tool for the early detection of breast cancer. They also intend to demonstrate that infrared imaging can be used to validate temperature profiles and to classify breast abnormalities.

In "The Efforts of Deep Learning Approaches for Breast Cancer Detection Based on X-Ray Images", Ismael and Gomes present deep learning-based approaches for deep feature extraction, fine-tuning of pre-trained convolutional neural networks (CNN) and end-to-end training of a developed CNN model to classify the malignant and normal breast X-ray images. For deep feature extraction, pre-trained deep CNN models such as ResNet18, ResNet50, ResNet101, VGG16 and VGG19 are used. For classification of the deep features, the support vector machines (SVM) classifier is used with various kernel functions namely linear, quadratic, cubic and Gaussian, respectively. The aforementioned pre-trained deep CNN models are also used in fine-tuning procedure. A new CNN model is also proposed in end-to-end training fashion. The experimental results point evidences of the potential of deep learning in detection of the breast cancer from the X-ray images.

We hope that the work presented in this collection will show some of the new trends on computational techniques based on the Fourth Industrial Revolution to support the detection and the diagnosis of breast cancer.

Enjoy your reading!

Wellington Pinheiro dos Santos

Maíra Araújo de Santana
June 2, 2020
Recife, Brazil

REFERENCES

Groot, M. T., Baltussen, R., Uyl-de Groot, C. A., Anderson, B. O., & Hortobágyi, G. N. (2006). Costs and health effects of breast cancer interventions in epidemiologically different regions of Africa, North America, and Asia. *The Breast Journal*, *12*(s1), S81–S90. doi:10.1111/j.1075-122X.2006.00206.x PMID:16430401

Shrivastava, S. R., Shrivastava, P. S., & Jegadeesh, R. (2017). Ensuring early detection of cancer in low- and middle-income nations: World health organization. *Archives of Medicine and Health Sciences*, *5*(1), 141.

Acknowledgment

We are grateful to our families, friends, and colleagues from the Research Group of Biomedical Computing of the Federal University of Pernambuco, Recife, Brazil, for their support in several stages of this work, especially for the elaboration of the chapters on the use of machine learning to aid breast cancer diagnosis.

We would like to thank the Brazilian research agencies CAPES, CNPq, and FACEPE, for the partial support on some of the researches presented in this book.

Last but not least, we also thank the authors for their kind contributions for this collection.

Chapter 1
Prototype of a Low-Cost Impedance Tomography Based on the Open-Hardware Paradigm

David Edson Ribeiro
Universidade Federal de Pernambuco, Brazil

Valter Augusto de Freitas Barbosa
Universidade Federal de Pernambuco, Brazil

Clarisse Lins de Lima
Universidade Federal de Pernambuco, Brazil

Ricardo Emmanuel de Souza
Universidade Federal de Pernambuco, Brazil

Wellington Pinheiro dos Santos
https://orcid.org/0000-0003-2558-6602
Universidade Federal de Pernambuco, Brazil

ABSTRACT

Electrical Impedance Tomography (EIT) is a noninvasive, painless, and ionizing radiation-free technique for image acquisition of a region of interest. It is performed through electrical parameters. The method is based on the application of an alternating electric current pattern of low intensity through electrodes arranged around the surface region in order to obtain the image and also to measure the excitation electrical potentials. The aim of this study is to develop a device based in open hardware. Furthermore, the authors aim to build a prototype of a data acquisition system based on EIT. This device is the first step to obtain a complete and portable tomography equipment at a low cost.

DOI: 10.4018/978-1-7998-3456-4.ch001

INTRODUCTION

Electrical Impedance Tomography (EIT) is a noninvasive and nonionizing technology for tomographic imaging. It is based on the application of a low amplitude, high frequency, alternating electric current pattern through electrodes (Tehrani, Jin, Mcewan & Schaik, 2010). These electrodes are arranged around the surface of the body section and the resulting potential in the electrodes is, then, measured. EIT images are the computational reconstruction of the estimated mapping of electrical conductivity or permittivity within the body section, calculated from the relationship between excitation data and response data. This imaging technique is starting to be used in the process of breast cancer diagnosis.

Breast cancer is the type of cancer that most affects women in the world (Walker & Kaczor, 2012;). The best strategy to fight this disease is still the early detection of the tumor. In other words, the best way to decrease the fatality rate associated to breast cancer is detecting it in early stages (Zou & Guo, 2003). As highlighted by Zou & Guo (2003), there is evidence that malignant tumors have lower electrical impedance value than neighboring tissues. Following from this premise, some studies have been pursued to evaluate if the EIT can be applied as a breast cancer detection method. Cherepenin et al. (2001) performed 3-D breast images to detect breast cancer through a planar array of electrodes arranged in a square shape. In 2002, he did the same procedure using a circular matrix (Cherepenin et al., 2002). Comparing his approaches, the circular matrix is more adequate rather than the square matrix because the electrodes on the square corners have low contact with the breast. This fact results in blurs on the reconstructed image corners, therefore, the central region of the image is the only region appropriate for analysis. The three-dimensional image of the breast is made from several images made in different slices at different distances from the electrode matrix (Cherepenin et al., 2001; Cherepenin et al., 2002). When applied to breast images, some authors also call the technique Electrical Impedance Mammography (EIM) (Trokhanova, Okhapkin, & Korjenevsky, 2008; Huber et al., 2010; Zhang, Wang, Sze, Barber, & Chatwin, 2014). Currently, the most widely accepted technique for early detection of breast cancer is mammography, which is a method that uses ionizing radiation and causes discomfort to the patient. So, in this case, EIT is a promising method, mostly because it is noninvasive and free of ionizing radiation.

In the medical field, EIT has several other applications, such as monitoring mechanical pulmonary ventilation in intensive care patients (Alves, Amato, Terra, Vargas, Caruso, 2014). In this case, the treatment efficiency is usually measured by blood tests. From samples taken throughout the day that evaluate the amount of oxygen and carbon dioxide present in the blood. With the use of EIT, it is possible to monitor the volume of injected air in real time. Furthermore, EIT can also be used to detect pulmonary embolism or blood clots in the lungs (Cheney, Isaacson, & Newell, 1999; Adler et al., 2009), to help in the prostate cancer detection (Wan et al., 2013), to monitor cardiac activity and blood flow in the heart (Eyuboglu, Brown, Barber & Seager, 1987). It can also be used to perform functional images of brain activity (Bayford, 2006) and to detect subdural hematomas (Dai et al., 2013). Besides the medical field, EIT also excels in geophysical and industrial applications. In geophysics, electrical impedance tomography is also known as electrical resistivity tomography (ERT) (Bouchette, Church, Mcfee, & Adler, 2014). Among its applications in geophysics, EIT can be used to find underground storage of minerals and different geological formations (Cheney, Isaacson, & Newell, 1999). It can help to detect buried objects and anti-tank mines in different soil types, especially for wet and submerged soils, where other mine detectors perform poorly (Church, Mcfee, Gagnon, & Wort, 2006; Bouchette et al., 2014). It can also be used to monitor in situ remediation processes for the removal of volatile organic compounds in groundwater or soil (Daily & Ramirez, 1995). In the industry field, EIT can be used to monitor biphasic or multiphase flows in pipes (Rolnik & Seleghim, 2006). According to Dong, Xu, Hua, and Wang (2006), besides the conductivity images, it is possible to estimate fluid flow rate and to measure some flow parameters. For example, it is possible to measure void fraction disperse phase, to investigate solid-liquid filtration processes, to measure the distribution of angular velocity in the mixture of miscible liquids. Hence, EIT is appropriate to monitor various types of biphasic flows such as gas-liquid. In this case, the liquid is the continuous phase and the gas is the dispersed phase (Dong et al., 2006), the oil-gas of the oil industry, the system gas-solid pneumatic conveying equipment (Huang, Wang, & Li, 2003). Other applications of EIT in the industry are: the imaging of the nylon polymerization process at elevated temperatures and pressures (Dyakowski et al., 2000), the leak detection in buried pipes (Jordana; Gasulla; Pallás-Areny, 1999), the monitoring of drug release in solution as a function of time (in this example the relationship between drug concentration and solution conductivity is explored) (Rimpiläinen et al., 2010).

Other techniques for medical imaging such as magnetic resonance imaging, ultrasound and computed tomography have a higher speed of reconstruction and image resolution with higher quality. However, the EIT does not use ionizing radiation, thus its harmless to the patient. Additionally, the associated low implementation cost and the small dimensions of the equipment, avoids the removal of the patient from his bed for the exam which makes this technique very promising to replace some existing technologies.

The EIT technique consists in the solution of the direct and the inverse problems (Tehrani et al., 2010; Kumar, Sriraam, Benakop, Jinaga, 2010). The direct problem is to determine the electrical potentials within the body section and the potentials measured at its contour from the current excitation pattern. This relationship is given by the Poisson Equation (Hua, Woo, Webster, & Tompkins, 1993; Barbosa et al., 2017; Santos et al., 2018). The estimation of the conductivity distribution and electrical permittivity of the interior of the body section from the measurements of the response to the electrical excitation is mathematically, an inverse, nonlinear and poorly conditioned problem (Yorkey, Webster, & Tompkins, 1987; Rolnik & Seleghim, 2006; Kumar et al., 2010). Because, the solution for the distribution of conductivities and permissivities may not be unique and unstable. Also, it has great sensitivity to numerical errors and experimental noise (Yorkey, Webster, & Tompkins, 1987; Rolnik & Seleghim, 2006). These characteristics make their solution very dependent on the reconstruction and regularization algorithm and can be obtained through non-iterative (linear) and interactive (nonlinear) methods.

Reconstruction methods based on computational intelligence have also been widely used in the state of the art (Adler, Lionheart, 2006; Liu, Sun, 2011; Price et al., 2006; Feitosa et al., 2014a; Feitosa et al., 2014b; Barbosa et al., 2017; Barbosa et al., 2018; Santos et al., 2018; Ribeiro et al., 2014a; Ribeiro et al., 2014b; Ribeiro et al., 2014c).

The proposal is to build a low-cost electrical impedance tomography using a project partitioning strategy. The data acquisition and conditioning system will be developed to preprocess and transfer the electrical potentials, from the edge of the area to be imaged to a computer, then performing image reconstruction with the proper reconstruction algorithms.

RELATED WORKS

The study of electrical impedance tomography for medical applications began in the 1980s. The pioneer related work is described in Brown, Barber & Seagar (1985), from Sheffield University Department of Medical Physics and Clinical Engineering (UK). The article brought the first images of EIT in humans. Also, it brought the use of 32 or 16 electrodes arranged in adjacent pairs. Its main importance was, however, the study of the biological tissue resistivity which is described in Table 1. Additionally, it showed that the reading and collection of the data took a very short time, 100 ms, and the time taken to generate the image relies in the data processing by the reconstruction software.

Table 1. Biological tissues resistivity values.

Tissue	Resistivity (Ωm)
Cerebrospinal fluid	0.65
Blood	1.5
Cardiac muscle	4.24
Neural tissue	5.8
Lung	7.2-23.6

Source: The authors

Since one of the fundamental steps for a good implementation of the EIT is the good quality of the data reading. Garcia, Souza & Pina (2013) brought in their work greater care with the hardware, so that the signal was treated before being sent to the reconstruction software. They used the PCI 6251 card, which features an A/D conversion capability, a sinusoidal current - with frequency of 50 kHz and amplitude of 1 mA - and a voltage to current converter based on OTA CA3080. This was possible through a PCI bus, a control through Labview software and the use of evolutionary and non-evolutionary algorithms. The evolutionary algorithms give more accurate results, but with more computational cost. In contrast, the non-evolutionary algorithms present opposite behavior.

The reading of the electrode pairs through multiplexers proposed in Bera et al. (2011), as well as the use of EIDORS, allows changes of techniques in their code. It also allows free modification using Gauss-Newton and Newton Modified Raphson algorithms (Vauhkonen, Lionheart, Heikkinen, Vauhkonen, & Kaipio, 2001; Adler & Lionheart, 2006). Its hardware architecture also brought better signal path visualization. Additionally, it guaranteed the pair sequence thanks to multiplexers. However, what really stood out in his work was the use of a 1 mA current source that has the signal defined through a multifrequency voltage-controlled oscillator, operating at 12.5 kHz, 25 kHz and 50 kHz. The advantage of this power supply is its ability to integrate with embedded systems, enabling the use of integrated circuits and shields for development kits.

Sing et al. (2015) were protagonist in the use of embedded systems. They proposed a prototype with more embedded elements and two microcontrollers: AVR ATMEGA 16 and the MSP430G2. The use of two microcontrollers has different functions. The ATMEGA 16 is responsible for the data acquisition and control system. On the other hand, the MSP430G2 is responsible for Analog / Digital conversion and sends the information to the PC through serial port for reconstruction.

MATERIALS AND METHODS

Electrical Impedance Tomography (EIT) is a technique for mapping conductivity or electrical permittivity of object or body section. The image is obtained by injecting alternating electric current through surface electrodes arranged around the body. The response to the electrical excitation is measured and, then, processed to form an image (Garcia et al., 2013; Tehrani et al., 2010), as outlined in Figure 1.

Figure 1. EIT schematization
Source: The authors

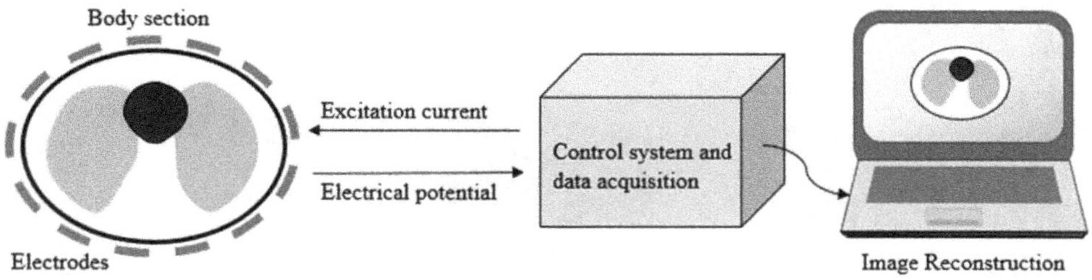

The possible forms of excitation of the body by injection of electric current can be: adjacent and diametrical. In the adjacent excitation pattern, the nearest electrode is taken as the reference point. On the other hand, the diametric pattern considers the diametrically opposite electrode as the reference point (Menin, 2009; Borcea, 2002). By alternating the electrode pair (injection and reference) around the body section, it is possible to obtain a linearly independent data. The result of the resolution of this data set is the map of electrical conductivity or permittivity.

The EIT image is obtained through a hardware and a software. The hardware is used to inject the electric current and measure the responses to this excitation, whereas the software to reconstruct the image. This reconstruction is performed by obtaining an approximate solution to the previously mentioned data set (Vallejo, 2007). In Figure 2, it is presented the block diagram which represents the proposed solution.

In this direction, we can analyze the features described in the block diagram as follows:

- **Imaged Area:** A phantom, consisting of a tank and 16 steel electrodes distributed around it, and an object in different positions. The electrodes are immersed in a normal NaCl (9 g / L) solution (Bera et al., 2012) and the object has a different conductivity than the solution conductivity.
- **Microcontroller Platform:** Based on low-cost open hardware, it is responsible for controlling the electrode excitation module and for reading the voltages from the pairs to be considered. These readings are made by analog input multiplexing and the data is, then provided to a software reconstruction system.
- **Alternating Current Source:** A 1 mA sinusoidal current source has been scaled to meet the needs of a signal with low amplitude and frequencies in the 10 KHz to 250 KHz range (Singh et al., 2015).
- **16-bit Analog Demultiplexer:** With this module it is possible to switch the current that excites the system to obtain the corresponding reading responses.
- **Acquisition and Preprocessing:** The signals collected from the electrodes are treated and amplified to be read through the multiplexers.
- **16-bit Analog Multiplexer:** It gives the microcontroller the output reading values of the voltages of a pair of electrodes following. The voltage reading follows the adjacent and diametrical current injection techniques.

- **Computer Communication:** The read data must be transmitted, through a communication port, to a computer to be processed by the reconstruction software.
- **Computational reconstruction:** On a computer, the impedance mapping data is processed by an algorithm that reconstructs the image.

Figure 2. Prototype EIT complete diagram
Source: The authors

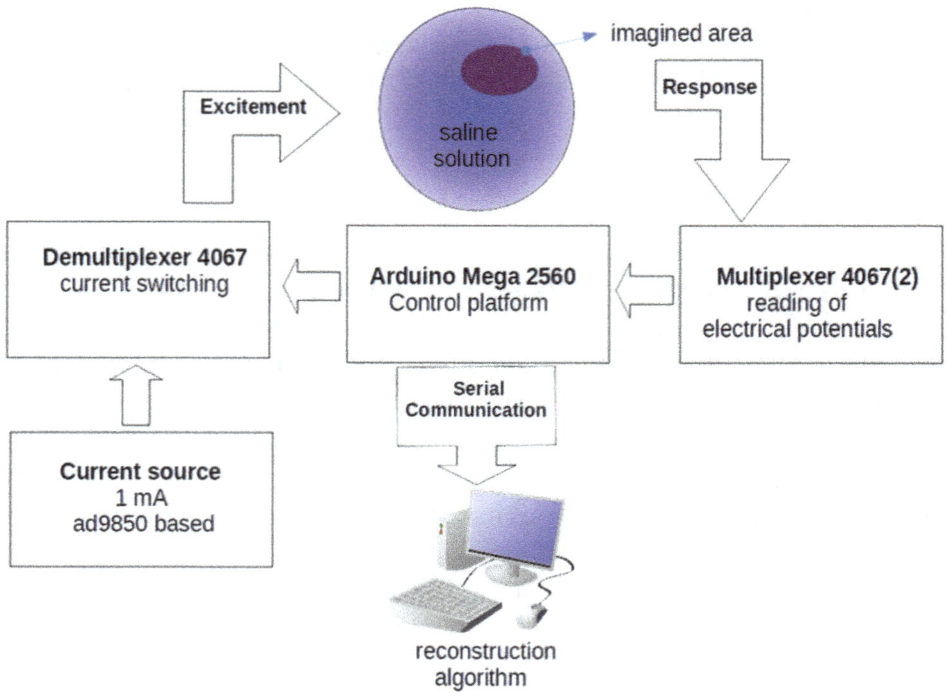

The proposed hardware for the EIT has to be calibrated and the way found for this was using the portable TH2821A LCR Meter. Among its functions, it measures the system impedance as well as resistance and reactances, separately. Thus, for the phantom system proposed conditions, we have the impedance of each electrode pair considered above. The Hantek 6022be oscilloscope interfaced with an Android tablet was also used. Analog and digital multimeters were also used to measure continuity, resistance and other circuit verification functions. The Figure 3 shows in details the experimental environment.

Figure 3. Experimental environment
Source: The authors

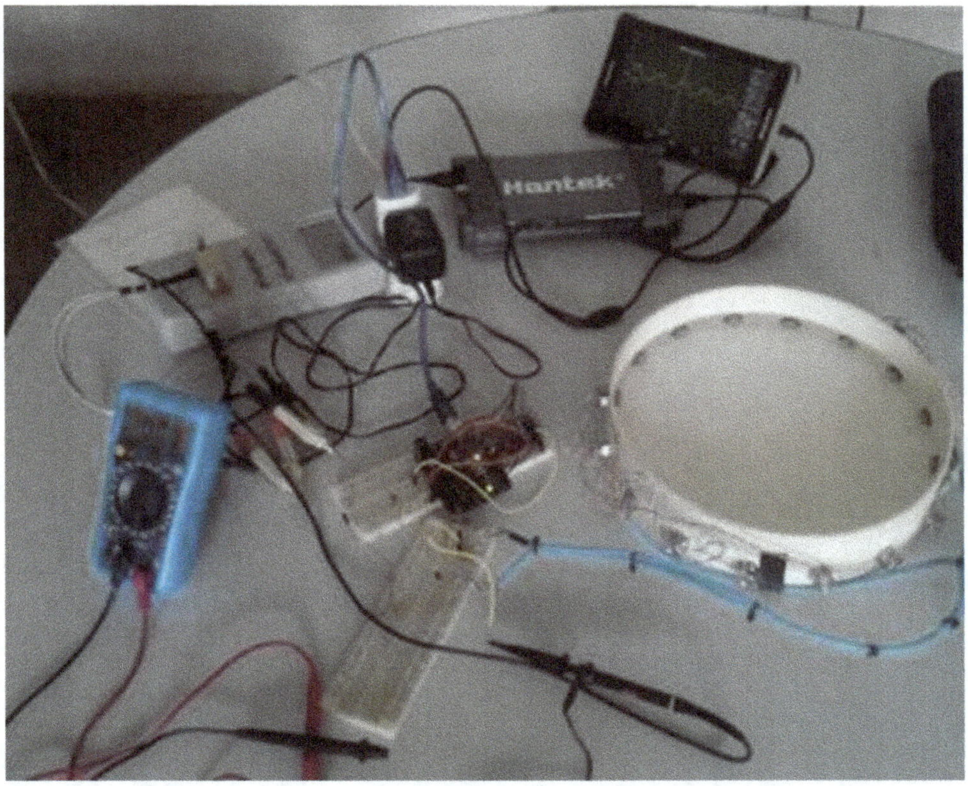

RESULTS

The tank used in the experiments has 16 electrodes around it. The electrodes are made with steel screws and fixed with screw nuts, and a rubber material is used to wrap the electrode hole in order to prevent leakage. The cables used for the signal bus were twisted pair used in communication networks with two four-wire pairs. Therefore, it totals 16 connections for the electrodes. The impedance of cables used is low and can be considered to decrease experimental distortion. To simulate a tissue, it was used an agar-agar based gelatinous disk, which had its conductivity controlled by the internal saline concentration. This concentration could be either the same or different from the aqueous medium in the tank, wherein it was immersed. The whole environment is shown in Figure 4.

In that direction, there is a small arduino-compatible shield-like card that offers an AD9850 (see Figure 5) reference function generator. When it is combined with an operational amplifier circuit, it provides a constant current of 1 mA. The AD9850 reference function generator can also vary the signal frequency via software. This signal is, thus, sent to a 16-bit demux and switched by all electrodes. For the excitation signal, the current source of the data acquisition system must be alternating, of low amplitude and power. Direct current should not be used because it generates electrolysis at the electrode poles. Hence it can cause skin surface damage if applied to humans (Bera et al., 2011). In the literature, voltage-controlled current sources are widely used, where this signal can be brought by an oscillator with low amplitude sinusoidal wave function.

Figure 4. phantom environment with the 16 electrodes
Source: The authors

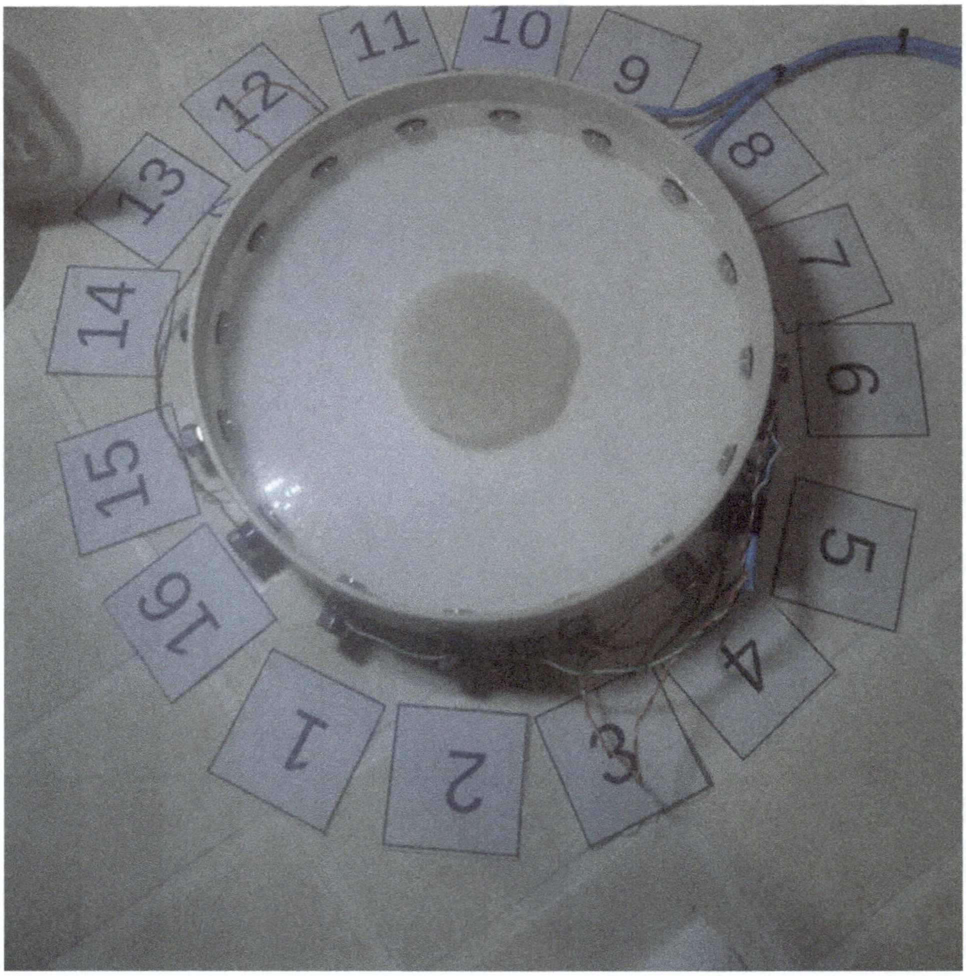

Figure 5. AD9850 current source based
Source: The authors

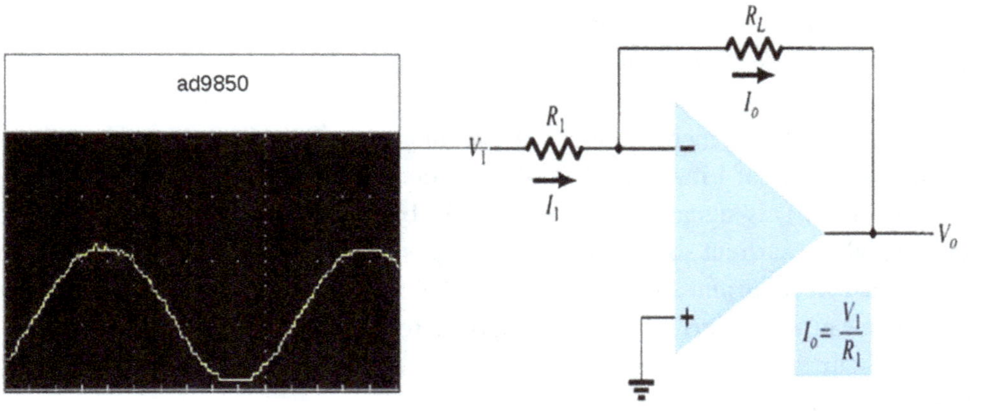

Figure 6. Boards used in the prototype
Source: The authors

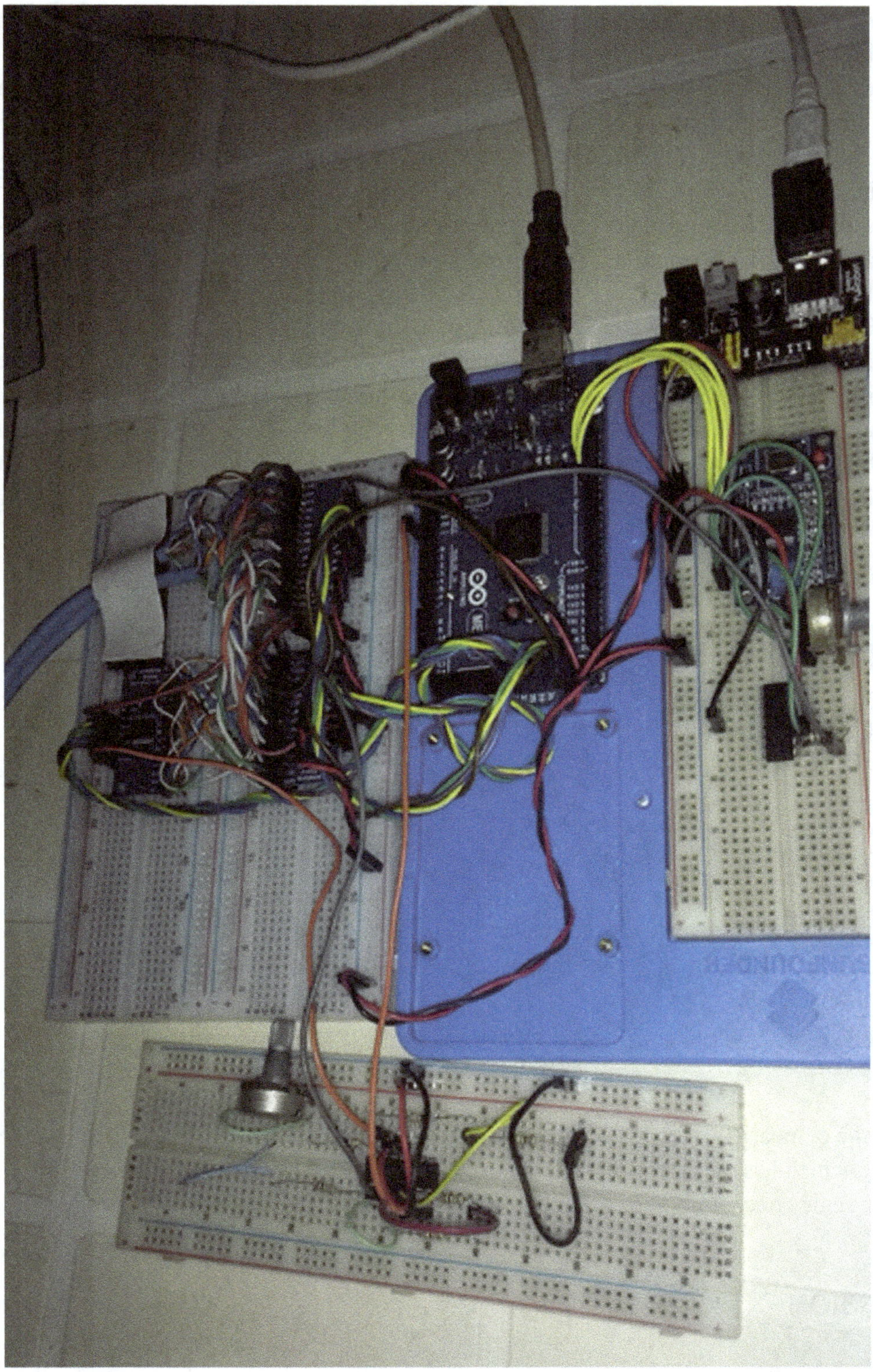

As for the potential readings, two 16-bit Multiplexers are used to bring the potential difference between two adjacent, interval or diametrical electrodes. Thus, for each potential read on one electrode, disregarding the electrodes of the current excitation and the one wherein the potential is being read, it remains thirteen electrodes for potential difference. This process returns the distribution of potentials that will be data to be sent for reconstruction. However, before being stored by the control platform, the potential signal is amplified by a circuit with a differential operational amplifier. So that, it is possible to digitize the signal on the internal circuit of the arduino digital analog converter.

Since inputs and outputs are needed, the development platform chosen was the arduino MEGA 2560. It has four serial USB-to-PC communication ports and can send information to real-time software reconstruction. This is an important step in prototyping. The prototype is organized into test contact matrices shown in Figure 6.

The USB communication available on the Arduino is used to send data to a PC running GNU Octave. GNU Octave is a development environment used by researchers from the biomedical computing research group to build reconstruction software. Like arduino is an open development platform, Octave is open source and installed on a computer running the ubuntu Linux operating system. Therefore, the project is free of charge for software licenses. Figure 7 shows the initial prototype of the tomograph. It is shown the main board, the simulation tank and the computer used for the reconstruction software.

Figure 7. EIT complete prototype
Source: The authors

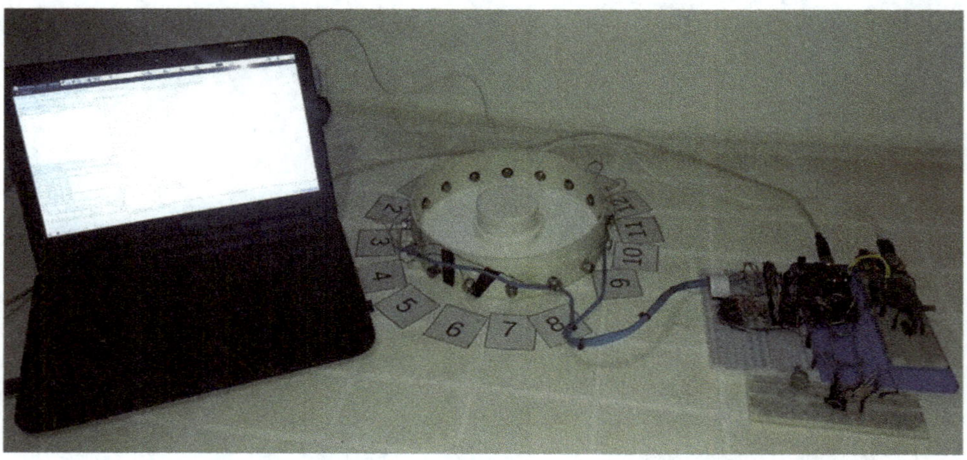

One of the comparisons made was the impedance measurements between the agar-agar gel disk and a PVC disk, which has dielectric characteristics. The agar-agar gel disc had its dissolution in water and NaCl at the same concentration of the solution that fills the tank.

CONCLUSION

The low cost prototype developed in this study enables an electrical potential mapping for the impedance measurement of a body. The authors achieved an impedance comparison of an agar-agar gel disk with a

PVC disk. The use of gel objects dissolved in saline liquids allows new experiments to be performed with resistivities similar to the biological tissues of Table 1. The calibration of the device for small impedance variations can reduce image reconstruction errors. Thus, it becomes an important tool to generate their own images other than those available in internationally recognized repositories. An important goal is the use of intelligent computation algorithms for the optimization of the EIT problem. Methods such as differential evolution, genetic algorithms, simulated annealing (Ribeiro et al., 2015) and fish school search (Barbosa et al., 2017) may optimize EIT image reconstruction. These algorithms aim to reduce reconstruction time and improve image resolution.

The strategy used to build the EIT tomograph prototype was based on the Open-Hardware design to allow the development of a low-cost and reproducible environment. Thus, the research group may be able to generate and calibrate its own data in order to obtain a user-friendly and portable device. Future approaches may improve the readability of biological devices. As a consequence, because of its modular design, it will independently enhance each function to bring the equipment closer to manufacturing and human testing.

ACKNOWLEDGMENT

The authors thank the brazilian research funding agencies Coordenação de Aperfeiçoamento de Pessoal de Nível Superior (CAPES) and Fundação de Amparo à Ciência e Tecnologia do Estado de Pernambuco (FACEPE) for the partial funding of this research.

REFERENCES

Adler, A., & Lionheart, W. R. B. (2006). Uses and abuses of EIDORS: An extensible software base for EIT. *Physiological Measurement*, *27*(5), S25–S42. doi:10.1088/0967-3334/27/5/S03 PMID:16636416

Adler, A., Arnold, J. H., Bayford, R., Borsic, A., Brown, B., Dixon, P., ... Grychtol, B. (2009). GREIT: A unified approach to 2D linear EIT reconstruction of lung images. *Physiological Measurement*, *30*(6), S35–S55. doi:10.1088/0967-3334/30/6/S03 PMID:19491438

Alves, S. H., Amato, M. B., Terra, R. M., Vargas, F. S., & Caruso, P. (2014). Lung reaeration and reventilation after aspiration of pleural effusions. A study using electrical impedance tomography. *Annals of the American Thoracic Society*, *11*(2), 186–191. doi:10.1513/AnnalsATS.201306-142OC PMID:24308560

Barbosa, V. A., Ribeiro, R. R., Feitosa, A. R., Silva, V. L., Rocha, A. D., Freitas, R. C., Souza, R. E., & Santos, W. P. (2017). Reconstruction of Electrical Impedance Tomography Using Fish School Search, Non-Blind Search, and Genetic Algorithm. *International Journal of Swarm Intelligence Research*, *8*(2), 17–33. doi:10.4018/IJSIR.2017040102

Barbosa, V. A., dos Santos, W. P., de Souza, R. E., Ribeiro, R. R., Feitosa, A. R. S., da Silva, V. L. B. A., & Valença, R. B. (2018). Image Reconstruction of Electrical Impedance Tomography Using Fish School Search and Differential Evolution. In *Critical Developments and Applications of Swarm Intelligence* (pp. 301–338). IGI Global. doi:10.4018/978-1-5225-5134-8.ch012

Bayford, R. H. (2006). Bioimpedance tomography (electrical impedance tomography). *Annual Review of Biomedical Engineering*, *8*(1), 63–91. doi:10.1146/annurev.bioeng.8.061505.095716 PMID:16834552

Bera, T. K., Biswas, S. K., Rajan, K., & Nagaraju, J. (2019). Improving image quality in electrical impedance tomography (EIT) using projection error propagation-based regularization (PEPR) technique: A simulation study. *Journal of Electrical Bioimpedance*, *2*(1), 2–12. doi:10.5617/jeb.158

Borcea, L. (2002). Electrical impedance tomography. *Inverse Problems*, *18*(6), R99–R136. doi:10.1088/0266-5611/18/6/201

Bouchette, G., Church, P., Mcfee, J. E., & Adler, A. (2013). Imaging of compact objects buried in underwater sediments using electrical impedance tomography. *IEEE Transactions on Geoscience and Remote Sensing*, *52*(2), 1407–1417. doi:10.1109/TGRS.2013.2250982

Brown, B. H., Barber, D. C., & Seagar, A. D. (1985). Applied potential tomography: Possible clinical applications. *Clinical Physics and Physiological Measurement*, *6*(2), 109–121. doi:10.1088/0143-0815/6/2/002 PMID:4017442

Cheney, M., Isaacson, D., & Newell, J. C. (1999). Electrical impedance tomography. *SIAM Review*, *41*(1), 85–101. doi:10.1137/S0036144598333613

Cherepenin, V., Karpov, A., Korjenevsky, A., Kornienko, V., Mazaletskaya, A., Mazourov, D., & Meister, D. (2001). A 3D electrical impedance tomography (EIT) system for breast cancer detection. *Physiological Measurement*, *22*(1), 9–18. doi:10.1088/0967-3334/22/1/302 PMID:11236894

Cherepenin, V. A., Karpov, A. Y., Korjenevsky, A. V., Kornienko, V. N., Kultiasov, Y. S., Ochapkin, M. B., Trochanova, O. V., & Meister, J. D. (2002). Three-dimensional EIT imaging of breast tissues: System design and clinical testing. *IEEE Transactions on Medical Imaging*, *21*(6), 662–667. doi:10.1109/TMI.2002.800602 PMID:12166863

Church, P., McFee, J. E., Gagnon, S., & Wort, P. (2006). Electrical impedance tomographic imaging of buried landmines. *IEEE Transactions on Geoscience and Remote Sensing*, *44*(9), 2407–2420. doi:10.1109/TGRS.2006.873208

Dai, M., Li, B., Hu, S., Xu, C., Yang, B., Li, J., Fu, F., Fei, Z., & Dong, X. (2013). In vivo imaging of twist drill drainage for subdural hematoma: A clinical feasibility study on electrical impedance tomography for measuring intracranial bleeding in humans. *PLoS One*, *8*(1), e55020. doi:10.1371/journal.pone.0055020 PMID:23372808

Daily, W., & Ramirez, A. (1995). Electrical resistance tomography during in-situ trichloroethylene remediation at the Savannah River Site. *Journal of Applied Geophysics*, *33*(4), 239–249. doi:10.1016/0926-9851(95)90044-6

Dong, F., Xu, Y., Hua, L., & Wang, H. (2006). Two methods for measurement of gas-liquid flows in vertical upward pipe using dual-plane ERT system. *IEEE Transactions on Instrumentation and Measurement*, *55*(5), 1576–1586. doi:10.1109/TIM.2006.881564

Eyuboglu, B. M., Brown, B. H., Barber, D. C., & Seager, A. D. (1987). Localisation of cardiac related impedance changes in the thorax. *Clinical Physics and Physiological Measurement*, *8*(4A), 167–173. doi:10.1088/0143-0815/8/4A/021 PMID:3568566

Feitosa, A. R., Ribeiro, R. R., Barbosa, V. A., de Souza, R. E., & dos Santos, W. P. (2014, May). Reconstruction of electrical impedance tomography images using particle swarm optimization, genetic algorithms and non-blind search. In *5th ISSNIP-IEEE Biosignals and Biorobotics Conference (2014): Biosignals and Robotics for Better and Safer Living (BRC)* (pp. 1-6). IEEE.

Feitosa, A. R., Ribeiro, R. R., Barbosa, V. A., de Souza, R. E., & dos Santos, W. P. (2014, October). Reconstruction of electrical impedance tomography images using chaotic ring-topology particle swarm optimization and non-blind search. In *2014 IEEE International Conference on Systems, Man, and Cybernetics (SMC)* (pp. 2618-2623). IEEE. 10.1109/SMC.2014.6974322

Dyakowski, T., York, T., Mikos, M., Vlaev, D., Mann, R., Follows, G., Boxman, A., & Wilson, M. (2000). Imaging nylon polymerisation processes by applying electrical tomography. *Chemical Engineering Journal*, *77*(1-2), 105–109. doi:10.1016/S1385-8947(99)00132-1

Dalvi-Garcia, F., Souza, M. N. D., & Pino, A. V. (2013). Algoritmo de reconstrução de imagens para um sistema de Tomografia por Impedância Elétrica (TIE) baseado em configuração multiterminais. *Rev. Bras. Eng. Bioméd., Rio de Janeiro, 29*(2), 133-143.

Huber, N., Béqo, N., Adams, C., Sze, G., Tunstall, B., Qiao, G., & Wang, W. (2010). Further investigation of a contactless patient-electrode interface of an Electrical Impedance Mammography system. *Journal of Physics: Conference Series*, *224*(1), 012166. doi:10.1088/1742-6596/224/1/012166

Hua, P., Woo, E. J., Webster, J. G., & Tompkins, W. J. (1993). Finite element modeling of electrode-skin contact impedance in electrical impedance tomography. *IEEE Transactions on Biomedical Engineering*, *40*(4), 335–343. doi:10.1109/10.222326 PMID:8375870

Huang, Z., Wang, B., & Li, H. (2003). Application of electrical capacitance tomography to the void fraction measurement of two-phase flow. *IEEE Transactions on Instrumentation and Measurement*, *52*(1), 7–12. doi:10.1109/TIM.2003.809087

Jordana, J., Gasulla, M., & Pallás-Areny, R. (1999, April). Leakage detection in buried pipes by electrical resistance imaging. In *Proc. 1st World Congress on Industrial Process Tomography (Buxton)* (pp. 28-34). Academic Press.

Kumar, S. P., Sriraam, N., Benakop, P. G., & Jinaga, B. C. (2010, July). Reconstruction of brain electrical impedance tomography images using particle swarm optimization. In *2010 5th International Conference on Industrial and Information Systems* (pp. 339-342). IEEE.

Liu, Y., & Sun, F. (2011). A fast differential evolution algorithm using k-Nearest Neighbour predictor. *Expert Systems with Applications*, *38*(4), 4254–4258. doi:10.1016/j.eswa.2010.09.092

Menin, O. H. (2009). *Método dos elementos de contorno para tomografia de impedância elétrica* (Doctoral dissertation). Universidade de São Paulo.

Price, K., Storn, R. M., & Lampinen, J. A. (2006). *Differential evolution: a practical approach to global optimization*. Springer Science & Business Media.

Ribeiro, R. R., Feitosa, A. R., Barbosa, V. A., da Silva, V. L., Rocha, A. D., Freitas, R. C., ... dos Santos, W. P. (2015). Reconstrução de Imagens de TIE usando Simulated Annealing, Evolução Diferencial e Algoritmos Genéticos. *XII Congresso Brasileiro de Inteligência Computacional*. 10.21528/CBIC2015-063

Ribeiro, R. R., Feitosa, A. R., de Souza, R. E., & dos Santos, W. P. (2014, May). A modified differential evolution algorithm for the reconstruction of electrical impedance tomography images. In *5th ISSNIP-IEEE Biosignals and Biorobotics Conference (2014): Biosignals and Robotics for Better and Safer Living (BRC)* (pp. 1-6). IEEE.

Ribeiro, R. R., Feitosa, A. R., de Souza, R. E., & dos Santos, W. P. (2014, April). Reconstruction of electrical impedance tomography images using genetic algorithms and non-blind search. In *2014 IEEE 11th International Symposium on Biomedical Imaging (ISBI)* (pp. 153-156). IEEE. 10.1109/ISBI.2014.6867832

Ribeiro, R. R., Feitosa, A. R., de Souza, R. E., & dos Santos, W. P. (2014, October). Reconstruction of electrical impedance tomography images using chaotic self-adaptive ring-topology differential evolution and genetic algorithms. In *2014 IEEE International Conference on Systems, Man, and Cybernetics (SMC)* (pp. 2605-2610). IEEE. 10.1109/SMC.2014.6974320

Rimpiläinen, V., Kuosmanen, M., Ketolainen, J., Järvinen, K., Vauhkonen, M., & Heikkinen, L. M. (2010). Electrical impedance tomography for three-dimensional drug release monitoring. *European Journal of Pharmaceutical Sciences*, *41*(2), 407–413. doi:10.1016/j.ejps.2010.07.008 PMID:20654713

Rolnik, V. P., & Seleghim, P. Jr. (2006). A specialized genetic algorithm for the electrical impedance tomography of two-phase flows. *Journal of the Brazilian Society of Mechanical Sciences and Engineering*, *28*(4), 378–389. doi:10.1590/S1678-58782006000400002

dos Santos, W. P., de Souza, R. E., Ribeiro, R. R., Feitosa, A. R. S., de Freitas Barbosa, V. A., da Silva, V. L. B. A., . . . de Freitas, R. C. (2018). Electrical Impedance Tomography Using Evolutionary Computing: A Review. In Bio-Inspired Computing for Image and Video Processing (pp. 93-128). Chapman and Hall/CRC.

Singh, G., Anand, S., Lall, B., Srivastava, A., & Singh, V. (2015, May). Development of a microcontroller based electrical impedance tomography system. In 2015 Long Island Systems, Applications and Technology (pp. 1-4). IEEE. doi:10.1109/LISAT.2015.7160174

Tehrani, J. N., Jin, C., McEwan, A., & van Schaik, A. (2010, August). A comparison between compressed sensing algorithms in electrical impedance tomography. In *2010 Annual International Conference of the IEEE Engineering in Medicine and Biology* (pp. 3109-3112). IEEE. 10.1109/IEMBS.2010.5627165

Trokhanova, O. V., Okhapkin, M. B., & Korjenevsky, A. V. (2008). Dual-frequency electrical impedance mammography for the diagnosis of non-malignant breast disease. *Physiological Measurement*, *29*(6), S331.

Montoya Vallejo, M. F. (n.d.). *Algoritmo de tomografia por impedância elétrica utilizando programação linear como método de busca da imagem* (Doctoral dissertation). Universidade de São Paulo.

Vauhkonen, M., Lionheart, W. R., Heikkinen, L. M., Vauhkonen, P. J., & Kaipio, J. P. (2001). A MATLAB package for the EIDORS project to reconstruct two-dimensional EIT images. *Physiological Measurement, 22*(1), 107–111. doi:10.1088/0967-3334/22/1/314 PMID:11236871

Walker, D., & Kaczor, T. (2012). Breast thermography: history, theory, and use. Is this screening tool adequate for standalone use. *Nat Med J, 4*(7).

Wan, Y., Borsic, A., Heaney, J., Seigne, J., Schned, A., Baker, M., Wason, S., Hartov, A., & Halter, R. (2013). Transrectal electrical impedance tomography of the prostate: Spatially coregistered pathological findings for prostate cancer detection. *Medical Physics, 40*(6Part1), 063102. doi:10.1118/1.4803498 PMID:23718610

Yorkey, T. J., Webster, J. G., & Tompkins, W. J. (1987). Comparing reconstruction algorithms for electrical impedance tomography. *IEEE Transactions on Biomedical Engineering, BME-34*(11), 843–852. doi:10.1109/TBME.1987.326032 PMID:3692503

Zhang, X., Wang, W., Sze, G., Barber, D., & Chatwin, C. (2014). An image reconstruction algorithm for 3-D electrical impedance mammography. *IEEE Transactions on Medical Imaging, 33*(12), 2223–2241. doi:10.1109/TMI.2014.2334475 PMID:25014954

Zou, Y., & Guo, Z. (2003). A review of electrical impedance techniques for breast cancer detection. *Medical Engineering & Physics, 25*(2), 79–90. doi:10.1016/S1350-4533(02)00194-7 PMID:12538062

Chapter 2
Using Extreme Learning Machines and the Backprojection Algorithm as an Alternative to Reconstruct Electrical Impedance Tomography Images

Juliana Carneiro Gomes
Escola Politécnica, Universidade de Pernambuco, Brazil

Maíra Araújo de Santana
Universidade Federal de Pernambuco, Brazil

Clarisse Lins de Lima
Universidade Federal de Pernambuco, Brazil

Ricardo Emmanuel de Souza
Universidade Federal de Pernambuco, Brazil

Wellington Pinheiro dos Santos
https://orcid.org/0000-0003-2558-6602
Universidade Federal de Pernambuco, Brazil

ABSTRACT

Electrical Impedance Tomography (EIT) is an imaging technique based on the excitation of electrode pairs applied to the surface of the imaged region. The electrical potentials generated from alternating current excitation are measured and then applied to boundary-based reconstruction methods. When compared to other imaging techniques, EIT is considered a low-cost technique without ionizing radiation

DOI: 10.4018/978-1-7998-3456-4.ch002

emission, safer for patients. However, the resolution is still low, depending on efficient reconstruction methods and low computational cost. EIT has the potential to be used as an alternative test for early detection of breast lesions in general. The most accurate reconstruction methods tend to be very costly as they use optimization methods as a support. Backprojection tends to be rapid but more inaccurate. In this work, the authors propose a hybrid method, based on extreme learning machines and backprojection for EIT reconstruction. The results were applied to numerical phantoms and were considered adequate, with potential to be improved using post processing techniques.

INTRODUCTION

Electrical Impedance Tomography (EIT) is a technique for imaging the interior of a body section based on the application of a low amplitude, high frequency alternating electric current. For this, electrodes are positioned on the surface of this body. They are responsible for sending this stimulus as well as for measuring the resulting electrical potentials. Thus, one can obtain images with estimates of the electrical conductivity or permittivity of the interior of a domain. Conductivity can be understood as the possibility of the medium to allow the displacement of electric charges, while permittivity is the measure of the ease of polarization of the material (Tehrani et al., 2010; Bera et al., 2011; Kumar et al., 2010).

EIT has applications in several areas: in geophysics, in industrial processes, in botany and medicine, for example. On the last, applications can be cited for detection of breast cancer (Pak et al., 2012), diagnosis of prostate cancer (Wan et al., 2013), monitoring of ventilator-imposed pulmonary ventilation (Alves et al., 2014; Adler et al., 2009) and in the measurement of intracranial bleeding.

EIT does not use ionizing radiation, which is harmful to human health. However, the technique still has low spatial resolution and a high computational cost in reconstructing its images compared to other medical imaging techniques, such as x-ray computed tomography (X-CT) and Nuclear Magnetic Resonance (NMR) and, therefore, is not yet strongly established. Hence, several methods have been studied and applied to solve these problems (Kumar et al., 2010).

For decades, breast cancer has been the most common type of cancer among women. In Brazil, the breast cancer mortality rates remain high, as the disease is still diagnosed in advanced stages. Even though Mammography, Ultrasonography, Magnetic Resonance and clinical breast examination (ECM) are the most widely used and indicated methods in mastology, there are still many problems associated to them. Sometimes they are not enough to identify breast lesions in women with dense and surgically altered breasts or in women under the age of 40 years old. In addition to it, some of these exams are extremely uncomfortable to the patient and there is concern about the risk associated to the use of ionizing radiation (Torre et al., 2015; Ministério da Saúde, 2017, Santana et al., 2018; de Lima et al., 2016; Cordeiro et al., 2017; Cordeiro et al., 2016a; Cordeiro et al., 2016b; Azevedo et al., 2015; Cordeiro et al., 2013; Cordeiro et al., 2012; Rodrigues et al., 2018; Oliveira et al., 2019; de Souza et al., 2019). Several works point out that electrical impedance tomography can be used successfully to aid at the diagnosis of breast cancer (Holder, 2004; Cherepenin et al., 2001; Halter et al., 2008; Choi et al., 2007; Zou & Guo, 2003; Hong et al., 2014; Soni et al., 2004).

In this work, the authors propose a new method for reconstruction of EIT images. They propose the use of the classic Backprojection Algorithm to obtain TIE images from sinograms. The sinograms, in turn, will be constructed from the data of electrical potential differences measured on the surface of the studied domain, using for this purpose Regression Extreme Learning Machine (R-ELM) Artificial

Neural Networks. Thus, they believed that a fast reconstruction method can be obtained due to the high speed of both chosen algorithms with still good image quality.

BACKGROUND

Electrical Impedance Tomography Image Reconstruction

The EIT technique consists of direct and inverse problem solving (Kumar et al., 2010; Ribeiro et al., 2014a; Ribeiro et al. 2014b; Feitosa et al., 2014a; Feitosa et al., 2014b; Barbosa et al., 2017; Barbosa et al., 2016; Barbosa et al., 2015). The inverse problem is the estimation of the electrical conductivity and permittivity distribution within the domain. However, besides the function that represents the potentials do not vary linearly with the applied current, there is not a single distribution of conductivity and permittivity corresponding to a given set of measured electrical potentials. The solution of the problem can still be unstable, presenting great sensitivity to numerical errors and experimental noises. From a mathematical point of view, the EIT problem is determined by the Poisson equation given in (1) (Dai et al., 2013):

$$)\nabla\bullet[\sigma(\vec{u})\nabla\phi(\vec{u})]=0,\ \forall\vec{u}\in\Omega, \quad (1)$$

with the boundary conditions in (2) and (3):

$$\phi\_ext\ (\vec{u})=\phi(\vec{u}),\ \forall\vec{u}\in\partial\Omega, \quad (2)$$

$$I(\vec{u})=-\sigma(\vec{u})\nabla\phi(\vec{u}),\ \forall\vec{u}\in\partial\Omega, \quad (3)$$

where $\vec{u}=(x,y,z)$ .is the position of the object under study, $\phi(\vec{u})$ .is the electrical potentials distribution, $\phi_{ext}(\vec{u})$ .is the electrical potentials distribution on the surface of the domain, $I(\vec{u})$ .is the alternate electrical current, $\tilde{A}(\vec{u})$ .is the distribution of electrical conductivity, i.e. the image of interest, Ω .is the domain, $\partial\Omega$ .is the border of the domain, $\hat{n}$ .is the normal vector, perpendicular to the border of the domain (Hamilton & Hauptmann, 2017; Santos et al., 2017).

When it comes to the direct problem, the electric potentials measured in its contour are determined from the current excitation pattern and the conductivity distribution. This relationship is given by the Laplace Equation. Thus, it is modeled by the relation given in (4):

$$\phi\_ext\ (\vec{u})=f(I(\vec{u}),\sigma(\vec{u})),\ \forall\vec{u}\in\partial\Omega, \quad (4)$$

with the boundary conditions in (5):

$$\sigma\frac{\partial\phi}{\partial\hat{n}}=\vec{J}, \quad (5)$$

where $\vec{J}$ .is the electrical current density (Ogava et al., 2017).

Radon Transform and Sinograms

The Radon transform (TR) is a line integral and thus the TR of a distribution $f(x,y)$ .is given by (6):

$$p(\xi,\phi) = \int f(x,y)\delta(x\cos\phi + y\sin\phi - \xi)\,dxdy, \tag{6}$$

where $\delta(\cdot)$ .is the Dirac's Delta function, ξ .is the vector perpendicular to the orientation of the injected current, considering in a simplified way that the electrical currents run in a straight trajectory between the electrodes. ϕ .is the angle between the vector ξ .and the axis x .(Leão & Macedo, 2014). The function $p(\xi,\phi)$ .s known as the *sinogram*, since the Radon Transform of a point out of the center is sinusoidal (Hiesh, 2009). The sinogram represents the alignment of all projections of a determined slice along a matrix. Thus, the Radon Transform models the projections of the object under study. On the contrary, the Inverse Radon Transform models the retroprojections, since the reconstruction of the slice image is the sum of all these retroprojections. In other words, the reconstruction by the backprojection algorithm has as its main goal to find a function $f(x,y)$ .given a sinogram $p(\xi,\phi)$. as depicted in Figure 1.

Figure 1. Example of computerized tomography image reconstruction based on the backprojection algorithm from sinograms.
Source: The Authors

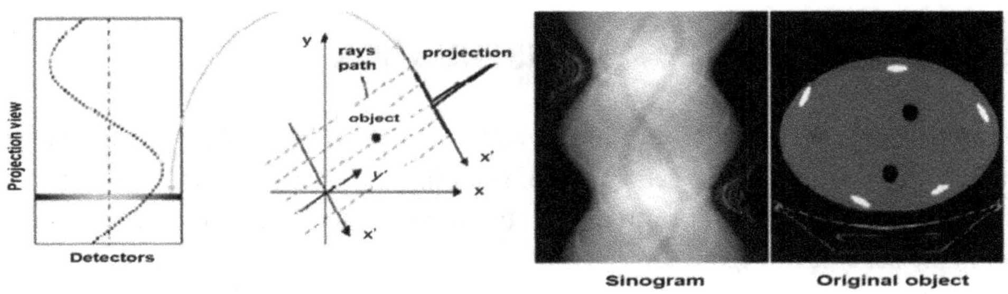

Backprojection Reconstruction Algorithm

The backprojection method is a simple and fast summation method commonly used in x-ray computed tomography image reconstructions (Hiesh, 2009; Wang et al., 2015; Guardo et al., 1991). This requires the collection of data that represents the sum of equally spaced 360-degree regions, and geometrically speaking, it turns the sinogram back into an image. Its operation is defined by (7):

$$f(x,y) = \int_0^{\pi} p(x\cos\phi + y\sin\phi)\,d\phi. \tag{7}$$

Extreme Learning Machines for Regression

Artificial neural networks are machines inspired by human brain functioning that seek to model how we respond to certain functions. These systems are naturally endowed with parallelism, and can be linear or nonlinear, with learning ability through observation of the environment. Due to this, they have generalization capacity, that is, they are able to generate appropriate outputs for situations that were not present in the learning process or that were not foreseen in the algorithm. This makes it possible to solve complex problems (Haykin, 2001).

A widely used neural network today is the extreme learning machine (ELM). It is a supervised hidden layered network known for its speed, less computational complexity in both training and execution, and good generalizability. In addition, all continuous functions can be used as activation function. Therefore, a single layer ELM network can be modeled as following (8):

$$\sum_{i=1}^{N_h} {}^{2}{}_{i} f\left(\acute{E}_i x_j + b_i\right) = t_i, j\epsilon\left[1, N\right]. \tag{8}$$

whilst N is the number of samples of the set of pairs $\left(x_i, t_i\right)$, N_h is the number of neurons in the hidden layer, $f\left(\cdot\right)$ is the activation function, ω_i are the input weights, b_i are the biases, β_i are the output weights, and t_i is the desired output. Then, the weights of the inputs of the hidden layer are randomly determined, independently from the training set, whilst the weights of the output layer are determined analytically by using the Moore-Penrose pseudoinverse, one-layered perceptron algorithm or simple linear regression (Huang et al., 2012; Huang et al., 2006; Qiong et al., 2017; Lei et al., 2017).

PROPOSAL: ELM-SINOGRAM RECONSTRUCTION

In this chapter the authors propose an innovative method for obtaining EIT images from backprojection reconstruction of sinograms. For the generation of sinograms, it is desired to train Regression ELMs to find a function that models the data from the electrical potentials measured at the domain surface, as summarized in the scheme of Figure 2.

For the development of a pilot test, synthetic EIT images and codes for reconstruction in the GNU Octave environment were developed. A grayscale image bank (128 x 128) was generated with circular domains, so that objects within the domain were represented by circles and ellipses of different sizes and intensities. Finally, 16 equidistant electrodes were simulated on the edge of the drawn object, and the path of the electric currents between the electrodes was considered as straight line. Thus, by summing the intensities of the pixels, the sum of the resistivities (inverse conductivity) between the electrodes can be obtained. Knowing the electric current of excitation, we obtained, thus, the values of electric potentials on the surface of the domain under study.

From the database, 100 synthetic images were randomly chosen. The program generated sinograms of these images as well as reconstructed them by backprojection. The reconstructions, therefore, serve as reference images for future reconstructions through the proposed method, while the sinograms serve as a training set for the neural networks.

In the case of artificial neural networks, the authors used ELM in the version for Maltab / GNU Octave, which was proposed by Huang et al. (2006). In order to find the best ELM configuration for image reconstruction, a scan between different configurations was performed. The sigmoid, sinusoidal and hard-limit activation functions were tested with the number of neurons in the hidden layer ranging from 50 to 500, with steps of 50. In addition to the above, ELMs using Kernel Wavelet, RBF, polynomial and linear were also included. All cases were tested using the 2/3 Percentage Division and 10-fold cross-validation algorithm sampling and validation methods. Thus, the best results presented were with higher number of neurons, as well as using cross-validation, being considered better after training with lower percentage error. A summary of these results can be seen in the graph in Figure 3.

Figure 2. Electrical impedance image reconstruction from sinograms
Source: The Authors

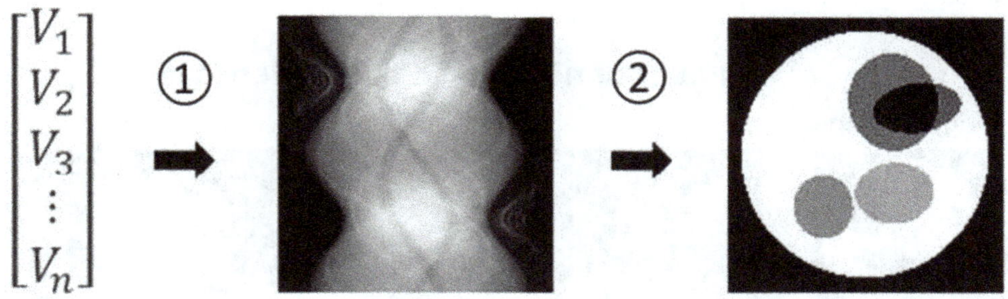

Figure 3. Evaluation of different ELM kernels
Source: The Authors

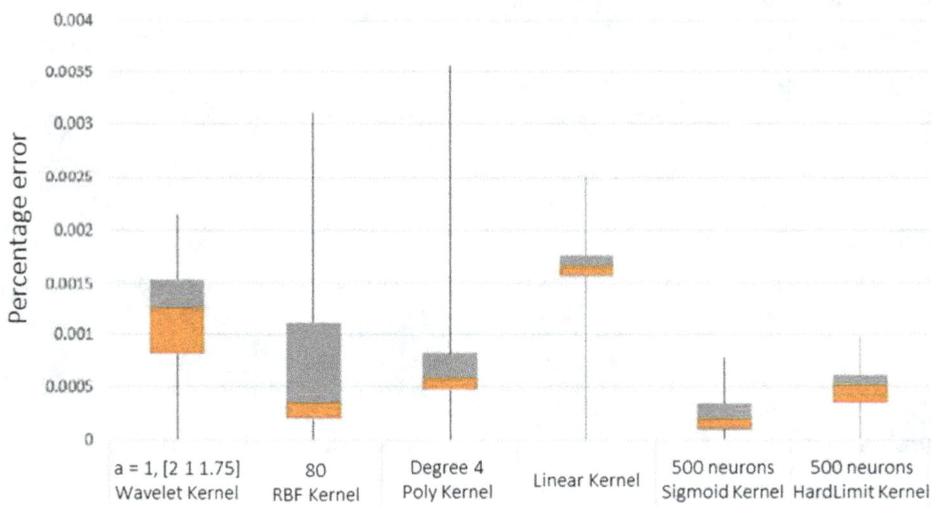

RESULTS AND DISCUSSION

In order to obtain the sinograms, 16 artificial neural networks were trained corresponding to the 16 electrodes positioned on the surface. We used the Sigmoidal activation function and the electrical potentials measured in the 100 EIT images selected as the sample, ie as the input set, while the sinograms of the original images were the expected outputs. Finally, the 16 trained neural networks generated the parameters input weights, output weights and bias, which were saved for later obtaining of each column of the sinograms. Finally, the sinograms were reconstructed by Backprojection and the result can be seen in Figure 4.

Figure 4. Images reconstruction from Backprojection using different amount of neurons in the hidden layer and different interior objects in the domain under study.
Source: The Authors.

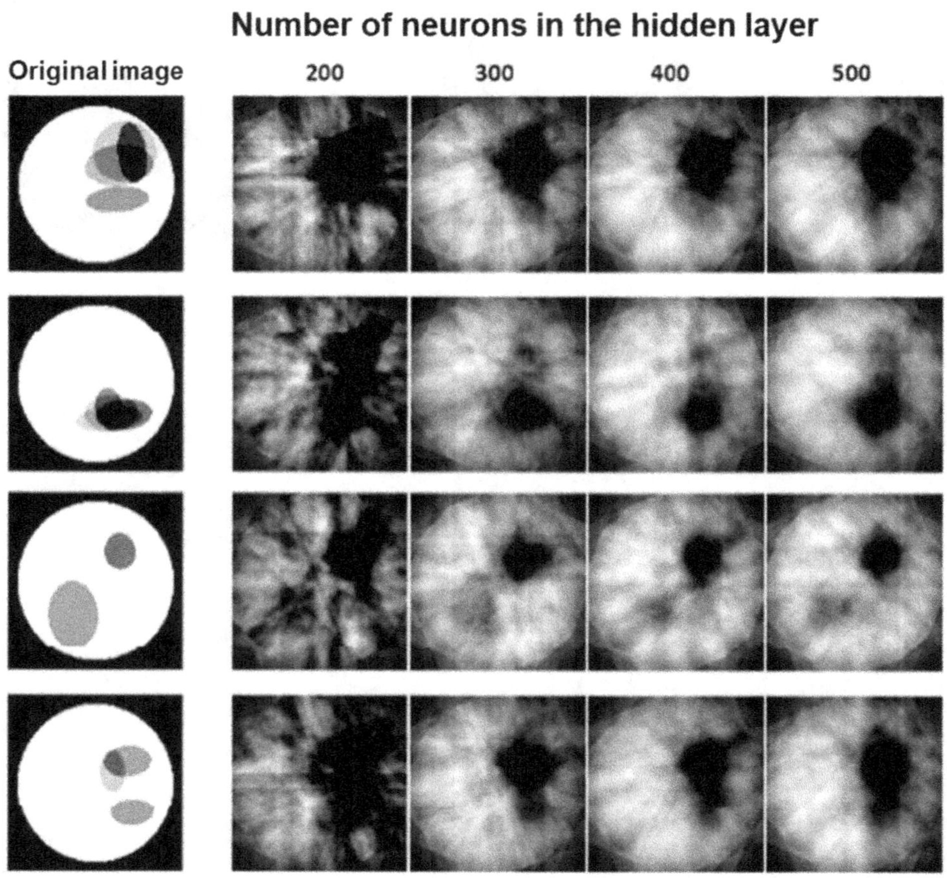

Finally, it can be seen that the images with larger number of neurons in the hidden layer presented higher quality in the reconstruction, in order to better visualize the domain under study, as can be seen in the images with 400 or 500 neurons.

CONCLUSION

In this work, the authors proposed a method for reconstruction of electrical impedance tomography images based on artificial neural networks for reconstruction of sinograms, thus generating a version of the backprojection algorithm.

All images obtained were consistent with the original reference image, indicating the presence of objects in similar regions. Nevertheless, it is not possible to define the number of objects present inside the domain. It is further suggested that the darker elements that are interior to the domain could be more easily reconstructed, in contrast to some of the lighter intensity that went unnoticed. Consequently, it is observed in the third image, for example, that the object of higher intensity was larger in dimensions than the lighter object, although the original image indicates the opposite.

Therefore, it was observed that errors decrease as the number of hidden layer neurons grows. In addition, as seen in the graph, the sigmoidal activation function performed better, probably constituting the best ELM configuration to obtain the sinograms.

In future works, the authors plan to use a larger number of images for the training of ELMs. By this way, the authors believe the artificial neural networks will present a better ability to generalize the problem. In the present work, 16 electrodes were also chosen to reduce the time of data acquisition and reconstruction, in order to simplify the preliminary results. However, it is still desired to perform reconstructions obtained with a larger number of electrodes positioned on the surface, preferably 32 electrodes, in order to obtain a better angular sampling and possible better image resolution.

Finally, the authors believe the present proposed method presented satisfactory and consistent preliminary results, constituting a promising method. It will be able to considerably reduce the time of reconstruction of TIE images, mainly due to the high speed of the Extreme Learning Machine (ELM) and the Backprojection algorithm, as well as to provide a reasonable image quality.

ACKNOWLEDGMENT

This research was supported by Conselho Nacional de Desenvolvimento Científico e Tecnológico, CNPq, Brazil [grant number DT-2 2019]; Coordenação de Apoio ao Pessoal de Ensino Superior, CAPES, Brazil [grant number BP-2017]; and Fundação de Apoio à Pesquisa do Estado de Pernambuco, Facepe, Brazil [grant number IBPG 2017].

REFERENCES

Adler, A., Arnold, J. H., Bayford, R., Borsic, A., Brown, B., Dixon, P., Faes, T. J. C., Frerichs, I., Gagnon, H., Garber, Y., Grychtol, B., Hahn, G., Lionheart, W. R. B., Malik, A., Paterson, R. P., Stocks, J., Tizzard, A., Weiler, N., & Grychtol, B. (2009). GREIT: A unified approach to 2D linear EIT reconstruction of lung images. *Physiological Measurement*, *30*(6), S35–S55. doi:10.1088/0967-3334/30/6/S03 PMID:19491438

Alves, S. H., Amato, M. B., Terra, R. M., Vargas, F. S., & Caruso, P. (2014). Lung reaeration and reventilation after aspiration of pleural effusions. A study using electrical impedance tomography. *Annals of the American Thoracic Society*, *11*(2), 186–191. doi:10.1513/AnnalsATS.201306-142OC PMID:24308560

Azevedo, W. W., Lima, S. M., Fernandes, I. M., Rocha, A. D., Cordeiro, F. R., da Silva-Filho, A. G., & dos Santos, W. P. (2015, August). *Fuzzy morphological extreme learning machines to detect and classify masses in mammograms. In 2015 IEEE international conference on fuzzy systems (fuzz-IEEE)*. IEEE.

Barbosa, V. A., Ribeiro, R. R., Feitosa, A. R., da Silva, V. L., Rocha, A. D., Freitas, R. C., Melo, M. F. B., da Silva, V. L. B. A., de Souza, R. E., & dos Santos, W. P. (2015). Reconstrução de imagens de tomografia por impedância elétrica usando cardume de peixes, busca não-cega e algoritmo genético. In *Anais do 12 Congresso Brasileiro de Inteligência Computacional* (pp. 1–6). ABRICOM. doi:10.21528/CBIC2015-043

Barbosa, V. A., Ribeiro, R. R., Feitosa, A. R., Silva, V. L., Rocha, A. D., Freitas, R. C., Souza, R. E., & Santos, W. P. (2017). Reconstruction of Electrical Impedance Tomography Using Fish School Search, Non-Blind Search, and Genetic Algorithm. *International Journal of Swarm Intelligence Research, 8*(2), 17–33. doi:10.4018/IJSIR.2017040102

Barbosa, V. A. F., Ribeiro, R. R., Feitosa, A. R. S., Freitas, R. C., Melo, M. F. B., da Silva, V. L. B. A., de Souza, R. E., & dos Santos, W. P. (2016). Reconstrução de imagens de TIE usando busca por cardume de peixes e density based on fish school search. *XXV Congresso Brasileiro de Engenharia Biomédica.*

Bera, T. K., Biswas, S. K., Rajan, K., & Nagaraju, J. (2019). Improving image quality in electrical impedance tomography (EIT) using projection error propagation-based regularization (PEPR) technique: A simulation study. *Journal of Electrical Bioimpedance, 2*(1), 2–12. doi:10.5617/jeb.158

Cherepenin, V., Karpov, A., Korjenevsky, A., Kornienko, V., Mazaletskaya, A., Mazourov, D., & Meister, D. (2001). A 3D electrical impedance tomography (EIT) system for breast cancer detection. *Physiological Measurement, 22*(1), 9–18. doi:10.1088/0967-3334/22/1/302 PMID:11236894

Choi, M. H., Kao, T. J., Isaacson, D., Saulnier, G. J., & Newell, J. C. (2007). A reconstruction algorithm for breast cancer imaging with electrical impedance tomography in mammography geometry. *IEEE Transactions on Biomedical Engineering, 54*(4), 700–710. doi:10.1109/TBME.2006.890139 PMID:17405377

Cordeiro, F. R., Bezerra, K. F. P., & dos Santos, W. P. (2017, June). Random Walker with Fuzzy Initialization Applied to Segment Masses in Mammography Images. In *2017 IEEE 30th International Symposium on Computer-Based Medical Systems (CBMS)* (pp. 156-161). IEEE. 10.1109/CBMS.2017.40

Cordeiro, F. R., Lima, S. M., Silva-Filho, A. G., & Santos, W. P. (2012, August). Segmentation of mammography by applying extreme learning machine in tumor detection. In *International Conference on Intelligent Data Engineering and Automated Learning* (pp. 92-100). Springer.

Cordeiro, F. R., Santos, W. P., & Silva-Filho, A. G. (2013). Segmentation of mammography by applying GrowCut for mass detection. *Studies in Health Technology and Informatics, 192*, 87–91. PMID:23920521

Cordeiro, F. R., Santos, W. P., & Silva-Filho, A. G. (2016). A semi-supervised fuzzy GrowCut algorithm to segment and classify regions of interest of mammographic images. *Expert Systems with Applications, 65*, 116–126. doi:10.1016/j.eswa.2016.08.016

Cordeiro, F. R., Santos, W. P., & Silva-Filho, A. G. (2016). An adaptive semi-supervised Fuzzy GrowCut algorithm to segment masses of regions of interest of mammographic images. *Applied Soft Computing, 46*, 613–628. doi:10.1016/j.asoc.2015.11.040

Dai, M., Li, B., Hu, S., Xu, C., Yang, B., Li, J., Fu, F., Fei, Z., & Dong, X. (2013). In vivo imaging of twist drill drainage for subdural hematoma: A clinical feasibility study on electrical impedance tomography for measuring intracranial bleeding in humans. *PLoS One*, *8*(1), e55020. doi:10.1371/journal.pone.0055020 PMID:23372808

de Lima, S. M., da Silva-Filho, A. G., & dos Santos, W. P. (2016). Detection and classification of masses in mammographic images in a multi-kernel approach. *Computer Methods and Programs in Biomedicine*, *134*, 11–29. doi:10.1016/j.cmpb.2016.04.029 PMID:27480729

de Oliveira, P. M., Silva, G. S., de Souza, G. M., Azevedo, W. W., de Santana, M. A., & dos Santos, W. P. (2019). Uso de classificadores na predição de lesões de mama a partir de imagens termográficas. *Anais do III Simpósio de Inovação em Engenharia Biomédica - SABIO 2019*, 69.

de Souza, T. K. S., de Santana, M. A., de Andrade, J. F. S., dos Santos, W. P., & de Almeida, M. B. J. (2019). Métodos Computacionais Aplicados ao Diagnóstico de Câncer de Mama por Termografia: uma revisão de literatura. *Anais do III Simpósio de Inovação em Engenharia Biomédica - SABIO 2019.*

dos Santos, W. P., de Souza, R. E., Ribeiro, R. R., Feitosa, A. R. S., de Freitas Barbosa, V. A., da Silva, V. L. B. A., Ribeiro, D. E., & de Freitas, R. C. (2018). Electrical Impedance Tomography Using Evolutionary Computing: A Review. In Bio-Inspired Computing for Image and Video Processing (pp. 93-128). Chapman and Hall/CRC.

Feitosa, A. R., Ribeiro, R. R., Barbosa, V. A., de Souza, R. E., & dos Santos, W. P. (2014, May). Reconstruction of electrical impedance tomography images using particle swarm optimization, genetic algorithms and non-blind search. In *5th ISSNIP-IEEE Biosignals and Biorobotics Conference (2014): Biosignals and Robotics for Better and Safer Living (BRC)* (pp. 1-6). IEEE.

Feitosa, A. R., Ribeiro, R. R., Barbosa, V. A., de Souza, R. E., & dos Santos, W. P. (2014, October). Reconstruction of electrical impedance tomography images using chaotic ring-topology particle swarm optimization and non-blind search. In *2014 IEEE International Conference on Systems, Man, and Cybernetics (SMC)* (pp. 2618-2623). IEEE. 10.1109/SMC.2014.6974322

Guardo, R., Boulay, C., Murray, B., & Bertrand, M. (1991). An experimental study in electrical impedance tomography using backprojection reconstruction. *IEEE Transactions on Biomedical Engineering*, *38*(7), 617–627. doi:10.1109/10.83560 PMID:1879853

Halter, R. J., Hartov, A., & Paulsen, K. D. (2008). A broadband high-frequency electrical impedance tomography system for breast imaging. *IEEE Transactions on Biomedical Engineering*, *55*(2), 650–659. doi:10.1109/TBME.2007.903516 PMID:18270001

Hamilton, S. J., & Hauptmann, A. (2018). Deep D-Bar: Real-time electrical impedance tomography imaging with deep neural networks. *IEEE Transactions on Medical Imaging*, *37*(10), 2367–2377. doi:10.1109/TMI.2018.2828303 PMID:29994023

Haykin, S. (2007). *Redes neurais: princípios e prática*. Bookman Editora.

Holder, D. (2004). *Electrical impedance tomography: methods, history and applications*. CRC Press. doi:10.1201/9781420034462

Hong, S., Lee, K., Ha, U., Kim, H., Lee, Y., Kim, Y., & Yoo, H. J. (2014). A 4.9 mΩ-sensitivity mobile electrical impedance tomography IC for early breast-cancer detection system. *IEEE Journal of Solid-State Circuits*, *50*(1), 245–257. doi:10.1109/JSSC.2014.2355835

Hsieh, J. (2009, November). *Computed tomography: principles, design, artifacts, and recent advances*. Bellingham, WA: SPIE.

Huang, G. B., Zhou, H., Ding, X., & Zhang, R. (2011). Extreme learning machine for regression and multiclass classification. *IEEE Transactions on Systems, Man, and Cybernetics. Part B, Cybernetics*, *42*(2), 513–529. doi:10.1109/TSMCB.2011.2168604 PMID:21984515

Huang, G. B., Zhu, Q. Y., & Siew, C. K. (2006). Extreme learning machine: Theory and applications. *Neurocomputing*, *70*(1-3), 489–501. doi:10.1016/j.neucom.2005.12.126

Kumar, S. P., Sriraam, N., Benakop, P. G., & Jinaga, B. C. (2010, July). Reconstruction of brain electrical impedance tomography images using particle swarm optimization. In *2010 5th International Conference on Industrial and Information Systems* (pp. 339-342). IEEE.

Leão, M. P. V., & Macedo, V. G. (2014). Comparação entre os métodos analítico e iterativo na reconstrução de imagens tomográficas. In *XXIV Congresso Brasileiro de Engenharia Biomédica. Uberlândia: Canal* (*Vol. 6*). Academic Press.

Lei, J., Mu, H. P., Liu, Q. B., Wang, X. Y., & Liu, S. (2018). Data-driven reconstruction method for electrical capacitance tomography. *Neurocomputing*, *273*, 333–345. doi:10.1016/j.neucom.2017.08.006

Li, Q., Zhao, T., Zhang, L., Sun, W., & Zhao, X. (2017). Ferrography wear particles image recognition based on extreme learning machine. *Journal of Electrical and Computer Engineering*, *2017*, 2017. doi:10.1155/2017/3451358

Ministério da Saúde. (2017). *Instituto Nacional de Câncer José Alencar Gomes da Silva*. Estimativa 2018: Incidência de Câncer no Brasil, Rio de Janeiro.

Ogava, R. L. T., Soares, N. S., Gomes, J. C., Barbosa, V. A. F., Ribeiro, R. R., Ribeiro, D. E., de Souza, R. E., & dos Santos, W. P. (2017). Algoritmo de Evolução Diferencial hibridizado e Simulated Annealing aplicados a Tomografia por Impedância Elétrica. *Anais do I Simpósio de Inovação em Engenharia Biomédica - SABIO 2017*, 65.

Pak, D. D., Rozhkova, N. I., Kireeva, M. N., Ermoshchenkova, M. V., Nazarov, A. A., Fomin, D. K., & Rubtsova, N. A. (2012). Diagnosis of breast cancer using electrical impedance tomography. *Biomedical Engineering*, *46*(4), 154–157. doi:10.100710527-012-9292-7 PMID:23035354

Ribeiro, R. R., Feitosa, A. R., de Souza, R. E., & dos Santos, W. P. (2014, May). A modified differential evolution algorithm for the reconstruction of electrical impedance tomography images. In *5th ISSNIP-IEEE Biosignals and Biorobotics Conference (2014): Biosignals and Robotics for Better and Safer Living (BRC)* (pp. 1-6). IEEE.

Ribeiro, R. R., Feitosa, A. R., de Souza, R. E., & dos Santos, W. P. (2014, April). Reconstruction of electrical impedance tomography images using genetic algorithms and non-blind search. In *2014 IEEE 11th International Symposium on Biomedical Imaging (ISBI)* (pp. 153-156). IEEE. 10.1109/ISBI.2014.6867832

Rodrigues, A. L., Bezerra, R. S., de Santana, M. A., dos Santos, W. P., Azevedo, W. W., & de Lima, R. C. (2018). Seleção de Atributos para Apoio ao Diagnóstico do Câncer de Mama Usando Imagens Termográficas, Algoritmos Genéticos e Otimização por Enxame de Partículas. *Anais do II Simpósio de Inovação em Engenharia Biomédica - SABIO 2018.*

Santana, M. A. D., Pereira, J. M. S., Silva, F. L. D., Lima, N. M. D., Sousa, F. N. D., Arruda, G. M. S. D., de Lima, R. C. F., da Silva, W. W. A., & Santos, W. P. D. (2018). Breast cancer diagnosis based on mammary thermography and extreme learning machines. *Research on Biomedical Engineering*, *34*(1), 45–53. doi:10.1590/2446-4740.05217

Soni, N. K., Hartov, A., Kogel, C., Poplack, S. P., & Paulsen, K. D. (2004). Multi-frequency electrical impedance tomography of the breast: New clinical results. *Physiological Measurement*, *25*(1), 301–314. doi:10.1088/0967-3334/25/1/034 PMID:15005324

Tehrani, J. N., Jin, C., McEwan, A., & van Schaik, A. (2010, August). A comparison between compressed sensing algorithms in electrical impedance tomography. In *2010 Annual International Conference of the IEEE Engineering in Medicine and Biology* (pp. 3109-3112). IEEE. 10.1109/IEMBS.2010.5627165

Torre, L., Siegel, R., & Jemal, A. (2015). *Global cancer facts & figures.* American Cancer Society.

Wan, Y., Borsic, A., Heaney, J., Seigne, J., Schned, A., Baker, M., Wason, S., Hartov, A., & Halter, R. (2013). Transrectal electrical impedance tomography of the prostate: Spatially coregistered pathological findings for prostate cancer detection. *Medical Physics*, *40*(6Part1), 063102. doi:10.1118/1.4803498 PMID:23718610

Wang, H., Xu, G., Zhang, S., & Yan, W. (2015). An implementation of generalized back projection algorithm for the 2-D anisotropic EIT problem. *IEEE Transactions on Magnetics*, *51*(3), 1–4. doi:10.1109/TMAG.2014.2356648

Zou, Y., & Guo, Z. (2003). A review of electrical impedance techniques for breast cancer detection. *Medical Engineering & Physics*, *25*(2), 79–90. doi:10.1016/S1350-4533(02)00194-7 PMID:12538062

Chapter 3
Classification of Breast Lesions in Frontal Thermographic Images Using a Diagnosis Aid Intelligent System

Maíra Araújo de Santana
Universidade Federal de Pernambuco, Brazil

Jessiane Mônica Silva Pereira
Universidade Federal de Pernambuco, Brazil

Clarisse Lins de Lima
Universidade Federal de Pernambuco, Brazil

Maria Beatriz Jacinto de Almeida
Universidade Federal de Pernambuco, Brazil

José Filipe Silva de Andrade
Universidade Federal de Pernambuco, Brazil

Thifany Ketuli Silva de Souza
Universidade Federal de Pernambuco, Brazil

Rita de Cássia Fernandes de Lima
Universidade Federal de Pernambuco, Brazil

Wellington Pinheiro dos Santos
https://orcid.org/0000-0003-2558-6602
Universidade Federal de Pernambuco, Brazil

ABSTRACT

This study aims to assess the breast lesions classification in thermographic images using different configuration of an Extreme Learning Machine network as classifier. In this approach, the authors changed the number of neurons in the hidden layer and the type of kernel function to further explore the network in order to find a better solution for the classification problem. Authors also used different tools to perform features extraction to assess both texture and geometry information from the breast lesions. During the study, the authors found that the results changed not only due to the network parameters but also due to the features chosen to represent the thermographic images. A maximum accuracy of 95% was found for the differentiation of breast lesions.

DOI: 10.4018/978-1-7998-3456-4.ch003

INTRODUCTION

Breast cancer is the most common type of cancer among women worldwide. According to the World Health Organization (WHO), 1.7 million people are affected by this disease each year. In Brazil, breast cancer corresponds to 28% of new cases of cancer per year. Even having a good prognosis, this disease is still responsible for the highest cancer fatality rate in the female population. According to WHO, early detection of tumors, which is the identification of cancer in early stages, is essential in order to reduce mortality from the disease (World Health Organization (WHO), 2014).

Nowadays, breast cancer screening is performed using many imaging techniques. The gold standard for the diagnosis of this disease is mammography. However, there are several limitations associated to it. This technique consists of an x-ray scanning of the breast, which is an ionizing radiation. Therefore, it already is a risk factor for the patient. Furthermore, mammography can only show anatomical changes in the region, which are usually only noticed when the disease is already in a more advanced stages. Thus, diagnosis at early stages becomes extremely difficult. To minimize the exposure of patients to ionizing radiation and seeking early identification of the disease, other techniques such as ultrasound, magnetic resonance imaging and thermography are being explored.

The thermography is based on the acquisition of images that present the temperature distribution of a surface. This imaging technique uses an infrared camera to acquire the images. In general, the camera captures infrared radiation emitted by the surface of interest. In breast thermography there is no need for invasive procedures or exposure of the patient to ionizing radiation. Moreover, the technique allows the investigation of physiological changes from the analysis of temperatures in the region. In the case of cancer cells, there is an increase in local metabolism, directly interfering on blood flow, and thus increasing the region temperature. In general, these physiological changes may appear up to 10 years before any anatomical change, favoring the diagnosis in early stages of the disease (Etehadtavakol & Ng, 2013).

One of the main challenges of imaging diagnosis is clinical variability. The fact that diseases behave differently in different individuals makes it difficult for professionals to extract useful information from the images. This fact leads to great variability in the diagnosis provided to the patient. So, the same case is often diagnosed differently by different professionals (McKinlay et al., 1998). Computer Aided Diagnosis (CAD) systems is a tool that has been explored worldwide to overcome this challenge. In these systems, computational tools are used to assist health professionals in the analysis of medical examinations in many areas (Acharya et al., 2012; Aguiar Junior et al., 2013; Andrade, Santana & Santos, 2018; Azevedo et al., 2015; Belfort, Silva & Paiva, 2015; Cheng et al., 2005; Cordeiro, Santos & Silva-Filho, 2016; Resmini et al., 2012; Rodrigues, et al., 2018; Santana, et al., 2018).

In this scenario, several groups are dedicated to the study of computational techniques for the identification of lesions in breast thermograms. Aguiar Junior et al. (2013) performed tests using multilayer perceptron as a classifier to detect the existence of lesions in breast thermographic images, obtaining accuracies of about 75%. Resmini et al. (2012), on the other hand, obtained results close to 90% of accuracy using other classifiers (SVM, KNN and Naive Bayes) to detect the existence of breast lesion. Belfort, Silva & Paiva (2015) introduced another method of breast lesion detection in thermographic images, wherein they obtained an accuracy of around 78% using Jaccard Similarity Index and Artificial Crawlers.

In the study of Martins et al. (2011), they used statistical attributes and texture descriptors to represent images. The authors tested the Support Vector Machine (SVM), Naive Bayes, Linear Discriminant Analysis (LDA), and K-Nearest Neighbor (kNN) classifiers. Using cross-validation and kNN, they achieved results of up to 92.5% accuracy. Burges (1998), on the other hand, used Fourier descriptors to evaluate differences between position and contrast of images with breast lesions. He used a sample of 146 images, with 46 diagnosed as malignant and the remaining benign, achieving an accuracy of up to 88.17% in the differentiation of lesions.

The method proposed here aims to specifically classify the type of lesion present in breast thermographic images. For this purpose, the authors used a very promising but not widely known classifier, the Extreme Learning Machines (ELM). Throughout the study, they sought to verify different ways of image representation, as well as different parameters for the ELM network, in order to improve the lesions classification. From the study, combinations of parameters allowed up to 95% of correct classification.

This chapter is organized in four sections. Initially, the authors present a background of the problematic approached and some theoretical concepts used in this chapter. Then, the proposed method is presented, as well as the tools used to develop it. The following section presents and discusses the results obtained through the proposed approach. Finally, the general conclusion reached is pointed out.

BACKGROUND

In this section, the authors introduce the main concepts explored along this chapter.

Anatomy and Physiology of the Breast

The breasts are the human reproduction auxiliary exocrine glands. Their main functions are the production, storage and release of milk. They are located on the anterior chest wall (outermost portion); are vertically positioned between the second and sixth ribs and horizontally positioned between the anterior axillary line and the edge of the sternum (Moore, Dalley & Agur, 2001). Its embryonic formation begins between the fifth and sixth weeks of gestation through the formation of the milk line (Menke, 2000).

The alveoli are the smallest forming units of the gland. They are organized similarly to grape clusters, in sets of 10 to 100 honeycomb units. The set of alveoli form the morphofunctional unit of the breast, the mammary lobes. In the lobes will occur the main chemical processes related to the breasts. Clusters of 20 to 40 lobes will constitute the mammary lobes. Then, there is the formation of the mammary parenchyma (the gland itself), consisting of the union of 15 to 20 lobes. Visually, the mammary parenchyma resembles an "inverted cauliflower". The parenchyma is surrounded by stroma, which is formed by fat, connective tissue, vessels and nerves (Menke, 2000).

Externally, the breast contains the areolomamilar complex, formed by areola and mammary papilla. In the areolas, there are elevations known as Morgagni tubers. These small prominences are caused by the opening of Montgomery's sebaceous gland ducts, which lubricate and protect the papilla during breastfeeding. The papillae (or nipples) are located in the center of the areolas and they are formed by smooth and circular muscle fibers without the presence of fat, hair or sweat glands.

In the breasts, there are "tubular" structures responsible for the drainage of the lobes. These ducts begin in the alveoli (with small intra and extralobular ducts) and extend into the mammary papillae. The lobes are drained by a main collecting duct that dilates near the areola. The dilated part of the ducts are called lactose sinuses or galactophore (Moore, Dalley & Agur, 2001).

During the female puberty (on average between 10 and 12 years), the maturation of the hypothalamus-pituitary-ovarian axis generates the production and release of hormones (Menke, 2000). The first hormones secreted during these years are estrogens. The ovaries secrete these hormones. In the breasts, estrogens are responsible for gland growth and development of milk-producing structures. These hormones actively participate in the development of mammary stroma, mammary duct growth and fat deposition, and, in part, in the development of lobes and alveoli (Guyton & Hall, 2011).

Throughout ovulatory cycles, progesterone hormone levels increase. This hormone is produced under the stimulus of hCG (chorionic gonadotropin) and is produced by the corpus luteum. Unlike estrogens, they act directly linked to reproduction. This feature is important for the fetus maintenance during pregnancy. It also causes alveolar cells to become secretory, aiding early breastfeeding. Moreover, it is responsible for breast enlargement due to the lobes and alveoli secretory development (Guyton & Hall, 2011).

During pregnancy, it is noticed the gradual increase of the prolactin hormone, which is released by the adenohypophyseal gland (Menke, 2000). During pregnancy, the large amount of progesterone inhibits the prolactin receptors. However, after delivery, and with decreasing progesterone levels, prolactin will act directly on lactogenesis (breast milk production by the mammary gland). Prolactin is not only important to provide the milk itself, but also to provide breast development during pregnancy in the preparation of the gland for milk production (Guyton & Hall, 2011).

Breast Cancer

The breast tissue is constantly changing, responding to environmental, dietary, hormone action stimuli. These actions cause cellular changes and thus preventing benign and malignant diseases (Saladin & Porth, 2010). Tumors are composed of masses of cells that do not have the ability to organize themselves, losing their functions (Weinberg, 2008). According to the International Agency for Research on Cancer (IARC), breast cancer is one of the three most prevalent cancers in the world. It is also responsible for a 6.6% fatality rate considering all types of diseases. This carcinoma may be clinically presented as a palpable nodule, as abnormalities on imaging exams, histologically and as metastases (Brasileiro Filho, 2011).

Breast cancer is a pathology with no defined etiology. However, it is possible to list some risk factors directly linked to the increase in their incidence (Barros, Pompei & Silveira, 2010). Risk factors for developing breast cancer are commonly hereditary or sporadic. Both are related to hormone exposure. The sporadic comprises sex, age, reproductive history and presence of exogenous estrogen. The major contributing factor is gender. The breast cancer in men comprises only 1% of cases, so, it mostly affects women. The occurrence of breast cancer increases with age. Starting at the age of 30, the chance of developing breast cancer grows considerably, with a peak at the ages between 50 and 60 years old. Women who have their first menstrual period before age 11 are about 20% more likely to develop this type of cell mutation when compared to women who have it after 14 years old. This also goes for a late menopause. Exposure to postmenopausal hormone replacement therapy also increases the risk of developing breast cancer. It also has a greater increase when added to progesterone. Estrogen metabolites can generate DNA-damaging mutations in cells, as well as some changes in the genes involved in their statistics and metabolism may increase the risk of breast cancer (Brasileiro Filho, 2011; Kumar et al., 2010).

On the hereditary factors, the probability of having breast cancer increases with the number of first-degree relatives affected with the same type of cancer. Approximately ⅓ of women with breast carcinoma had or have a relative with the same condition. Gene inheritance is the cause of about 5 to 10% of breast cancers. Mutations in the BRCA1 and BRCA2 genes also leads to a greater predisposition to the development of breast cancer, usually when there is the inactivation of these genes. (Brasileiro Filho, 2011; Kumar et al., 2010). These genes are classified as tumor suppressors and are associated to cell metabolism, cell cycle control, DNA damage repair, and gene expression regulation (Coelho et al., 2018).

Thus, the neoplasm process is initiated with mutations that deregulate the function of these genes that act, directly or indirectly, on cell proliferation or survival. When its functioning is altered, the result is abnormal stimulation in cell division and its proliferation (Brasileiro Filho, 2011; Kumar et al., 2010).

About 95% of mammary carcinomas can be classified into two types: *in situ* or invasive carcinomas. *In situ* carcinoma comprises a neoplastic proliferation bound to the ducts and lobes by the basement membrane without invading the stroma. It can be divided into two types, ductal or lobular carcinoma *in situ*, where they differ in both their cells and their clinical behavior. The ductal usually presents in the same quadrant, with calcifications that can be identified by imaging exams and expression of Estrogen Receptor (ER) and of Human Epidermal growth factor Receptor 2 (HER2/neu). The development rate for invasive cancer is very small (about 1% per year). Lobular cancer *in situ* is hardly associated with calcifications, and it has some morphological changes, similar to invasive lobular carcinoma. Their cells may be ER-negative and some overexpress HER2/neu (Brasileiro Filho, 2011; Kumar et al., 2010).

The invasive carcinoma infiltrates the stroma and, in most cases, presents itself as a palpable mass. If it involves the central part of the breast, it may have nipple retraction. When it also covers lymphatic vessels it may occur skin blockage drainage with consequent lymphedema and thickening of the skin. Invasive cancer can be grouped into some types and subtypes. The invasive ductal carcinoma is classified as the most frequent type of breast cancer and it has a more aggressive behavior with heterogeneous lesions. This type of cancer can not be categorized into special subtypes due to its morphology. It shows up as a palpable mass with irregular density and microcalcifications. The invasive lobular carcinoma also has the presence of a mass with irregular borders. Yet, they are more difficult to feel on self-examination, because the tumor may infiltrate the tissue. It has a greater tendency towards bilaterality and a considerably large rate for late recurrence with metastases (Brasileiro Filho, 2011; Kumar et al., 2010).

Some subtypes of breast carcinoma are relevant to mention. The tubular carcinoma is characterized by the formation of tubules in which tumor cells are in direct contact with the stroma. It also appears as a palpable and detectable nodule in mammography. They are usually ER-positive and HER2/neu negative, linked to the type of hereditary cancer with mutations in the BRCA2 gene. Mucinous breast cancer, also called colloid, has a jelly-like tumor and commonly affects older women. It accounts for only about 2-3% of breast carcinomas and is ER-positive. Medullary carcinoma has a well-circumscribed soft tumor and is often associated with abnormalities in the BRCA1 genes, mainly occurring in women of ages around 60 years. Typically, these three types of invasive carcinoma have a good prognosis and a good survival rate (Brasileiro Filho, 2011; Kumar et al., 2010).

Metaplastic carcinoma accounts for less than 1% of breast cancers, with a rare tumor (presence of squamous and fusiform cells) and heterogeneous behavior. In most cases, this subtype is aggressive and susceptible to metastasis. They are ER-PR-HER2/neu triple negative. Inflammatory breast cancer differs from other types of breast cancer. In addition to being rare, it spreads much faster than the others. It does not commonly manifest with the presence of nodules, making its diagnosis difficult. Its main characteristics are breast swelling and skin thickening, resulting from embolization of the lymphatic vessels of the dermis (caused by cancer cells). Its signs and symptoms, such as redness, tenderness and itching, are common to benign conditions such as inflammation of the breast (mastitis), often leading to misdiagnosis. These last two subtypes have a poor prognosis in general (Brasileiro Filho, 2011; Kumar et al., 2010).

It is very important to know about the prognostic marker of carcinomas. It helps to understand tumor growth and biological characteristics. When predictive, it provides information that mediates how the patient's response to therapeutic intervention will be (Brasileiro Filho, 2011). Some factors that greatly influence the prognosis of breast carcinoma are: classification in *in situ* or invasive, tumor size, axillary involvement (lymph nodes), the histological grade and subtype. Hormone receptors are a factor of tumor type differentiation. They are also considered an important predictor of hormone treatment. The cell type that is most common in cancer origin is the ER-expressive and PR-expressive luminal cell. Most cancers are ER-positive and PR-positive (estrogen and progesterone receptors). In such cases, hormone treatment usually provides good results and a positive short-term prognosis. The hormone treatment acts either reducing or blocking progesterone and estrogen. There are also cancers that express HER2/neu protein, which promotes the growth of breast cells. These types of cancers are usually associated to poor prognosis. However, there are treatments that directly act on this protein, increasing the chances of success (Brasileiro Filho, 2011; Kumar et al., 2010).

Thermography and Breast Cancer Diagnosis

There are several tests for early diagnosis of breast cancer. The most accessible one is the self-examination. The self-examination consists in the patient's act of palpating their own breasts in order to verify the existence of some abnormality in this region. When an anomaly is found, it is advisable for the patient to seek medical attention to confirm a diagnosis (WHO, 2018). In other cases, the patient themselves seek a health institution and undergoes examinations (WHO, 2018). Generally, to confirm the existence of any breast disorder, the doctor asks the patient to perform one or some of the imaging screening tests. The most common is the mammogram exam. However, in some specific cases, magnetic resonance imaging, ultrasonography and thermography are also used (Instituto Nacional de Câncer (INCA), 2002).

Breast thermography is a non-invasive, fast, safe and totally painless diagnostic exam. It does not emit ionizing radiation and has no side effects. It simply acquires the infrared radiation emitted by the skin of the patient, creating a temperature map of the region for further analysis (Ring & Ammer, 2012). The human body regulates heat transfer to the environment through a system called thermoregulation. It can change the cross section of blood vessels by modifying tissue irrigation and, thereby, modifying temperature. Thermoregulation depends on the autonomic nervous system (Sessler, 1994). Therefore, in the presence of pathologies, there will be a strong blood supply in the affected region in order to feed the enlarged amount of cells and to deliver antibodies to fight the disease. Thermography would, then, be able to detect these irregularities due to temperature changes present in this region (Ring & Ammer, 2012). This exam consists of three main stages: the preparation of the patient and the environment, the acquisition of images and the identification of the cancer (Araújo, 2009).

During the first stage, the procedure consists on the regularization of the thermal conditions of the examination room. At this step, it is also important to take specific measures to the patient comfort. First, the examination room must be large enough to accommodate patient and professional. There must be an appropriate space for the camera transition in order to record the specific body part to be diagnosed. Second, the room temperature and humidity must remain stable. Therefore, the room needs to be fully enclosed so that there is no airflow interfering on these variables. The temperature should be adjusted so the patient is comfortable, neither sweating nor feeling cold. These small details can interfere on the diagnosis, affecting the veracity of temperatures in the images collected from the tissue (Cockburn, 2018).

At least 24 hours before the examination, it is extremely important that the patient receives instructions for a better imaging result. The protocols should be followed and confirmed before the examination. There are some restrictions that the patient must follow. For example, not to bathe in hot water at least two hours before the examination. It is also recommended not to shave their armpits or other parts of the body that will be examined. The patient should avoid the consumption of caffeinated or alcoholic beverages 24 hours before the examination . Lotions, creams, antiperspirants deodorants, perfumes or talcum powder should not be used. Moreover, the patient should not have a sunburn nor physical exercise nor physical therapy activities at least 24 hours before the test, except under medical advice. Throughout the whole process, it is highly suggested that the patients inform the doctor about all the medications they are taking. Therefore, it is strongly recommended for them not to stop taking their medications without medical supervision (Cockburn, 2018).

At the beginning of the exam, the patient must complete a report regarding their health history, birth history and menstrual cycle. The patient must sign a statement confirming that they followed the protocols which are prerequisites for the exam. After this step, the patient is transferred to a changing room, where they undress from the waist up and wear a robe. Then, she may not touch her breasts until the body temperature and the room temperature are balanced. This last process is called acclimatization. In most axams, the patients place their hands on their heads with their elbows extended outward to lift the breast and cool the armpit region. Other exam environments have bars for the patient to hold. Both methods are acceptable (Cockburn, 2018). After this, a set of images is acquired. These images are, then, analyzed in the most appropriate way chosen by the specialist or defined by the health institution.

To obtain the patient thermograms, an infrared camera is used, which is able to identify temperature levels at different points on the body. The discovery and use of these cameras began during World War II (1939-1945) (Tyson, 2001). The military used binocular and sensors as cameras for night conflicts. The heat emitted by the human body was recorded in these tools and, thus, improved the attacking strategies of the soldier who had these instruments. In 1957, these cameras were first used for medicinal purposes by Dr. R. Lawson (Lawson, 1957). He found a noticeable rise in temperature in cancerous breast tissue compared to healthy ones (Lawson, 1957). Only in later years, this technique started being highly used to support breast cancer detection.

The infrared cameras capture images by a temperature sensor, in a spectral range different from visible light (Araújo, 2009). The electromagnetic spectrum is a scale of electromagnetic radiation. It is obtained by the set of electromagnetic waves formed by the propagation of electric fields and magnetic fields in space (Halliday, Resnick & Walker, 2009). Infrared radiation has a lower frequency than visible light. Which means it belongs to a level that is invisible to human vision on the electromagnetic scale. This radiation is emitted by any body that is at a temperature above absolute zero. Its use is based on the fact that its intensity is proportional to the fourth power of its absolute temperature, the so-called Stefan-Boltzmann Law (Bohren & Huffman, 1998). Therefore, the temperature sensors allocated to the cameras capture the electrical signals of the radiation intensity and convert them to digital signals. These electrical signals are amplified and then processed to a visual display, where the image shows a heatmap that encodes each temperature in a specific color by using the pseudo-coloring technique.

There are essential parameters for accurate temperature measurement by infrared cameras on an object, because the radiation that reaches the camera is not entirely from the body itself (Araújo, 2009). The measured radiation will vary according to some factors of the object:

- **Distance:** the distance between the camera and the object.
- **Body Emissivity:** this parameter is based on the comparison between the radiation emitted by the body and the radiation emitted by the black body (a theoretical object that absorbs all electromagnetic radiation that hits it). The human skin has an emissivity close to 1.

- **Reflected Temperature:** is used to compensate for radiation from the body and radiation from external sources in the camera.
- **Relative humidity:** since the transmittance (heat transfer rate through matter) partially depends on atmospheric humidity, the humidity must be regulated by the camera.

Calibrating the camera with these parameters is essential for more accurate measurement. Because the camera receives some information from the atmosphere around the body, and atmospheric factors interfere in the results accuracy (Araújo, 2009).

These images may be assessed in laboratories by software that determines the existence of cancer (Souza et al., 2019). Thermography has given accurate results in different methods used to classify cancer in the collected images. Furthermore, the development of various analytical techniques using artificial intelligence is on the rise (Souza et al., 2019).

Artificial Intelligence for Breast Cancer Detection

Artificial intelligence is a multidisciplinary science that seeks to develop and apply computational techniques that attempts to simulate human behavior in specific activities (Goldschmidt, 2010). This field provides solutions for countless applications. The intelligent algorithms allow computers to have a large capacity to process and store knowledge in many fields. So they became able to recognize patterns that would normally be difficult for human perception (Pontes, 2011).

An alternative to achieve artificial intelligence is through machine learning. This approach gives the machine an autonomy to perform a task without manual software routine implementations. Algorithms are used, at first, to collect a range of data and their patterns are modeled according to the experience obtained by the algorithms. The process of gaining this experience is commonly known as data training. There are two main types of training algorithms: supervised and unsupervised (Jordan & Mitchell, 2015). The choice of which algorithm to use depends on the application.

For diagnosis, as in thermographic assessment, the supervised method is the most used to identify pathologies, so the system undergoes training based on predefined data. In this case, the data is a bank of breast images in different health conditions. A subcategory of supervised learning and widely used in this occasion is classification which consists of assigning labels to the entry data, which are called classes.

During the data training, several tests are performed aiming the correctly classification of the instances. The metrics used to evaluate these results are the accuracy, which represents the sum of all expected values divided by the total values; and the kappa statistic, that measures the agreement level between the results. Accuracy ranges from 0% to 100%, while kappa maximum value is 1, indicating full agreement. Kappa values that are close to or below 0 (zero) shows no agreement or total dissociation between the obtained and the expected results.

Basically, there are two ways to improve classification performance. The first one is to choose the most suitable method to represent the data through a process called features extraction. The second one is to find the algorithm the has the best ability to learn and differentiate the patterns of this data. There are several possible ways to perform features extraction and classification. Some researchers are being successful on detecting breast cancer in thermographic images by using well established computational techniques (Pereira et al., 2017; Santana et al., 2018; Souza et al., 2019).

Haralick and Zernike Moments for Features Extraction

Haralick descriptor extracts texture-based features from statistical calculations between neighboring pixels of the image (Haralick, Shanmugam & Dinstein, 1973). These features are obtained through co-occurrence matrices. The co-occurrence matrix has the color occurrence values at a given image and represents the spatial distribution and dependence of gray levels within a local area. From Haralick descriptor it is possible to differentiate textures that do not follow a certain pattern of repetition in the image (Haralick, Shanmugam & Dinstein, 1973). This study used 32 texture features.

Zernike descriptor, on the other hand, is an effective tool for extracting shape information from a given image. Zernike moments captures global shape of an image while being rotation invariant and robust to noise (Kan & Srinath, 2001). To calculate these moments, the center of an image is considered as a center of an unitary disk. Each of the 64 moments are calculated from a Zernike polynomial, which are divided into low and high order (Azevedo et al., 2015).

Extreme Learning Machine (ELM)

The Extreme Learning Machine (ELM) is a training approach for single hidden layer feedforward networks. ELM was first proposed to overcome some issues from the learning algorithm used in feedforward neural networks. Some of these issues are the presence of local minima, network over-training and the time-consuming learning. This classifier randomly assign input weights and bias. The output weights are estimated using analytical methods based on Moore-Penrose generalized inverse. Therefore, it is usually associated with fast learning phases (Huang, Zhu & Siew, 2006).

As shown in Huang, Zhu and Siew (2006), ELM algorithm works for any infinitely differential activation function. In the study presented in this chapter, the authors chose to test ELM classification performance using different configuration of activation function (kernels). They performed experiments using linear, polynomial and radial basis (RBF) functions.

PROPOSED METHOD

The thermographic images used in this study were acquired through a FLIR S45 infrared camera. The access to the images was provided through a collaboration with the breast thermography research group of the Department of Mechanical Engineering of the Federal University of Pernambuco (UFPE). The breast images were acquired for each patient in eight different positions (see Figure 1). Two of the images are frontal images of both breasts (T1 and T2). The other images are from each breast individually in three different views: frontal (MD, for right breast, and ME, for left breast), external lateral (LEMD and LEME) and internal lateral (LIMD and LIME) (Oliveira, 2012).

As mentioned before, some preparations are required before performing images acquisition. Regarding the room, it is important not open and close the door very frequently in order to avoid the airflow. Moreover, the room temperature and humidity were periodically measured using a THAL-300 thermo-hygro-anemometer-luxmeter. A mechanical device was also used to provide greater standardization of patient positioning, such as shown in Figure 2. For the patients, they underwent a 10-minute acclimatization period. During this period, they were asked to sit still, without touching their breasts. Their body body temperature were also measured using a clinical thermometer.

Figure 1. Examples of images acquired in the exam. In the superior left corner is the frontal images of both breasts (T1 and T2), in T1 the arms are on the waist, while in T2 the patient is holding a bar above her head. Still in the superior portion of this figure is MD, the frontal image of the right breast alone, and ME, the frontal image of the left breast. In the bottom are the four images of lateral views of each breast.
Source: The authors

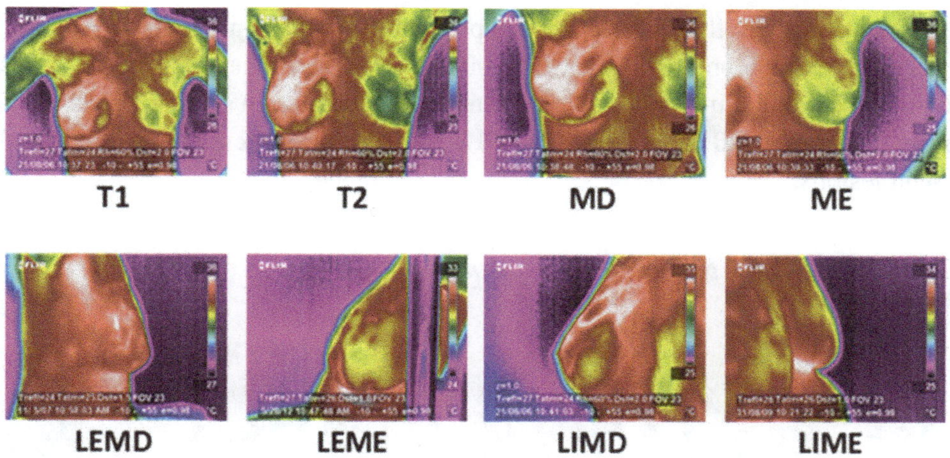

Figure 2. Acquisition room with the mechanical device built for acquisition of breast thermography
Source: The authors

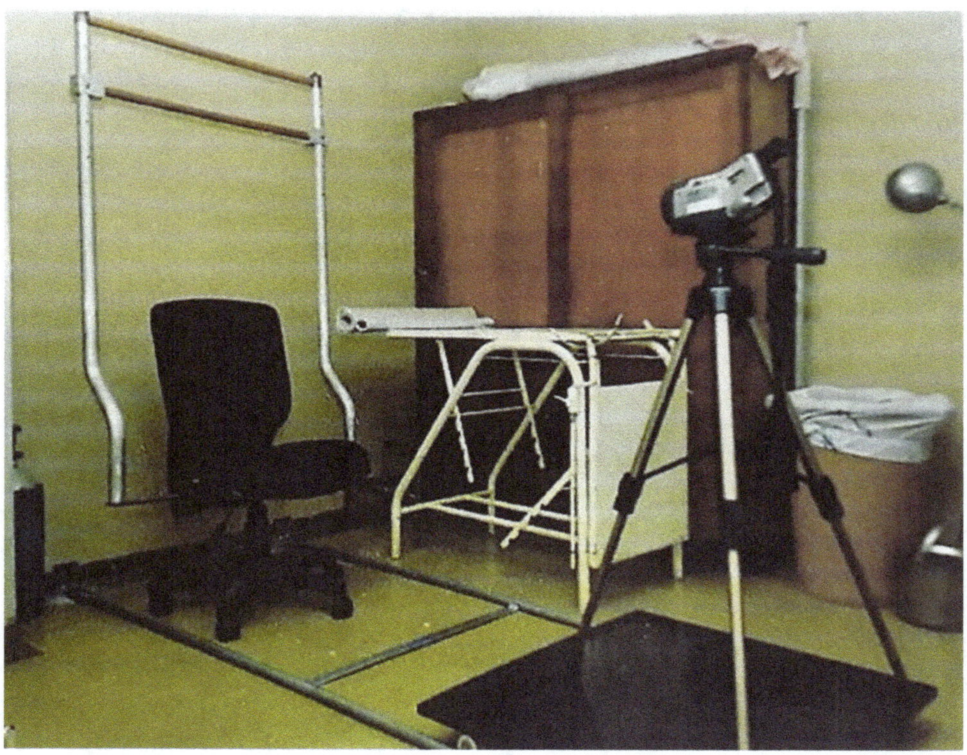

The image database was also organized according to the types of diagnoses. Each type of diagnose were previously established based on specific methods for each case, such as clinical examinations, biopsies, mammograms and breast ultrasounds (Dourado Neto, 2014). In this study, the authors used images where there was cystic lesions, benign lesions or malignant lesions. Figure 3 shows examples of images from each of these groups. These classes were chosen to verify the effectiveness of the system in classifying the images into their respective groups. Moreover, the experiments were performed only using frontal images of both breasts (T1 and T2), since these conditions eases the identification of the region of interest. The diagram on Figure 4 presents a brief description of the method used to perform the experiments. A total of 270 images participated in this study: 73 of cysts, 121 of benign lesions and 76 of malignant lesions.

Figure 3. Examples of images of each class of diagnosis
Source: The authors

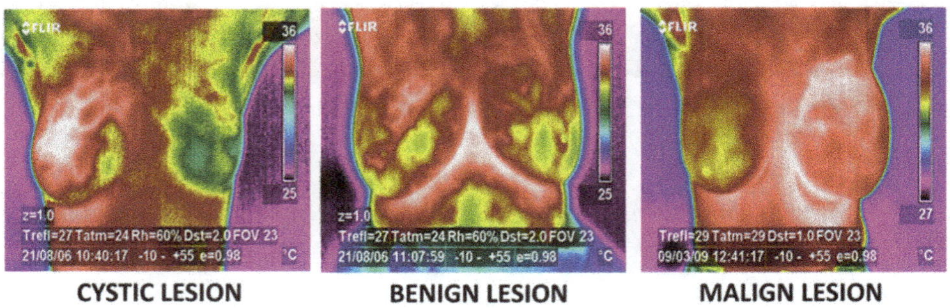

Figure 4. Brief description of the proposed method
Source: The authors

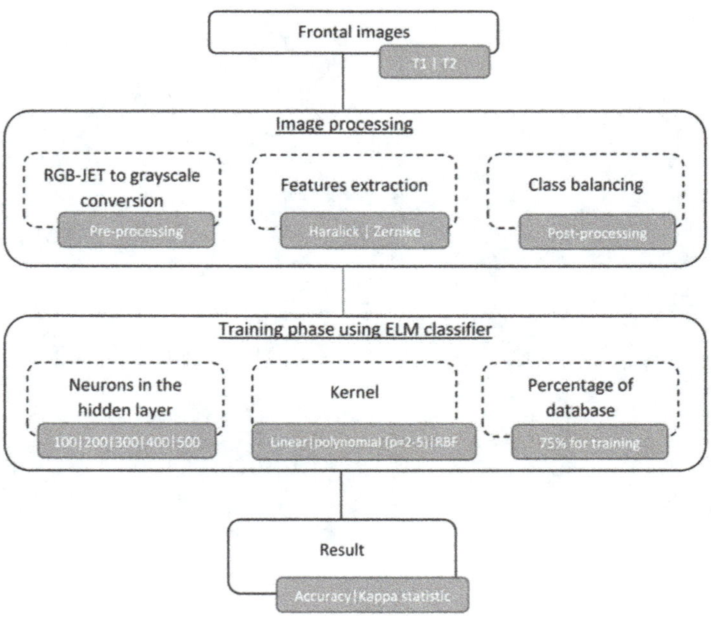

Initially, the images were submitted to a preprocessing step, which consisted in converting the images from RGB-JET pseudo-color to grayscale images. As mentioned before, since thermal images use the principle of pseudo-coloring, the colors shown in the images are actually associated with the temperature of the region. Thus, in conversion process, this principle was respected, so lighter shades of gray indicate higher temperatures, while the darker ones are associated to lower temperatures.

The method also proposes the use of Haralick moments and Zernike moments to perform features extraction, to represent the dataset. These extractors were chosen because the texture and shape characteristics have been relevant for the differentiation of these types of lesions in clinical practice (Ribeiro et al., 2008; Rodrigues, 2008; Azevedo et al., 2015).

As previously mentioned, the number of images in each class is different, which may lead to a biased result during training. The algorithms may interpret that the lesions should be more commonly classified as of the class with more instances. To overcome this problem, the authors performed a class balancing by inserting synthetic instances. These instances were created from a linear combinations of features vectors of real instances of the same class (Lima, Silva-Filho & Santos, 2016).

The following step was training the data with Extreme Learning Machines (ELM). During the tests, some classifier parameters were modified. The first one was the number of hidden layer neurons, which are especially important in cases where the problem is nonlinear. In general, the larger the number of neurons in the layer the higher is the network fitness. Different configurations were also tested for the kernel function, which is responsible for establishing the decision boundary of the problem. The linear, polynomial, with exponent (P) ranging from 2 to 5, and Radial Basis Function (RBF) kernels were tested. For the hidden layer the authors verified the use of 100, 200, 300, 400 and 500 neurons.

Furthermore, the tests were performed under three different conditions for the features: using only Haralick moments, only Zernike moments and both at the same time. To perform each test, the percentage division method was applied to randomly split the dataset into 75% for training and 25% for test. To evaluate the configurations, the authors compared the results of accuracy and kappa statistic metrics for each case.

SOLUTIONS AND RECOMMENDATIONS

Initially, it was used the database obtained through the Haralick extractor. Figure 5a shows the accuracy values achieved by each configuration. In Figure 5b are the results for kappa statistic for this dataset. From Figure 5, it is possible to notice a minimum variation of the results when the authors changed the amount of neurons in the hidden layer. However, the best results were obtained when using 300, 400 or 500 neurons in the hidden layer. As for the kernels, the linear kernel showed the best results, while the worst results appeared when the RBF kernel was used. Polynomial kernels showed similar results. Overall, the best accuracy obtained for this case was slightly over 80%, and kappa around 0.75, using linear kernel and 400 neurons. The worst result was around 70% of accuracy and 0.55 of kappa, using RBF kernel and 100 hidden layer neurons.

The second database was built using only the features extracted by Zernike moments. The results of accuracy and kappa statistic are shown in Figure 6. From the results of Figure 6, it is possible to see an improvement in the differentiation of lesions when using the Zernike features. The use of polynomial kernels, from second to fourth degree, also provided better results than with linear kernel. On the other hand, the fifth degree polynomial kernel and the RBF kernel accounted for the worst results. Regarding

Figure 5. Results using the database from Haralick moments alone. In (a) are the results of accuracy, (b) shows the kappa statistics.
Source: The authors

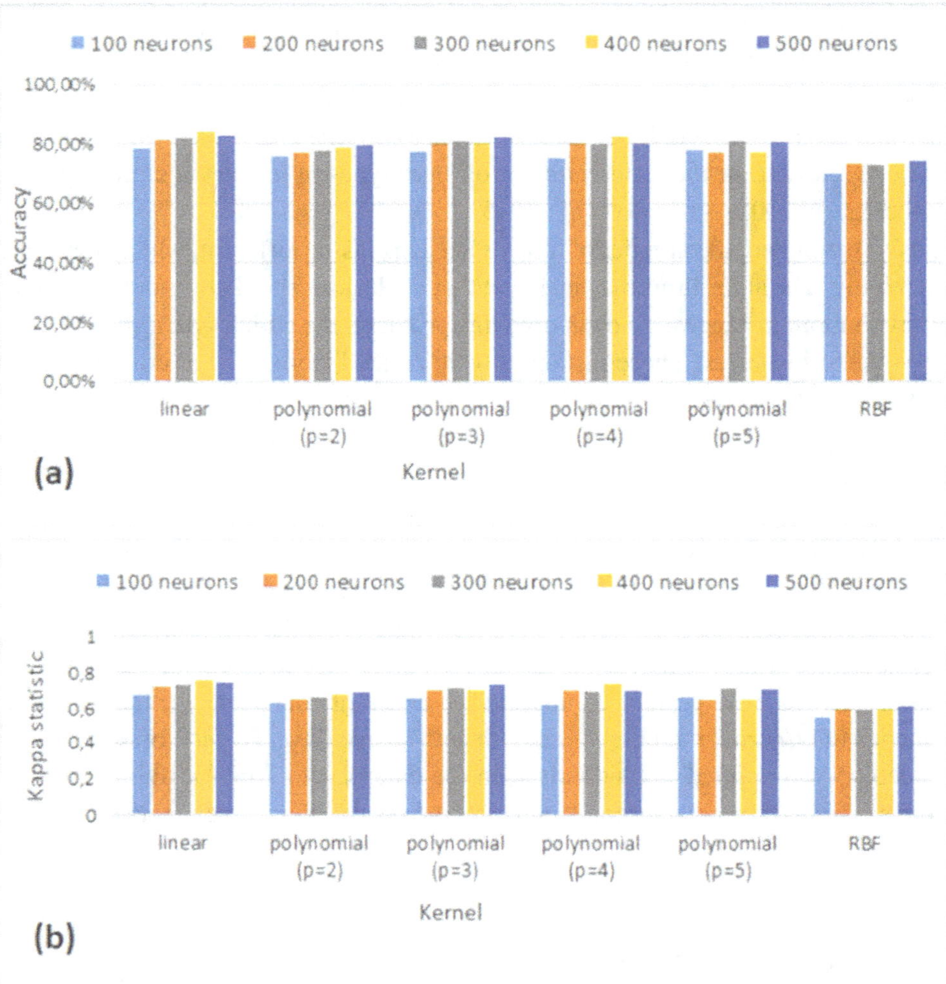

the amount of neurons, the worst results were obtained when using 100 neurons in the hidden layer. Furthermore, the use of 400 and 500 neurons increased the accuracy and kappa values. For this database, where the images were represented by Zernike moments, the best result was obtained with the second degree polynomial kernel and 500 neurons. This configuration achieved more than 90% of accuracy and kappa around 0.90. The worst result was obtained when using the fifth degree polynomial kernel and 100 neurons, with accuracy around 75% and kappa slightly over 0.60. However, this result was still higher than the worst result when the images were represented only by Haralick features.

After the individual evaluation of the features extraction techniques studied in this chapter, the descriptors were combined. In this step, the authors represented the images using both Haralick and Zernike features. This combination was used to access more information from the images, in an attempt to provide a better differentiation of the types of lesions. The results from this dataset are shown in Figure 7. The results from Figure 7 show that the combination of Haralick and Zernike features was positive in

Figure 6. Results using the database from Zernike moments alone. In (a) are the results of accuracy, (b) shows the kappa statistics.
Source: The authors

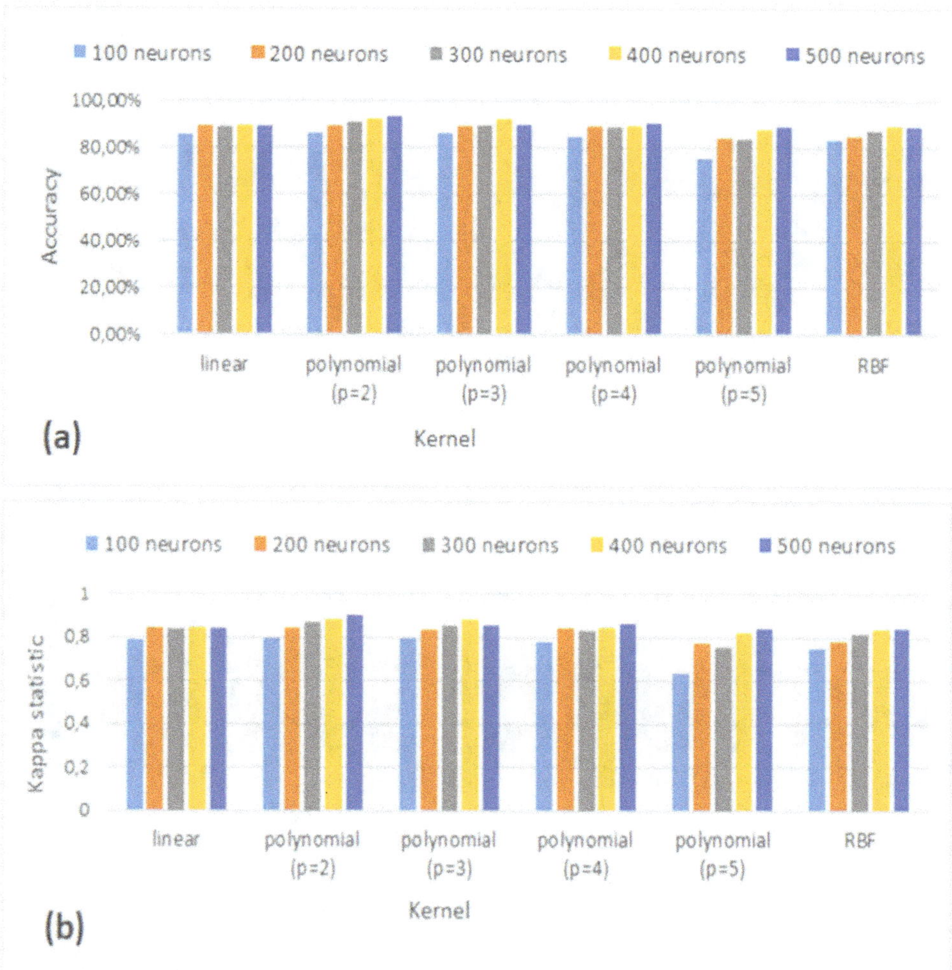

order to provide a better representation of the breast thermographic images. This combination favored the differentiation of breast lesions in this images, when using ELM as classifier. The authors found an accuracy around 95%, with kappa statistic close to 0.95, when using linear kernel and 500 neurons in the hidden layer. Similar results were obtained with the polynomial kernel of exponent 2 and 300 neurons. Again, the worst results was reached when they used polynomial kernel of exponent 5 and RBF kernel, with accuracy of 80% and 0.70 for kappa statistic.

CONCLUSION

From the results obtained in this chapter, it was possible to verify a more suitable configuration for ELM to differentiate cystic, benign and malignant lesions from breast thermography. Overall, the linear kernel

Figure 7. Results using the database from the combination of both Haralick and Zernike moments. In (a) are the results of accuracy, (b) shows the kappa statistics.
Source: The authors

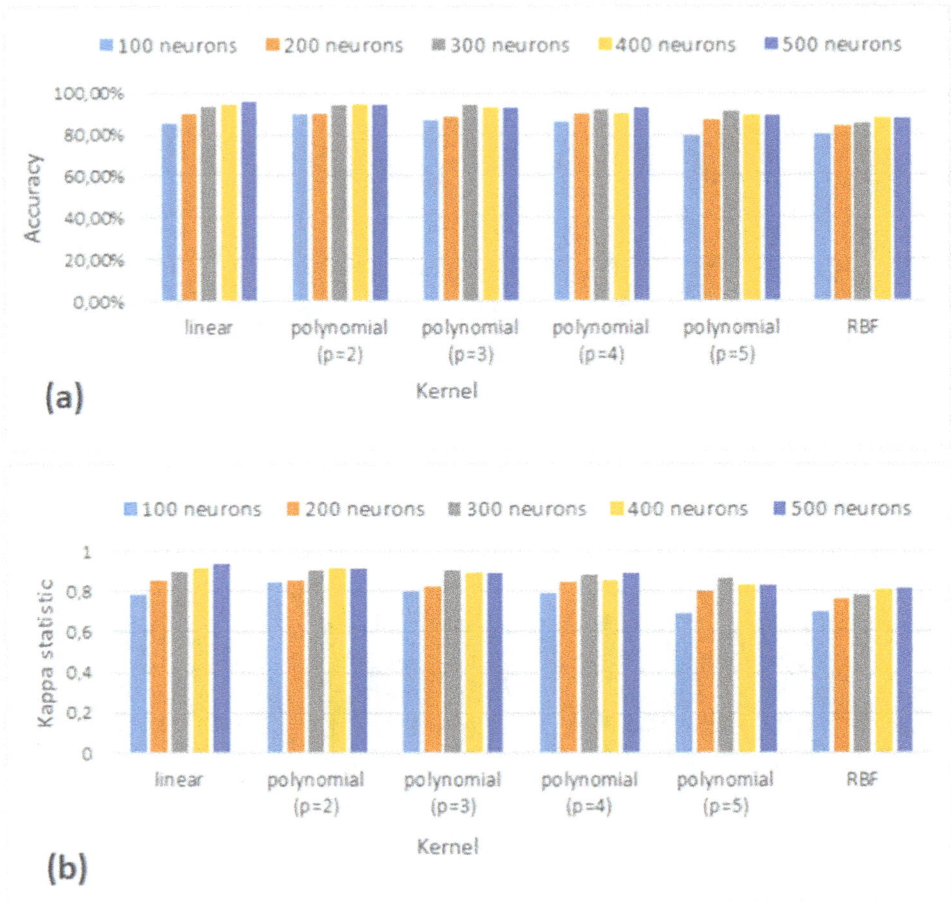

with 500 neurons showed more expressive results than the other configurations. This scenario indicates that the problem is relatively easy to solve, since the best performing kernel was using a linear function. However, it was necessary to use more agents (neurons) to obtain better classification rates.

Regarding the features extraction techniques, the best results were obtained using the combination of features from Haralick and Zernike moments. This agrees with the idea that both shape and texture characteristics are relevant for the differentiation of breast lesions. The least satisfactory results were obtained under the conditions where only Haralick features were used. So, the results also demonstrated that the form seems to be more deterministic to differentiate cystic, benign and malignant lesions than the texture in this type of images.

Overall, the Extreme Learning Machine proved to be an effective tool for classifying breast lesions in thermographic images when acquired in frontal position. The use of this network is interesting given the low computational cost associated to it. Minimizing computational costs is important for such applications, so it is possible to develop tools to be used in mobile devices for screening procedures in clinical practice. Future studies may optimize the results obtained from this approach and evaluate results using other classification methods. Other techniques of features extraction and selection may also be assessed.

ACKNOWLEDGMENT

The authors thank to Coordenação de Aperfeiçoamento de Pessoal de Nível Superior (CAPES), Brazil, and to Fundação de Amparo à Ciência e Tecnologia de Pernambuco (FACEPE), Brazil, for the partial financial support to the research.

REFERENCES

Acharya, U. R., Ng, E. Y. K., Tan, J.-H., & Sree, S. V. (2012). Thermography Based Breast Cancer Detection Using Texture Features and Support Vector Machine. *Journal of Medical Systems, 36*(3), 1503–1510. doi:10.100710916-010-9611-z PMID:20957511

Aguiar, P. S. Junior, Belfort, C. N. S., Silva, A. C., Diniz, P. H. B., Lima, R. C. F., Conci, A., & Paiva, A. C. (2013). Detecção de Regiões Suspeitas de Lesão na Mama em Imagens Térmicas Utilizando *Spatiogram* e Redes Neurais. *Cadernos de Pesquisa, 20*(2), 56–63. doi:10.18764/2178-2229.v20n2p56-63

Andrade, M. K. S., Santana, M. A., & Santos, W. P. (2018). Avaliação do Desempenho de Classificadores Inteligentes na Detecção da Doença de Alzheimer em Imagens de Ressonância Magnética Utilizando Extratores de Forma e Textura. In II Simpósio de Inovação em Engenharia Biomédica (SABIO 2018), Recife, Brazil.

Araújo, M. C. (2009). *Utilização de Câmera por Infravermelho para Avaliação de Diferentes Patologias em Clima Tropical e Uso Conjunto de Sistemas de Banco de Dados para Detecção do Câncer de Mama* [dissertation]. Recife: Universidade Federal de Pernambuco.

Azevedo, W. W., Lima, S. M. L., Fernandes, I. M. M., Rocha, A. D. D., Cordeiro, F. R., Silva-Filho, A. G., & Santos, W. P. (2015). *Morphological extreme learning machines applied to detect and classify masses in mammograms*. In *2015 International Joint Conference of Neural Networks (IJCNN)*, Killarney, Ireland. 10.1109/IJCNN.2015.7280774

Barros, A. C. S. D., Pompei, L. M., & Silveira, J. B. M. (2010). *Manual de Orientação Mastologia*. Federação Brasileira das Associações de Ginecologia e Obstetrícia.

Belfort, C. N. S., Silva, A. C., & Paiva, A. C. (2015). *Detecção de lesões em imagens termográficas de mama utilizando Índice de Similaridade de Jaccard e Artificial Crawlers*. In *XV Workshop de Informática Médica*, Recife, Brazil.

Bohren, C. F., & Huffman, D. R. (1998). *Absorption and scattering of light by small particles*. John Wiley & Sons. doi:10.1002/9783527618156

Brasileiro Filho, G. (2011). *Bogliolo Patologia* (8th ed.). Guanabara Koogan.

Burges, C. J. C. (1998). A Tutorial on Support Vector Machines for Pattern Recognition. *Data Mining and Knowledge Discovery*, *2*(2), 121–167. doi:10.1023/A:1009715923555

Cheng, H. D., Shi, X. J., Min, R., Hu, L. M., Cai, X. P., & Du, H. N. (2005). Approaches for automated detection and classification of masses in mammograms. *Pattern Recognition*, *39*(2006), 646-668.

Cockburn, W. (2018). *The Truth About Breast Thermography*. Retrieved from https://www.healingwell.com/articles/post/the-truth-about-breast-thermography

Coelho, A. S., Santos, M. A. S., Caetano, R. I., Piovesan, C. F., Fiuza, L. A., Machado, R. L. D., & Furini, A. A. C. (2018). Predisposição hereditária ao câncer de mama e sua relação com os genes BRCA1 e BRCA2: Revisão da literatura. *Revista Brasileira de Análises Clínicas*, *50*(1), 17–21.

Cordeiro, F. R., Santos, W. P., & Silva-Filho, A. G. (2016). A semi-supervised fuzzy GrowCut algorithm to segment and classify regions of interest of mammographic images. *Expert Systems with Applications*, *65*, 116–126. doi:10.1016/j.eswa.2016.08.016

Dourado Neto, H. M. (2014). *Segmentação e análise automática de termogramas: um método auxiliar na detecção do câncer de mama* [dissertation]. Recife: Universidade Federal de Pernambuco.

Etehadtavakol, M., & Ng, E. Y. K. (2013). Breast Thermography As a Potential Non-Contact Method in the Early Detection of Cancer: A Review. *Journal of Mechanics in Medicine and Biology*, *13*(02), 1330001. doi:10.1142/S0219519413300019

Goldschmidt, R. R. (2010). *Uma Introdução à Inteligência Computacional: fundamentos, ferramentas e aplicações*. IST-Rio.

Guyton, A. C., & Hall, J. E. (2011). *Tratado de fisiologia médica* (12th ed.). Elsevier Brasil.

Halliday, D., Resnick, R., & Walker, J. (2009). *Fundamentos de Física* (8th ed.). LTC.

Haralick, R. M., Shanmugam, K., & Dinstein, I. (1973). Textural Features for Image Classification. *IEEE Transactions on Systems, Man, and Cybernetics*, *3*(6), 610–621. doi:10.1109/TSMC.1973.4309314

Huang, G.-B., Zhu, Q.-Y., & Siew, C.-K. (2006). Extreme learning machine: Theory and applications. *Neurocomputing*, *70*(1-3), 489–501. doi:10.1016/j.neucom.2005.12.126

Instituto Nacional de Câncer. (2002). *Falando sobre câncer de mama*. INCA.

Jordan, M. I., & Mitchell, T. M. (2015). Machine learning: Trends, perspectives, and prospects. *Science*, *349*(6245), 255–260. doi:10.1126cience.aaa8415 PMID:26185243

Kan, C., & Srinath, M. D. (2001). Combined Features of Cubic B-Spline Wavelet Moments and Zernike Moments for Invariant Character Recognition. In *IEEE International Conference on Information Technology: Coding and Computing (ITCC'01)*. IEEE.

Kumar, V., Abbas, A. K., Fausto, N., & Aster, J. C. (2010). *Robbins & Cotran Patologia Bases Patológicas das Doenças* (8th ed.). Elsevier.

Lawson, R. (1957). Thermography: A new tool in the investigation of breast lesions. *Canadian Services Medical Journal*, *8*(8), 517–524. PMID:13460932

Lima, S. M. L., Silva-Filho, A. G., & Santos, W. P. (2016). Detection and classification of masses in mammographic images in a multi-kernel approach. *Computer Methods and Programs in Biomedicine, 134*, 11–29. doi:10.1016/j.cmpb.2016.04.029 PMID:27480729

Liu, J. G., & Mason, P. J. (2016). *Image Processing and GIS for Remote Sensing: Techniques and Applications* (2nd ed.). Wiley-Blackwell. doi:10.1002/9781118724194

Martins, J. G., Costa, Y. M. G., Gonçalves, D. B., & Oliveira, L. E. S. (2011). Uso de descritores de textura extraídos de GLCM para o reconhecimento de padrões em diferentes domínios de aplicação. In *XXXVII Conferencia Latinoamericana de Informática*. Elsevier.

McKinlay, J. B., Burns, R. B., Feldman, H. A., Freund, K. M., Irish, J. T., Kasten, L. E., Moskowitz, M. A., Potter, D. A., & Woodman, K. (1998). Physician Variability and Uncertainty in the Management of Breast Cancer: Results from a Factorial Experiment. *Medical Care, 36*(3), 385–396. doi:10.1097/00005650-199803000-00014 PMID:9520962

Menke, C. H. (2000). *Rotinas em Mastologia* (2nd ed.). ArtMed Editora.

Moore, K. L., Dalley, A. F., & Agur, A. M. R. (2001). *Anatomia orientada para a clínica* (6th ed.). Guanabara Koogan.

Norvig, P., & Russell, S. (2014). *Inteligência Artificial* (3rd ed.). Elsevier.

Oliveira, M. M. (2012). *Desenvolvimento de protocolo e construção de um aparato mecânico para padronização da aquisição de imagens termográficas de mama* [dissertation]. Recife: Universidade Federal de Pernambuco.

Pereira, J. M. S., Santana, M. A., Lima, N. M., Sousa, F. N., de Lima, R. C. F., & dos Santos, W. P. (2017) *Método para Classificação do Tipo da Lesão na Mama Presentes nas Imagens Termográficas utilizando Classificador ELM*. Paper presented at the I Simpósio de Inovação em Engenharia Biomédica (SABIO 2017), Recife, PE, Brazil.

Pontes, R. (2011). *Inteligência Artificial nos Investimentos*. Joinville: Clube dos Autores Publicações.

Resmini, R., Conci, A., Borchartt, T. B., Lima, R. C. F., Montenegro, A. A., & Pantaleão, C. A. (2012). Diagnóstico Precoce de Doenças Mamárias Usando Imagens Térmicas e Aprendizado de Máquina. *Revista Eletrônica do Alto Vale de Itajaí, 1*(1), 55–67.

Ribeiro, P. B., Schiabel, H., Patrocinio, A. C., & Romero, R. A. F. (2008). Análise da Variação de Textura em Imagens Mamográficas para Classificação de Massas Suspeitas. In 4o Workshop de Visão Computacional, 2008, São Paulo, Brazil.

Ring, E. F., & Ammer, K. (2012). Infrared thermal imaging in medicine. *Physiological Measurement, 33*(3), 33–46. doi:10.1088/0967-3334/33/3/R33 PMID:22370242

Rodrigues, A. L., Santana, M. A., Azevedo, W. W., Bezerra, R. S., Santos, W. P., & Lima, R. C. F. (2018). *Seleção de Atributos para Apoio ao Diagnóstico do Câncer de Mama Usando Imagens Termográficas, Algoritmos Genéticos e Otimização por Enxame de Partículas*. Paper presented at the II Simpósio de Inovação em Engenharia Biomédica (SABIO), Recife, Brazil.

Rodrigues, C. I. H. (2008). *Sistemas CAD em Patologia Mamária* [dissertation]. Porto: Universidade do Porto.

Saladin, K. S., & Porth, C. (2010). *Anatomy & physiology: the unity of form and function* (Vol. 5). McGraw-Hill.

Santana, M. A., Pereira, J. M. S., Silva, F. L., Lima, N. M., Sousa, F. N., Arruda, G. M. S., Lima, R. C. F., Silva, W. W. A., & Santos, W. P. (2018). Breast cancer diagnosis based on mammary thermography and extreme learning machines. *Research on Biomedical Engineering*, *34*(1), 45–53. doi:10.1590/2446-4740.05217

Sessler, D. I. (1994). Consequences and treatment of perioperative hypothermia. *Anesthesiology Clinics of North America*, *12*, 425–456.

Souza, T. K., Andrade, J. F. S., Almeida, M. B. J., Santana, M. A., & Santos, W. P. (2019). *Métodos Computacionais Aplicados ao Diagnóstico de Câncer de Mama por Termografia: uma revisão de literatura*. Paper presented at the III Simpósio de Inovação em Engenharia Biomédica (SABIO 2019), Recife, Brazil.

Tyson, J. (2001). *How Night Vision Works*. Retrieved from https://electronics.howstuffworks.com/gadgets/high-tech-gadgets/nightvision.htm

Weinberg, R. A. (2008). *A biologia do câncer*. Artmed.

World Health Organization. (2014). *WHO position paper on mammography screening*. WHO.

World Health Organization. (2018). Early Detection. In Cancer control: knowledge into action: WHO guide for effective programmes. Geneva: WHO.

Chapter 4
Feature Selection Based on Dialectical Optimization Algorithm for Breast Lesion Classification in Thermographic Images

Jessiane Mônica Silva Pereira
Universidade Federal de Pernambuco, Brazil

Maíra Araújo de Santana
Universidade Federal de Pernambuco, Brazil

Clarisse Lins de Lima
Universidade Federal de Pernambuco, Brazil

Rita de Cássia Fernandes de Lima
Universidade Federal de Pernambuco, Brazil

Sidney Marlon Lopes de Lima
https://orcid.org/0000-0002-4350-9689
Universidade Federal de Pernambuco, Brazil

Wellington Pinheiro dos Santos
https://orcid.org/0000-0003-2558-6602
Universidade Federal de Pernambuco, Brazil

ABSTRACT

Breast cancer is the leading cause of death among women worldwide. Early detection and early treatment are critical to minimize the effects of this disease. In this sense, breast thermography has been explored in the process of diagnosing this type of cancer. Furthermore, in an attempt to optimize the

DOI: 10.4018/978-1-7998-3456-4.ch004

diagnosis, intelligent pattern recognition techniques are being used. Features selection performs an essential task in this process to optimize these intelligent techniques. This chapter proposes a features selection method using Dialectical Optimization Method (ODM) associated to a KNN classifier. The authors found that this combination proved to be a good approach showing a low impact on breast lesion classification performance. They obtained around 5% decrease in accuracy, with a reduction of about 46.80% of the features vector. The specificity and sensitivity values they found were competitive to other widely used methods.

INTRODUCTION

Cancer is one of the leading causes of death and has become one of the biggest public health problems in the world. For decades, breast cancer has been the most common type of cancer among women and is currently ranked among the top five causes of cancer death worldwide (American Cancer Society, 2019). Several studies have shown that in the case of breast cancer, the early detection raises the possibility of cure to 85%. When detected at an advanced stage this percentage reduces to 10% (Ng & Sudharsan, 2001).

Nowadays, some imaging techniques are used to detect breast cancer. The most common techniques are mammography, ultrasonography, magnetic resonance imaging, x-ray tomography and thermography. The combination of these techniques is also assessed to provide a robust and more accurate diagnosis. Among these screening tools, mammography is the most widely used. It is a low-dose x-ray procedure and is considered the gold standard for breast cancer diagnosis. Yet, mammography has some limitations. Among its main limitations are the cost of the exam and the exposure to cumulative ionizing radiation, which is a risk factor for cancer. Another important concern is the high false negative rates among young women, since their breasts tend to have mostly dense tissue, which appear on the same color of a lesion in mammographic image (American Cancer Society, 2019).

These limitations of mammography, in parallel with the increasing number of cases of breast lesions in younger patients (dense breasts), lead to the search and development of new techniques for the early detection of breast lesions. Among which, the thermography is evident.

Thermography began to be used in mastology in 1959. But, the existing technology at the time made the method discredited and not recommended for the diagnosis of breast lesions. With the technological advancement of the new thermographic cameras, new methodologies using image processing and analysis techniques can be developed. These techniques can help the detection of breast alterations by thermographic images. Thus, these new methodologies aim to verify the possibilities of using thermography as a screening exam in mastology.

Thermography is being used as an auxiliary screening tool for breast cancer. In this technique, the image is acquired by an infrared camera. The camera captures infrared radiation emitted by the surface of interest. The resulting image shows the surface temperature distribution. Therefore, there is no need for invasive procedures or exposure to ionizing radiation. In addition, this technique provides physiological information, since damaged areas show increased metabolic activity. More cellular activity increases the temperature around the area, so breast lesions can be seen as warmer spots. Considering that physiological alterations precede anatomical alterations, the use of this technique is a great step for early diagnosis (Ng & Sudharsan, 2001).

Despite being a promising technique, the interpretation of thermographic images is often difficult. It becomes more difficult when the lesions are far from the surface of the skin. In these cases, changes in temperature occur in a diffuse and non-punctual manner. Thus, pattern recognition techniques are being explored as an important tool to support diagnosis.

When using pattern recognition algorithms, images are represented by features vectors. In the approach presented in this chapter, the authors chose to use Haralick moments and Zernike moments as features extractors. Zernike moments extract geometry information, while Haralick is associated to texture characteristics.

Another important step in optimizing the performance of intelligent systems is the features selection. This step plays a key role in reducing computational costs and increasing accuracy as it seeks to remove irrelevant and redundant features. In this study, the authors propose a feature selection approach combining the Dialectical Optimization Method (ODM) and the K-nearest neighbors (KNN) algorithms.

The ODM is an evolution and revolution based tool to perform search and optimization tasks (Santos & de Assis, 2009). Such as Genetic Algorithms (GA), the bee colony-based algorithm and the Particle Swarm Optimization (PSO) methods are bioinspired.

Compared to the optimization and search methods present in the literature, ODM has the advantage that new individuals are generated at each historical phase, just as similar individuals are merged into a single individual.

Given this, this study proposes to model the features selection method based on the dialectical method of optimization. The authors chose to use KNN as the objective function of the ODM, since the KNN classifier is a basic learning method based on instances. This type of learning consists of storing training samples without, however, generating a rule as in most conventional learning methods (Galvão & Júnior Hruschka, 2004).

This chapter is organized as follows: in the background section the authors introduce some concepts and definition for theoretical background of the study. In the methods section they present the proposed methodology, a brief description of the image database and the tools used. After this, in the results section, they present and discuss the results from the experiments, performing a qualitative and quantitative analysis of the findings. Finally, the authors summarize the scientific contribution of this study, show some potential future work and present their conclusion.

BACKGROUND

Next, we will demonstrate the concepts and definition for the theoretical basis of this chapter and a brief literature review.

Anatomy and Physiology of the Breast

The female breast is composed of lobes, ducts and stroma, and it is located in the anterior chest wall. The lobes are the glands which are responsible for the milk producing while the ducts are small tubes which function is to carry the milk from the lobes to the nipple. And the stroma is the adipose and the connective tissue surrounding the ducts and lobes, and the blood vessels. The mammary gland, also called parenchyma, is formed by lobes and ducts and is the functional structure of the gland. Younger women have breasts with larger amounts of glandular tissue, making these organs firmer and increasing their density. It also represents great psychological importance for women, playing an important role in the constitution of their self-esteem and self-image (MS & INCA, 2002).

At a young age, girls have slight elevation in the mammary region due to the existence of rudimentary breast tissue. In the pubertal phase, the pituitary gland (a gland located in the brain), secretes the follicle-stimulating and luteinizing hormones. These hormones are responsible for the ovarian production of estrogen. (MS & INCA, 2002).

Thus, the breasts begin their development with the multiplication of lobes and acini. When menstrual cycles become ovulatory, the progesterone produced depends on the previous action of estrogen. It, then, differentiates the mammary duct-lobular tree (Davidson, 1997).

As menopause approaches, the breast tissue atrophies and is gradually replaced by fatty tissue. This replacement progresses until the breast is almost exclusively composed of fat and remnants glandular tissue. Thus, in the postmenopausal phase, the breast tissue consists of fat and remnants of glandular tissue (Spritzer, 2003).

Methods for Breast Cancer Diagnosis

Breast cancer represents a higher frequency in incidence and mortality in females rather than in males. It shows an ascending curve from the age of 25, with greater concentration between women from 45 and 50 years old. The analysis of the fatality rate due to breast cancer in Brazil, points to a progressive increase. It increases even more in the age group from 50 years. The increased incidence of breast cancer in Brazil has been accompanied by increased fatality rate, which can be attributed to the diagnosis of the disease in advanced stages. Thus, the earlier it is detected, the more successful it can be in the treatment provided, reducing fatality rate (Nascimento, Pitta, & Rêgo, 2015).

As for diagnosis, the main allies of breast cancer detection are the low-cost self-exam and mammography. Mammography is the main exam used for the diagnosis in early stages of breast cancer. In search for other complementary techniques to early diagnosis of breast cancer, thermography is evident (Traldi, Galvão, de Morais, & Fonseca, 2016).

Breast Thermography

Thermography has become an auxiliary tool in the process of diagnosing breast cancer. This technique uses an infrared camera to acquire images that present the temperature distribution in the region. The camera captures the infrared radiation emitted by the surface of interest. It is a non-invasive process where the patient is not exposed to any ionizing radiation. This technique access metabolic changes resulting from the appearance of altered cells in the breast tissue. Cancer cells increased activity leads to changes in temperature distribution in the breast surface, thus allowing a better visualization of the physiological changes caused by the disease (da Silva, et al., 2018).

Features selection

For machine learning field, an important step is the features selection. This step aims to rank the features according to some criteria of importance. So, it is possible to reduce the dimensionality of the features search space and remove noisy data. Thus, features selection may be seen as a search process where an algorithm must find the smallest subset of features that result in the best classification performance (Pappa, Freitas, & Kaestner, 2002).

There are basically two different approaches to handle features selection: Wrapper and Filter. The first approach deals essentially with the use of the classifier system itself as a metric to check the performance of many features subsets. In the second approach, heuristic metrics are used to try to find a subset that meets some criterion or metrics (Rocha, 206). The features selection method used in this chapter uses the Wrapper approach and it will be further detailed in the following section. The Wrapper approach e briefly explained in Figure 1.

Figure 1. Flowchart of wrapper-based approach to feature subset selection
Source: Kohavi & John, 1997

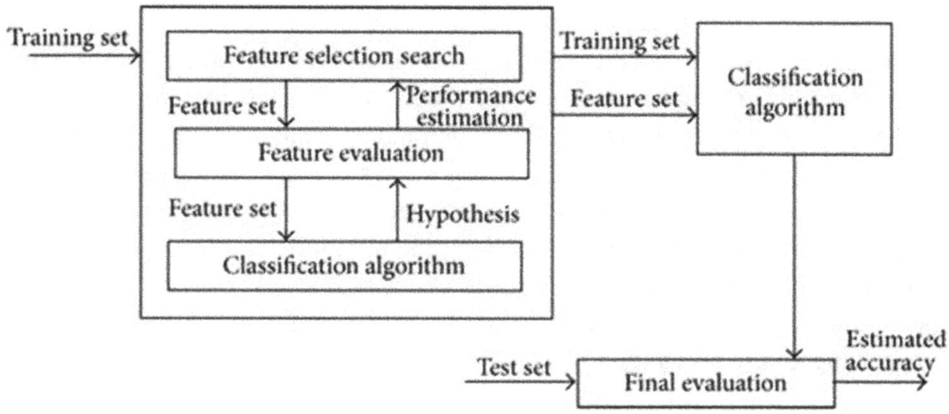

Dialectical Optimization Method

Dialectical Optimization Method (ODM) is a class of evolutionary algorithm to be adapted to search and optimization problems. It is based on the concepts of evolution and revolution (Santos & de Assis, 2009).

The origin of the word "dialectic" comes from the original Greek dialetiké. The prefix "dia" corresponds to interaction, while "letiké" stands for knowledge. Thus, for Socratic philosophers, dialectics are seen as "the art of dialogue". In this way, dialectics is seen as the free interaction between contrary ideas about an object, and it is possible to obtain information about the truth of an object (Vázquez, 2007; Santos & Assis, 2009).

The dialectical method and its modern definition began in the late 18th and early 19th centuries through the works of the German philosopher George Wilhelm Friedrich Hegel (1770-1831). This definition was developed with influence on the Eastern dialectical conceptions brought from China by the Jesuits and on the Heraclitus' thinking of reality as a process of eternal modification (Santos W. P., 2009; Santos W., et al., 2009).

The ODM is based on the conception of parts of reality, or phenomena, as systems. The systems consist of several poles. Each pole has a force or power. The system is then characterized by its correlation of forces, that is, by the grouping of the forces of its component poles. This interaction follows the model conceived by Hegel and based on three fundamental concepts. The first concept is the contradiction, which is the basis of dialectic and is defined by the correlation between the forces of the poles over time. The second concept is the principle of totality, which defines that a totally isolated system cannot be conceived, but in its various relations and dependencies with other systems. The third is the endless movement, which, as the name implies, expresses the fundamental dialectic hypothesis that there is nothing eternal, nothing fixed, nothing absolute. In this way, the dialectic and the movement of contradictions (Santos & De Assis, 2013)

The dialectical method adapted to search and optimization problems considers each pole as a possible candidate for the problem. Thus, it is necessary to associate the objective function of the optimization problem to the social force of each pole. So the dynamics of the optimization method is governed by the poles fight. These struggles consist of the movement of the poles, which happens due to the present hegemonic pole and the historical hegemonic pole. The present hegemonic pole is the one with the largest social force in the current correlation of forces, whereas the historical hegemonic pole is the one with the greatest historical force to date (Santos & De Assis, 2013).

The search for possible solutions is intrinsically associated with the pole movement and its contradictions in the various historical phases, which are involved in periods of revolutionary crisis. In this period occurs the fusion of poles with low levels of contradiction, the creation of new poles by synthesis in order to solve high levels of contradiction and also the formation of absolute antithesis of the poles thesis. Still, at this stage, there is a process to generate diversity in the search process that corresponds to adding disturbances to the surviving poles, which is a process similar to mutation in evolutionary-based computational approaches (Santos & De Assis, 2013).

To understand the goal of the dialectical method for search and optimization, it is necessary to understand the following general definition.

General Definition

The basic concepts of dialectics were mathematically defined as follows (Santos dos, de Souza, Santos Filho, Lima Neto, & de Assis, 2008).

Pole: It is a candidate for the solution of the problem and also the fundamental unit of the dialectical system. Given a set of poles $\Omega = \{w_1, w_2, \ldots, w_m\}$ one pole w_i is associated to a weight vector $w_i = \left(w_{i,1}, w_{i,2}, \ldots, w_{i,n}\right)_T$ where $w_i \in s$, m is the number of poles and n is the dimensionality of the system.

Social force: Evaluation through the objective function for a pole. Each w_i pole has a social force that equals the evaluation of the objective function f at pole w_i.

Hegemony: In the process of pole fighting, it is said that a pole k exerts hegemony at time t if:

$$f(w_k(t)) = f_C(t) = max\, f\left(w_j(t)\right), 1 \leq j \leq m(t)$$

The vector $w_c(t) = w_k(t)$ is called present hegemonic pole or contemporary hegemonic pole, while $f_C(t)$ is the present hegemonic force or contemporary hegemonic force. The historical hegemonic force at the instant t so, $f_H(t)$ is expressed by:

$$f_H(t) = max\, f_C(t'), \text{onde } w_H = w_H, \text{ para } f(w_C(t')) = f_H(t) e 0 \leq t' \leq t$$

Absolute antithesis: The absolute antithesis vector of the pole w is defined as the opposite vector to w and can be expressed as: $w = s_i - x_i + r_i$, where $i = 1, 2, \cdots, n$. Thus assuming $x = (x_1, x_2, \ldots x_n)^T$ and that $x \in s \Rightarrow r_i \le x_i \le s_i$, and r_i and s_i correspond to the lower and upper limits of the i-th dimension of s.

Contradiction: Contradiction can be calculated from a distance function, which in this case is the Euclidean distance. Thus we can mathematically define the distance between two poles w_p and w_q through:

$$\delta_{p,q} = d(w_p, w_q)$$

Synthesis: Based on the dialectical conception, synthesis is the answer to the contradiction between two poles where one plays the role of thesis and the other of antithesis. Given a pole $w_r \in s$ whose synthesis between poles w_p and w_q can be obtained through the expression: $w_r = g(w_p, w_t)$, where $g : S^2 \to S$ there are possible synthesis days:

$$w_{u,i} = \{w_{p,i}, i\, mod\, 2 = 0\; w_{q,i}, i\, mod\, 2 = 1, i = 1, 2, \ldots, n$$

$$w_{u,i} = \{w_{p,i}, i\, mod\, 2 = 1\; w_{q,i}, i\, mod\, 2 = 0, i = 1, 2, \ldots, n$$

Based on these definitions it is possible to build the dialectical method as the search and optimization algorithm that will be shown in the following section.

Dialectic Method as Search and Optimization Algorithm

To use the dialectical method in a search and optimization problem (such as features selection), it is necessary to understand the adaptation that is shown below and proposed by Santos and Assis (2013) (Santos & De Assis, 2013).

First of all, we define the fundamental parameters, which are the initial number of poles, $m(0)$, number of historical phases, n_p, nd duration of each historical phase, n_H. Thus, the system will be started with $m(0)$ poles and will last n_p historical phases with n_H generations per phase. The number of poles $m(0)$ corresponds to the concept of initial population when compared to evolutionary approaches, it must be even so that half of the poles are randomly generated and the other half is obtained by generating the absolute antithesis poles. This process generates a more intense pole fight, generating a greater initial dynamic.

The phase of poles generation is performed according to the following expression:

$$w_{i,j}(0) = \begin{cases} U(r_j, s_j), 1 \le i \le m(0) \\ w_{i',j}(0), 1 + \frac{1}{2}m(0) \le i \le m(0) \end{cases}$$

$$w_{i',j} = s_j - w_{i,j} + r_j$$

For $i' = 1 + \frac{1}{2}m(0) \le i \le m(0)$, $1 \le i \le m(0)$ and $1 \le j \le n$, where n is the dimensionality of the optimization problem, $U(r_j, s_j)$ is a random number evenly distributed over the range $[r_j, s_j]$ and $S = [r_1, s_1] \times [r_2, s_2] \times \ldots \times [r_n, s_n]$, since $s_j > r_j$ and $s_j, r_j \in R$.

While it does not reach the number of historical phases n_p and the historical hegemonic force is not higher than the given upper force threshold (initial estimate of the maximum objective function value), $f_H(t) < f_{sup}$ ((criterion to consider the maximum objective function achieved), there is the stage of evolution and revolutionary crisis. Evolution occurs until the total of n_H iterations and $f_H(t) < f_{sup}$, is reached, thus the poles are adjusted as follows.

$$w_i(t+1) = w_i(t) + \Delta w_{C,i}(t) + \Delta w_{H,i}(t),$$

to

$$\Delta w_{C,i} = \eta_{C,i}(t)(1 - \mu_C(t))^2 (w_C(t) - w_i(t)), 0 < \eta_C(t), 1,$$

$$\Delta w_{H,i} = \eta_{H,i}(t)(1 - \mu_H(t))^2 (w_H(t) - w_i(t)), 0 < \eta_H(t), 1,$$

Where $\eta_C(0) = \eta_H(0) = \eta_0$ and $0 < \eta_0 < 1$. The influences of present and historical hegemonies are modeled by the following terms $\Delta w_{C,i}(t)$ and $\Delta w_{H,i}(t)$ respectively, on the i-th pole. The present and historical poles update step are represented by $\eta_C(t)$ and $\eta_H(t)$. This update occurs at each historical phase as defined in the expression below.

$$\eta_C(t+1) = \alpha \eta_C(t)$$

And for every interaction occurs:

$$\eta_H(t+1) = \alpha \eta_H(t)$$

At the end of each historical phase, to $\alpha < 1$ (typically, $\alpha = 0.9999$). The present pertinence degree and the historical relevance degree correspond to the terms $\mu_{C,i}(t)$ and $\mu_{H,i}(t)$, these terms are based on the pertinence functions according to the expressions described below.

$$\mu_{C,i}(t) = \sum_{j=1}^{m} \left(\frac{\left| f\left(w_i(t) - f_C(t)\right) \right|}{\left| f\left(w_j(t) - f_C(t)\right) \right|} \right)^{-1}, \text{ where } 1 < i < m(t)$$

$$\mu_{H,i}(t) = \sum_{j=1}^{m} \left(\frac{\left| f\left(w_i(t) - f_H(t)\right) \right|}{\left| f\left(w_j(t) - f_H(t)\right) \right|} \right)^{-1}, \text{ where } 1 < i < m(t)$$

Where these expressions are based on the membership functions of the classical version of the unsupervised fuzzy c-average classifier. Thus, when the social force of the i-th pole, $f\left(w_i(t)\right)$ is close to the present hegemonic force $f_C(t)$, the term of $\mu_{C,i}(t)$ is close to 1 making the influence of present hegemony $\Delta w_{C,i}(t)$ approaches zero and practically student its effect and similar behavior happens when $f\left(w_i(t)\right)$ approaches the value of historical hegemonic force $f_H(t)$.

In the revolutionary crisis stage all contradictions are evaluated and contradictions smaller than a minimal contradiction (δmin) imply fusion between the poles. From the contradictions evaluated in the previous step, those greater than one maximum contradiction (δmax) are found. These contradictions will be considered the main contradictions of the dialectic system. The thesis-antithesis pairs are involved, whose synthesis poles also pass to belong to the new set of poles (Santos, Souza, Santos Filho, Lima neto, & Assis, 2008).

Additionally there is the effect of the crisis given by the maximum crisis ($Xmax$), to all poles belonging to the dialectic system, thus generating a new set of poles, according to the following expression.

$$w_{k,i}(t+2) = w_{k,i}(t+1) + Xmax\,G(0,1),$$

To $1 \le k \le m(t+1)$ and $1 \le i \le n$, where $G(0,1)$ is a random number from a gaussian distribution with hope 0 and variance 1.

If the stopping criterion has not yet been met (maximum number of historical phases reached or another stopping criterion to be defined), a new set of poles is generated. This is a step called antagonistic poles generation that is given by the expression below:

$$w_i(t+2) \in \Omega(t+2) \Rightarrow w(t+2) + \in \Omega(t+2),$$

to $1 \le i \le m(t+2)$, where $m(t+2) = 2m(t+1)$.

In this direction, it is possible to enlarge the set of poles by adding the antithetical poles to the existing poles.

Figure 2 shows the general flowchart of the dialectical optimization method adapted for search and optimization tasks. In summary, it can be stated that the pole evolution phase is composed of the hegemony search and weight update stages that model the iterations between the poles and the information exchange over time. While the crisis phase is composed of the stages of evaluation, fusion, synthesis, revolutionary crisis and generation of antithesis pairs (Santos, Assis, Souza, Santos Filho, & Lima Neto, 2009). It is also understood that the stage of synthesis occurs the separation of groups of poles that are between two ideological extremes during the crisis, while the generation stage of the antagonistic poles models the emergence of groups with ideas totally contrary to those of the current group. The fusion stage of low contradictions shapes the union of poles that have similar thinking in times of crisis (Feitosa, 2015).

In this study, the objective function, which calculates the social force of each pole of this method, was applied a classifier in order to minimize the error rate in the classification process. The authors used the k-Nearest Neighbors (KNN) classifier.

K-Nearest Neighbors

The K-Nearest Neighbors is one of the oldest and simplest classification method to implement (Cover & Hart, 1967). Although it has a simple implementation, this method has performed well in different scenarios (Wilcox, 1961; Simard, Le Cun, & Denker, 1992). The KNN uses supervised learning. The training set consists in n-dimensional vectors and each element of this set represents a point in the n-dimensional space. To determine the class of an element that does not belong to the training set, the KNN classifier searches for K training set elements that are closest to this unknown element, ie, which have the shortest distance.

The most common metric for calculating the distance between two points is the Euclidean distance. These K elements are called the nearest K-neighbors. So, it is checked what are the K-neighbors classes, and the most frequent class will be assigned to the unknown element class. Thus, KNN has only one parameter to configure, which is the number of K-neighbors that can be adjusted to obtain a better rating (Cover & Hart, 1967). In this work we tested values of $K = 3$, $K = 5$ and $K = 7$.

Literature Review

Following there is a brief literature review of breast thermography for detection of breast lesion classification.

Nowadays, there is a lot of studies regarding to breast thermography as a complementary tool for the diagnosis of breast cancer. Aguiar et al. (2013) performed tests using multilayer perceptron as a classifier to detect the existence or not of lesions in breast thermographic images, obtaining accurate ratings of about 75%. In the work of Resmini et al. (2012), it was obtained results close to 90% of accuracy using other classifiers (SVM, KNN and Naive Bayes) to also detect the existence of breast lesion. In Belfort, Silva, & de Paiva (2015), another detection method was introduced, from which an accuracy of around 66% was obtained using the SVM classifier.

Vasconcelos, Santos, & de Lima (2018) reported an accuracy around 63.46% in the classification of lesions using thermography after automatic total segmentation of the region of interest.

In Santana et al. (2018), it was obtained an accuracy around 73% in the classification of breast lesions in frontal and lateral thermographic images using conventional extreme learning machines. In De Santana et al. (2018), it was obtained an accuracy around 95.19% in the classification of breast lesions

Figure 2. General flowchart of the dialectical optimization method adapted to search and optimization tasks.
Source: Adapted from Santos & De Assis, 2013

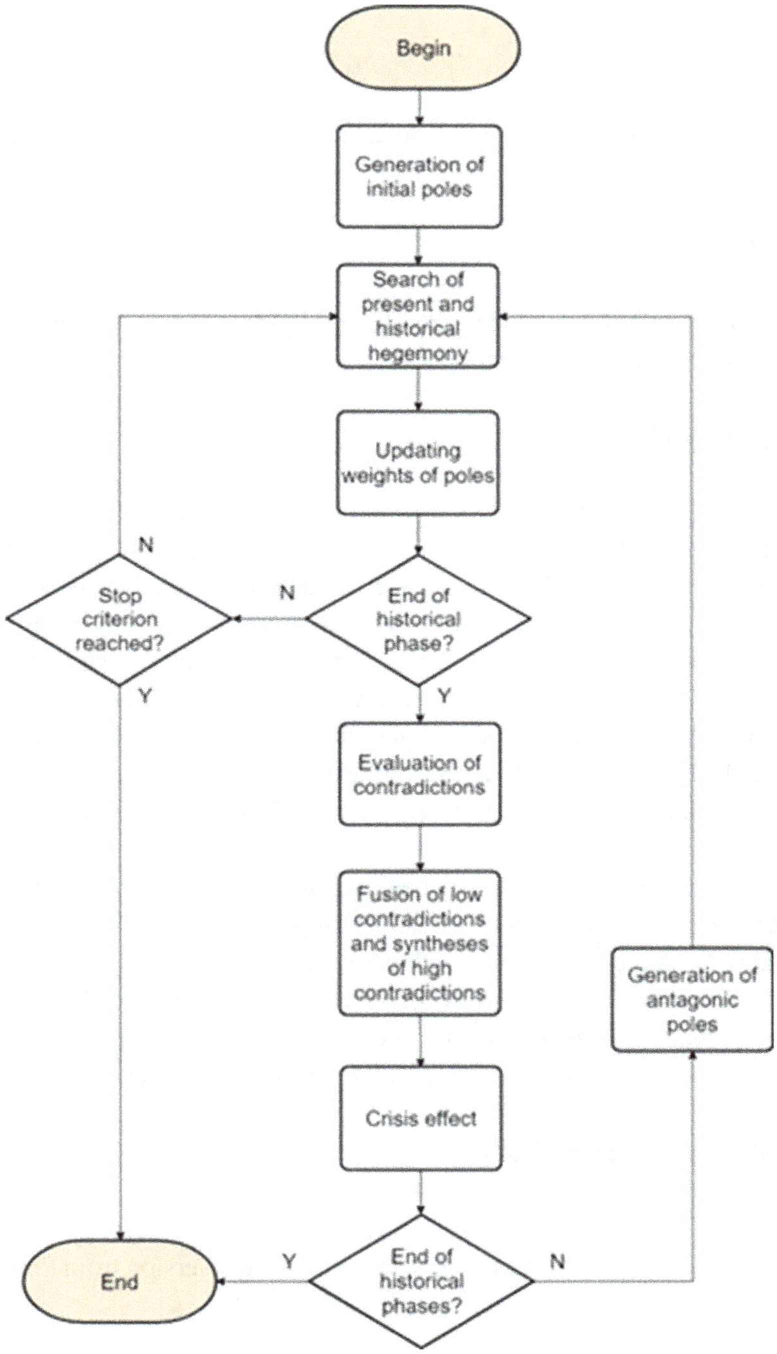

into two classes: with and without lesion. For the classification, De Santana et.al (2018) used frontal thermographic images and used the morphological ELM with dilatation kernel as a classifier.

METHOD

The following will be demonstrated the proposed methodology, image database description and the tools used.

Proposed Method

This section presents the method from this approach, highlighting how the study will be conducted, as shown in Figure 3. The steps will be further described in the following subsections.

Breast Thermography Database

The thermographic images used in this study follow the acquisition protocol proposed in Oliveira (2012) and were acquired at Hospital das Clínicas (HC) - UFPE. According to Silva (2015)the thermographic images were obtained from a FLIR S45 infrared camera and the method adopted in the image acquisition process was the static one, in the static acquisition the patient is in thermal equilibrium with the environment. Eight (8) images were obtained from each patient in JPG format, each image being named: T1 (frontal with hands on waist), T2 (frontal with hands raised holding a bar above the head), internal side of breast right breast (LIMD), left breast internal lateral (LIME), right breast external lateral (LEMD) and left breast external lateral (LEME). Example of the eight images obtained from each patient can be seen in Figure 4. In this chapter, only frontal images T1 and T2 were used, as this condition is considered to benefit the identification of the region of interest.

The database has been labeled using established diagnostic methods as described by Dourado Neto (2014). The database is separated into four classes: Malignant Lesion, Benign Lesion, Cyst and No Lesion. The Malignant Lesion class comprises all cases of biopsy-proven malignant breast injury. The Benign Lesion class refers to cases of tumors with benignity, also confirmed by biopsy. The Cyst class includes cases with this diagnosis proven by fine needle aspiration (FNA) or ultrasound (da Silva, 2015). The No Lesion class is composed of all images that did not present an injury.

Preprocessing and Features Extraction

Thermographic images use pseudo-coloring techniques. For this database, the JET color palette was used in the acquisition process. Therefore, it was necessary to use the conversion from RGB-JET to grayscale,

Figure 3. Flowchart of the proposed method
Source: The authors

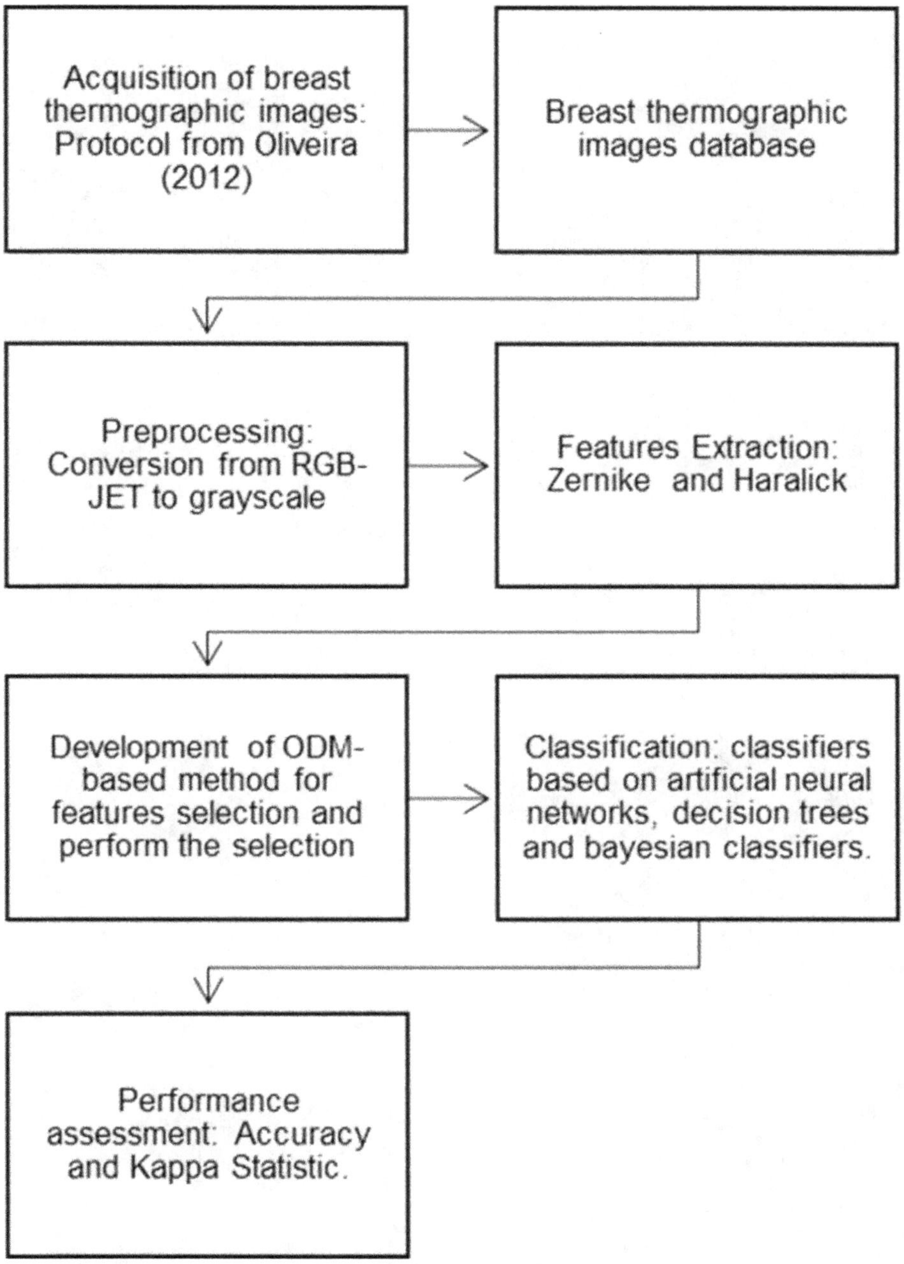

in order to reduce the amount of information to be processed. Grayscale images have less detail but retain the important features of objects or regions of interest (Pedrini & Schwartz, 2008).

The definition of the feature extraction method is one of the most important factors for the satisfactory performance of a computer system for diagnosis support (Cheng, et al., 2006).

So, regarding to image representation, the features in this chapter were based on geometry or texture. The authors used the Zernike moments features extractor, that extracts geometry-based information and

Figure 4. Positions for the eight images acquired from each patient
Source: The authors

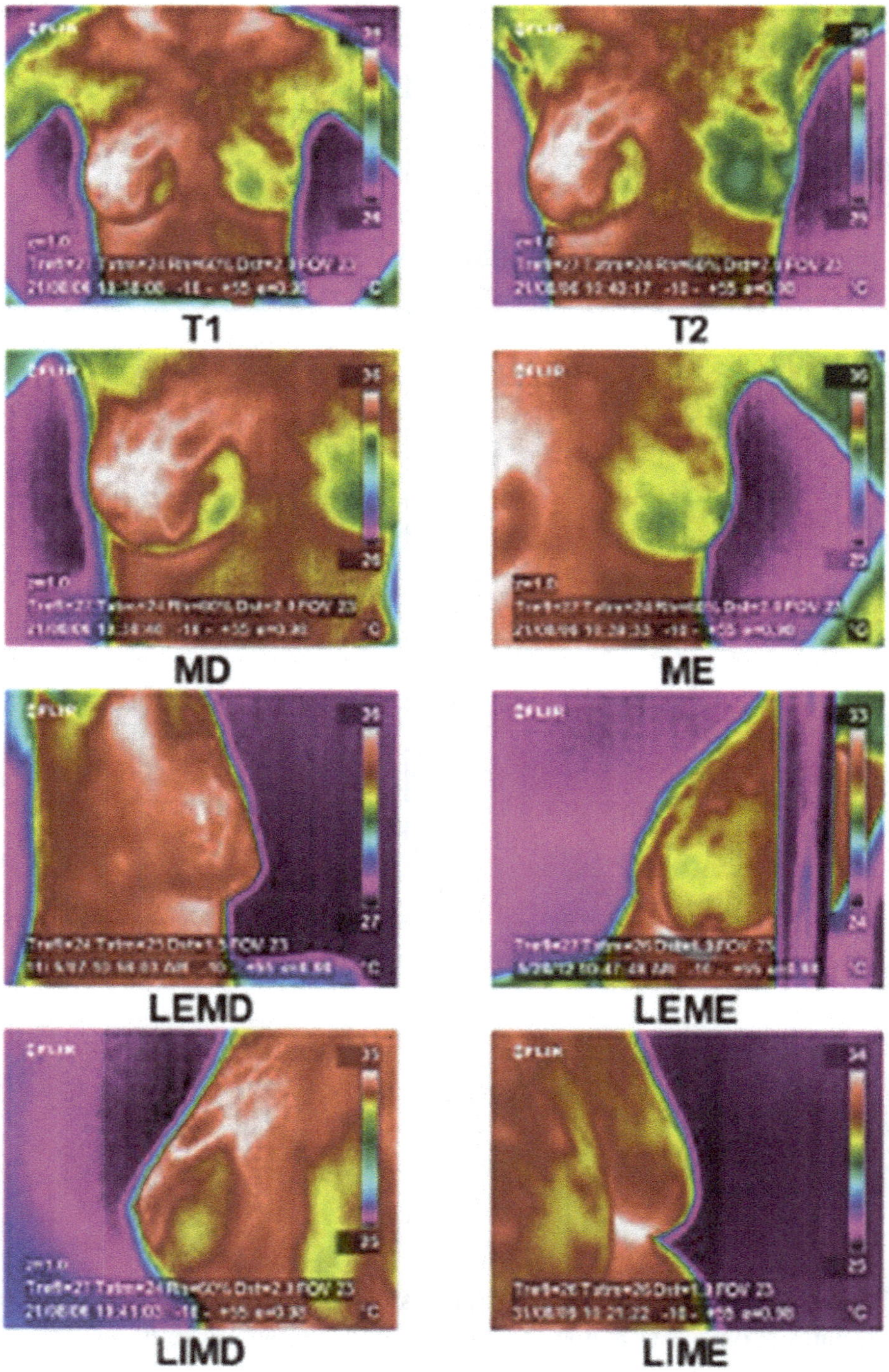

the Haralick moments extractor, which is based on texture features. The first one is from projections of the image function on orthogonal base functions and only rotation invariants (Shanthi & Bhaskaran, 2013). The second calculates texture information from the co-occurrence matrix of the image, which quantifies some characteristics from gray level variation of these images (Cheng, et al., 2006; Shanthi & Bhaskaran, 2013).Thus, the extracted features were organized in an .arff format file, in which a total of 168 attributes and 968 instances were counted.

The number of images per class in the database is different, which may lead to biased result during training, in a way that injuries could be more often classified in the class that has the most number of instances. In order to solve this problem, the authors performed a class balancing by inserting synthetic instances through the linear combination of features vectors of the same class (Cheng, et al., 2006).

Features Selection Based on ODM

As earlier stated, the dialectical method can be used in a search and optimization problem, such as features selection. Features selection plays an essential role within machine learning process. Its goal is to reduce the computational cost of the system, but always taking into account the need to maintain high performance rates during the classification (Pappa, Freitas, & Kaestner, 2002).

When using ODM for features selection, the poles were represented by numerical vectors containing their binary values dimensions using a threshold of 0.5. In the dialectical method, as already described, half of the poles are created with random values and the other half is generated by the poles that are antagonistic to the first half of poles already initialized. The aptitude values are obtained by defining the objective function, which in this case will be the minimum error rate of the KNN classifier.

The parameters used for this approach were obtained by successive executions of the algorithm, changing the parameters and, thus, saving the parameter values from where the authors found the lowest error rate at the end of each execution. Table 1 shows the ODM parameters for the lowest error rate in this study.

Table 1. Parameters used for ODM

Parameter	Value
Initial amount of poles	10
Pole Dimension	168
Number of Historical Phases	1
Duration of each Historic Phase	500
Superior Range	1
Inferior Range	0
Alpha	0.999
Eta L	0.999
Eta H	1.001
Maximum contradiction	0.0005
Minimal Contradiction	0.001
Maximum Crisis Effect	0.005

Source: The authors

Classification

The authors performed classification before and after the features selection step to assess the efficiency of the features selection process. Thus, these features are used as input for classifiers who will be trained and will later perform classification of breast lesions (malignant, benign and cyst) or no lesion. This experiment was performed with seven classifiers to compare their ability to detect and classify breast lesions in thermographic images. The classifiers used were: Bayes Net, Naive Bayes, Support Vector Machine (SVM), J48, Multilayer Perceptron (MLP), Random Forest and Random Tree.

Naive Bayes and Bayes Net are Bayes theory-based classifiers that use conditional probability to create a data model. BayesNet builds a complete Bayesian network and then searches that network according to any search algorithm and its main parameter is the type of search performed. Naive Bayes assumes that all features are independent, given the class variable so it is considered naive (Cheng & Greiner, 2001).

The support vector machine (SVM) classifier performs a nonlinear mapping of the dataset in a larger dimension space, and then a hyperplane is created to separate the distinct classes. SVM is based on the Statistical Learning Theory (Haykin, 2003).

J48 classifier configures itself by creating a decision tree from a database for gaining knowledge, and thereby creating a decision making tool. This method has the goal to build a decision tree where the most significant feature is called the root of the tree (Librelotto & Mozzaquatro, 2014).

The Multilayer Perceptron (MLP) consists of a tightly connected network with feedforward connections. This neural network is a perceptron type that has a set of sensory units that make up the input layer, an intermediate or hidden layer. Its output layer consists of a layer of neurons that generate the network output. Learning in this type of network is usually performed through the backpropagation algorithm (Haykin, 2003).

The Random Forests (RF) are decision tree combinations that hierarchically splits the data. In this method, after a certain number of trees are generated, each one casts a vote for a problem class, considering an input vector. Then, the most voted class will be chosen in the prediction of the classifier (Breiman, 2001). The Random Tree classifier is a decision tree that considers only a few randomly selected features for each tree node (Geurts, Ernst, & Wehenkel, 2006).

For all classifiers the training step was performed with 75% of the database and the remaining was used for test. Bayes Net, Naive Bayes, SVM, J48, MLP, Random Forest, Random Tree were also tested for the k-fold cross-validation method, with k equal to 10.

Finally, the authors assessed the different classifiers performances through the accuracy, kappa statistic, sensitivity and specificity. Accuracy is a percentage of correctly classified data (Landis & Koch, 1977). Kappa statistic is a statistical method to evaluate the level of agreement or reproducibility of classification; it can vary between -1 and 1. Sensitivity measures the proportion of positive diagnoses that are correctly identified, while specificity measures the proportion of negative diagnoses that are correctly classified (Resmini, et al., 2012).

Materials

The authors used GNU/Octave, an open source environment that uses Matlab programming language. The classification step was performed with the Waikato Environment for Knowledge Analysis (WEKA) tool, version 3.8, also available for free.

RESULTS AND DISCUSSION

Initially, the classification results were obtained with the 168 attributes extracted using Haralick and Zernike moments. The evaluation metrics used to measure the performance of the classification were the accuracy values, Kappa index. The results are shown in Table 9 and Table 10. One of the proposals to be analyzed by this work is the reduction of attributes by analyzing the optimization technique ODM + KNN in the configurations K = 3, K = 5 and K = 7 and simulating 20 (twenty) times each configuration. Table 2 shows the averages of the number of attributes selected for each configuration.

Table 2. Features selection average using ODM and KNN with K = 3, K = 5 and K = 7

K configuration	Average amount of selected features	Reduction percentage
K=3	85.85	48.90%
K=5	86.05	48.80%
K=7	86	48.80%

Source: The authors

Considering that initially the attribute vector had a dimension 168 attributes and after the selection step resulted a dimension attribute vector 86 attributes. This is equals to percentage reduction of 48.80% in the original attribute vector. It is also observed that for any value of K the number of attributes selected and the percentage value of attribute reduction are close. Thus, the hypothesis is that the database classes are quite distinct and therefore the value of K did not influence so much on the attribute selection process.

In the sequence, it will be presented and analyzed the average values of accuracy and Kappa index of the various classifiers with the attributes selected in the previous step. These results will be compared with the results of the classifiers before the selection process, ie with all 168 attributes. For the training, it will be used the techniques of data percentage split (75% for training and 25% for testing) and cross validation with k = 10 folds. Each simulation of the classification process with or without attribute selection was performed 20 (twenty) times. The values presented in the tables below (Table 3, 4, 5, 6, 7, 8, 9 and 10) are the arithmetic means.

Table 3. Average accuracy and kappa values from the classification process after features selection using ODM + KNN with K = 3 and using 75% of the database for training and 25% for testing.

	BayesNet	NaiveBayes	MLP	SVM linear	J48	RandomTree	RandomForest
Accuracy	49.666%	48.032%	**74.916%**	68.528%	52.463%	49.238%	67.985%
Kappa statistic	0.360	0.337	**0.718**	0.627	0.400	0.355	0.617

Table 4. Average accuracy and kappa values from the classification process after features selection using ODM + KNN with K = 5 and using 75% of the database for training and 25% for testing.

	BayesNet	NaiveBayes	MLP	SVM linear	J48	RandomTree	RandomForest
Accuracy	50.558%	50.536%	**74.731%**	66.914%	51.260%	47.024%	67.038%
Kappa statistics	0.373	0.373	**0.717**	0.604	0.384	0.326	0.603

Table 5. Average accuracy and kappa values from the classification process after selection using ODM + KNN using K= 7 and using 75% of the database for training and 25% for testing.

	BayesNet	NaiveBayes	MLP	SVM linear	J48	RandomTree	RandomForest
Accuracy	48.388%	46.278%	**75.160%**	63.111%	51.634%	46.322%	65.077%
Kappa statistics	0.342	0.315	**0.720**	0.550	0.392	0.322	0.578

Table 6. Average accuracy and kappa values from the classification process after selection using ODM + KNN using K= 3 and using 10-folds cross-validation.

	BayesNet	NaiveBayes	MLP	SVM linear	J48	RandomTree	RandomForest
Accuracy	52.203%	50.649%	**81.084%**	71.671%	55.395%	51.921%	71.461%
Kappa statistics	0.361	0.340	**0.744**	0.620	0.403	0.358	0.617

Table 7. Average accuracy and kappa values from the classification process after selection using ODM + KNN using K= 5 and using 10-folds cross-validation.

	BayesNet	NaiveBayes	MLP	SVM linear	J48	RandomTree	RandomForest
Accuracy	52.115%	53.143%	**80.351%**	71.298%	54.329%	50.879%	70.916%
Kappa statistics	0.360	0.373	**0.735**	0.614	0.389	0.344	0.609

Table 8. Average accuracy and kappa values from the classification process after selection using ODM + KNN using K= 7 and using 10-folds cross-validation.

	BayesNet	NaiveBayes	MLP	SVM linear	J48	RandomTree	RandomForest
Accuracy	52.124%	48.020%	**80.561%**	66.618%	54.270%	49.239%	69.281%
Kappa statistics	0.360	0.306	**0.737**	0.552	0.388	0.322	0.587

Next, the authors will present the results of the classification with all extracted attributes. And, then, the results with or without attribute selection will be compared.

Table 9. Average accuracy and kappa values from the classification process using all features and 75% of the database for training and 25% for testing.

	BayesNet	NaiveBayes	MLP	SVM linear	J48	RandomTree	RandomForest
Accuracy	50.866%	48.592%	**80.107%**	73.139%	54.093%	48.118%	67.348%
Kappa statistics	0.376	0.347	**0.792**	0.693	0.427	0.341	0.610

Table 10. Average accuracy and kappa values from the classification process using all features and 10-folds cross-validation.

	BayesNet	NaiveBayes	MLP	SVM linear	J48	RandomTree	RandomForest
Accuracy	52.61%	51.63%	**85.79%**	78.65%	57.88%	50.97%	71.28%
Kappa statistics	0.367	0.353	**0.809**	0.712	0.436	0.345	0.614

Comparing the accuracy and kappa index values, it is observed that the best result, considering before and after the attribute selection process, the classifier that presented the best result was the MLP classifier. After the attribute selection step, we can observe a reduction of around 5% in the average accuracy considering the results with percentage split and cross validation.

Analyzing the mean values of accuracy and kappa index, it is noticeable that the Bayesians or tree-based classifier did not have significant reductions. The hypothesis that these classifiers already consider the relevance of each attribute when setting up their nets or trees. In the case of tree-based classifiers, the most relevant attributes are located in tree roots whereas the least relevant ones are located in the leaves.

As it is an application to aid medical diagnosis, the sensitivity and specificity metrics will also be analyzed. Thus, the results presented in the tables below shows the specificity and sensitivity values for the classification process using MLP networks with cross-validation with k = 10. The results shown are for the classification before and after the attribute selection process.

Table 11. Sensibility and specificity for the dataset with all features (168 features), using MLP classifier and 10-folds cross-validation.

CLASS	SPECIFICITY (%)	SENSITIVITY (%)
Cyst	94.63	90.08
Benign Lesion	74.59	71.90
Malignant Lesion	94.49	89.26
No Lesion	96.56	89.67

Table 12. Sensibility and specificity for the dataset with features selection (86 features), using K=5, MLP classifier and 10-folds cross-validation.

CLASS	SPECIFICITY (%)	SENSITIVITY (%)
Cyst	94.63	86.78
Benign Lesion	74.16	72.31
Malignant Lesion	94.35	83.06
No Lesion	94.08	82.23

Only the sensitivity and specificity metrics of the classifier that presented the best accuracy will be analyzed. For this analysis, it was considered the percentage split techniques (75% training and 25% tests) and cross validation with k = 10 folds. In this case, the classifier selected was the MLP with cross validation (k = 10 folds).

Using the original attribute vector (168 features) the best result of the tests performed showed 85.79% accuracy, 96.59% specificity for non-lesion images, 74.59% specificity for benign lesions, 94.49% specificity for malignant lesions and 94.63% cyst sensitivity. This result was obtained using the MLP network classification and the cross-validation technique. When reducing the attribute vector by about 48.80% (86 attributes), the best result was: 81.094% accuracy, 94.08% specificity for non-lesion images, 74.19% specificity for benign lesions, 94.35% specificity for malignant lesions and 94.63% sensitivity for cyst. The results were obtained using the MLP network classification with the cross-validation technique and the ODM + KNN selection and attributes technique. A comparative analysis between these metrics shows that the values were either stable or slightly reduced after the attribute selection step.

FUTURE RESEARCH DIRECTIONS

After data analysis it was concluded that the proposed method is a promising technique for attribute selection. Therefore, further exploration of the parameters of the search algorithms used is suggested. The authors also suggest comparing the proposed method of attribute selection in relation to the methods consolidated in the literature. Such as genetic algorithms and particle swarm optimization. Thus, the aim is to consolidate the dialectical method of optimization and search for attribute selection.

The results analysis also showed that the Haralick and Zernike attribute extractors represent well each class of the problem. However, it is suggested to test other attribute extraction techniques that might improve the accuracy of the classifiers.

In order to validate one of the hypotheses that emerged after analyzing the results in this work, it is necessary to change the evaluation function (fitness function) of the proposed methods and to observe the influence on a particular architecture type of the classifier. Thus, it is intended to perform tests using as a function of evaluation the tree-based classifier as the decision tree structure C4.5.

CONCLUSION

The use of breast thermography for breast cancer classification and detection is a promising technique to be used as a screening test for the diagnosis of breast lesions. Therefore, it can be an helpful tool in breast cancer diagnosis. This technique has some advantages. For example, it is a non-invasive, painless examination that enables the detection and classification of the lesion in dense breasts. In these type of breasts, other techniques such as mammography have difficulty in detection. Thermography also does not emit ionizing radiation and is a low cost technique. In addition to the advantages mentioned above, breast thermography may enable breast lesions to be diagnosed at an early stage. This may lead to a reduction in the fatality rate due to breast cancer.

From a database with thermal images, the authors performed features extraction using Haralick and Zernike moments. In this study, they performed features selection using the Dialectical Optimization Method combined to KNN classifier. Later, they performed classification using seven different classifiers, in an attempt to classify the images into one of the four possible classes: no lesion, benign lesion, malignant lesion or cyst.

The results were promising and confirmed that breast thermography may help in the detection of breast cancer. Using the original attribute vector (168 attributes), the best result of the tests performed showed 85.79% accuracy. After reducing the attribute vector by 48.80% (86 attributes) the best result showed 81.094% accuracy. Considering what was mentioned above and the analysis of the results, it is observed that the approach to attribute selection was positive. It was characterized by a significant reduction in the number of attributes without considerable decrease in accuracy or other metrics used in comparison to the classification with all attributes.

Thus, the results of the present research regarding breast thermography performance are consistent with several studies cited in the literature. Those studies evaluated the breast thermography performance effectiveness in helping to diagnose breast cancer, which may reduce fatality due to the disease or diagnosis in early stages of the disease.

The attribute selection technique used in this work was able to simplify the classification models by reducing the computational cost of creating and executing these models. It provided a better understanding of the results obtained as well as the reduction of the database size.

Regarding the difficulties found in this work, we highlight, mainly, the difficulty in adjusting the parameters of the search and optimization algorithms used. Mainly due to the empirical character of determination of a satisfactory set of parameters.

ACKNOWLEDGMENT

The authors thank the Brazilian research agencies: Coordenação de Aperfeiçoamento de Pessoal de Nível Superior (CAPES), Conselho Nacional de Desenvolvimento Científico e Tecnológico (CNPq) and Fundação de Amparo à Ciência e Tecnologia de Pernambuco (FACEPE), for the partial financial support of this research.

REFERENCES

Aguiar, P. S., Belfort, C., Silva, A., Diniz, P., De Lima, R., Conci, A., & de Paiva, A. (2013). Detecção de Regiões Suspeitas de Lesão na Mama em Imagens Térmicas Utilizando Spatiogram e Redes Neurais. *Cadernos de Pesquisa, 20*(2), 56–63. doi:10.18764/2178-2229.v20n2p56-63

American Cancer Society. (2019). Cancer Facts & Figures 2019. *CA: A Cancer Journal for Clinicians*, 1–71.

Belfort, C. N., Silva, A. C., & de Paiva, A. C. (2015). *Detecção de lesões em imagens termograficas da mama utilizando Índice de Similaridade de Jaccard e Artificial Crawlers.* XXXV CONGRESSO DA SOCIEDADE BRASILEIRA DE COMPUTAÇÃO.

Breiman, L. (2001). Article. *Machine Learning, 45*(1), 5–32. doi:10.1023/A:1010933404324

Cheng, H., Shi, X., Min, R., Hu, L., Cai, X., & Du, H. (2006). Approaches for automated detection and classification of masses in mammograms. *Pattern Recognition, 39*(4), 646–668. doi:10.1016/j.patcog.2005.07.006

Cheng, J., & Greiner, R. (2001). *Learning Bayesian Belief Network Classifiers: Algorithms and System.* Advances in Artificial Intelligence - Springer Berlin Heidelberg. doi:10.1007/3-540-45153-6_14

Cover, T., & Hart, P. (1967). Nearest neighbor pattern classification. *IEEE Transactions on Information Theory, 13*(1), 21–27. doi:10.1109/TIT.1967.1053964

da Silva, A. L., de Santana, M. A., Azevedo, W. W., Bezerra, R. S., dos Santos, W. P., & de Lima, R. C. (2018). *Seleção de Atributos para Apoio ao Diagnóstico do Câncer de Mama Usando Imagens Termográficas, Algoritmos Genéticos e Otimização por Enxame de Partículas.* II Simpósio de Inovação em Engenharia Biomédica - SABIO.

da Silva, A. S. (2015). *Classificação e segmentação de termogramas de mama para triagem de pacientes residentes em regiões de poucos recursos médicos.* Federal University of Pernambuco.

Davidson, N. (1997). Diseases of the Breast. *Journal of the National Cancer Institute, 89*(1), 85–85. doi:10.1093/jnci/89.1.85

Dourado Neto, H. (2014). Egmentação e análise automática de termogramas: um método auxiliar na detecção do câncer de mama. *Dissertation Respomse to the Graduate Program in Mechanical Engineering*. Federal University of Pernambuco.

Feitosa, A. S. (2015). Reconstrução de imagens de tomografia por impedância elétrica utilizando o método Dialético de otimização. *Dissertation Response to the Graduate Program in biomedical engineering*. Federal University of Pernambuco.

Galvão, S. D., & Júnior Hruschka, E. R. (2004). Ponderação do knn utilizando-se de métodos. *da Vinci, Curitiba, 1*(1), 115-125.

Geurts, P., Ernst, D., & Wehenkel, L. (2006). Extremely randomized trees. *Machine Learning, 63*(1), 3–42. doi:10.100710994-006-6226-1

Haykin, S. (2003). Redes neurais, Princípios e Prática. *The Bookman*.

Kohavi, R., & John, G. (1997). Wrappers for feature subset selection. *Artificial Intelligence, 97*(1-2), 273–324. doi:10.1016/S0004-3702(97)00043-X

Ladis, R. J., & Koch, G. G. (1977). The Measurement of Observer Agreement for Categorical Data. *Biometrics, 33*(1), 159–174. doi:10.2307/2529310 PMID:843571

Landis, J. R., & Koch, G. G. (1977). The Measurement of Observer Agreement for Categorical Data. *Biometrics, 33*(1), 33. doi:10.2307/2529310 PMID:843571

Librelotto, S. R., & Mozzaquatro, P. (2014). Análise dos algoritmos de mineração j48 e apriori aplicados na detecção de indicadores da qualidade de vida e saúde. *Revista Interdisciplinar de Ensino, Pesquisa e Extensão - RevInt*.

MS & INCA. (2002). *Falando sobre câncer de mama*. Rio de Janeiro: Instituto Nacional de Câncer. Coordenação de Prevenção e Vigilância – (Conprev).

Nascimento, F. B., Pitta, M. G., & Rêgo, M. J. (2015). Análise dos principais métodos de diagnóstico de câncer de mama como propulsores no processo inovativo. *Arquivos de Medicina, 29*(6).

Ng, E. K., & Sudharsan, N. M. (2001). Numerical computation as a tool to aid thermographic interpretation. *Journal of Medical Engineering & Technology*, 53–60. doi:10.1080/03091900110043621 PMID:11452633

Oliveira, M. M. (2012). *Desenvolvimento de protocolo e construção de um aparato mecânico para padronização da aquisição de imagens termográficas de mama*. Federal University of Pernambuco.

Pappa, G. L., Freitas, A. A., & Kaestner, C. A. (2002). Attribute Selection with a Multi-objective Genetic Algorithm. *Advances in Artificial Intelligence: 16th Brazilian Symposium on Artificial Intelligence, SBIA*, 280-290. doi:10.1007/3-540-36127-8_27

Pedrini, H., & Schwartz, W. (2008). *Análise de Imagens Digitais: Princípio, Algoritmos e aplicações*. Cengage Learning.

Resmini, R., Conci, A., Borchartt, T. B., de Lima, R. d., Montenegro, A. A., & Pantaleão, C. A. (2012). Diagnóstico precoce de doenças mamárias usando imagens térmicas e aprendizado de máquina. *Revista Eletrônica do Vale do Itajaí*, 55-67.

Rocha, A. D. (2006). Detecção e classificação de lesões em imagens de mamografia usando classificadores SVM. *Dissertation Response to the Graduate Program in Biomedical Engineering*. Federal University of Pernambuco.

Santana, M. A., da Silva, W. W., da Silva, A. L., Pereira, J. M., Barbosa, V. A., Diniz, C. A., ... dos Santos, W. P. (2018). Desempenho de máquinas de aprendizado extremo com operadores morfológicos para identificação e classificação de lesões em imagens frontais de termografia de mama. *XXII Congresso Brasileiro de Automática. SBA Sociedade Brasileira de Automática*. doi:10.20906/CPS/CBA2018-0202

Santana, M. A., Pereira, J. M., Silva, F. L., Lima, N. M., Sousa, F. N., Arruda, G. M., Lima, R. C. F., Silva, W. W. A., & Santos, W. P. (2018). Breast cancer diagnosis based on mammary thermography and extreme learning machines. *Research on Biomedical Engineering*, *34*(1), 45–53. doi:10.1590/2446-4740.05217

Santos, W., Assis, F., Souza, R., Mendes, P., Monteiro, H., & Alves, H. (2009). Dialectical Non-Supervised Image Classification. *IEEE Congress on Evolutionary Computation*, 2480-2487.

Santos, W., Assis, F., Souza, R., Santos Filho, P. B., & Lima Neto, F. B. (2009). Dialectical multispectral classification of diffusion-weighted magnetic. *Computerized Medical Imaging and Graphics*, *33*(6), 442–460. doi:10.1016/j.compmedimag.2009.04.004 PMID:19446434

Santos, W. P. (2009). Método Dialético de Busca e Otimização para Análise de Imagens de Ressonância Magnética. *Master Thesis Response to the Graduate Program in Electrical engineering*. Federal University of Pernambuco.

Santos, W. P., & Assis, F. (2009). Optimization based on Dialectics. *International Joint Conference on Neural Networks*, 2804-2811.

Santos, W. P., & de Assis, F. M. (2009). Método Dialético de Otimização usando o Princípio da Máxima Entropia. *Learning and Nonlinear Models – Revista da Sociedade Brasileira de Redes Neurais (SBRN)*, *7*(2), 54-64. doi:10.21528/CBRN2009-010

Santos, W. P., & De Assis, F. M. (2013). *Algoritmos dialéticos para inteligência computacional*. Universitária da UFPE.

Santos, W. P., Souza, R., Santos filho, P., Lima neto, F., & Assis, F. (2008). A Dialectical Approach for Classification of DW-MR Alzheimer's. *IEEE Congress on Evolutionary Computation*, 1728-1735.

Santos dos, W. P., de Souza, R. E., Santos Filho, P. B., Lima Neto, F. B., & de Assis, F. M. (2008). A dialectical approach for classification of DW-MR Alzheimer. *IEEE Congress on Evolutionary Computation (IEEE World Congress on Computational Intelligence)*. doi:10.1109/CEC.2008.4631023

Shanthi, S., & Bhaskaran, V. (2013). A Novel Approach for Detecting and Classifying Breast Cancer in Mammogram Images. *International Journal of Intelligent Information Technologies*, *9*(1), 21–39. doi:10.4018/jiit.2013010102

Simard, P., Le Cun, Y., & Denker, J. (1992). Efficient Pattern Recognition Using a New Transformation Distance. *Proceedings of the 5th International Conference on Neural Information Processing Systems*, 50-58.

Spritzer, P. (2003). TRHM e proliferação do tecido mamário normal: O debate continua. *Brasileiros de Endocrinologia & Metabologia*, *5-6*(1), 5–6. Advance online publication. doi:10.1590/S0004-27302003000100003

Traldi, M., Galvão, P., de Morais, S., & Fonseca, M. (2016). Demora no diagnóstico de câncer de mama de mulheres atendidas no Sistema Público de Saúde. *Cadernos Saúde Coletiva*, *24*(2), 185–191. doi:10.1590/1414-462X201600020026

Vasconcelos, J., Santos, W., & de Lima, R. (2018). *Analysis of Methods of Classification of Breast*. IEEE Latin America Transactions. doi:10.1109/TLA.2018.8444159

Vázquez, A. (2007). *Filosofia da práxis*. Expressão Popular.

Wilcox, R. H. (1961). Adaptive control processes - A guided tour. *Naval Research Logistics Quarterly*, *8*(3), 315–316. doi:10.1002/nav.3800080314

Chapter 5
Computer Techniques for Detection of Breast Cancer and Follow Up Neoadjuvant Treatment:
Using Infrared Examinations

Adriel dos Santos Araujo
Fluminense Federal University, Brazil

Roger Resmini
Federal University of Rondonópolis, Brazil

Maira Beatriz Hernandez Moran
Fluminense Federal University, Brazil

Milena Henriques de Sousa Issa
Federal Hospital of Servants of Rio de Janeiro, Brazil

Aura Conci
Fluminense Federal University, Brazil

ABSTRACT

This chapter explores several steps of the thermal breast exams analysis process in detecting breast abnormality and evaluating the response of pre-surgical treatment. Topics concerning the process of acquiring, storing, and preprocessing these exams, including a novel segmentation proposal that uses collective intelligence techniques, will be discussed. In addition, various approaches to calculating statistical and geometric descriptors from thermal breast examinations are also considered of this chapter. These descriptors can be used at different stages of the analysis process of these exams. In this sense, two experiments will be presented. The first one explores the use of genetic algorithms in the feature selec-

DOI: 10.4018/978-1-7998-3456-4.ch005

tion process. The second conducts a preliminary study that intends to analyze some descriptors, already used in other works, in the process of evaluating preoperative treatment response. This evaluation is of fundamental importance since the response is directly associated with the prognosis of the disease.

INTRODUCTION

Cancer is characterized by uncontrolled growth of cells genetically altered that can be treated when correctly diagnostic is done. This situation expands to various types of cancer, including breast cancer. After the malignancy of breast cancer is indicated (by some method of tissue analysis, such as a core biopsy or mammotomy, for example), the patient in the nowadays neoadjuvant follow-up is treated in order to promote a process to encapsulate it reducing its size and especially its activity before the removal of cancerous tissues by surgery. This process is done to prevent the blood and lymphatic stream on carrying and distributing malignant cells to other parts of the body (causing metastasis or cancer in other organs).

In this sense, the use of imaging to follow this process of treatment of patients whose breast cancer has already been diagnosed can be a vital ally. The use of thermography certainly causes less discomfort in patients, who often have hypersensitivity in the breast region, and organ pain caused by the disease or forms of treatments. Digital Infrared Thermal Examination (DITE) appears as a possibility for follow up that has been recently studied and applied in research for detection and clinical monitoring of different diseases. The camera used for DITE allows capturing infrared radiation emitted by objects and converts this radiation to temperature values when environmental conditions are well known. This is a noninvasive and inexpensive technique that has recently been applied to the study of various diseases (Polidori et al., 2017; Staffa et al., 2017; Etehadtavakol and Ng, 2017; Moran et al., 2018).

The temperature acquired at each point can be analyzed in its original form, that is, a set of temperatures arranged in a bidimensional matrix represented by M(x,y), where x e y represents the indexes in that matrix. Another approach converts the range of temperature into a generic image I, represented by the function I (x, y) = i, being I a color that represents a temperature value and x e y the indexes in that image.

DITEs are characterized as functional exams and could be able to detect changes by the thermal pattern earlier than other exams since most of those exams are structural rather than physiological. There are reports in the literature mentioning that this type of test can help detect cancer up to ten years before being observed in other approaches. Besides, unlike other tests, DITE does not use ionizing radiation, are not harmful to the patient and are completely noninvasive (Gautherie, 1983; Keyserlingk et al., 1998).

MAIN FOCUS OF THE CHAPTER

The process of DITE analysis can be divided into several stages. Some of the most common could include activities inherent in exam acquisition, preprocessing, segmentation, the definition of the Region of Interest (ROI), feature computation, feature selection, and classification. In this chapter, several important points that go through all these steps will be discussed.

Some protocols used in the process of acquiring thermographic exams, will be discussed, pointing out the main differences and similarities between them. Moreover, a public dataset with over 7000 DITE and over 2500 users will be presented. The exams in this repository have helped thousands of institutions in their research around the world. Additionally, such a large number of users presents an opportunity for the development of several kinds of research involving the use of collective intelligence in order to assist the process of breast DITE segmentation.

The preprocessing step will also be discussed, in particular, the segmentation approaches, ROI identification, and registration of already segmented breasts will be addressed. Automatic and semi-automatic techniques for preprocessing activities that involve computer vision, crowdsourcing, and machine learning will be discussed (Resmini et al., 2018).

Another critical phase in the DITE analysis process involves feature computation. These features could help to obtain indicators capable of measuring the evolution of the clinical condition of a patient already diagnosed with breast cancer in the neoadjuvant treatment phase. Considering the many features that can be computed to aid breast cancer DITE analysis process, those related to texture are particularly interesting. Imaging analysis and processing activities routinely use texture information in their processes because this information can especially contribute to the process of identifying objects and patterns. This chapter will cover some approaches to computing such features that can be divided into statistical and geometric approaches.

Measurements based on statistical approaches represent general properties of texture, describing the distributions and relationship between the pixels of an image. The statistical features that will be discussed in this chapter are calculated from Simple Statistics, Thermographic Index, Asymmetry Parameter, Moments, and texture descriptors from Grayscale Co-occurrence Matrix (GLCM) (Haralick, Shanmugam & Distein, 1973), and Sum and Difference Histograms (SDH)(Unser, 1986). Additionally, the similarities between the last two approaches will be discussed, highlighting works in the literature that investigate the equivalence between approaches in the computation for a significant number of texture descriptors.

The geometric approach calculates features that understand texture as composed of well-defined primitives (micro-texture) and a hierarchy of spatial arrangements (macro-texture). Unlike the statistical approach, this approach defines texture events according to their shape. This chapter will discuss measures extracted using rules to describe the spatial position and the relationship between primitives. In particular, the use of Number of Texture Unit (NTU) to calculate features from texture spectrum. (Resmini et al., 2018).

Several papers in the literature discuss the performance of different approaches and algorithms of machine learning to improve the classification process. However, sometimes, the performance of these algorithms can be improved, finding the features of breast cancer DITEs that are most important to the classification process. In this sense, this chapter will discuss approaches to feature selection. The purpose of this step is to find the smallest feature set that can result in satisfactory prediction performance in breast cancer analyze.

The literature exposes several heuristic measures to estimate the relative importance or relative contribution of the feature vector for Breast Cancer classification system, i. e. quality of attributes. A solution is to select features by some techniques, like Principal Components Analysis (PCA). Another strategy is using the classifier to select texture features, that can be implemented using a Genetic Algorithm (GA). GA is a kind of evolutionary algorithm, or a meta-heuristic algorithm, that generates search solutions to optimize results that have concepts biologically inspired on natural evolution. Besides, a study exploring a GA in this feature selection process will be conducted. This experiment intents to show that the GA with a correct performance measure can act as a judge for choosing the best DITE features from different datasets.

In the literature, several studies explore the use of thermography to increase the accuracy of an early breast cancer diagnosis. However, few studies are devoted to investigating the use of DITEs in the process of evaluating preoperative treatment response. This evaluation is of fundamental importance since the response is directly associated with the prognosis of the disease. The identification of changes in the thermal pattern of the tissue can contribute to the monitoring of breast cancer and will be discussed in this chapter. Moreover, a preliminary study that intents to analyze some descriptors, already used in other works, in the process of evaluating preoperative treatment response will be performed.

The next sections of this chapter will discuss several concerns inherent in the DITE evaluation process. Essential aspects will be punctuated regarding the multiple stages and their consequences, contemplating approaches that can be used not only for detecting abnormalities but also to evaluate the response of breast cancer treatment.

EVALUATING NEOADJUVANT TREATMENT THROUGH INFRARED EXAMINATIONS

Currently, breast cancer treatment could be performed by combining several variables, the most common of which are: a) surgery; b) radiotherapy; c) hormone therapy; and d) chemotherapy. Treatment of the disease, regardless of the form chosen, should be started, individualized.

Factors such as disease staging or histological/immunohistochemical type of cancer are documented using the definition of approach to be used in the treatment process. Of these, both hormone therapy and chemotherapy can be strategically inserted as a first approach to combat the tumor. The use of chemotherapy as neoadjuvant treatment (i.e., preoperative) has become one of the most used and indicated for patients with locally advanced disease. Besides, the use of this approach has been seen as an alternative to extensive operational diseases without converting radical surgery to conservative surgery (Mamounas, 2015).

These treatment approaches may observe, in vivo, an action of the administered drug on the tumor. This phenomenon is commonly called response to treatment. Response to treatment can take different outcomes, including: a) entirely positive responses: where the disease has been eliminated; b) partial: representing positive results, but without tumor eradication; c) null: when the treatment shows no effects on the tumor; or even d) progressive: when disease progresses during treatment surveillance.

Histopathology of the surgical specimen, obtained through biopsy, is the gold standard method for assessing complete pathological response, i.e., the absence of any disease residue after neoadjuvant treatment in breast cancer (Kong, Moran, Zhang, Haffty, & Yang, 2011). It is expected that patients with a complete pathological response after neoadjuvant therapy have a better outcome compared with those who did not have a good response (Cortazar et. al., 2014).

However, several imaging modalities are used to evaluate, before surgery, the response to the treatment. The most routinely used are mammography, ultrasound, and breast magnetic resonance imaging. The first two are exams that evaluate the morphology and size of the tumor. Nuclear magnetic resonance evaluates both the morphology and the tumor vascularization, thus being considered a functional examination. Although several studies have attempted to determine an optimal imaging modality for assessing response to therapy before surgery, there are still discussions about the most accurate method for detecting complete pathological response (Sheikhbahaei et. al, 2016).

Tumor growth is dependent on the angiogenesis process. This means that without continuous recruitment of new capillary blood vessels, the tumor tends to be unable to grow beyond two cubic millimeters. Tumor treatment can reduce or interrupt this process, causing vascularization also to be reduced. The absence of vascularization limits the growth of solid tumors. (Folkman J, 1971).

In this context, the thermographic exam may also potentially act as a new functional exam in the process of evaluating treatment response, since increased vascularization alters the temperature pattern of the region (Ng, 2009). The fact that it allows the identification of changes in the thermal pattern of the breast may contribute to the monitoring of breast cancer (Raj, et al., 2018) and can be used to detect changes resulting from pre-surgery treatments. Interestingly, the use of thermography causes less discomfort in patients, who often have hypersensitivity in the region, and organ pain caused by the disease, forms of diagnosis, and treatments. The authors of this chapter have explored this new application of DITEs: assisting in the treatment response evaluation process.

This research has potential in health, as it can directly impact the lives of thousands of patients diagnosed with breast cancer, assisting in the evolutionary follow-up of the treatment of the disease. In the future, the results of this research may potentially assist in the constitution of a computational methodology that will be delivered to the physician via a mobile device with a thermal camera attached, providing a quick preliminary opinion on the evolutionary situation of cancer during treatment.

ACQUISITION PROCESSES

Medical thermography is an exam under study. This implies that this exam is the main target of studies investigating its use in several health areas. In this chapter, we present some discussions and studies regarding the use to aid in the diagnosis and monitoring of breast cancer.

Borchartt et al. (2013) carry out a survey that includes the main approaches used in the process of thermal imaging of the breast. This study explored the different variables, such as the type of acquisition, recommended ambient temperature, and even particular recommendations for moments before the start of capture.

Silva et al. (2014), proposed a comparative study in which four new approaches to DITE capture protocols were explored. These proposals were built, observing some perceived inconsistencies between the various capture protocols existing. In this study, the protocols were divided into two categories: static and dynamic.

In both static protocols, the patient was put to rest for a while. The purpose of this rest is to make the breast temperature stabilize concerning the ambient temperature. The difference between the two is regarding the time: one consider 10-minute to rest and the other to 15 minutes. The two dynamic protocols, on the other hand, the patient's breasts is exposed to a cooling process and subsequently the sequence of captures starts. The difference between these two dynamic approaches was the method used for cooling: one considered cooling using an electric fan aimed at the breasts, and the other, the application of alcohol in the breast region.

The results of this study supported the consolidation of two protocols for the acquisition of breast DITEs. Each of these protocols has indications for static and dynamic captures. These new protocols seek to correct errors and problems found in the protocols presented in the literature.

Static captures include five DITE acquisitions, with the patient in the following positions in relation to the equipment: a) left side 90º; b) left side 45º; c) frontal; d) right side 45º; and e) right side 90º. In all positions, the patient is positioned with his hands over his head. Figure 1 illustrates these acquisitions.

Figure 1. Static captures from Silva et al. (2014) protocol

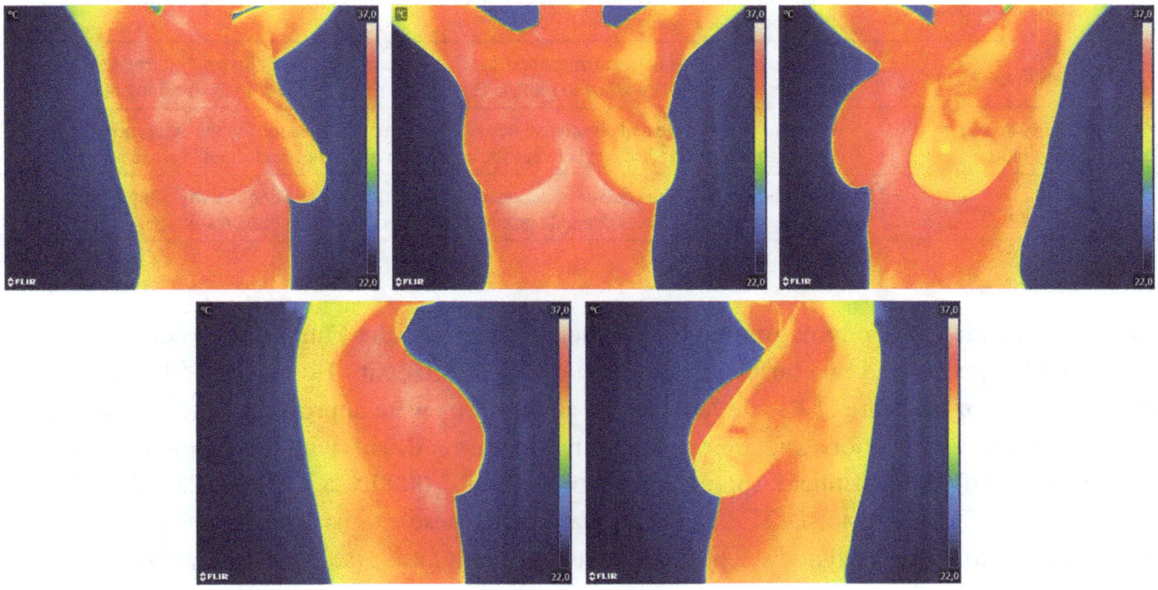

Dynamic captures occur after a patient's breast cooling process. This cooling is induced by an electric fan pointing to the breasts. The entire cooling process takes place for 5 minutes or until the patient's breasts reach an average temperature of 30.5 ° C. After this process, 20 captures are performed every 15 seconds, thus totaling 5 minutes of capture. These captures occur with the patient in the front position and with the hands on the head. The protocol proposed by Silva et al. (2014) contemplates five phases, as shown in Table 1.

To support the investigations regarding the treatment response, new DITE sessions are being performed in patients already diagnosed with breast cancer, following Silva Protocol. For these acquisitions, volunteer patients with neoadjuvant treatment indication are selected. It is essential to mention that the patient's treatment routine is not changed.

In this study, each patient will go through two acquisition sessions at different times. The first acquisition (Visit 1 - V1) happens during the mastology consultation, that is, before the referral to oncology, responsible for the execution of neoadjuvant treatments. The second acquisition (Visit 2 - V2) happens when the patient is referred back to mastology, that is, after the end of treatment. This period usually has an average duration of 6 months. The agreement between the histopathological and the DITEs obtained after neoadjuvant treatment will subsidize the inclusion of thermographic exams in the arsenal of imaging exams used to evaluate treatment response.

Table 1. Silva Protocol Steps

	Phase	Description
1	Patient Recommendations	Recommends that the patient avoid caffeine, alcohol and nicotine consumption within two hours of the test. In addition, the patient should not apply creams or deodorants to the breast and armpit area and should not exercise.
2	Environment Recommendations	The room to be used must have a temperature between 20° and 22°, without windows and openings. The ambient airflow should not be pointing at the patient. Fluorescent lamps should illuminate the environment.
3	Patient Preparation	Patients should remove earrings, necklaces, scarves, or any other elements attached to their bodies. Also, they are asked to remove clothes that cover the waist to the head region.
4	Exam Parameter Configuration	Patient temperature and air relative humidity information are added in the equipment configuration. The distance between the equipment and the patient should be one meter.
5	DITEs Capture	At this stage, DITE acquisitions are made. It is essential to mention that the equipment is configured so that these dynamic protocol acquisitions occur automatically.

These acquisitions are ongoing through a partnership between the Fluminense Federal University Institute of Computing and two hospitals: a) Antônio Pedro University Hospital; and b) Federal Hospital of Servants of the State of Rio de Janeiro. All acquisitions were approved by the Research Ethics Committee of these institutions and are registered in Plataforma Brasil, with the following numbers of Presentation Certificate for Ethical Appreciation: a) 04134918.7.0000.5252; b) 01042812.0.0000.5243; and c) 04134918.7.3002.5243. DITEs and other data from these exams will be stored anonymously and be available to the clinical and scientific community through the Database for Mastology Research (DMR, 2019) platform.

DATABASE FOR MASTOLOGY RESEARCH: STORING AND DISTRIBUTING BREAST EXAMS

Almost all scientific research, using clinical data from medical examinations, needs at some point a significant amount of data. In general, to meet this demand, researchers have two options: to provide this data autonomously or to use data provided in benchmarks or open-access repositories on the Internet.

Providing this data needed for research is not an easy task. This implies, mainly, the rescheduling of the research plan, since a considerable slice of time should be allocated to the acquisition of the necessary clinical exams. This stage involves, indirectly, a series of variables, such as: a) acquisition of the necessary equipment; b) the preparation of an appropriate environment for the examinations; c) definition of an acquisition protocol; d) approval of research in ethics management committees; e) participation of volunteer patients; f) interdisciplinary involvement of professionals and researchers to perform the acquisitions. Besides the obvious need for time to perform and adjust these steps, sometimes the challenge is also financial.

The use of a repository or benchmarks can meet many of these needs and help the researcher focus his efforts on the activities directly inherent to their research. For this chapter, we could mention the DMR. This repository concentrates data from various breast exams for the clinical and scientific community, providing an open-access database for the interested community (DMR, 2019). This represents a valuable resource of data that can be used in many kinds of research around the world.

The DMR is accessible through a user-friendly online interface (http://visual.ic.uff.br/dmi) for managing and retrieving information from breast exams and clinical data from patients. It provides thermal imaging of the breast, mammograms, magnetic resonance imaging, and ultrasound images for patients who agree to be a volunteer for breast cancer research.

All exams in this repository contain data that support the community in the activities inherent in their research and analysis. These can be exam images, patient reports, and reports on exams, or even medical record details. This record is a crucial element in care and gathers the information that summarizes the history and ensures continuity of treatment (e.g., age, race, complaints, symptoms, eating habits, personal and family history, medical history). It is essential to mention that all this data is stored anonymously.

Using DMR, the interested community can conduct research that seeks to provide mechanisms to assist in obtaining more accurate diagnoses or even in monitoring the evolution of the clinical condition of patients. This enables the same set of exams to be used on different research fronts — each of these, observing, in different ways, problems and characteristics inherent in breast cancer. The DITEs stored in the DMR uses the static and dynamic acquisition protocols.

The first exam was made available to the scientific community through the DMR platform are dated 2013. In these six years, there has been a substantial increase in the volume of exams available by the repository — especially concerning the number of DITEs. Table 2 summarizes the main actual DMR numbers.

Table 2. DMR Usage Statistics

Patients	291
Thermographic exam	289
Thermal images	7289
Registered users	2564

These numbers allow new research perspectives involving breast cancer to be considered. The large number of registered users, in contrast to the substantial volume of exams, especially DITEs, sets precedents for various computational approaches to be used. Research involving collective intelligence and crowdsourcing techniques can bring new approaches to life that assist in preprocessing, segmentation, and classification. Some of these perspectives will be discussed and exemplified in later sessions of this chapter.

PREPARING BREAST THERMAL EXAMINATIONS FOR ANALYSIS

One of the essential activities inherent in preprocessing concerns obtaining the region of interest for each DITE capture. This step is vital as it defines the limits of the DITEs to be observed in subsequent steps of the exam analysis process.

Several papers explore this need by providing and discussing different approaches to segmenting and obtaining ROI. These approaches range from manual segmentation techniques to those involving fully automated solutions. In this way are also found approaches categorized as semi-automatic, involving human activity. The participation of the human being in the process of obtaining the ROI in a breast DITE can conceive the participation of several actors: doctors, specialists, and even laypeople.

Using an automatic approach, Motta (2010) presents an automatic solution for obtaining the ROI in frontal breast DITEs. In his work, infra-mammary folds and armpits are used as reference points in the automatic segmentation process. For this, traditional image processing techniques and mathematical morphology were used in this process. Figure 2 illustrates the steps of this methodology.

Figure 2. Motta Segmentation Process

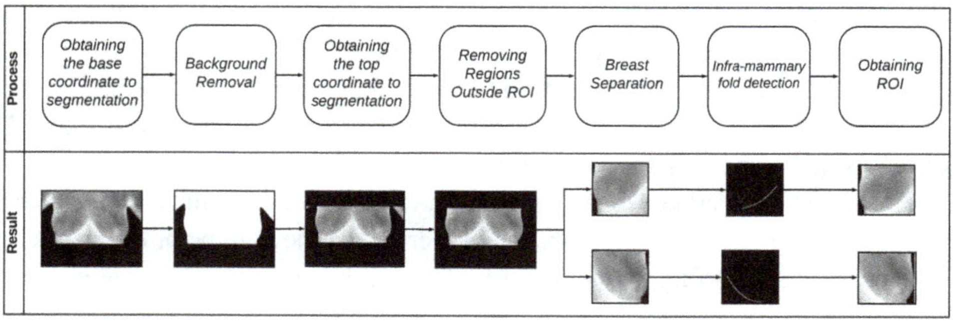

In this proposal, DITEs were used whose patients hands were placed at the waist. The captures of these exams took place at the Clinical Hospital of the Federal University of Pernambuco and were made available in a PROENG image bank (Dean & Ilventom, 2006)

Subsequently, Maques (2012), develops a proposal for automatic segmentation using images where patients follow another capture protocol. In this paper, DITEs are captured with patients placing their hands over their heads. These images were taken from DMRI. Breast segmentation in this approach is performed in three stages: lateral contour detection; b) obtaining the upper limits; and c) identification of the lower bounds, as illustrated in Figure 3.

Marques used several image processing techniques, such as thresholding, contour detection, morphological operations, region growth, and clustering. (Haralick et al. 1987, Adans & Bischof, 1994, Coleman & Andrews, 1979). Besides, numerical methods of approximation and interpolation curve adjustments were used by the author to assist in the process of defining the lower edge of the lady.

Figure 3. Marques Segmentation Process

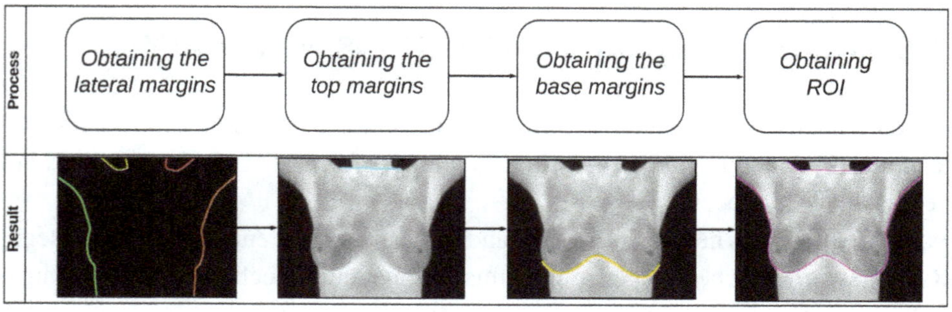

In scenarios where automated solutions do not effectively contribute to the process of segmentation and ROI definition, manual segmentation is a viable solution. Resmini (2016), in his work, used this approach to segment and obtained the ROIs of images for which automatic proposals did not produce consistent results. Although manual, this segmentation considered the same output patterns assumed by automatic segmenters.

As seen, fully automatic approaches could not always perform well, resulting in not adequately segmented images. Like most fully automated computer systems, the results may eventually be inconsistent with the expected result. This means that in most cases, even having a fully automated segmentation process, sometimes the result needs to be validated, and this validation is usually performed by one of the actors mentioned earlier: doctors, specialists, and even laypeople. Therefore, involving the human factor in part of the process.

In this sense, other solutions, which explore different types of approaches, are beginning to emerge in the process of segmenting and obtaining ROIS from DITEs. Thus approaches, whether automatic or semi-automatic, begin to incorporate techniques based on other principles, such as collective intelligence. These techniques often involve the community (crowd) in the process of automating or validating an activity.

As the volume of DITEs grows, manual segmentation and validation become unfeasible. Large databases make the manual process costly and extremely stressful, requiring a massive effort of the analyst. On the other hand, it subsidizes and drives the use of collective intelligence techniques. With the use of these techniques, individual effort tends to decrease substantially as the number of human actors involved in this process grows.

In this sense, Moran et al. (2019), propose a novel approach for the segmentation of DITEs, which combines image processing and collective intelligence. They propose a process where the crowd plays an essential role in validating the segmentation and, eventually, breast re-segmentation. They argue that this approach can help to maximize the quality of the segmentation process of DITEs, and, at the same time, minimize the need for expert intervention in this stage of the process.

Figure 4. Evaluation of the consistency of this segmentation

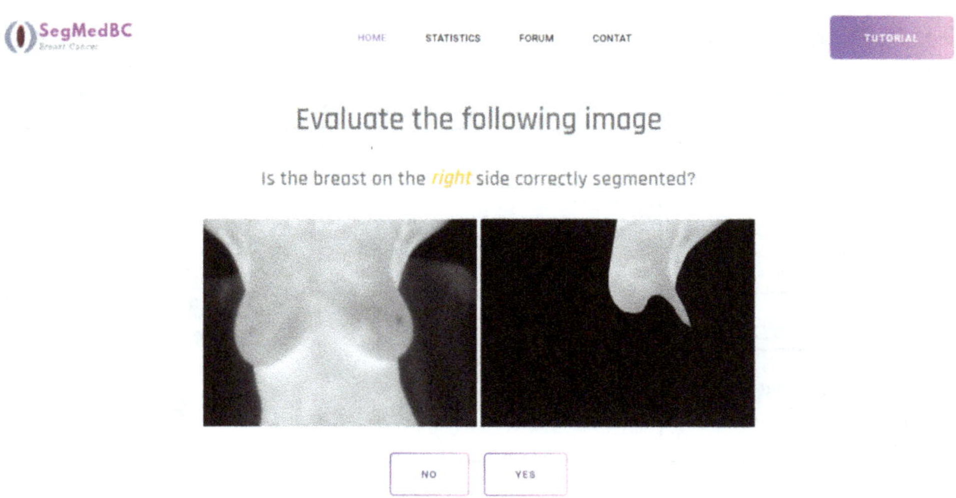

Figure 5. Re-segmentation process

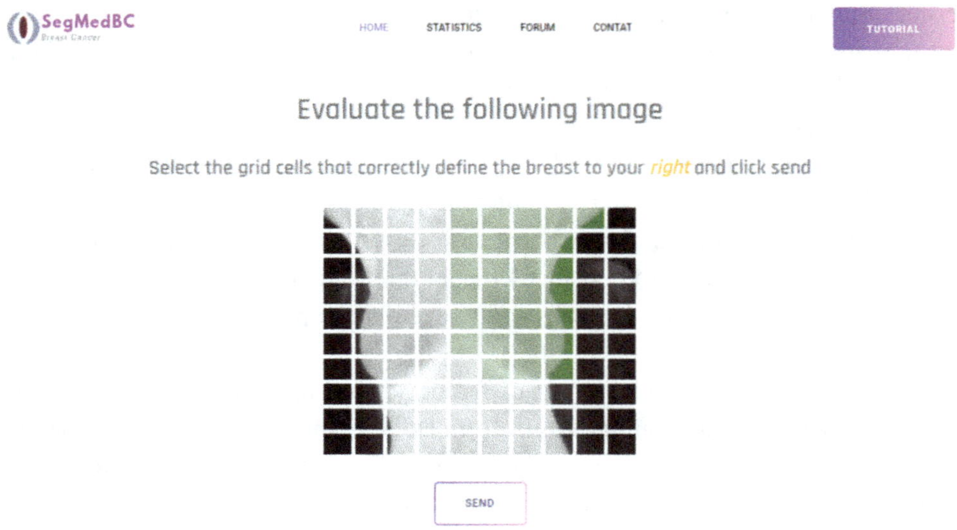

In their proposal, the authors make use of the three approaches: automatic, semi-automatic, and manual. The automatic segmentation obtained is then presented to the crowd, which plays two fundamental roles: a) evaluates the consistency of this segmentation; and b) submit a proposal for re-segmentation if the automatic result is inconsistent. To support this process, the authors built an interface capable of receiving user inputs a) and b), as shown in Figure 4 and Figure 5, respectively.

Note that the re-segmentation process receives manual indications of the correct segmentation points from the user. Thus, semi-automatic algorithms can make use of this input and process over the DITEs to generate a more appropriate segmentation. This entire process can be repeated iteratively, as often as the community user is interested in contributing. Figure 6 illustrates the flow of this process.

Also in this research, the authors developed the SegMedBC prototype (an acronym for Segmentation of Medical Images for Breast Cancer) and, on it, conducted an experimental study that assessed community capacity on two points: a) contributing to the validation of the quality of breast DITE seg-

Figure 6. SegMedBC Operating Flow

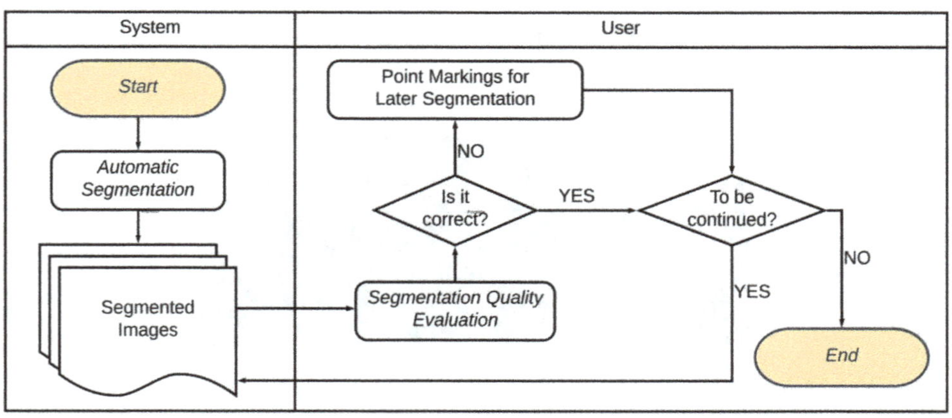

mentation; and b) contribute to the re-segmentation process, informing the essential points of ROI. The results showed that users could perform both activities properly, providing substantially better results than those obtained from the single application of traditional techniques. The authors also concluded that about 80% of the re-segmentation points presented by users are the same, thus presenting a high rate of similarity between them.

In addition to segmenting and obtaining ROI, other activities can also compose the preprocessing of an image to aid the handling of DITEs in subsequent analysis steps. An activity commonly performed in the preprocessing of DITEs concerns the registration of images (Borchartt, 2013; Galvão, 2015). This task allows two images, captured at different time points or different points of view, to be aligned. Therefore, with the registration, the breast DITEs can be aligned, facilitating the subsequent comparison process between the right and left breasts.

REPRESENTING BY DESCRIPTORS THE PROPERTIES OF EXAMS

Following preprocessing activities from DITEs, a pattern detection system can be used in the process of analysis of these images providing a specialized support tool (Gan, Ma & Wu, 2007). One of the possible flows in the pattern recognition process from DITEs concerns the computation of features that can numerically translate specific properties of these images. A feature in this context is a value calculated from the image, according to a descriptor. The set of some of these features can then be used in the pattern recognition process by artificial intelligence algorithms.

Of the information that can be computed, texture-related features are particularly relevant. Image analysis and processing activities routinely use this information in their processes. Texture analysis is a generic term that describes several techniques used to quantify the spatial variation of image color tones.

Several authors define textures from different perspectives, and there is no single formal definition of the term. Gonzales & Wood (2000) present them as the information capable of quantifying properties such as smoothness, roughness, and regularity in an image. Watt & Policarpo (1998) define textures as a region capable of presenting a set of similar elements, arranged in a partially ordered way. Pedrini & Schwartz (2008), similarly, define it as a set of repetitive pixel variations, which usually has a pattern, whether regular or random. Ebert & Musgrave (2003) describes the texture of an image as a set of features directly related to the surface properties of objects. In general, the term refers to a set of patterns that tend to repeat on a given surface.

Computing this information becomes an essential task in order to support the pattern recognition process in DITEs. In this sense, such information can be grouped according to the approach used in the computing process. The most common classifications are a) Statistics: those that use spatial relationship and tone variation; (b) Structural: relating to information calculated from geometric shapes; and c) Spectrals: relating to techniques that operate in the frequency domain (e.g., Fourier). (Parker, 1997). In this chapter, we will discuss the statistical and structural techniques used in breast DITE processing.

Features Based on Statistical Approaches

The statistical methods employed in computing the texture information of DITEs essentially use properties that define the distribution of tones in an image. Moreover, these methods usually quantify certain properties taking into account the spatial relationship between the elements of this image. (Materka & Strzelecki, 1998; Pedrini & Schwartz, 2008).

In this chapter, we will discuss four statistical approaches to computing texture descriptors from DITEs: Simple Statistics, Thermographic Index, Asymmetry Parameter, Moments, Grayscale Co-occurrence Matrix (GLCM), and Sum and Difference Histograms (SDH). The latter is presented as an alternative to GLCM, able to compute the same descriptors using less computational resources (Unser, 1986; Araújo et. al, 2018).

Using Simple Statistics_

Thermographies are used in the diagnostic process of several diseases, in which qualitative forms of diagnosis are most often used, and more rarely, approaches based on data analysis, i.e. using a quantitative way. The most commonly quantitative descriptors are: minimum, maximum and average values, both based on the ROI area temperatures (Brioschi et al., 2010). These descriptors are commonly described in the literature as basic statistical measures. (Schaefer, Záviŝek & Nakashima, 2009; Resmini, 2011; Borchartt, 2013). Such information is defined because it is based on basic statistical notions, which tend not to involve complex calculations. Also, these descriptors often do not consider the neighborhood of a pixel in the calculation process.

Thermographic Index

The Thermographic Index (TI) was initially defined by Collins et al. (1974). It is based on regions called isothermal areas, here named ISO. To find these areas in each ROI, the temperatures in M (x, y) of the points belonging to ROIp, are separated in intervals of 0.50 °C starting at *minROI* and *ending at maxROI,* as shown Equation (1). For each of these intervals there is a corresponding isothermal area, which is defined by the points whose temperature lies within this range.

$$n_{interval} = \frac{max_{ROI} - min_{ROI}}{0,50} \quad (1)$$

Note that the number of elements in each ISOq ∈ ISO, with q ∈ [1, 2, ..., n intervals], can be determined through the histogram of the set of temperatures given by M (x, y) considering the points p = (x, y) that belong to ROIp. Considering the number of elements of each set in ISO, the TI is given by the Equation 2

$$TI = \sum_{q=1}^{N\,intervals} \frac{D(ISOq)}{ROIq} \quad (2)$$

Where:

$$D(ISOq) = \prod_{i=1}^{ISOq} ISOq \times \Delta t(p) \quad (3)$$

p = (xp, yp) ∈ ISOq

Δt = M(x, y) - C,

C = 26 (Collins et al., 1974)

Thus, in any thermographic profile, the thermographic index was the summation of the products of difference in temperature from 26°C. to each isothermal temperature, and the areas of each isothermal area, divided by the total area measured. For similar studies, considering other parts of the body, the use of TI allowed differentiating healthy regions from regions that have some dysfunction (Moran, Conci & Araujo, 2019; Moran et al., 2019, Brioschi et al., 2010).

Asymmetry Parameter

It is also possible to compare points with others of a region considering an equivalent region, which in the case of symmetrical organs, corresponds to the same region on the opposite side considering an axis of symmetry. This analysis can be done through the named Asymmetry Parameter (AP).

According to Brioschi et al. (2010), the asymmetry parameter is defined by the temperature difference of a region relative to its contralateral side, considering a vertical axis of symmetry of the body. Values of AP above 0.3 C can indicate some dysfunction, and in general, if the value exceeds 1°C some significant problem may be occurring in the region (Brioschi, 2010). Yaneli et al. (2013) and Nicandro et al. (2013), on the other hand, group the thermal asymmetry into three ranges: a) Less than 1ºC; b) Between 1° C and 2 ° C; and c) Exceeding 2 ° C .

Considering only the ROI of each patient, the vertical axis used for the calculation of PA was established based on the ROI geometric center O, which is defined by the coordinates O (ox, oy), being ox and oy defined by the Equations (4) and (5).

$$o_x = \frac{\sum_{u=0}^{A}\sum_{v=0}^{B} uROI(u,b)}{I(u,v)} \quad (4)$$

$$o_y = \frac{\sum_{u=0}^{N}\sum_{v=0}^{M} uROI(u,b)}{I(u,v)} \quad (5)$$

Where A and B represent the number of line and rows, respectively, of image or matrix values.

After defining the vertical axis, the AP of each point in ROIp can be calculated. AP considers the temperature difference of points at the same y coordinate on opposite sides of the e axis. To perform this calculation, we consider only the points belonging to ROIp, as well as their symmetric points. The PA of a point is given by Equation (6):

$$PA(x,y)=\begin{cases} M(x,y)-M(x+(2o_x-x),y), if\ x<o_x \\ M(x,y)-M(x-(2x-o_x),y), if\ x\geq o_x \end{cases} \tag{6}$$

Where (x, y) are the coordinates of points belonging to ROIp.

Note that the value of AP indicates the hottest side. If the value is positive, the point p1 defined by the coordinates (x, y) is the hottest one. If the value is negative, the point p2 opposite to p1 is the hottest one.

Geometric Moments

The moment technique has been used in many cases to compute image features. In general, the moments and functions derived from them are used to describe the spatial distribution in an image or DITEs. For this, the spatial relationship between the tones of an image or a region is considered. The most commonly geometric moments are defined in Equation 7.

$$m_{pq}=\sum_{x=0}^{A-1}\sum_{y=0}^{B-1}x^p y^q (x,y) \tag{7}$$

Where m_{pq} is the order moment $p + q$; and $f(x, y)$ is the intensity of the tone at the x, y coordinates of the image. In the case of binary images, $f(x, y)$ takes the values 0 or 1. A and B are the number of line and rows, respectively, of image or matrix values. Moment *m00* represents the area in a binary image or the sum of all elements in grayscale images. The second-order moments (m_{02}, m_{11} *and* m_{20}) are called moments of inertia.

From the geometric moments, some measurements on objects can be defined. These measurements are essential in representing shapes in images. The geometric moments of order 0 and 1 are used to calculate the centroid or center of mass (barycenter) of the object (Equations 8 and 9).

$$x_c=\frac{m_{10}}{m_{00}} \qquad y_c=\frac{m_{01}}{m_{00}} \tag{9}$$

In this case, *xc* and *yc* are the ROI centroid coordinates.

Haralick Descriptors

Haralick et al. (1973) proposed a set of mathematical methods capable of describing 14 texture properties. This set of descriptors are able of presenting different aspects related to the way pixels are arranged in the image. In their calculation, these descriptors use grayscale co-occurrence to represent texture properties.

In addition to applications in the processing of breast DITEs, several studies make use of the Haralick descriptors in other health areas. Wibmer et al. (2015), shows that the analysis of these descriptors, calculated from magnetic resonance imaging (MRI), may help in the detection of prostate cancer. Still using magnetic resonance imaging, Soomro et al. (2017), presents contributions in the study of the evolution of colon cancer from Haralick's texture descriptors.

In this chapter, two ways to compute these descriptors are discussed, one using the GLCM e the another using SDH. The second approach optimizes the calculation for theses descriptors, once it has a linear cost, O(N), instead a quadratic cost from GLCM, O(N^2), where N represent the number of elements in a image, in this case, in a M(x,y) (Araújo et. al, 2018).

Gray Level Co-occurrence Matrix

One of the most extensively statistical approaches in the literature for computing texture descriptors is the Gray Level Co-occurrence Matrix (GLCM), also known as Simultaneous Occurrence Matrix.

GLCM consists of quantifying the gray level transitions between two pixels in an image, taking into account two parameters: distance and angle between these pixels. This matrix can also be viewed as a probability matrix since it computes and stores the probability that these two pixels perform simultaneously, given a distance and angle setting. These pixels are referred to as a reference and neighbor pixels.

The interval between the reference pixel and the neighboring pixel is given by: $P(i,j)d,\theta$ .Where $P(i,j)$ .s the reference pixel, *i* is the row ID and *j* the column ID to which the reference pixel is associated in the image. The elements of set *d* and θ .represent, respectively, the distance and angle of the reference pixel to the neighboring pixel. These values could change so that each set of these parameters generates a new probability matrix.

In the initial proposal (Haralick et al., 1973), any angle value could be used to establish the direction of calculation between the two pixels. Subsequently, a study that looked at various angle configurations concluded that the 0 °, 45 °, 90 °, and 135 ° angles adequately represent all other options (Haralick, 1979) thereby decreasing processing time (Pedrini & Schwartz, 2008).

Sum and Difference Histograms

Sum and Difference Histograms (SDH) are an alternative to computing the co-occurrence between the tones of an image. For this, these histograms also observe the relationship between two pixels, that is, reference and neighbor, given a spatial configuration (distance and angle) (Unser, 1986; Araújo et. al, 2018).

Similar to GLCM, Sum and Difference Histograms also use the entire image in their calculation process. Therefore, iteratively, the algorithms run through the image and, in each iteration, there is a summation or subtraction operation, respectively relative to the sum histogram and difference histogram. These operations occur between the reference pixel and the neighboring pixel, with the results computed in the corresponding histogram.

The SDH calculation process may involve the same parameters used in GLCM computing. In this sense, two distance configurations, one horizontal and one vertical, can represent the same angle configurations adopted in the calculation of the co-occurrence matrix (0, 45, 90, 135°). Figure 7 illustrates this representation, considering the four angles of calculations.

In Figure 7, the distance adopted between the reference pixel and the neighboring pixel is 1 unit. However, other settings of these parameters may occur. To do this, multiply the values of the parameters *di* and *dj* by the desired new distance. Another way to get distance parameters properly is to change their values equal to 1 by the desired distance values, paying attention to the signals of each parameter. Thus, the calculation of the sum and difference histograms can be expressed by the sum or difference of the reference pixel and the neighboring pixel, given by the *di* and *dj* distance and angle settings. The Equations (10) and (11) denote these calculations:

$$Sum\ Histogram = P_{(i,j)} + P_{(i+di,j+dj)}\ (1. \tag{10}$$

$$Difference\ Histogram = P_{(i,j)} - P_{(i+di,j+dj)}\ (1. \tag{11}$$

Where $P_{(i,j)}$ .s the reference pixel, *di* is the horizontal distance, and *dj* is the vertical distance.

Unser (1986) discusses the calculation of some of Haralick's descriptors, based on the information computed in the SDH. In this study, a set of equations to express the same properties of the descriptors

Figure 7. Representation of angle and distance from parameters di and dj.

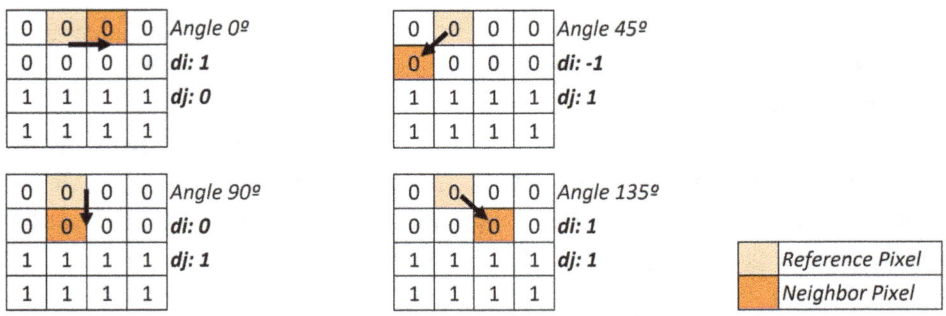

based on GLCM is proposed. Some of these equations were able to yield similar but not numerically identical results. Subsequently, Araujo et al. (2018) explore these descriptors, proposing adaptations in the calculation equations and new equations for the other descriptors. These studies concluded that the descriptors calculated from SDH are capable of presenting the same behavior pattern as those obtained from GLCM. Moreover, they are more computationally efficient, since those based on SDH have linear O (N) complexity while those based on GLCM have quadratic O (N^2) complexity.

Geometric Approaches

The descriptors defined in this approach (also called the structural approach) understand texture as composed of primitives (Gonzalez & Woods, 2002). Unlike the statistical approach, this approach defines texture events according to their shape.

The structural approach represents the texture by well-defined primitives (micro texture) and hierarchy of spatial arrangements (macro texture) of these primitives (Haralick, 1979). To describe texture, two strategies can be adopted: defining the primitives that make up the texture or defining the positioning and relationship rules. The advantage of the second strategy is that it provides good symbolic representation of the texture (Materka & Strzelecki, 1998). The focus of this work is on the second strategy.

Number of Texture Unit

At the same time that the pixel is the basic unit of an image, He and Wang (1990) formulated a concept that texture also has its basic unit and considers the pixel and its neighborhood. The authors called this unit the "Texture Unit" (TU). According to this concept, a texture can be described as a set of TUs or Number of Texture Units (NT U). To formalize the concept, it is described:

Let be a 3x3 pixel neighborhood formed by the elements $[g_0, g_1, \ldots, g_8]$, where g_0 is the gray scale value of the center pixel and the other g_i are the gray scale values of the neighboring pixels, g_1 through g8. Thus, TU = [e1, e2,. . ., e8] and is formed by values ranging from 0 to 2, according to Equation (12):

$$N_{TU} = \sum_{i=0}^{7} e_i * 3^i \; (1. \qquad (12)$$

Where $\{0, if\ g_i < g_0\}.\ \{1, if\ g_i = g_0\}.\ \{0, if\ g_i > g_0\}.$

Based on Equation (12), $N_{TU} = 3^0 * e^{0,0} + 3^1 * e^{0,1} + 3^2 * e^{0,2} + 3^3 * e^{1,2} + 3** e^{2,2} + 3^5 * e^{2,1} + 3^6 * e^{2,0} + 3^7 * e^{1,0}$. Then, $N_{TU} = 1 * 0 + 3 * 2 + 9 * 2 + 27 * 1 + 81 * 0 + 243 * 0 + 729 * 2 + 2187 * 0 = 0$

Figure 8. Example N_{TU} operations: a) original image (g_0 = 40); b) N_{TU} e_i calculation; c) N_{TU} 3^i calculation; d) multiplication results. N_{TU} code = 1509.

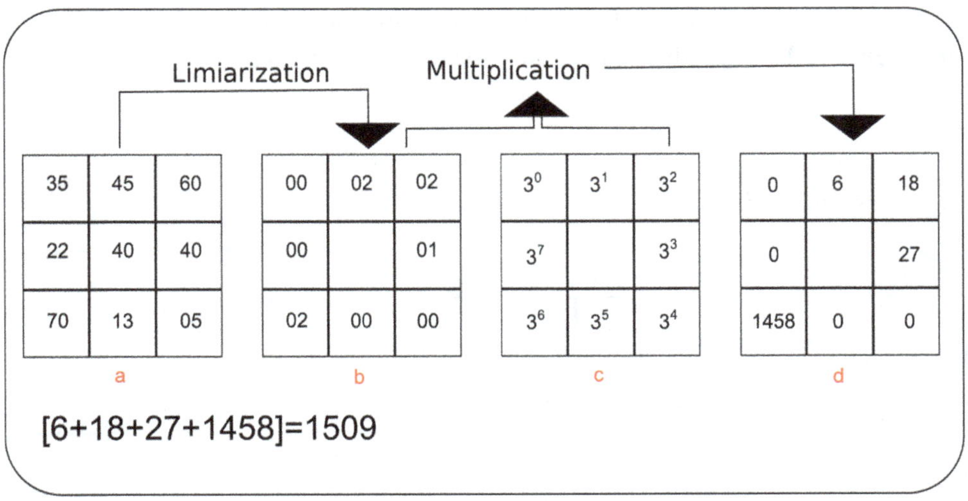

$+ 6 + 18 + 27 + 0 + 0 + 1458 + 0$. The final code for this configuration (Figure 8 c) is 1509.

Others seven configurations are possible changing start point of N_{TU} 3^i calculation (Figure 9).

For example, in this demonstration start point (3^0) is in position $e^{0,0}$. In next configuration the start point will be in position $e^{0,1}$. In a vector with 6560 positions, this code (1509) is marked, the spectrum. The seven other codes are calculated and marked in the vector. After that the window navigate changing g_0 pixel until entire image be covered. At the end, eight spectrum are calculated. Next step is to calculate features from these spactrums.

Feature Computation From N_{TU}

Black-White Symmetry (BWS), Equation 2.32, calculates the symmetry between the two halves of the spectrum resulting in normalized values between zero and one hundred.

$$BWS = \left| 1 - \frac{\sum_{1=0}^{3279} \left| S(i) - S(3281+i) \right|}{\sum_{i=0}^{6560} S(i)} \right| * 100(1. \tag{13}$$

where BWS is the symmetry value, the higher the BWS values, the greater the similarity between the left and right sides of the texture spectrum; *S(i)* is the frequency that signature values *i* occur in the spectrum. In practice, BWS measures the ability to change between *0* and *2* in the spectrum calculation, Equation (13).

Geometric Symmetry (GS) quantifies the shape regularity of the image and is defined in Equation (12).

$$GS = \left| 1 - \frac{1}{4} \sum_{j=1}^{4} \frac{\sum_{i=0}^{6560} \left| S_j(i) - S_{j+4}(i) \right|}{2 * \sum_{i=0}^{6560} S_j(i)} \right| (1. \tag{14}$$

where GS is the value of geometric symmetry; $S_j(i)$ is the frequency that the value *i* (for *i* from 0 to 6560) occurs in the N_{TU} spectrum under an order *j* (for *j* from 1 to 8). Each value of *j* represents a calculation order of the N_{TU} spectrum. High GS values indicate that when rotating the image 180°, the spectrum will remain similar. Possible values are between zero and one hundred.

Direction Degree (DD) is another feature and is shown in Equation (15).

Figure 9. N_{TU} codes calculations.

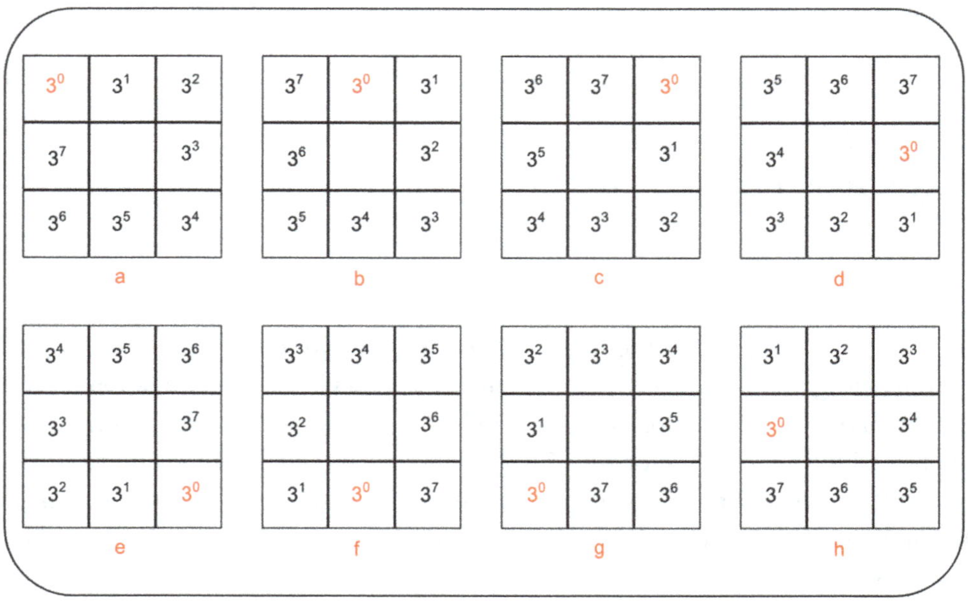

Figure 10. Window orientation for calculating micro texture measurements

a	b	b
h		d
g	f	e

$$DD = \left| 1 - \frac{1}{6} \sum_{m=1}^{3} \sum_{n=m+1}^{4} \frac{\sum_{i=0}^{6560} \left| S_m(i) - S_n(i) \right|}{2 * \sum_{i=0}^{6560} S_m(i)} \right| * 100(1. \tag{15}$$

where *DD* is the Degree of Direction; $S_m(i)$ and $S_n(i)$ represent the order of creation of the texture spectra. This measurement is also normalized between zero and one hundred and quantifies how linear the image structures are.

The previous three measurements quantify the geometric appearance of the texture and therefore measure the macro texture of the original image and are invariant to rotation. To measure the micro texture, four more rotation-sensitive measurements were defined. Figure 10 provides guidance for calculating measurements.

Micro Horizontal Structure (MHS):

$$MHS = \sum_{i=0}^{6560} S(i) * P(a,b,c) * P(f,g,h)(1. \tag{16}$$

Micro Vertical Structure (MVS):

$$MVS = \sum_{i=0}^{6560} S(i) * P(a,d,f) * P(c,h,e)(1. \tag{17}$$

First Micro Diagonal Structure (MDS1):

$$MDS1 = \sum_{i=0}^{6560} S(i) * P(d,a,b) * P(g,h,e)(1. \tag{18}$$

Second Micro Diagonal Structure (MDS2):

$$MHS = \sum_{i=0}^{6560} S(i) * P(b,c,e) * P(d,f,g)(1. \tag{19}$$

where $S(i)$ is the frequency of the texture unit at position i; $P(k,l,m)$ represents the amount of elements with the same value at positions e^k, e^l and e^m of the window represented in Figure 10.

One last measure, regardless of the form of ordering is called Central Symmetry (CS), defined below.

$$CS = \sum_{i=0}^{6560} S(i) * [K(i)]^2 (2 \tag{20}$$

where CS represents the Central Symmetry; $S(i)$ is the frequency of TU at position i; and $K(i)$ is the number of pairs having the same value, considering (e^a, e^h), (e^b, e^g), (e^c, e^f) and (e^e, e^d).

Local Binary Pattern and Local Ternary Pattern

Ojala et al. (1996) proposed a variation of the NTU, in which each spectrum value could only contain two possible values, the Local Binary Pattern (LBP).

TAN et al. (2007), extended the LBP approach by inserting a ternary code into the texture spectrum, similar to the initial proposal of the N_{TU}, but with some modifications: Ei values may vary between -1, 0 and 1; the calculation has received a constant k that is the degree of relaxation that influences mainly when the result is 0, for example, if $k = 5$ and $g^0 = 40$, g^i values less than 35 will receive the code $\neq$ 1, g^i values between 40, inclusive and 45, exclusive, will receive code 0, and g^i with values equal to or greater than 45 will receive code 1. In addition, neighbors of g^0 could have distances greater than 1, that is, neighborhood greater than 8.

CHOOSING THE PROPERTIES THAT BEST REPRESENT EACH EXAM

After the feature computation step, the feature dataset and the supervised learning algorithm are used for the classification of breast abnormality. This step is responsible for providing classification models that can operate on these data in the pattern identification process. As a result, it can potentially predict specific scenarios, such as breast cancer abnormality.

Several papers in the literature discuss the performance of different approaches and algorithms of machine learning to improve the classification process. However, sometimes the performance of these algorithms can be improved, finding the features of breast cancer DITEs that are most important to the classification process. In this sense, this chapter will discuss approaches to feature selection.

Common sense tends to believe that the existence of a large number of characteristics results in higher discriminating power. In many supervised learning tasks, the input variables represent a large attribute vector. However, in practice, adding irrelevant attributes to the dataset confuses the machine learning system (Witten, Frank, Hall, & Pal, 2016). Few of them are needed or relevant to classify instances.

This problem is commonly called the dimensionality curse (Bellman, 1961). Also, multiple algorithms become impractical with increasing dimensionality. On the other hand, if the selected attribute set is very relevant, even the simplest classifier can achieve high performance (Guyon, Gunn, Nikravesh, & Zadeh, 2008). Thus, the performance can be improved using a small subset of attributes from the entire base (Chica-Olmo & Abarca-Hernandez, 2000).

Another reason for feature selection is the decreased processing cost. Additionally, by reducing the number of features, the classification process can improve results (Kuncheva, 2014). In feature extraction, redundant attributes are often extracted, with no influence on learning or even contradictory (Witten et al., 2016).

In this sense, feature selection algorithms are designed to learn what are the most appropriate attributes to use for making decisions. These algorithms aim to obtain the smallest possible set of attributes capable of resulting in a relevant prediction. One of the possible solutions to act in this scenario concerns the application of genetic algorithms in the process of choosing the attributes.

A genetic algorithm is an evolutionary (or bioinspired) algorithm that generates search or optimization solutions using techniques inspired by the natural evolution of species. These algorithms tend to initially use random representations of a population in the exploration for a set that best represents it. The evolution of this initial population then characterizes the search for better solutions through several generations. In each generation, the individuals are evaluated in order to know which ones best represent the population. Some of these individuals are selected for the next generation. Others are recombined or mutated to form a new group of individuals. This process forms a new generation, which in turn will also have its individuals evaluated and recombined or mutated to form new generations.

A genetic algorithm is usually composed of the following steps: a) Generate Population; b)Evaluate; c) Selection; d) Crossover; e) Mutation; and e) Stopping Criteria. The general flow is illustrated in Figure 11.

The first stage is responsible for establishing, based on some criterion, the generation of the initial population. The Evaluate step is used to analyze the performance of the population. The Selection step is where a strategy for selecting the individuals that best individuals, is performed. In the Reproduction stage, individuals are combined, based on some predetermined approach, creating new individuals. The

Figure 11. Genetic Algorithm Operating Flow

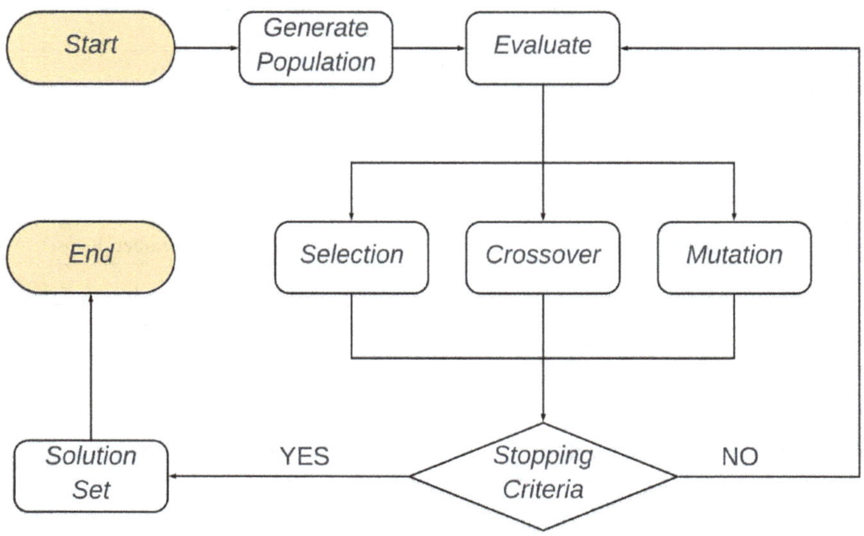

Mutation refers to the generation of new individuals from changes in their design. Moreover, finally, Stopping Criteria is responsible for defining when the algorithm should stop generating new generations. The individuals that best represent the last population compose the Solution Set.

EXPERIMENT FOR CHOOSING THE BEST DITE FEATURES FROM DIFFERENT DATASETS

This experiment intends to show that the GA with a correct performance measure can act as a judge for choosing the best DITE features from different datasets, whether unbalanced or not. For this, Resmini (2016) performs this experiment using two different DITEs datasets, one being balanced and one not. For each dataset, a feature set is computed. The following sections detail this study.

Datasets Distribution

In this experiment, were used DITEs from two different datasets: Proeng and DMR, respectively Datasets 1 and 2, each one composing examinations made by different protocols . The first, used DITES cases that represent three different diagnostic possibilities: normal, benign tumor, and cancer. For the second dataset, the diagnostic classes represent normal and cancer. Tables 3 and Table 4 show the diagnostic distribution of the DITEs.

The "normal" and "benign" classes, from Dataset 1, have a higher number of instances compared to the number of DITEs representing the amount of cases with "cancer". Therefore, the bases are unbalanced. To deal with this problem, were used performance evaluation measures of classification algorithms that do not favor the majority class. Measures such as Area Under the Curve ROC (AUC), F1,

Table 3. Diagnostic distribution of Dataset 1

Diagnosis	Number of cases
Normal	60
Benign Tumor	66
Cancer	38

Table 4. Diagnostic distribution of Dataset 2

Diagnosis	Number of cases
Normal	40
Cancer	40

Sensitivity and Specificity are indicated to deal with this problem, as they can discern between the two classes analyzed (Resmini, 2016).

Features Computed

In the literature can be found several references of works that make use of the descriptors of Haralick et al. (1973), or derivations based on these descriptors. However, Baraldi and Parmiggiani (1995) points out that the properties expressed by six descriptors is the most relevant than others: Second Angular Moment, Entropy, Contrast, Variance, Correlation, and Homogeneity

In this sense, to perform this experiment, were computed these six features from segmented DITEs for each patient's breast. This process also included the four angles for the calculation, that is, the angles 0°, 45°, 90°, and 135°. For all calculations, the distance value used was 1. Consequently, in this process, a group of 48 features (6 descriptors * 4 calculation angles * 2 breasts) was composed for each DITE dataset.

Classification Process

This work uses a supervised method of machine learning to acquire rules for classification from each dataset. Support Vector Machines (SVM) with an implementation based on the LibSVM version were used. It is essential to mention that the main objective of this experiment is not to find the best classification model, but rather to evaluate GA performance in the selection process of DITEs feature. For this reason, the best classifier settings are not discussed at this time.

Preconfigured classifiers based on tests using the SVM classifier were used for validation of the Acquired Knowledge using used two techniques: a) a holdout technique with 70% of the dataset in training step end 30% of the dataset in test, and b) a stratified cross-validation technique with 4-folds.

Genetic Algorithm Configuration

In this algorithm, each individual was composed of a sequence of features that were extracted from the breast DITEs. To compose the initial population, 140 individuals were randomly generated. To evaluate each individual in the population, 10 preconfigured classifiers. For each classifier, was computed performance considering the AUC for it.

The Selection, Crossing, and Mutation steps are responsible for composing the new generation of individuals. Therefore, each new generation was created following elitist, reproductive, or mutant criteria, as follows:

a) The selection of the 20 individuals that best represent the current generation. These individuals are chosen to remain in the population because, as they are the best performers, they tend to continue contributing or even generating better results by mixing with other individuals.
b) The Crossings that generate new 40 individuals, where:
    - Twenty are generated from an elitist strategy with crosses among the top 20 individuals. Each crossing generates two new individuals.
    - Twenty are generated from a strategy where the top 10 individuals are crossed with the 10 worst. Although it seems contradictory, the use of the worst individuals can help to avoid the occurrence of local minimums.
    - Seventy-four are generated from random crossings among the entire population.
c) The Mutations, responsible for generating 6 new individuals. These mutations alter some of the features that form the individual.

The Stopping Criteria is used by Resmini concerns the number of generations the genetic algorithm will make, which in his study were 100 generations. After operating for 100 different generations, composed of individuals formed by different approaches, the set of individuals that best defines the last generation is chosen. These individuals represent the best performing features in the Evaluate process.

This study also includes disturbance events in the generations. This disturbance, from a conceptual point of view, can be assimilated as some catastrophic event, responsible for eliminating most of the population. In the context of that work, if performance remained constant for five consecutive generations, the disturbance selected the individual who best represents such generation, and the rest are eliminated. The next generation, therefore, has 139 randomly generated new individuals.

Results for DITEs Captured Under two Different Capture Protocols

The use of a genetic algorithm in the feature selection process brought a significant performance increase regarding the assertiveness of the classifiers. The analyses were performed in different groups of DITEs, based on the diagnosis of patients: a) Normal vs. Cancer; b) Normal vs. Benign; and c) Benign vs. Cancer. Each one of these groups has segmented DITEs following different approaches: a) with the presence of the armpit region; and b) without the presence of the armpit region. In all these groups, there was a significant increase in classification performance after the use of the genetic algorithm in the feature selection process. Table 5 illustrates these results.

The results show a substantial improvement in classification after using GA in the feature selection process. In all diagnostic combinations, these results were superior compared to not using this technique. Through Table 5, it is possible to observe that, even being unbalanced concerning the number of cases representing the "Cancer" class, the quality of the classification increased significantly. From the results, it is also possible to observe that the different types of DITE capture protocols can potentially influence the analysis process. In this study, even using the same set of classifiers and selection techniques, the results tend to differ among themselves.

Table 5. Results before and after application of feature selection technique

Dataset	Armpit	Diagnosis	Feature Selection	
			Before (%)	After (%) *(Genetic Algorithm)*
1	With	*Normal* x *Benigno*	75.79	**87.30**
		Normal x *Cancer*	80.20	**91.14**
		Benigno x *Cancer*	74.01	**81.86**
	Without	*Normal* x *Benigno*	70.63	**86.90**
		Normal x *Cancer*	80.72	**92.70**
		Benigno x *Cancer*	74.19	**91.17**
2	With	*Normal* x *Cancer*	80.12	**94.87**
	Without	*Normal* x *Cancer*	83.97	**94.87**

These results meet the purpose of this experiment, confirming GA as an interesting approach to the feature selection process. Besides, the results also allow us to point out that this approach can be applied even to datasets with irregularities in the number of instances in each class, i.e., unbalanced or not.

EXPERIMENTS FOR FOLLOW-UP

This experiment is a preliminary study and intents to analyze some descriptors already used in other works (Moran et al., 2018, 2019) to evaluate which of them could be used the identification of Breast Cancer evolution. More specifically, the feasibility of the use of descriptors based on thermograms in the process of evaluating preoperative treatment response.

Patients Group

To perform this study was selected a set of four patients who already have DITEs captured in two visits, i.e., in V1 (pre-treatment) and V2 (post-treatment). The first capture of the dynamic protocol of each visit, used in these preliminary analyses of this study.

In this study, each breast was considered an ROI (Motta, 2010). Therefore, from each capture, there are two ROIs, one referring to the left breast and another to the right breast. In this sample, only one breast presents cancer for each patient, therefore there are 2e ROIs one for each breast. Table 6 summarizes the cancerous breast for each patient. It is necessary to mention that the exact position of the tumor is unknown, the indications presented in Table 6 is approximate area in the breast.

Features Computed

In order to verify if the temperatures in the thyroid region are influenced by the presence of malignant or benign nodules, the following statistical descriptors were calculated for each ROI: minimum, maximum, average temperatures, TI and AP. Previous studies, considering other parts of the body, show that the values of these descriptors differ for healthy regions and regions that present some anomalies. In this study will be investigated if theses descriptors could provide some indication of evolution of breast cancer caused by treatment.

Table 6. Patients details

<table>
<tr><th>Patient</th><th>Breast with cancer</th><th>Tumor Region</th></tr>
<tr><td>P1</td><td>Left</td><td>Center</td></tr>
<tr><td>P2</td><td rowspan="3">Right</td><td rowspan="3">Upper Inner</td></tr>
<tr><td>P3</td></tr>
<tr><td>P4</td></tr>
</table>

Besides, a gray level re quantization of the ROI, called posterization by some authors (Conci, Azevedo & Leta, 2009) is applied to each ROIp in order to visually assess temperature groups. If there is a visual pattern of tones that correspond to nodular regions, then there could be a temperature pattern that would indicate the presence of abnormality. Thus, quantifications were generated in the ROIs patients using 8 gray levels. Thus, the temperatures would be visually grouped in 8 groups. This technique is also based on the qualitative analysis that the physicians do in the visual exams of the thermal images

Statistical Tests

Although the patient's sample number of this preliminary study has small proportions, the Pearson Correlation test is used to investigate the relationship between the features in question. This test evaluates the linear relationship in data. By linear relationship, it is understood that the change in the value of one variable may change the value of another proportionally.

In this sense, the Null Hypothesis (H0) is used when there is no difference between the groups analyzed. The Alternative Hypothesis (HA) is used when there is a significant difference between the data of each group. In this study, a confidence level of 95% was used, with a significance level $\alpha = 0.05$. So, only p-values $<\alpha$ prove HA.

Results

To verify the hypothesis that descriptors based on thermograms could provide some information regarding the preoperative treatment response, they were computed and tested by the statistical tests previously mentioned. These descriptors were calculated from the DITEs performed at both patient visits to the hospital (V1 and V2), representing the pre and post-treatment moments, respectively. Figure 12 illustrates the values of these descriptors for each patient's diseased breast in V1 and V2.

Figure 12. Descriptors values for Maximum, Minimum, and Average temperature

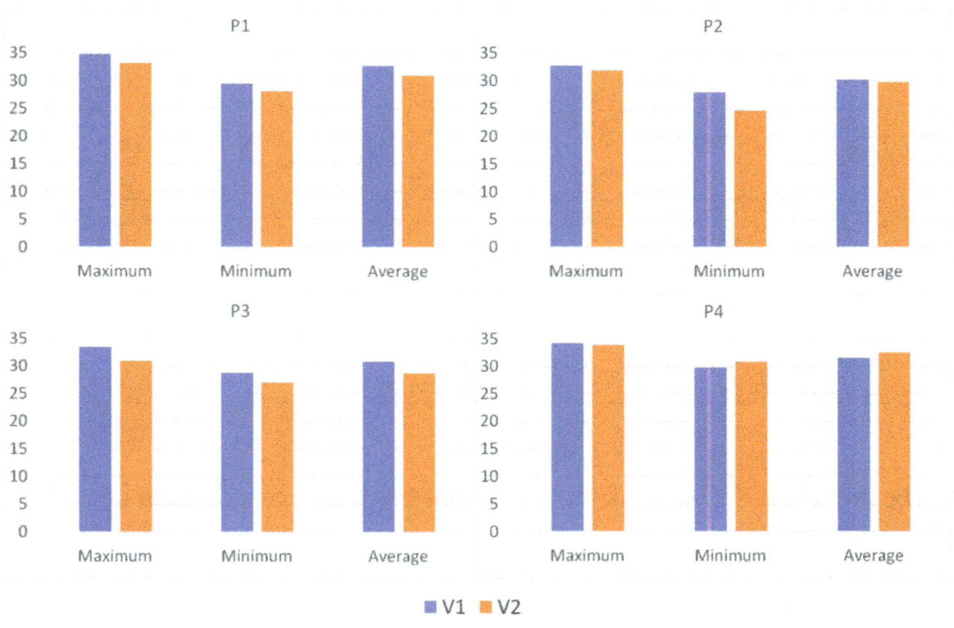

It is possible to notice that the values for patients P1, P2, and P3 present a decreasing relation between V1 and V2. In these patients, both descriptors, maximum, minimum, and average temperatures, decreases from V1 to V2. In contrast, the values for P4 do not indicate a notable change in the thermal pattern between pre and post-treatment visits.

At each patient visit, the approximate tumor size was also collected. Table 7 presents these results. It can be observed that, as pointed out by the DITEs of patients P1, P2, and P3, tumor volume decreased after neoadjuvant treatment. Regarding patient P4, it is also possible to observe that, although the thermography does not show a considerable variation in the thermal pattern, tumor volume was decreased by about 27%.

One of the possible clinical explanations for contradictory tumor warming with tumor reduction could be given by Chung et al. (2011). According to them, the increase in temperature and oxygen saturation in early phases of neoadjuvant treatment can potentially cause mitochondrial thermogenesis, thus interfering with the organ's thermal pattern. Although patient P4 has reached the end of treatment, tumor size, computed on V1, probably could have influenced this change in thermal pattern.

For the analysis of these values, the Pearson test was used with a confidence level of 95% in order to verify if the values obtained from the sick breast are significantly different from the healthy breast.

Table 7. Approximate tumor size for each patient

Patient	*Approximate Tumor Size (mm)*		*Approximate Reduction (%)*
	V1	*V2*	
P1	60	20	66.6
P2	60	30	50
P3	60	20	66.6
P4	110	80	29.27

Table 8 shows that the maximum and average descriptors have a p-value below 0.05, indicating a significant difference.

Another test was performed, considering the TI. This descriptor also was calculated for DITEs from V1 and V2 for each patient included in this study. The same observed patterns of the descriptors maximum, minimum, and average temperatures were observed through the TI. Patients P1, P2, and P3 had a reduction in the thermal index of the diseased breast after the end of treatment. Alternatively to these patients, the P4 temperature rise also resulted in a higher value TI at V2 than at V1. Figure 13 illustrates these values.

Table 8. P-values from Maximum, Minimum, and Average temperature descriptors

Descriptor	*P-value*
Maximum	0.034
Minimum	0.265
Average	0.023

Pearson's statistical test also showed that there is a significant difference between the TI values calculated from the sick breast and the healthy breast of the patients in this study. The p-value obtained was 0.041. Statistical analyses between the differences between V1 and V2 could be performed as the sample size increases.

The results obtained by grouping the temperature by posterization also show differences between visits V1 and V2. For patients P1, P2, and P3, the tumor region in V2 has a lower concentration of hot spots, suggesting a decrease in tumor size. On the other hand, as expected, the thermal behavior of the patient in V2 does not allow to recognize the tumor reduction. Figure 14 illustrates the posterization made from the DITEs of each patient in V1 and V2.

Figure 13. Descriptors values for TI

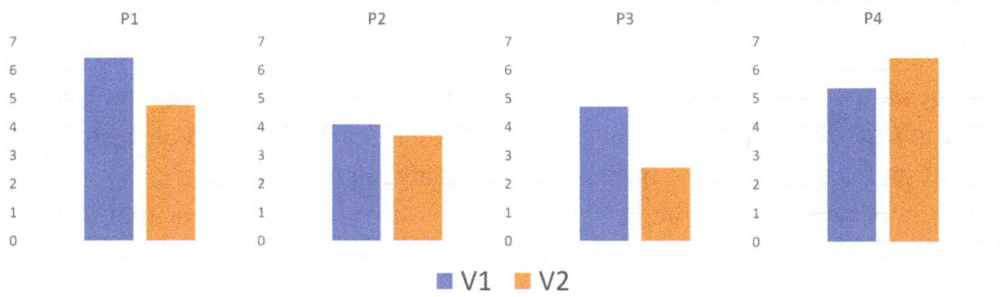

Figure 14. Posterization results from 8 gray-levels.

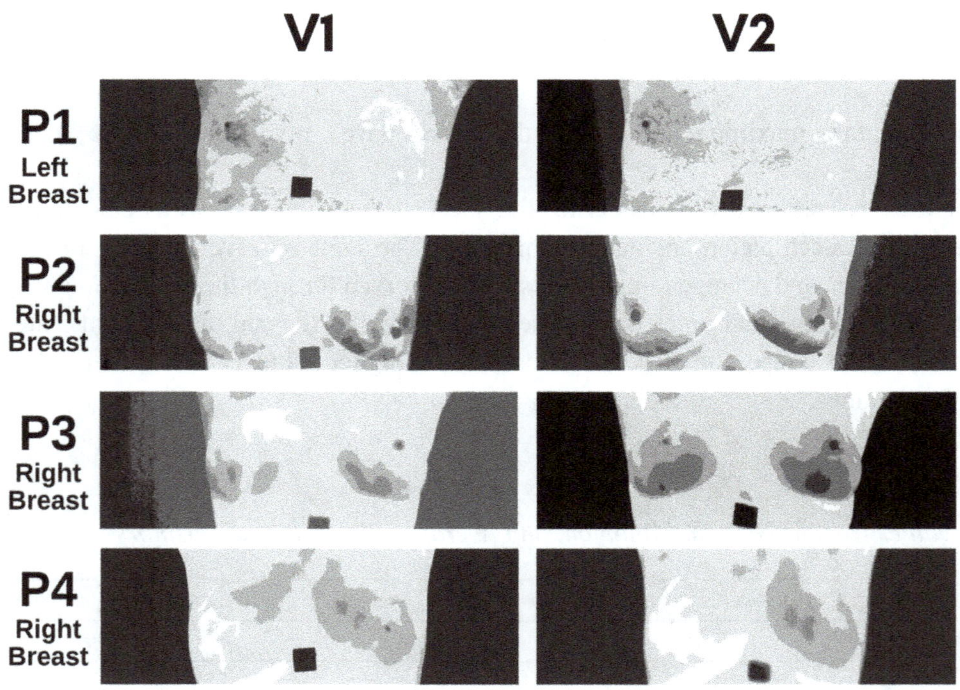

Finally, the asymmetry between the thermograms obtained from the exams V1 and V2 was calculated. Except for patient P4, a minor asymmetry in the tumor region (see Table 8) can also be observed in V2. Figure 15 shows the asymmetry calculation view. For this visualization, the 1.5° C threshold was considered. Note that although P2 - V2 appears to have more asymmetry when compared to the entire breast region, the Right Breast-Upper Inner area has a lower asymmetric index.

The analyses performed in this experiment represent the initial steps in investigating the response to neoadjuvant breast cancer treatment from DITEs. This experiment made it possible, although preliminarily, to understand the thermal behavior of the breast after treatment. The behavior of the maximum, average, and TI descriptors suggests that this thermal change is related to the treatment response. Besides, the posterization of regions and calculation of asymmetry contributed to observe these changes visually.

Figure 15. Visualization of asymmetry parameter

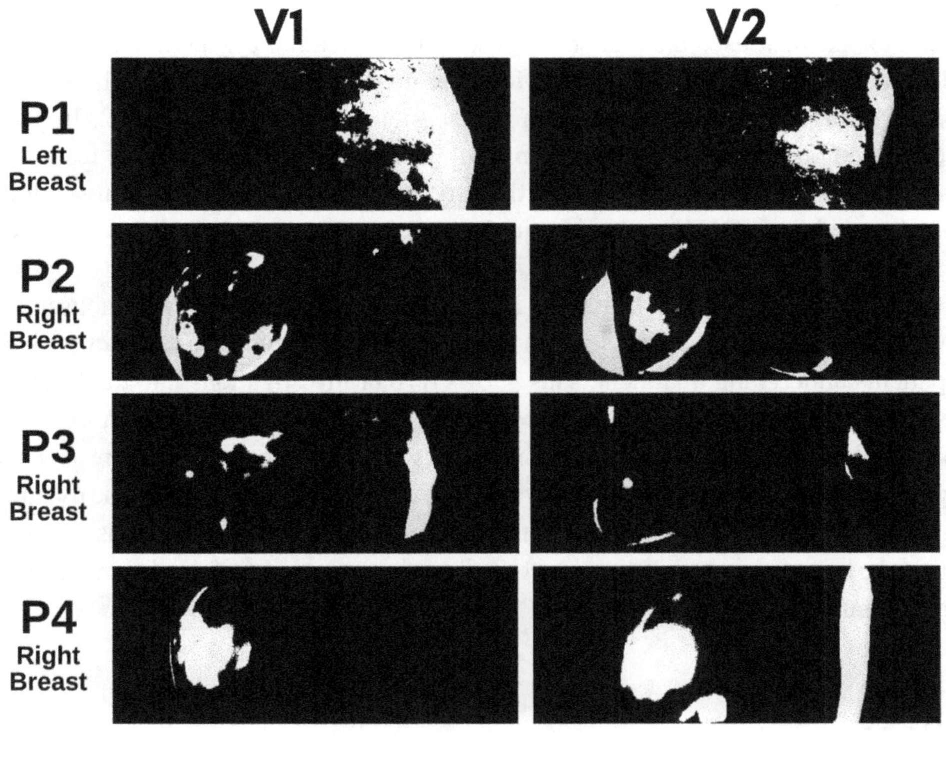

CONCLUSION

This book chapter has discussed the essential steps in the process of analyzing thermal breast images. Several computational techniques were presented to support the execution of these analyzes, both to detect breast abnormality and to follow the evolution of the tumor after neoadjuvant treatment.

The process of acquisition of DITEs was discussed, punctuating studies on the problem and discussing some differences in protocols commonly used in the literature. Still, in this context, a repository of mastology images, especially thermal examinations, was discussed and presented, discussing its importance in the conception of new approaches to the preprocessing process of these exams. In this sense, collective intelligence techniques could provide an alternative to the thermal image segmentation process through community collectivity. Besides, other approaches used in this segmentation process were also discussed, including automatic solutions.

A large and relevant set of descriptors for feature computation of DITEs has been discussed in this chapter, classified as statistical and geometric. All of them are used in studies involving the analysis of medical images. The computation of these descriptors is a vital step in the computational evaluation process of the exams since they allow to represent several exam properties numerically. All of these properties expressed as features are fundamentally important for classification activities involving machine learning algorithms.

Two sets of these features were used in experiments performed and discussed in this chapter. The first of these experiments investigated the use of a GA in feature selection activities. This experiment used DITEs available in two different repositories, which, in turn, have different acquisition protocols. The results confirm the study hypothesis, showing that GA can act as a judge for choosing the best DITE features from different datasets, under different protocols.

The second experiment used another set of descriptors in feature computation. In this experiment, descriptors were used to evaluate breast behavior after neoadjuvant treatment preliminarily. Analyzes were performed using a set of 4 patients with two sessions of DITE: V1 and V2. In addition, these analyses were based on tumor mass volume (in mm), as measured by the medical team at each of the different patient visits. The results suggest that the variations resulting from neoadjuvant forms of treatment can be observed from DITEs, allowing, in the next steps, to perform analyzes that seek to relate these indicators with tumor volume.

All this research has potential in health, as it can directly impact the lives of thousands of patients diagnosed with breast cancer. The next steps in these studies are intended to conduct studies in a larger volume of patients undergoing treatment. This allows further investigations into the thermal pattern of pre and post-treatment patients to be performed. Also, this will enable the exploration of more robust descriptors in the thermal breast imaging analysis process to monitor treatment progress. Another important activity will be the use of time series through the use of DITEs captured under the dynamic protocol. All these investigations aim to provide computational methodologies capable of assisting doctors and patients during the breast cancer treatment process, obtaining an opinion of the thermal situation capable of assisting the analysis process.

REFERENCES

Adams, R., & Bischof, L. (1994). Seeded region growing. *IEEE Transactions on Pattern Analysis and Machine Intelligence*, *16*(6), 641–647. doi:10.1109/34.295913

Araújo, A. S., Conci, A., Moran, M. B., & Resmini, R. (2018, July). Comparing the Use of Sum and Difference Histograms and Gray Levels Occurrence Matrix for Texture Descriptors. In *2018 International Joint Conference on Neural Networks (IJCNN)* (pp. 1-8). 10.1109/IJCNN.2018.8489705

Baraldi, A., & Parmiggiani, F. (1995). An Investigation of the Textural Characteristics Associated with Gray Level Cooccurrence Matrix Statistical Parameters. *IEEE Transactions on Geoscience and Remote Sensing*, *33*(2), 293–304. doi:10.1109/TGRS.1995.8746010

Bellman, R. (1961). *Adaptive control processes: A guided tour*. Princeton University Press. doi:10.1515/9781400874668

Borchartt, T. B. (2013). *Análise de imagens termográficas para a classificação de alterações na mama* (M Sc. Dissertation). Computer Institute, Universidade Federal Fluminense, Niterói, RJ, Brazil.

Brioschi, M., Teixeira, M. J., Silva, F., & Colman, D. (2010). *Medical thermography textbook: principles and applications*. Andreoli.

Chica-Olmo, M., & Abarca-Hernandez, F. (2000). Computing geostatistical image texture for remotely sensed data classification. *Computers & Geosciences*, *26*(4), 373–383. doi:10.1016/S0098-3004(99)00118-1

Chung, S. H., Mehta, R., Tromberg, B. J., & Yodh, A. G. (2011). Non-invasive measurement of deep tissue temperature changes caused by apoptosis during breast cancer neoadjuvant chemotherapy: A case study. *Journal of Innovative Optical Health Sciences*, *4*(04), 361–372. doi:10.1142/S1793545811001708 PMID:22408653

Coleman, G. B., & Andrews, H. C. (1979). Image segmentation by clustering. *Proceedings of the IEEE*, *67*(5), 773–785. doi:10.1109/PROC.1979.11327

Collins, A. J., Ring, E. F., Cosh, J. A., & Bacon, P. A. (1974). Quantitation of thermography in arthritis using multi-isothermal analysis. I. The thermographic index. *Annals of the Rheumatic Diseases*, *33*(2), 113–115. doi:10.1136/ard.33.2.113 PMID:4821383

Conci, A., Azevedo, E., & Leta, F. R. (2008). *Computação Gráfica (in portuguese)*. Campus/Elsevier.

Cortazar, P., Zhang, L., Untch, M., Mehta, K., Costantino, J. P., Wolmark, N., Bonnefoi, H., Cameron, D., Gianni, L., Valagussa, P., Swain, S. M., Prowell, T., Loibl, S., Wickerham, D. L., Bogaerts, J., Baselga, J., Perou, C., Blumenthal, G., Blohmer, J., ... von Minckwitz, G. (2014). Pathological complete response and long-term clinical benefit in breast cancer: The CTNeoBC pooled analysis. *Lancet*, *384*(9938), 164–172. doi:10.1016/S0140-6736(13)62422-8 PMID:24529560

Dean, J. C., & Ilvento, C. C. (2006). Improved cancer detection using computer-aided detection with diagnostic and screening mammography: Prospective study of 104 cancers. *AJR. American Journal of Roentgenology*, *187*(1), 20–28. doi:10.2214/AJR.05.0111 PMID:16794150

DMR, Database For Mastology Research. (2020). Retrieved from http://visual.ic.uff.br/dmi/

Ebert, D. S., & Musgrave, F. K. (2003). *Texturing & modeling: a procedural approach*. Morgan Kaufmann.

Etehadtavakol, M., & Ng, E. Y. (2017). Potential of thermography in pain diagnosing and treatment monitoring. In *Application of infrared to biomedical sciences* (pp. 19–32). Springer. doi:10.1007/978-981-10-3147-2_2

Folkman, J. (1971). Tumor angiogenesis: Therapeutic implications. *The New England Journal of Medicine, 285*(21), 1182–1186. doi:10.1056/NEJM197111182852108 PMID:4938153

Galvão, S. D. S. L. (2015). *Registro de imagens térmicas da mama adquiridas dinamicamente. Doctoral dissertation* (PhD thesis). Computer Institute, Universidade Federal Fluminense, Niterói, RJ, Brazil.

Gan, G., Ma, C., & Wu, J. (2007). Data clustering: Theory, algorithms, and applications. *International Statistical Review, 76*(1), 141–141.

Gautherie, M. (1983). Thermobiological assessment of benign and malignant breast diseases. *American Journal of Obstetrics and Gynecology, 147*(8), 861–869. doi:10.1016/0002-9378(83)90236-3 PMID:6650622

Gonzalez, R. C., & Woods, R. E. (2002). *Digital image processing*. Pearson.

Guyon, I., Gunn, S., Nikravesh, M., & Zadeh, L. A. (2008). *Feature extraction: foundations and applications*. Springer.

Haralick, R. M. (1979). Statistical and structural approaches to texture. *Proceedings of the IEEE, 67*(5), 786–804. doi:10.1109/PROC.1979.11328

Haralick, R. M., Shanmugam, K., & Distein, I. H. (1973). Textural features for image classification. *IEEE Transactions on Systems, Man, and Cybernetics, SMC-3*(6), 610–621. doi:10.1109/TSMC.1973.4309314

Haralick, R. M., Sternberg, S. R., & Zhuang, X. (1987). Image analysis using mathematical morphology. *IEEE Transactions on Pattern Analysis and Machine Intelligence, PAMI-9*(4), 532–550. doi:10.1109/TPAMI.1987.4767941 PMID:21869411

He, D. C., & Wang, L. (1990). Texture unit, texture spectrum, and texture analysis. *IEEE Transactions on Geoscience and Remote Sensing, 28*(4), 509–512. doi:10.1109/TGRS.1990.572934

Keyserlingk, J. R., Ahlgren, P. D., Yu, E., & Belliveau, N. (1998). Infrared Imaging of the Breast: Initial Reappraisal Using High-Resolution Digital Technology in 100 Successive Cases of Stage I and II Breast Cancer. *The Breast Journal, 4*(4), 245–251. doi:10.1046/j.1524-4741.1998.440245.x PMID:21223443

Kong, X., Moran, M. S., Zhang, N., Haffty, B., & Yang, Q. (2011). Meta-analysis confirms achieving pathological complete response after neoadjuvant chemotherapy predicts favourable prognosis for breast cancer patients. *European Journal of Cancer, 47*(14), 2084–2090. doi:10.1016/j.ejca.2011.06.014 PMID:21737257

Kuncheva, L. I. (2014). *Combining pattern classifiers: methods and algorithms*. John Wiley & Sons.

Mamounas, E. P. (2015). Impact of neoadjuvant chemotherapy on locoregional surgical treatment of breast cancer. *Annals of Surgical Oncology, 22*(5), 1425–1433. doi:10.124510434-015-4406-6 PMID:25727558

Marques, R. S. (2012). *Segmentação automática das mamas em imagens térmicas* (M Sc. Dissertation). Computer Institute, Universidade Federal Fluminense, Niterói, RJ, Brazil.

Materka, A., & Strzelecki, M. (1998). Texture analysis methods–a review. Technical university of lodz, institute of electronics, COST B11 report.

Moran, M. B., Apostolo, G. H., Araujo, A., Andrade, E., Viterbo, J. V., & Conci, A. (2019). A novel approach for the segmentation of breast thermal images combining image processing and collective intelligence. In *IEEE 19th International Conference on Bioinformatics and Bioengineering (BIBE)*. 10.1109/BIBE.2019.00099

Moran, M. B., Conci, A., & Araujo, A. S. (2019). Evaluation of quantitative features and convolutional neural networks for nodule identification in thyroid thermographies. In *IEEE 19th International Conference on Bioinformatics and Bioengineering (BIBE)*. 10.1109/BIBE.2019.00140

Moran, M. B., Conci, A., Gonzalez, J. R., Araujo, A. S., Fiirst, W., Damiao, C., Lima, G., & Filho, R. (2018). Identification of thyroid nodules in infrared images by convolutional neural networks. In *31st International Joint Conference on Neural Networks (IJCNN)*. 10.1109/IJCNN.2018.8489032

Moran, M. B., Conci, A., González, J. R., Araújo, A. S., Fiirst, W. G., Damião, C. P., Lima, G., & da Cruz Filho, R. A. (2018). Identification of thyroid nodules in infrared images by convolutional neural networks. In *2018 International Joint Conference on Neural Networks (IJCNN)* (pp. 1-7). 10.1109/IJCNN.2018.8489032

Motta, L. S. (2010). *Obtenção automática da região de interesse em termogramas frontais da mama para o auxílio à detecção precoce de doenças* (M Sc. Dissertation). Computer Institute. UFF, Niteroi, Brazil.

Ng, E. K. (2009). A review of thermography as promising non-invasive detection modality for breast tumor. *International Journal of Thermal Sciences*, *48*(5), 849–859. doi:10.1016/j.ijthermalsci.2008.06.015

Ojala, T., Pietikäinen, M., & Harwood, D. (1996). A comparative study of texture measures with classification based on featured distributions. *Pattern Recognition*, *29*(1), 51–59. doi:10.1016/0031-3203(95)00067-4

Parker, J. R. (1997). *Algorithms for image processing and computer vision*. John Wiley & Sons.

Pedrini, H., & Schwartz, W. R. (2008). *Análise de imagens digitais: princípios, algoritmos e aplicações*. Thomson Learning.

Polidori, G., Renard, Y., Lorimier, S., Pron, H., Derruau, S., & Taiar, R. (2017). Medical Infrared Thermography assistance in the surgical treatment of axillary Hidradenitis Suppurativa: A case report. *International Journal of Surgery Case Reports*, *34*, 56–59. doi:10.1016/j.ijscr.2017.03.015 PMID:28359047

Resmini, R. (2011). *Análise de imagens térmicas da mama usando descritores de textura* (M Sc. Dissertation). Computer Institute, Universidade Federal Fluminense, Niterói, RJ, Brazil.

Resmini, R. (2016). *Classificação De Doenças Da Mama Usando Imagens Por Infravermelho* (Doctoral dissertation). Instituto de Computação, Universidade Federal Fluminense, Brazil.

Resmini, R., Araujo, A., Conci, A., Silva, L., & Moran, M. (2018). Number of Texture Unit as Feature to Breast's Disease Classification from Thermal Images. In *2018 IEEE/ACS 15th International Conference on Computer Systems and Applications (AICCSA)* (pp. 1-6). IEEE. 10.1109/AICCSA.2018.8612826

Schaefer, G., Závišek, M., & Nakashima, T. (2009). Thermography based breast cancer analysis using statistical features and fuzzy classification. *Pattern Recognition*, *42*(6), 1133–1137. doi:10.1016/j.patcog.2008.08.007

Sheikhbahaei, S., Trahan, T. J., Xiao, J., Taghipour, M., Mena, E., Connolly, R. M., & Subramaniam, R. M. (2016). FDG-PET/CT and MRI for evaluation of pathologic response to neoadjuvant chemotherapy in patients with breast cancer: A meta-analysis of diagnostic accuracy studies. *The Oncologist*, *21*(8), 931–939. doi:10.1634/theoncologist.2015-0353 PMID:27401897

Silva, L. F., Saade, D. C. M., Sequeiros, G. O., Silva, A. C., Paiva, A. C., Bravo, R. S., & Conci, A. (2014). A new database for breast research with infrared image. *Journal of Medical Imaging and Health Informatics*, *4*(1), 92–100. doi:10.1166/jmihi.2014.1226

Soomro, M. H. (2017). Haralick's texture analysis applied to colorectal T2-weighted MRI: A preliminary study of significance for cancer evolution. In *2017 13th IASTED International Conference on Biomedical Engineering (BioMed)* (pp. 16-19). IEEE. 10.2316/P.2017.852-019

Staffa, E., Bernard, V., Kubicek, L., Vlachovsky, R., Vlk, D., Mornstein, V., Bourek, A., & Staffa, R. (2017). Infrared thermography as option for evaluating the treatment effect of percutaneous transluminal angioplasty by patients with peripheral arterial disease. *Vascular*, *25*(1), 42–49. doi:10.1177/1708538116640444 PMID:26993145

Tan, X., & Triggs, B. (2007). Enhanced local texture feature sets for face recognition under difficult lighting conditions. In *International workshop on analysis and modeling of faces and gestures* (pp. 168-182). Springer. 10.1007/978-3-540-75690-3_13

Unser, M. (1986). Sum and difference histograms for texture classification. *IEEE Transactions on Pattern Analysis and Machine Intelligence*, *PAMI-8*(1), 118–125. doi:10.1109/TPAMI.1986.4767760 PMID:21869331

Watt, A., & Policarpo, F. (1998). *The computer image*. Academic Press.

Wibmer, A., Hricak, H., Gondo, T., Matsumoto, K., Veeraraghavan, H., Fehr, D., Zheng, J., Goldman, D., Moskowitz, C., Fine, S. W., Reuter, V. E., Eastham, J., Sala, E., & Vargas, H. A. (2015). Haralick texture analysis of prostate MRI: Utility for differentiating non-cancerous prostate from prostate cancer and differentiating prostate cancers with different Gleason scores. *European Radiology*, *25*(10), 2840–2850. doi:10.100700330-015-3701-8 PMID:25991476

Witten, I. H., Frank, E., Hall, M. A., & Pal, C. J. (2016). *Data Mining: Practical machine learning tools and techniques*. Morgan Kaufmann.

Chapter 6
Breast Cancer Diagnosis With Mammography: Recent Advances on CBMR-Based CAD Systems

Abir Baâzaoui
https://orcid.org/0000-0001-7206-3842
SIIVA, LIMTIC Laboratory, Institut Supérieur d'Informatique El Manar, Université de Tunis El Manar, Tunisia

Walid Barhoumi
https://orcid.org/0000-0003-2123-4992
Ecole Nationale d'Ingénieurs de Carthage, Université de Carthage, Tunisia & SIIVA, LIMTIC Laboratory, Institut Supérieur d'Informatique El Manar, Université de Tunis El Manar, Tunisia

ABSTRACT

Breast cancer, which is the second-most common and leading cause of cancer death among women, has witnessed growing interest in the two last decades. Fortunately, its early detection is the most effective way to detect and diagnose breast cancer. Although mammography is the gold standard for screening, its difficult interpretation leads to an increase in missed cancers and misinterpreted non-cancerous lesion rates. Therefore, computer-aided diagnosis (CAD) systems can be a great helpful tool for assisting radiologists in mammogram interpretation. Nonetheless, these systems are limited by their black-box outputs, which decreases the radiologists' confidence. To circumvent this limit, content-based mammogram retrieval (CBMR) is used as an alternative to traditional CAD systems. Herein, authors systematically review the state-of-the-art on mammography-based breast cancer CAD methods, while focusing on recent advances in CBMR methods. In order to have a complete review, mammography imaging principles and its correlation with breast anatomy are also discussed.

DOI: 10.4018/978-1-7998-3456-4.ch006

INTRODUCTION

The tremendous amount of data became readily available in various application domains, especially in the medical field. This field contains many imaging modalities (such as magnetic resonance imaging (MRI), X-ray computed tomography (CT), digital radiography, mammography and ultrasound), multidimensional images, as well as co-registered multimodality images. These image collections are produced in ever increasing quantities and offer the opportunity for diagnosis, for treatment planning, and for assessing response to treatment (Barhoumi & Baâzaoui, 2014). For breast cancer diagnosis, mammography is the main screening tool for radiologists to visually analyze and evaluate breast density. However, visual diagnosis and mammography interpretation entail several errors in decision-making since it is subjective and thus it is dependent on the physicians' experience. In addition, the breast cancer detection rate improves by about 15% using a second reading. Faced with the increase in the number of mammograms in recent decades, various research studies make the effort either to detect automatically breast lesions through Computer Assisted Detection systems (CADe) or to interpret automatically mammograms through Computer Assisted Diagnostic Systems (CAD). CAD systems can be a great helpful tool to replace the second reader by analyzing a mammogram and making a decision about its abnormality. Besides, they can assist radiologists in their interpretation. However, the major limit of these systems is the black-box outputs, which decrease the radiologists' confidence. To tackle this problem, content-based mammogram retrieval (CBMR) systems, which display similar mammograms, relatively to a query mammogram, with their corresponding similar images, are more and more adopted as an alternative to traditional CAD systems.

All relevant studies, published in Springer Link, Elsevier, IEEE Xplore and pubmed from 2010 to middle of October 2019, were investigated herein to elucidate to the readers the terminologies, various subfields of computer-aided diagnosis based on breast cancer mammography, and the clinical potential. However, unintentionally there is some relevant studies, which can be skipped. Totally, 155 full papers studies were retrieved (abstracts, books, letters, and reports are excluded). All retrieved papers (journal or proceedings) are relevant to the inclusion search criteria, which is "breast cancer diagnosis from mammography". Figure 1 shows a flow diagram, which summarizes the breast cancer diagnosis selection of the retrieved studies. From this figure, it should be noted that the most current CADx systems aim to classify mammogram breast cancer using only a single view, and a few recent studies use breast multi-views (*e.g.* bilateral views (the same view of the two breast), ipsilateral views (two views of the same breast) and four views).

Figure 1. The chronological evolution of the published papers for mammogram breast cancer diagnosis using CADx and CBMR from 2010 to 2019

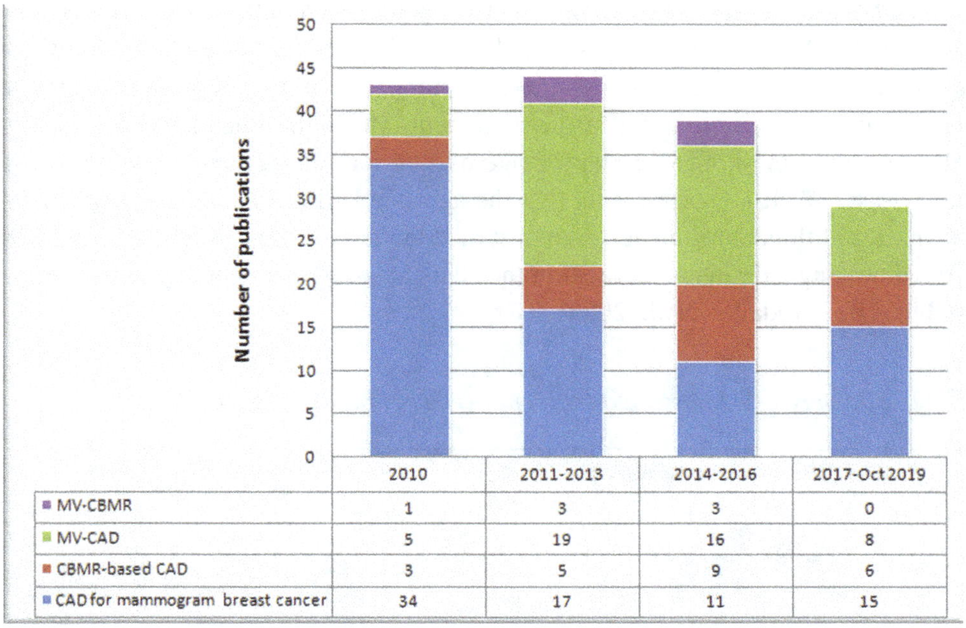

The rest of this paper is organized as follows. In Section II, authors introduce some basic concepts on breast cancer and the principles of breast imaging. They also discuss the correlation between mammography and breast anatomy. In Section III, some existing types of CAD systems are reviewed. In Section IV, they review in details the recent advances CBMR systems for breast cancer diagnosis with mammography. The scalability of CBMR systems on large-scale datasets is discussed in Section V. When concluding the paper in section VI, some issues concerning the future of CBMR-based CAD systems for breast cancer diagnosis are detailed.

BACKGROUND ON BREAST CANCER AND MAMMOGRAPHY

1. Breast Cancer Definition

Breast cancer is the commonly occurring cancer and the major concern among women. In both sexes combined, it is the second-most common and leading cause of cancer deaths after lung cancer. According to the most recent data from the World Health Organization (WHO), breast cancer accounts 11.6% of the total cancer deaths (WHO, 2019). In the same report, 2.088.849 of breast cancer new cases were recorded worldwide in 2018. Therefore, this challenging cancer has recently attracted increasing interest. In this context, several hospitals and institutions have studied the evolution of standardized breast cancer incidence and mortality to the world population (Bray et al., 2018). Incidence refers to measuring the frequency of new cancer cases occurring each year, whilst mortality indicates the number of deaths per year. In Figure 2, beginning by top left authors specially mention the Age-Standardized Incidence (ASI) in north Africa for 105 women. The general remark in this study that the second highest ASI rate is for Tunisia after Algeria (Belkacémi et al., 2010). More particularly, in Tunisia, three regional cancer registries were set up in 1998, respectively in Tunis for the northern region, in Sousse for the central region and in Sfax for the southern region. The coordination of these registries is ensured by the National Institute of Public Health, and this with the aim of describing the epidemiological situation of cancers throughout Tunisia. From these registries, the authors unanimously analyzed five age groups to identify the most attacked age group for further treatment. The highest incidence was observed among women in the age group of 40-44 years with a rate of 52% for 105 women, while the ASI for women under 40 years was 27%. It is worth noting that the age-standardized incidence ranged from 30 to 45 for 105 women. In addition, unfortunately demonstrated in the Tunisian ASI curves from 1980 to 2013, ASI rates are witnessing a dramatic increase in the statistics over years notably in the last years, when the rates doubled (Ben Abdallah et al., 2009).

Figure 2. The trends in Age-Standardized Incidence (ASI) of breast cancer

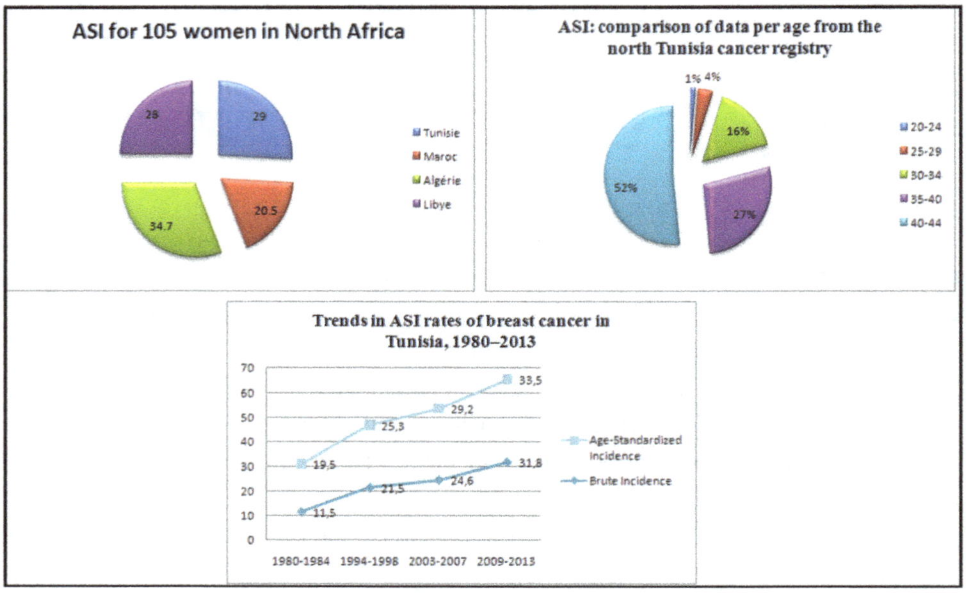

Against this backdrop and since that up to now, breast cancer cause is unknown and there is no effective way to prevent it, and thus its early detection is becoming a necessity in order to increase the survival chances of patients and to decrease its morbidity and mortality. Unlike its early diagnosis based on biopsy, which generates sorrowful consequences for the patient and is useless in many cases, there are many imaging modalities used for breast cancer diagnosis/detection.

2. Breast Cancer Imaging Modalities

For breast cancer diagnosis, medical image examination is the most effective method. Different medical imaging tools can be used for the screening as well as for the diagnosis of breast cancer, such as mammography (X-ray imaging), Ultrasound(US), Magnetic Resonance Imaging (MRI) and Molecular Breast Imaging (MBI).

Figure 3. Illustration of the different incidences (a) MLO, (b) CC and the positioning of the X-ray tube and detector in both incidences

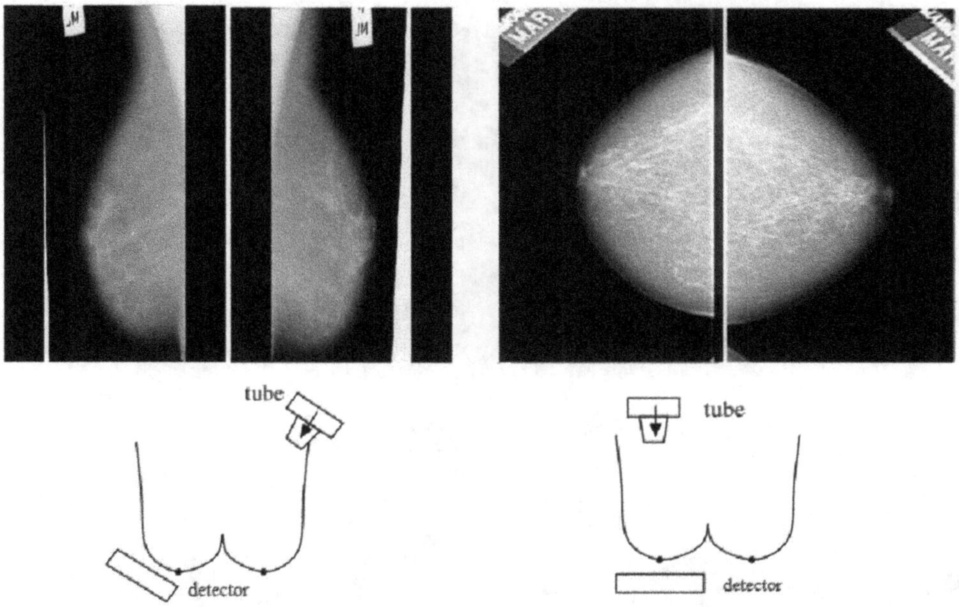

a. Mammography: is a radiological X-ray examination, particularly suitable for women breasts. Its purpose is to detect abnormalities as early as possible before they cause clinical symptoms. In particular, mammography (Figure 3) is widely used for screening or diagnosing breast cancer (Jouirou et al., 2015; Dhahbi et al., 2015; Kumar et al., 2017). During the acquisition of mammograms, the two breasts are compressed in turn between two plates. This compression allows the spreading of the mammary tissues, which facilitates the visualization of the structures of the breast and the reduction of the delivered X-rays dose. Subsequently, both breasts are exposed to a low dose of X-rays from the low-energy X-ray generator tube (between 20 and 50 keV). Breast projection on a planar detector is therefore obtained. Radiography is performed on silver film or high quality digital radiology systems. The mammary gland analysis is ensured by the differences of the different tissue types' attenuation. The strength of such an examination is that it allows to examine all breast tissues with only one or two incidences. Given the complexity of breast anatomy, mammography is usually taken in different directions called incidences. Depending on the examined breast part, different incidences are used. In the standard protocol of screening, a front incidence also called Cranio-Caudal (CC) and external oblique incidence appointed MedioLateral-Oblique (MLO) are performed on each breast. In the case of CC incidence, the detector and the X-ray tube are horizontal. This incidence explores the central and the internal breast regions well. In the case of the MLO incidence, the detector is inclined from 40° to 60° depending on the morphology of the patient. This incidence partly takes the pectoral muscle and allows to explore almost the entire mammary gland on a single incidence. In Figure 3, the positioning of the X-ray tube and detector as well as the different incidences are shown.

Figure 4. Ultrasound image of left breast containing a lesion (BUS, 2019)

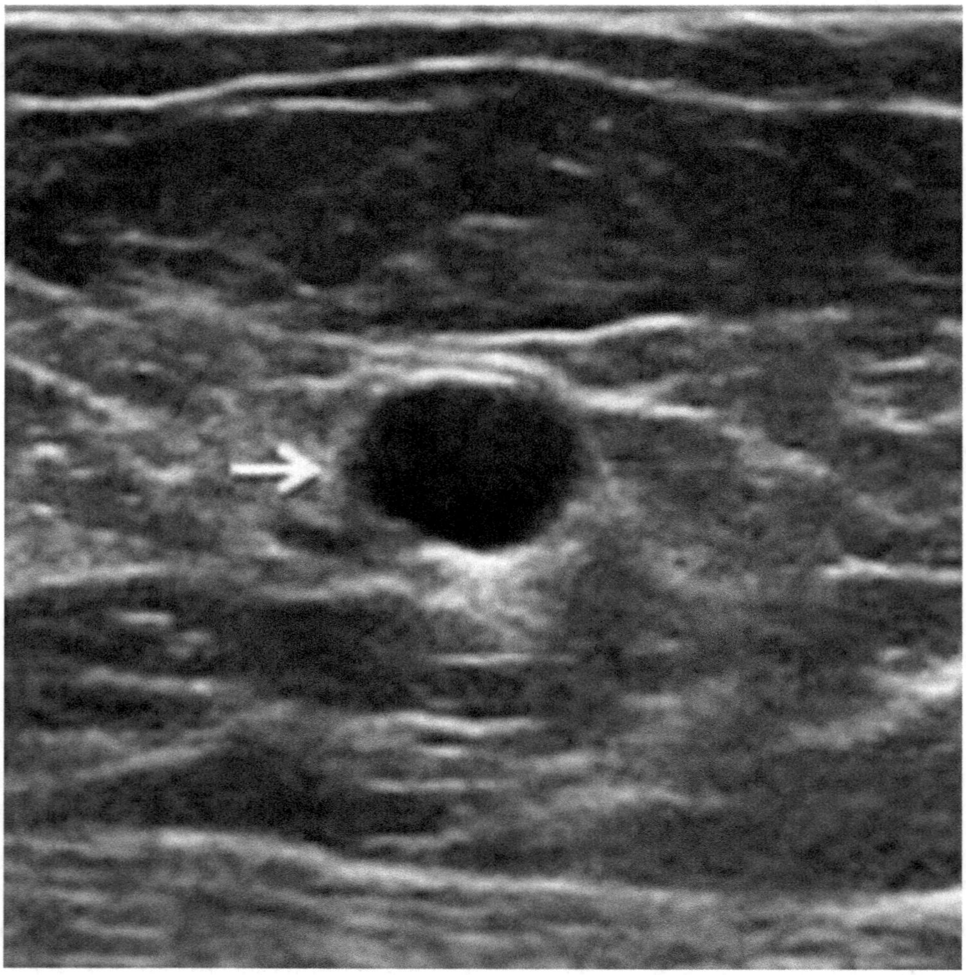

b. Ultrasound(US): For breast cancer screening, ultrasound (Figure 4), which is the second intention examination compliant with mammography when it revealed an anomaly, is carried out with 7.5 to 13 MHz probes. It uses ultrasound applied against the breast skin after having coated it with a gel. These emitted ultrasounds are echoed to each obstacle they encounter, while crossing the tissues of the breast. This signal is analyzed by a computer system that retransmits, in real time, the image of the breast on a video screen. The radiologist can thus consistently compare what he/she feels with the palpation of the breast and axillary hollows (ganglion, nodule, cyst ...) and the images that appear on the screen. In general, US is useful notably in three cases (Han et al., 2017): for dense breast tissue, for pregnant woman (since that mammography uses radiation) and for younger woman (less than 25). However, its efficiency is limited for several reasons such as the partial views, the difficulty to reproduce the results accurately by the same ultrasonographer (character operator-dependent exam) and the complexity of giving a quantitative character to the images (Murtaza et al., 2019).

c. Magnetic Resonance Imaging (MRI): Breast MRI is considered as a supplemental tool along with ultrasound and mammography (Warner et al., 2001). It is mainly used for breast cancer diagnosed women in order to measure the size of the cancer, and to check for other tumors in the same breast or in the opposite one. The main advantage of this technique is the absence of the use of ionizing radiation. In addition, it is characterized by a millimetric spatial resolution. In particular, it offers very marked contrasts between the different breast tissues that outline abnormalities more easily thanks to the injected contrast into a vein in the arm before or during the procedure. During this procedure, woman lies face down, with her breasts positioned through openings in the table, which are surrounded by special coils. The table is then moved inside the MRI machine that creates a strong magnetic field around the patient. The magnetic field, along with radio waves transmitted by coils, alters the hydrogen atoms' natural alignment in the breast tissues. As the nuclei realign into proper position, they send out radio signals. These signals are received by a computer that analyzes and converts them into an image of the breast tissues. Recently, breast MRI (Figure 5) has been extensively used in high risk screening in order to distinguish between benign and cancerous lesion, in dense breast tissue and in small abnormalities (Yassin et al., 2018). In spite of its distinct advantages over mammography and US, breast MRI also has potential limits such as the high false positive (normal tissue assimilated to a lesion) rate and its inability for identifying calcifications or tiny calcium deposits that can indicate breast cancer.

Figure 5. Woman positioning and breast magnetic resonance image

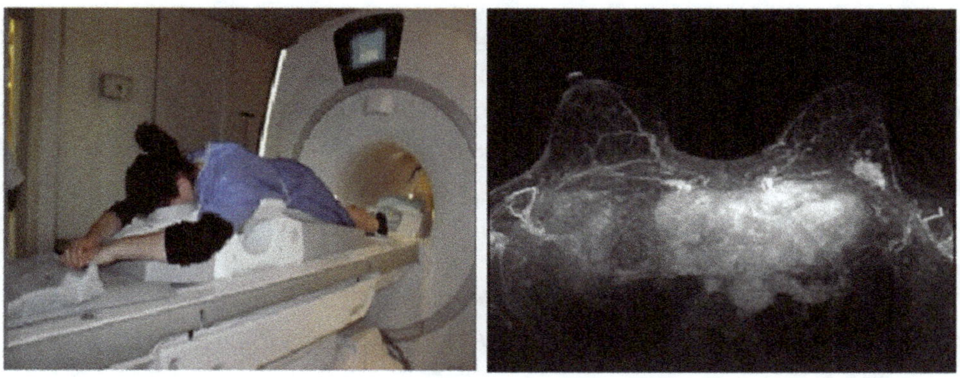

d. Molecular Breast Imaging (MBI): It is a test that uses a radioactive tracer that lights up breast cancer tissues, visualized by a small semiconductor-based γ-cameras (Figure 6). This technique; which is also called Miraluma test, specific gamma imaging, cintimammography and sestamibi test; provides high-resolution functional images of the breast. Current studies on MBI utilize a single injection of 20 mCi Tc-99m sestamibi, which is an approved agent for breast imaging. The MBI test starts approximately 5 min postinjection. The compression force, performed over breast tissues using the two detectors, is approximately a third that of mammography. Each breast is obtained in the CC and MLO projections. The key benefit of MBI is the high sensitivity for small lesions. Indeed, it has a sensitivity of 82% for all lesions less than 10 mm in size. Comparatively to MRI and mammography, it has comparable sensitivity and recall rates to MRI and rather a higher specificity that can detect small breast lesions. However, the recall rates are slightly lower for MBI compared with mammography (O'Connor et al., 2009).

Figure 6. The special-MBI camera and the right MLO view obtained by molecular breast imaging of a patient with confirmed invasive ductal carcinoma

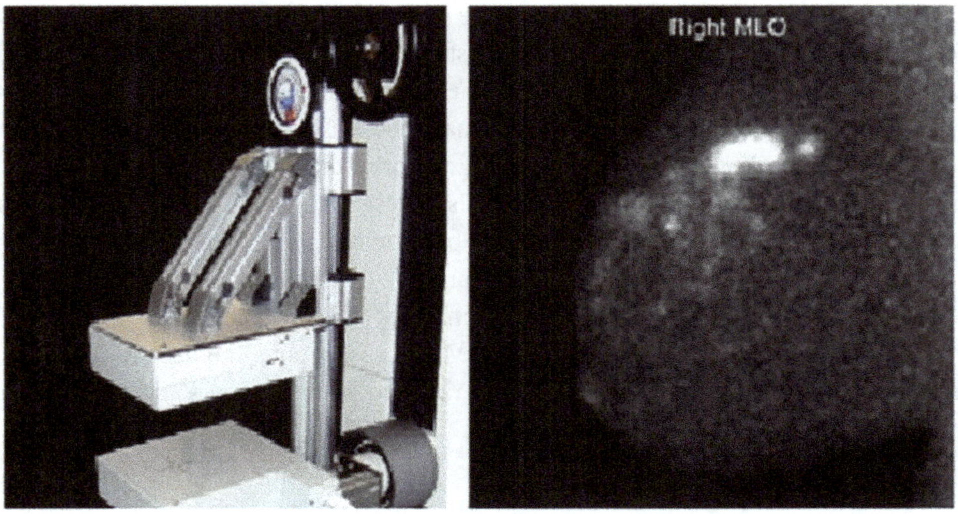

All of these promising tools, which assist radiologists and physicians in identifying abnormalities, can effectively reduce the mortality rates by 30–70% (Baeza-Yates & Ribeiro-Neto, 1999).The interpretation of these tools is performed in accordance with American College of Radiology (ACR) standard lexicon BIRADS (Breast Imaging-Reporting And Data System). This interpretation is radiologist-dependent, while requiring expertise. Therefore, computational methods based on CAD systems are a necessity to support and optimize the diagnosis, while providing a second opinion to the expertise.

Table 1. Radiological attenuation of breast components

Breast Component	Frequency (%)	Radiological attenuation	Mammography appearance
Fat	7.1	Transparent radio	Very dark
Water	25	Slightly opaque radio	Dark
Fibroglandular tissue	46.4	Opaque radio	Clear
Calcium	21.4	Very radio opaque	Very clear

3. Correlation between breast anatomy and mammography

Mammography is the result of the attenuation of a low-dose X-ray passing through the different mammary tissues. This attenuation depends essentially on the breast tissue composition (Table1). Since that mammogram is the reflection of breast anatomy, the fat is considered as a transparent radio zone since it has a very light physical density. Thereby, it appears very dark on a mammogram. On the other hand, the opaque radio zones appear clear and correspond to the fibroglandular tissue and the calcium, which are the essential components of the mammary lesions. By gathering the information about anatomy and radio transparency (Figure 7), authors can confirm that the general appearance of a mammogram is dark while the areas containing microcalcifications or masses (composed of calcium) are clearer.

Furthermore, fatty breast is mostly fat and dense breast is mostly breast and connective tissues. Dense breast mammogram is harder to read than fatty breast mammogram. In other words, in high breast density there is a greater amount of breast and connective tissue compared to fat, contrary to the fatty breast (low breast density) the amount of fat is high compared to breast and connective tissue.

Figure 7. Breast anatomy with mammography correlation

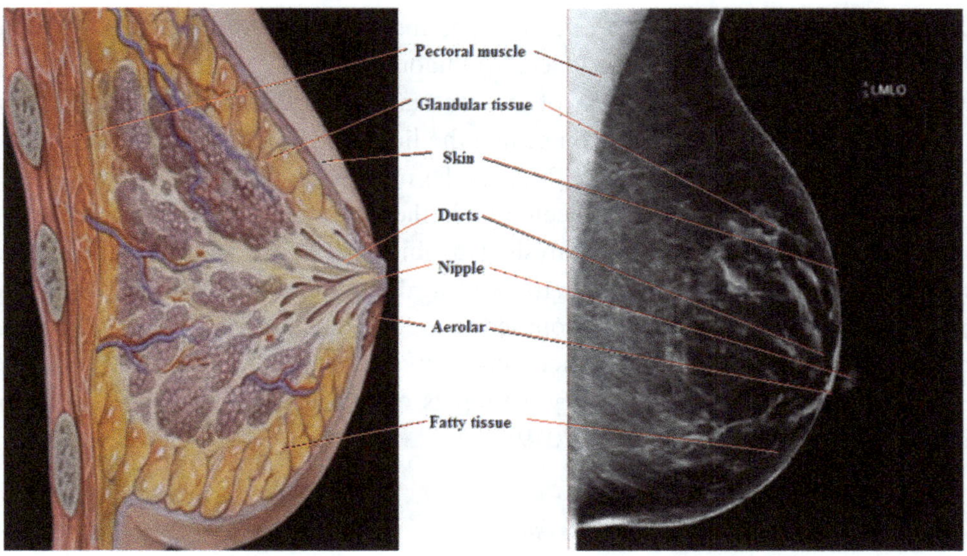

COMPUTER AIDED DIAGNOSIS (CAD) SYSTEMS

Computer-Aided Diagnosis systems use image processing techniques, pattern recognition tools and artificial intelligence in order to detect abnormal areas of density, mass, or calcification that may indicate the presence of cancer. The aim of these systems is to serve as an objective second opinion to radiologists, while assisting them in their clinical routines (e.g. lesion detection, lesion classification, recognition of malignant breast cancer, visualization…). The general scheme of a CAD system is composed of four stages; including preprocessing, segmentation, feature extraction and selection, and classification. The first stage allows to emphasize the appearance of the mammogram, while removing noise effects from it using image preprocessing operations. In fact, the main objective is to facilitate the subsequent stage, which is the segmentation. The later aims to divide the input mammogram into different regions to distinguish the Region Of Interest (ROI) from others. It is widely confirmed that the segmentation of mammary masses is much more difficult than the segmentation of calcifications (Oliver et al., 2010). This difficulty is due not only to the wide variation in sizes and possible shapes of masses that may be present in mammograms, but also because the masses often have poor contrast within mammograms. Thus, breast mass segmentation was largely studied in recent works and several methods have been proposed (thresholding, region growing, watershed, active contours, level sets...). In fact, thresholding methods have been widely used for mass segmentation. These methods can operate directly on the intensities of the mammogram (Abdel-Dayem & El-Sakka, 2005) or on a pre-processed version of the mammogram (Varela et al., 2007). These methods are generally fast, but they are inaccurate. Thus, thresholding is typically performed only to obtain an initial segmentation, which can then be improved using, for example, region growing or active contours. It is worth noting that since segmentation is a very difficult task, and thus its errors can degrade the global performance of the diagnosis, this segmentation stage is more and more avoided in the recent works. The third stage, which is feature extraction and selection, intends to extract visual features from ROI (or from the mass and surrounding tissues in the case of absence of the segmentation stage). Then, the selection of the most discriminative features is performed in order to differentiate between normal and cancerous regions. Indeed, as a mass of round shape is typically benign, whereas a lobulated form is more likely to be malignant, many shape descriptors have been proposed to describe a breast mass. For instance, (Mudigonda et al., 2001) proposed to describe masses by the coefficient of variation of the power of the contour, which is defined based on the variance of the values of the intensities of the pixels composing the line perpendicular to the contour of the mass. Thereafter, Principal Component Analysis (PCA) is the most widely used technique of feature selection in many areas. For example, ACP has been used in the field of curvelet to extract multi-resolution texture characteristics for mammography analysis (Dhahbi et al., 2016). The last stage is classification, where labels/classes are assigned to different groups using different machine learning techniques. Generally, various related techniques have been proposed in the recent years for abnormalities detection and classification. In particular, different classifiers (e.g. Naïve Bayes, SVM, random forest, KNN, neural networks, C4.5…) were employed to classify the inputs mammograms into normal or abnormal, and again benign or malignant (Mohanty et al., 2019).

Figure 8. Bloc diagram of a generic CBMR system

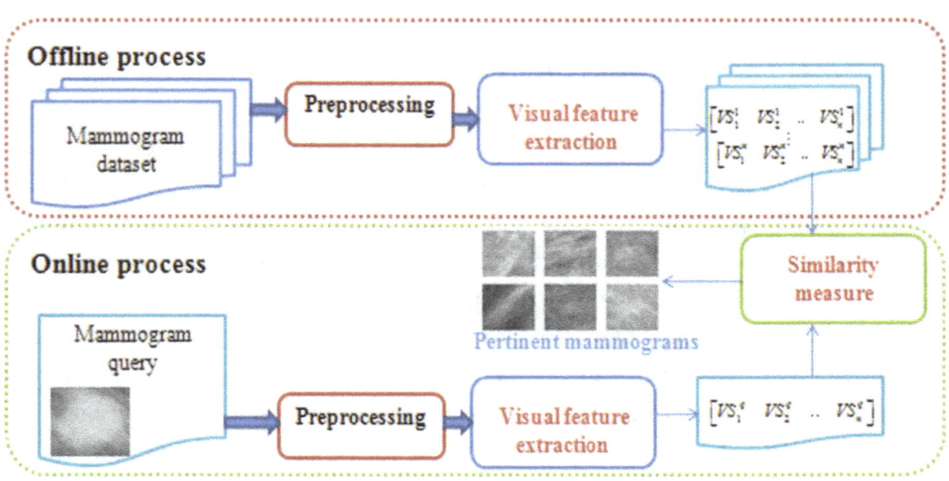

Table 2. Examples of SV-CBMR methods presented in the last three years.

Ref.	Mammogram features	Similarity metric	Used dataset	Accuracy
(Jouirou et al., 2015; Dhahbi et al., 2016)	Curvelet moments	Euclidean distance	DDSM	Precision=84.43%
(Chandy et al., 2017)	grey level co-occurrence matrix, Daubechies-4 wavelet, Gabor, Cohen–Daubechies–Feauveau 9/7 wavelet and Zernike moments	Neighbourhood structure	MIAS	Mean precision rate (MAP)= 76.2
(Kulshreshtha et al., 2017; Singh et al., 2017)	Local binary pattern (LBP) and k-means clustering	Euclidean distance	MIAS	Precision=85%, Precision=78%
(Zhiqiong et al., 2018)	Standard location feature, Histogram of Oriented Gradients, the Edge Direction Histogram, the Local Binary Pattern and the Gray Level Histogram	Earth Mover's Distance	440 mammograms, which are from Chinese women in Northeast China	Precision=0.83, Recall=0.76, Comprehensive indicator=0.79, Satisfaction=96.0%
(Baâzaoui et al., 2018)	Med-level features based on the clinician medical-knowledge	Mahalanobis Distance	MIAS	MAP= 0.9530
(Muramatsu et al., 2018)	CNN features	Similarity space modeling using CNN	MIAS	Average precision= 0.852
(Jiang et al., 2018)	SIFT features	discriminative learning and similarity maps	DDSM	Area under ROC curve = 0.89

CBMR-BASED CAD SYSTEMS

Since that CAD systems suffer from the black-box outputs, what increases the false positive rates and decreases the radiologists' confidence, CBMR is developed to tackle this problem, while it serves as an alternative to classic CAD system. In general, CBMR systems aim to retrieve similar images based on the visual content of a query mammogram (Figure 8) after extracting their content, known as signature. It can gather radiologists' confidence by displaying similar mammograms with their corresponding information, since that it can provide experts image-guided avenues to access relevant cases. Indeed, breast cancer clinical decisions based on such cases offer a reliable and consistent supplement for experts.

In this context, many frameworks on mammogram retrieval have been proposed, dealing with feature extraction, similarity measure, multi-view information fusion, scalability and relevance feedback (Dhahbi et al., 2016). Aside from CBMR scalability, which is treated separately in the next section, and the relevance feedback, which is not investigated in this work, CBMR systems can be further divided into two groups: single-view CBMR, and multi-view CBMR.

1. Single-View CBMR (SV-CBMR)

Figure 9. The proposed classification of existing methods for mammogram dataset indexing

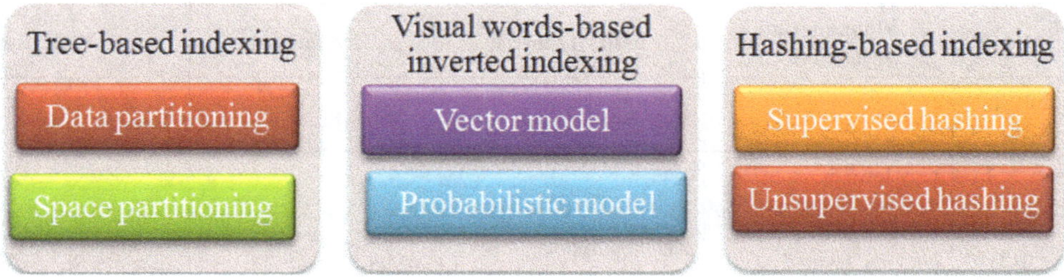

In SV-CBMR, as its name implies, the user submits in the online seeking process only one view of the query mammogram. This one view may be given as left MLO, right MLO, left CC, or right CC. Herein, an underlying assumption of the most SV-CBMR is that the selected mammogram features and the selected similarity metric are sufficient enough to describe the mammogram accurately, and choose the most similar mammograms to the query one, respectively. In other words, in many clinical studies, efforts have been made to improve feature extraction in order to select the most discriminative mammogram features [Dhahbi et al., 2016; Singh et al., 2017). Similarly, several studies focus on the choice of similarity measure to distinguish between mammograms that are dissimilar (Chandy et al., 2017; Muramatsu et al., 2018). Table 2 briefly presents the notable studies in the literature that used SV-CBMR. It lists the chosen feature extraction, the chosen similarity metric, the used dataset, and the accuracy reported in the study. Since there is no consensus and a common goal as discussed above on SV-CBMR as shown in Table 2, variable SV-CBMR results were reported even for similar mammogram dataset.

2. Multi-view CBMR (MV-CBMR)

Since that screening mammography provides two views for each breast (LMLO, RMLO, LCC, and RCC) and radiologists use both views in breast cancer diagnosis before making decision to interpret the undiagnosed mammogram, multi-view CBMR has been widely applied in the recent years. This class may be divided into two categories, including early fusion-based MV-CBMR, and late fusion-based MV-CBMR. The former consists on merging both views' features into one vector, which is used afterwards as input for the retrieval process. The second one consists on treating each view separately, and the final retrieval is carried out through the fusion of the obtained results of each view. Among early fusion-based MV-CBMR methods, authors cited those that automatically describe masses through the combination of the CC and MLO view features in mammograms with the Breast Imaging Reporting And Data System (BIRADS) lexicon (Narvaez, 2011). Compared to SV-CBMR, MV-CBMR helps to further improve the retrieval performance. Nonetheless, its main disadvantage is that it does not offer scalability. To overcome this limit, late fusion-based MV-CBMR was recently proposed. For instance, in (Dhahbi et al., 2015) the couples of the MLO and CC views of mammogram ROIs are used in the mammogram retrieval context. In fact, a MV-CBMR system is generally composed of the CBMR-MLO and the CBMR-CC. By analyzing the recorded results presented in the literature, late fusion-based MV-CBMR is more efficient than early fusion-based MV-CBMR. Readers are referred to (Jouirou et al., 2018) for a more comprehensive review on multi-view CBMR.

Figure 10. Sample of M-tree and slim-down application: a) construction of M-tree, b) M-tree before applying slim-down algorithm, c) M-tree after applying slim-down algorithm

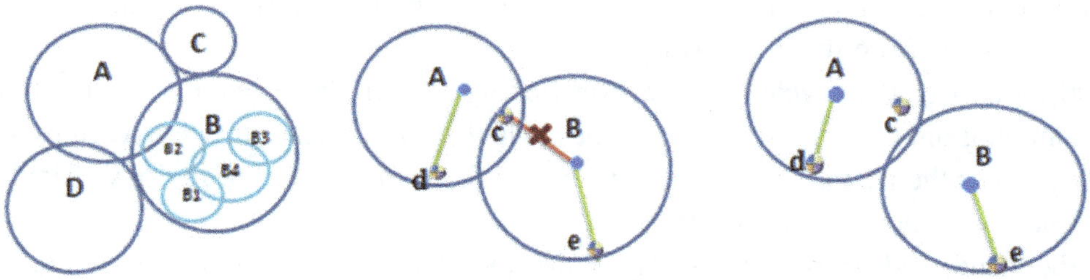

CBMR SCALABILITY ON LARGE-SCALE DATASETS

Among the variety of multidimensional index structures, authors classified mammogram indexing methods into three main classes: tree-based indexing methods, visual words-based inverted indexing methods and hashing-based indexing ones (Figure 9) (Ai et al., 2013). As conventional indexing, tree-based indexing methods allow to encompass the vectors, after regrouping them in packages, in simple geometric shapes forming a tree of hierarchical structure. Indeed, these methods can reduce the search path to a subset of packets, while selecting the most relevant ones and only accessing the vectors that belong to the selected packets. These methods can be classified into two main categories including data partitioning methods and space partitioning-based ones (Gallas et al., 2015).

On the one hand, the data-partitioning-based methods, which are classified in their turn into two sub-classes, consist on partitioning data space according to the data distribution. Indeed, the first sub-class is based on static trees, whilst the second sub-class is based on dynamic trees. Inasmuch as static tree methods suffer from overlapping between static hierarchical data structure, dynamic tree methods are applied in the mammogram context. More specifically, the most commonly used technique is M-tree and the slim-down algorithm (Zhang et al., 2008). In fact, M-tree groups the data into fixed-size disk pages that correspond to the nodes of the tree in order to form a multi-layered M-tree structure. The vectors stored in the leaves of the tree are organized as a hierarchical structure through a data representative, which is the center of the smallest region that covers the objects in a sub-tree. During the search, M-tree uses the triangular inequality and the distance of the representative to eliminate irrelevant sub-trees. The index structure of M-tree is constructed by the successive insertion of the different vectors. The insertion algorithm firstly searches, from the root node, the node that can contain the vector to be inserted. If no node is found, the algorithm chooses the node whose center is closest to the vector. If several nodes, which may contain the vector, are identified, the algorithm chooses the node either in a random manner, or the node that has the minimum of vectors, or the node that has a minimal distance between the node center and the vector. To divide the data, M-tree uses the method of the minimum bounding circle, and each node corresponds to a hyper sphere in the multi-dimensional feature space. In order to be able to cover every point in the multidimensional feature data space, when the amount of data is relatively large, M-tree will inevitably generate node overlap. How to reduce the node overlap rate is the key to improve the efficiency of M-tree indexing. The Slim-down algorithm is a post-processing algorithm that optimizes the structure of the established tree to reduce the node coverage radius, reduce the node overlap rate, and improve the retrieval efficiency. Indeed, the "Slim-down" algorithm consists of three main steps.

Firstly, it computes for each node the vector VS_1 furthest from its representative vector VS_0. Secondly, the algorithm identifies the nodes that cover the vector VS_1. Finally, the algorithm moves the vector VS_1 to the nearest node and corrects the resulting node radius. Figure 10 further explains the optimization of the M-tree using the Slim-down algorithm.

In general, the two major drawbacks of data-partitioning-based indexing methods, notably the dynamic tree in the mammogram case, are the trivial nodes, which may contain either few vectors or be empty. This greatly reduces the performance of the index and the large number of regions visited during the search that leads to an increase in response time.

On the other hand, aside from mammography, the space partitioning-based indexing methods, which split the multidimensional space into disjoint regions and store the data according to this division, are developed in the literature for many medical image indexing. Among these methods, KD-tree is presented in (Robinson et al., 1996). The major problem of most of these methods is the frequent need of backtracking in the trees in order to find the optimal solution, what causes a long processing time. Besides, although that conventional indexing methods are effective in small size spaces, their performance degrades rapidly when the data size increases. Thus, this class fails in high-dimensional feature spaces due to the curse of dimensionality.

The second class of mammogram indexing is based on Bag-of-features (BOF), also known as bag-of-visual-words (BOVW). BOVW are the first visual words based inverted indexing methods. These methods are introduced from text retrieval systems to content-based image retrieval (Sivic et al., 2003). They intend to shorten the semantic gap by partitioning a low-level feature space into regions of the features space, which correspond to visual concepts. Indeed, the construction of the visual vocabulary takes place in four stages. Firstly, the images are represented by sets of local low-level descriptors calculated on regions of interest, which are extracted using an invariant primitive to the affine transformations. Secondly, classes of similar descriptors are created using a clustering technique. The representation of each descriptor by the centroid of the cluster that contains is called quantification and the visual words are the quantization indices of these descriptors. Then, each image is represented by the histogram of the visual words appearance frequencies. Finally, the indexing is done by an inverted file, such that each element in the inverted file list indicates the images where this word appeared. Therefore, the relevant images for a given query are those containing at least one word of the query. BOVW methods can be categorized into two categories: BOVW methods based on the vector model and those based on the probabilistic model. Traditionally, BOVW indexing methods based on conventional models (Baeza-Yates & Ribeiro-Neto, 1999), which assume that the descriptors of an image have equal importance, is not general enough to be used in clinical applications and especially in mammography, since that the descriptors do not all have the same importance in mammograms (*e.g.* the descriptors of muscle or breast tissues are much less important than mass or calcification descriptors). In BOVW indexing methods based on vector models, the descriptors are weighted according to their representations of the content of the image, whereas in BOVW indexing based on the probabilistic model the importance of words in the images is expressed in terms of the probability of belonging to the image and looking for similar images in terms of probability of relevance of the image to the query. With the vector model, an image is represented by a vector of frequencies weighted according to the appearance of the words with k components. Each component of the vector brings a compromise between two factors: the word appearance frequency in the image (tf, for term frequency) and the estimation of the degree of importance of this word to distinguish a relevant image from the non relevant one (idf, for inverse document frequency). As an example of indexing methods based on the vector model, authors cite the vocabulary tree method

(Jiang et al., 2015), which quantifies and indexes the image characteristics from the DDSM dataset of 11553 mammogram ROIs. Firstly, the k-means algorithm is applied to the set of learning data to define clusters with their centers. The same algorithm is applied recursively on all clusters to divide each cluster into sub-clusters. Thus, after a few iterations, the vocabulary tree is constructed with a depth *Pf* and a branch factor *fb*. Each node of the tree corresponds to a cluster center and the nodes are weighted using the tf-idf scheme. In Figure 11, the SIFT characteristics of the query are quantized in the same way but they are not indexed. Each leaf node in the tree has an inverted file (illustrates with solid lines), which records the identifiers of the ROIs of the image dataset containing an instance of the node. Each internal node has an inverted virtual file (shown in dotted lines) which is defined as the concatenation of the files associated with its nodes of the descending leaves. The obtained results seem to achieve an accuracy of 88.4% for a number of returned images equal to 5. However, this method is highly sensitive to the choice of weighting coefficients that are set empirically.

Figure 11. Quantification and indexing of mammograms based on SIFT characteristics and the vector model (Jiang et al., 2015)

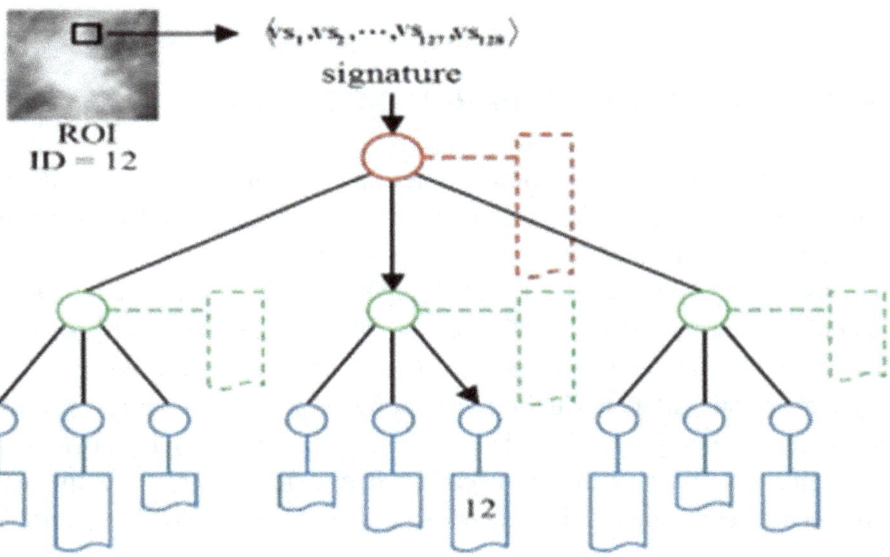

Noteworthy is that the BOVW indexing methods based on the probabilistic model are not applied in the mammogram context and despite that this class of indexing methods give good results, the major disadvantage is the large required vocabularies and thus the high-dimensional feature space, which leads to the curse of dimensionality and increases the computational time. To address the problem of the curse of dimensionality and to improve the accuracy of the retrieval, hashing-based methods have been widely used in the last years for indexing large datasets. The intuition behind hashing-based indexing is straightforward: withstand the curse of dimensionality and accelerate the search of the nearest neighbors, while introducing a certain degree of imprecision during the search. Indeed, instead of performing a sequential search based on the descriptive vectors, the search will be performed on a compressed representation of these vectors. These methods allow to perform a quick search for relevant image while preserving the semantic similarity. These methods can be subdivided into three categories: supervised, semi-supervised and unsupervised hashing methods. Supervised hashing methods integrate information on the label. Differently, semi-supervised methods use both labeled and unlabeled data, whilst the unsupervised hashing-based ones use the unlabeled data. However, in the medical field and notably in the mammography context, authors identify only two categories, supervised and unsupervised hashing methods. For instance, kernel-based supervised hashing (KSH) algorithm is presented in (Lv et al., 2016) combined with multiple-features. Despite their effectiveness to greatly improve the detection performance, the performance evaluation results are more sensitive to the modulus and the bias values, which are the most essential parameters to obtain the final prediction function. To tackle this limit, unsupervised hashing-based methods were developed for generating the binary code for each point. Locality Sensitive Hashing (LSH) (Jouirou et al., 2015) is arguably the most notable unsupervised hashing method. It consists on projecting the data in the Hamming space to generate a binary code for each data, named the hash key, where the nearest data have the possibility of having similar hash keys. Then, this method optimizes the search to find the relevant images using the hash functions (Figure 12).

In the same context, for compressing the mammogram features into compact binary codes, and performing the search in the Hamming space, Anchor Graph Hashing (AGH) is recently applied in (Liu et al., 2017).

CONCLUSION AND FUTURE RESEARCH DIRECTIONS

Authors proposed in this chapter an overview of relevant CAD and CBMR methods in order to assist radiologists in making decision. In fact, after citing breast imaging principles and demonstrating the correlation between breast anatomy and mammography, several CAD methods are studied to detect/classify input mammograms. Although the usage of single-view CAD systems has steadily increased and widespread, studies demonstrate that MV- CADx systems recorded higher performances. Then, recent methods based on CBMR are described since that CBMR is serving as an encouraging alternative to classic CAD systems. Lastly, after concluding, some of future perspectives are deeply discussed. In fact, since the ultimate goal in this systematic review is the help of researchers in innovating and developing CBMR-CAD systems to assist the radiologists/experts in decision making for early treatment of breast cancer, authors discuss herein some of issues concerning the future of CBMR systems:

- In light of the heterogeneous shape and size presented in mammograms, deep learning-based CAD system is affected. CBMR system depends heavily on radiologist-specified suspicious
- regions. To overcome the drawbacks of both kinds of methods, deep learning was recently investigated in CBMR systems and this combination presents an active research topic.
- In parallel to the development of mammography scanners, there have been recent attempts in the literature to develop CAD systems using 3D mammography, which has a higher cancer detection rate compared with conventional 2D mammography.
- Clinically, experts start the analysis of the four views obtained by mammography by firstly looking at left CC view and if they did not find abnormality in this view, they prefer after that to check left MLO, right CC and right MLO views of the mammogram, respectively. This point should be considered to develop four views-CBMR systems in the future.

Figure 12. Example of LSH mammogram indexing

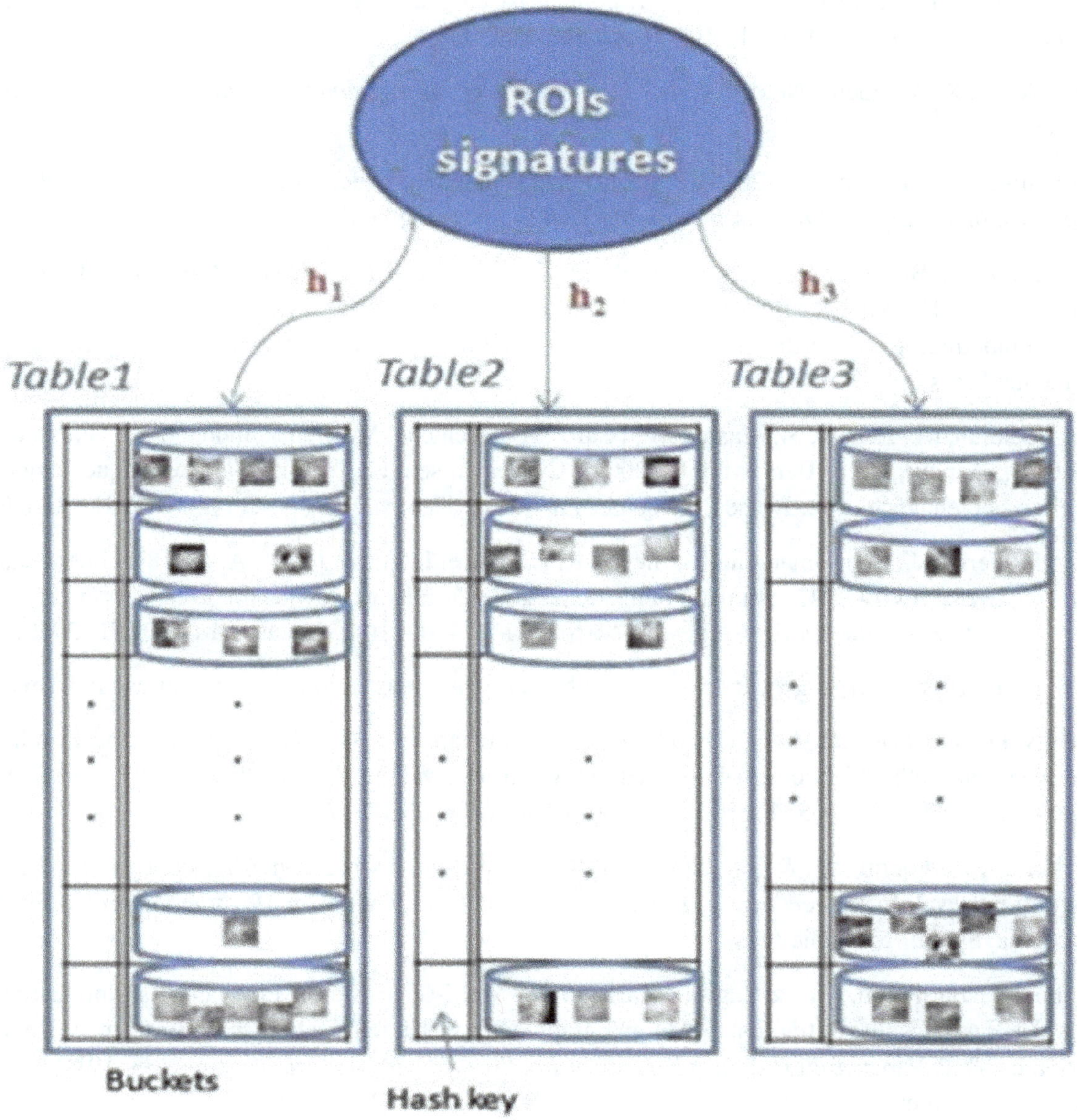

REFERENCES

Abdel-Dayem, A. R., & El-Sakka, M. R. (2005). Fuzzy entropy based detection of suspicious masses in digital mammogram images. *In Proceedings of 27th IEEE Engineering Annual Conference in Medicine and Biology* (pp. 4017-4022). Shanghai, China. 10.1109/IEMBS.2005.1615343

Ai, L., & Yu, J., & He, Y., & Guan, T. (2013). High-dimensional indexing technologies for large scale content-based image retrieval: a review. *Journal of Zhejiang University SCIENCE C (Comput & Electron),* 14 (7), 505-520.

Baâzaoui, A., Barhoumi, W., Ahmed, A., & Zagrouba, E. (2018). Modeling clinician medical-knowledge in terms of med-level features for semantic content-based mammogram retrieval. *Expert Systems with Applications*, *94*(1), 11–20. doi:10.1016/j.eswa.2017.10.034

Baeza-Yates, R., & Ribeiro-Neto, B. (Eds.). (1999). *Modern Information Retrieval*. ACM Press/Addison-Wesley.

Barhoumi, W., & Baâzaoui, A. (2014). Pigment network detection in dermatoscopic images for melanoma diagnosis. *Innovation and Research in BioMedical Engineering, 35*(3), 128-138.

Belkacémi, Y., Boussen, H., Hamdi-Cherif, M., Benider, A., Errihani, H., Mrabti, H., Bouzid, K., Bensalem, A., Fettouki, S., Ben Abdalah, M., Abid, L., & Gligorov, J. (2010). Young women breast cancer epidemiology in North Africa. In Proceedings of thirty two SFSPM days (pp. 56-68), Strasbourg: Academic Press.

Ben Abdallah, M., Zehani, S., Maalej, M., Hsairi, M., Hechiche, M., Ben Romdhane, K., Boussen, H., Saadi, A., Achour, N., & Ben Ayed, F. (2009). Cancer du sein en Tunisie: Caractéristiques épidémiologiques et tendance évolutive de l'incidence. *La Tunisie Medicale*, *87*(7), 417–425. PMID:20063673

Bray, F., Ferlay, J., Soerjomataram, I., Siegel, R. L., Torre, L. A., & Jemal, A. (2018). Global cancer statistics 2018: GLOBOCAN estimates of incidence and mortality worldwide for 36 cancers in 185 countries. *CA: a Cancer Journal for Clinicians*, *68*(6), 394–424. doi:10.3322/caac.21492 PMID:30207593

BUS. (n.d.). *Breast ultrasound*. Retrieved from https://densebreast-info.org/breast-ultrasound.aspx

Chandy, D. A., Christinal, A. H., Theodore, A. J., & Selvan, S. E. (2017). Neighbourhood search feature selection method for content-based mammogram retrieval. *Medical & Biological Engineering & Computing*, *55*(3), 493–505. doi:10.100711517-016-1513-x PMID:27262458

Dhahbi, S., Barhoumi, W., & Zagrouba, E. (2015). Multi-view score fusion for content-based mammogram retrieval. In *Proceedings of Eighth International Conference on Machine Vision* (*vol. 9875*). Barcelona, Spain: Academic Press.

Dhahbi, S., Barhoumi, W., & Zagrouba, E. (2016). Multi-scale Kernel PCA and Its Application to Curvelet-Based Feature Extraction for Mammographic Mass Characterization. In H. Boström, A. Knobbe, C. Soares, & P. Papapetrou (Eds.), *Advances in Intelligent Data Analysis XV* (pp. 183–191). Lecture Notes in Computer Science. Springer. doi:10.1007/978-3-319-46349-0_16

Gallas, A., & Barhoumi, W. (2015). Locality-sensitive hashing for region-based large-scale image indexing. *IET Image Processing*, *9*(9), 804–810. doi:10.1049/iet-ipr.2014.0910

Han, S., Kang, H. K., Jeong, J. Y., Park, M. H., Kim, W., Bang, W. C., & Seong, Y. K. (2017). A deep learning framework for supporting the classification of breast lesions in ultrasound images. *Physics in Medicine and Biology*, *62*(19), 7714–7728. doi:10.1088/1361-6560/aa82ec PMID:28753132

Jiang, M., Zhang, S., Li, H., & Metaxas, D. (2015). Computer-aided diagnosis of mammographic masses using scalable image retrieval. *IEEE Transactions on Biomedical Engineering*, *62*(2), 783–792. doi:10.1109/TBME.2014.2365494 PMID:25361497

Jiang, M., Zhang, S., & Metaxas, D. N. (2018). Detecting Mammographic Masses via Image Retrieval and Discriminative Learning. In K. Suzuki & Y. Chen (Eds.), *Artificial Intelligence in Decision Support Systems for Diagnosis in Medical Imaging*. Springer. doi:10.1007/978-3-319-68843-5_5

Jouirou, A., Baâzaoui, A., & Barhoumi, W. (2019). Multi-view information fusion in mammograms: A comprehensive overview. *Information Fusion*, *52*, 308–321. doi:10.1016/j.inffus.2019.05.001

Jouirou, A., Baâzaoui, A., Barhoumi, W., & Zagrouba, E. (2015). Curvelet-based locality sensitive hashing for mammogram retrieval in large-scale datasets. In *Proceedings of 12th IEEE/ACS International Conference of Computer Systems and Applications* (pp. 1-8). IEEE. 10.1109/AICCSA.2015.7507106

Kulshreshtha, D., Singh, V. P., Shrivastava, A., Chaudhary, A., & Srivastava, R. (2017). Content-based mammogram retrieval using k-means clustering and local binary pattern. In *Proceedings of 2nd International Conference on Image, Vision and Computing* (pp. 634-638). Academic Press. 10.1109/ICIVC.2017.7984633

Kumar, I., Bhadauria, H. S., Virmani, J., & Thakur, S. (2017). A classification framework for prediction of breast density using an ensemble of neural network classifiers. *Biocybernetics and Biomedical Engineering*, *37*(1), 217–228. doi:10.1016/j.bbe.2017.01.001

Liu, J., Zhang, S., Liu, W., Deng, C., Zheng, Y., & Metaxas, D. N. (2017). Scalable Mammogram Retrieval Using Composite Anchor Graph Hashing With Iterative Quantization. *IEEE Transactions on Circuits and Systems for Video Technology*, *27*(11), 2450–2460. doi:10.1109/TCSVT.2016.2592329

Lv, X., & Wang, Y. (2016). Multiple-Feature Kernel Hashing for Mass Detection. In *Proceedings of the International Conference on Internet Multimedia Computing and Service* (pp. 99-104). Xi'an, China: Academic Press.

Mohanty, F., Rup, S., Dash, B., Majhi, B., & Swamy, M. N. S. (2019). Digital mammogram classification using 2D-BDWT and GLCM features with FOA-based feature selection approach. *Neural Computing & Applications*, 1–15. doi:10.100700521-019-04186-w

Mudigonda, N. R., Rangayyan, R. M., & Desautels, J. L. (2001). Detection of breast masses in mammograms by density slicing and texture flow-field analysis. *IEEE Transactions on Medical Imaging*, *20*(12), 1215–1227. doi:10.1109/42.974917 PMID:11811822

Muramatsu, C., Higuchi, S., Morita, T., Oiwa, M., Kawasaki, T., & Fujita, H. (2018). Retrieval of reference images of breast masses on mammograms by similarity space modeling. In *Proceedings of Fourteenth International Workshop on Breast Imaging* (Vol. 1071809). Atlanta, GA: Academic Press.

Murtaza, G., Shuib, L., Wahab, A. W., Mujtaba, A. G., Mujtaba, G., Nweke, H. F., Al-garadi, M. A., Zulfiqar, F., Raza, G., & Azmi, N. A. (2019). Deep learning-based breast cancer classification through medical imaging modalities: State of the art and research challenges. *Artificial Intelligence Review*, 1–66.

Narvaez, F., Diaz, G., & Romero, E. (2011). Multi-view information fusion for automatic BI-RADS description of mammographic masses. In Proceedings of SPIE 7963, Medical Imaging 2011: Computer-Aided Diagnosis (pp. 84–89). Academic Press.

O'Connor, M., Rhodes, D., & Hruska, C. (2009). Molecular breast imaging. *Expert Review of Anticancer Therapy*, *9*(8), 1073–1080. doi:10.1586/era.09.75 PMID:19671027

Oliver, A., Freixenet, J., Marti, J., Perez, E., Pont, J., Denton, E. R., & Zwiggelaar, R. (2010). A review of automatic mass detection and segmentation in mammographic images. *Medical Image Analysis*, *14*(2), 87–110. doi:10.1016/j.media.2009.12.005 PMID:20071209

Robinson, G. P., Tagare, H. D., Duncan, J. S., & Jaffe, C. C. (1996). Medical image collection indexing: Shape-based retrieval using KD-trees. *Computerized Medical Imaging and Graphics*, *20*(4), 209–217. doi:10.1016/S0895-6111(96)00014-6 PMID:8954229

Singh, V. P., & Srivastava, R. (2017). Content-based mammogram retrieval using wavelet based complete-LBP and K-means clustering for the diagnosis of breast cancer. *International Journal of Hybrid Intelligent Systems*, *14*(1-2), 31–39. doi:10.3233/HIS-170240

Sivic, J., & Zisserman, A. (2003). Video google: a text retrieval approach to object matching in video. In *Proceedings of Ninth IEEE International Conference on Computer Vision* (Vol. 2, pp. 1470-1477). 10.1109/ICCV.2003.1238663

Varela, C., Tahoces, P. G., Mendez, A. J., Souto, M., & Vidal, J. J. (2007). Computerized detection of breast masses in digitized mammograms. *Computers in Biology and Medicine*, *37*(2), 214–226. doi:10.1016/j.compbiomed.2005.12.006 PMID:16620805

Warner, E., Plewes, D. B., Shumak, R. S., Catzavelos, G. C., Di Prospero, L. S., Yaffe, M. J., Goel, V., Ramsay, E., Chart, P. L., Cole, D. E. C., Taylor, G. A., Cutrara, M., Samuels, T. H., Murphy, J. P., Murphy, J. M., & Narod, S. A. (2001). Comparison of Breast Magnetic Resonance Imaging, Mammography, and Ultrasound for Surveillance of Women at High Risk for Hereditary Breast Cancer. *Journal of Clinical Oncology*, *19*(15), 3524–3531. doi:10.1200/JCO.2001.19.15.3524 PMID:11481359

WHO. (2019). *Global Health Observatory.* Geneva: World Health organization. Retrieved from who.int/gho/database/en/

Yassin, N. R., Omran, S., El Houby, E. M. F., & Allam, H. (2018). Machine learning techniques for breast cancer computer aided diagnosis using different image modalities: A systematic review. *Computer Methods and Programs in Biomedicine*, *156*, 25–45. doi:10.1016/j.cmpb.2017.12.012 PMID:29428074

Zhang, L. F., & Zhang, L. (2008). Study of index for mammogram database. *Journal of Shanghai Jiaotong University*, *28*(5), 548–551. doi:10.100711741-008-0615-2

Zhiqiong, W., Junchang, X., Yukun, H., Chen, L., Ling, X., & Yang, L. (2018). A similarity measure method combining location feature for mammogram retrieval. *Journal of X-Ray Science and Technology*, *26*(4), 553–571. doi:10.3233/XST-18374 PMID:29865106

KEY TERMS AND DEFINITIONS

BIRADS (Breast Imaging-Reporting and Data System): Standard and complete lexicon that takes into account the different malignancy factors for characterization of mammography, ultrasound and MRI as defined by the American College of Radiology (ACR) in 1998. It classifies mammograms into six categories according to the degree of suspicion of their pathological character.

Calcification (CALC): Is a deposit of calcium salts composed of chemical substances $Ca_3\,(PO_4)_2$, $CaCO_3$ and $Mg_3\,(PO_4)_2$. These substances are very radio-opaque and present in the mammographic images, by small clear dots. There are two types of CALC, namely microcalcifications (Mcs) which are of high contrast and small size (<0.5mm) and macrocalcifications once the size exceeds 1mm and they are often benign.

Chapter 7
The Evolution of New Trends in Breast Thermography

Marcus Costa de Araújo
https://orcid.org/0000-0002-1818-5686
Universidade Federal de Pernambuco, Brazil

Luciete Alves Bezerra
https://orcid.org/0000-0002-5363-7545
Federal University of Pernambuco, Brazil

Kamila Fernanda Ferreira da Cunha Queiroz
https://orcid.org/0000-0003-4257-5155
Federal Institute of Rio Grande do Norte, Brazil

Nadja A. Espíndola
https://orcid.org/0000-0003-1080-2173
Universidade Federal de Pernambuco, Brazil

Ladjane Coelho dos Santos
https://orcid.org/0000-0001-9239-8746
Federal Institute of Sergipe, Brazil

Francisco George S. Santos
Universidade Federal de Pernambuco, Brazil

Rita de Cássia Fernandes de Lima
DEMEC, Federal University of Pernambuco, Brazil

ABSTRACT

In this chapter, the theoretical foundations of infrared radiation theory and the principles of the infrared imaging technique are presented. The use of infrared (IR) images has increased recently, especially due to the refinement and portability of thermographic cameras. As a result, this type of camera can be used for various medical applications. In this context, the use of IR images is proposed as an auxiliary tool for detecting disease and monitoring, especially for the early detection of breast cancer.

DOI: 10.4018/978-1-7998-3456-4.ch007

INTRODUCTION

In this chapter, the theoretical foundations of Infrared Radiation Theory and the principles of the infrared imaging technique are presented.

The use of infrared (IR) images has increased recently, especially due to the refinement and portability of thermographic cameras. As a result, this type of camera can be used for various medical applications.

In this context, the use of IR images is proposed as an auxiliary tool for detecting disease and monitoring, especially for the early detection of breast cancer.

Thermal Radiation: Some Theoretical Considerations

"Thermal radiation (radiative heat transfer) is the science of transferring energy in the form of electromagnetic waves". It does not require a medium for propagation and is the dominant mode in outer-space applications or in a vacuum (Modest, 2013).

According to Incropera and DeWitt (1996), radiation begins by being emitted from a body. But this radiation does not require the presence of any material for it to be transported. There is a theory that considers that radiation is the propagation of particles termed photons or quanta. Another theory considers that radiation is the propagation of electromagnetic waves that travel at the speed of light.

Planck stated that electromagnetic radiation, including thermal radiation, is emitted as discrete quanta of energy E,

$$E = h\nu \tag{1}$$

where h = 6.625 x 10^{-34} J.s is Planck's constant and ν is the frequency of the radiation.

A few years later, Einstein proved that electromagnetic radiation behaves like a collection of quanta with energy equal to h ν. In 1905, he used the concept of the quantum nature of light to explain some particular properties of metals (Gasiorowicz, 1979).

All electromagnetic radiation obeys similar laws of reflection, refraction, diffraction and polarization. This radiation propagates at the speed of light.

As bodies emit or absorb electromagnetic waves, their internal energy changes, at a molecular level. The process depends on the temperature and the wavelength.

The spectrum of thermal radiation ranges from 0.1 μm to 100 μm and includes almost all the infrared part of the spectrum, the visible light and a small part of the ultraviolet spectrum. The infrared portion of the electromagnetic spectrum begins at a wavelength of 0.7 and extends to 1000 μm (Figure 1).

In the early 1900s, thermal radiation included the part mentioned above because the known engineering applications at that time occurred at that interval. Nowadays, it is considered that all bodies above 0K emit thermal radiation. This radiation can be used to obtain IR images of an object by using IR detectors.

In our considerations here, radiation is a surface phenomenon because, in most solids and liquids, the radiation emitted from interior molecules is absorbed by the adjacent molecules. However, the radiation emitted from a body originates from molecules located at 1 μm below the outer surface (Modest, 2013).

According to Incropera and DeWitt (1996), a blackbody has the following properties:

Figure 1. Part of the electromagnetic spectrum (HyperPhysics, 2019).

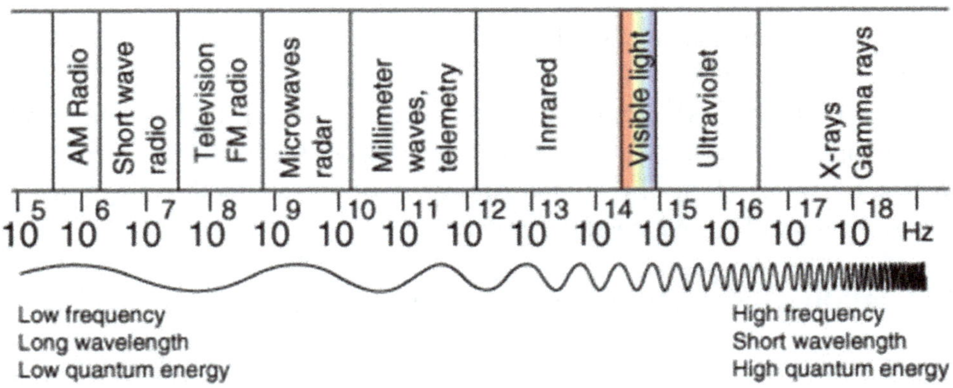

a) It absorbs all the incident radiation, regardless of wavelength and direction;
b) No surface can emit more energy than a blackbody at the same temperature;
c) A blackbody is a diffuse emitter.

The amount of radiation can be calculated if we define the spectral emissive power, E_{λ}, which is equal to the rate at which radiation of wavelength λ is emitted in all directions from a surface, per unit of wavelength dλ, per unit surface area. $I_{\lambda}(\lambda)$ is the spectral intensity of the radiation emitted (Incropera & DeWitt, 1996).

Planck first determined the spectral distribution of blackbody emission, $I_{\lambda b}$:

$$I_{\lambda b}(\lambda,T)=\frac{2hc^2}{\lambda^5\left\{exp(hc/\lambda kT)-1\right\}} \quad (2)$$

where:

h= 6.6256 x 10^{-34} J.s (Planck's constant);
k= 1.385 x 10^{-23} J/K (Boltzmann's constant);
c= 2.998 x 10^{8} m/s (the speed of light in a vacuum);
T= the absolute temperature of the blackbody (K).

For a blackbody, the Planck distribution can be calculated as:

$$E_{b\lambda}=\pi I_{b\lambda}(\lambda) \quad (3)$$

Using Eq. (2), Boltzmann demonstrated that the emissive power of a blackbody E_b is equal to:

$$E_b = \int_0^\infty E_{b\lambda} d\lambda = \sigma T^4 \tag{4}$$

where σ= 5.67 x 10^{-8} W/m^2 K^4 (the Stefan-Boltzmann constant).

It is important to emphasize that the same law was obtained empirically by Stefan a few years earlier.

For real bodies, the total hemispherical emissive power E can be calculated by:

$$E = \int_0^\infty E_\lambda(\lambda) d\lambda \tag{5}$$

where $E_\lambda = \pi I_\lambda(\lambda)$.

and E_λ is the spectral emissive power of a real body. For further details, see Incropera and DeWitt (1996).

Emissivity is a function of material and can vary with the wavelength and with the temperature. Thus, spectral emissivity $\varepsilon(\lambda)$ can be used to calculate the total emissivity of a real body ε, which is defined as its total hemispherical emissive power at temperature T, compared with the total hemispherical emissive power of a blackbody at the same temperature:

$$\varepsilon(T) = \frac{E(T)}{E_b(T)} = \frac{\int_0^\infty \varepsilon(\lambda) E_{b\lambda}(\lambda) d\lambda}{\sigma T^4} \tag{6}$$

Infrared Portion of the Electromagnetic Spectrum

In 1800, Sir William Herschel was the first to detect and announce the existence of the infrared portion of the spectrum. He did not use the term infrared region but referred to "invisible rays" or "the rays that occasion heat". In 1840, Herschel's son, John, developed a radiation-detection process based on the differential evaporation of a thin film of oil. He also showed that optical materials had a different transparency to infrared radiation. Conventional optical glass had a limited transparency in infrared radiation. But he also discovered that rock salt is almost transparent to infrared. Today we know that over 100 optical materials have useful transparency in parts of this section of the spectrum, amongst which are germanium and some fine plastics (Hudson, 1969).

John Herschel also "showed that there was a satisfactory detector for investigating the new region of the spectrum; raised provocative questions concerning the basic similarity between light and heat; and showed that there were significant differences in the way various materials transmit light and heat" (Hudson, 1969).

In 1860, Kirchhoff proposed that good absorbers are good radiators. He was also the first to propose the term blackbody (Hudson, 1969).

As cited above, the infrared portion of the electromagnetic spectrum begins at a wavelength of 0.7 and extends to 1000 μm.

The IR part of the electromagnetic spectrum can be divided into four regions:

- NIR – *Near Infrared*, from 0.75 to 3 μm;
- MIR – *Middle Infrared*, from 3 to 6 μm;
- FIR – *Far Infrared*, from 6 to 15 μm;
- XIR - *Extreme Infrared*, from 15 to 1000 μm.

The first three regions are regions in which the Earth's atmosphere is relatively transparent. In the last one, the atmosphere is essentially opaque.

The region from 8 to 14µm is normally called thermal infrared, as it contains the region where we find the peak emission from a body with a temperature of between -50°C to 50°C.

The energy of the IR part of the spectrum can produce molecular vibrations that result in heating the body caused by the vibrational activity of the molecules (HyperPhysics, 2019) (Fig.2).

Figure 2. Influence of IR radiation (HyperPhysics, 2019)

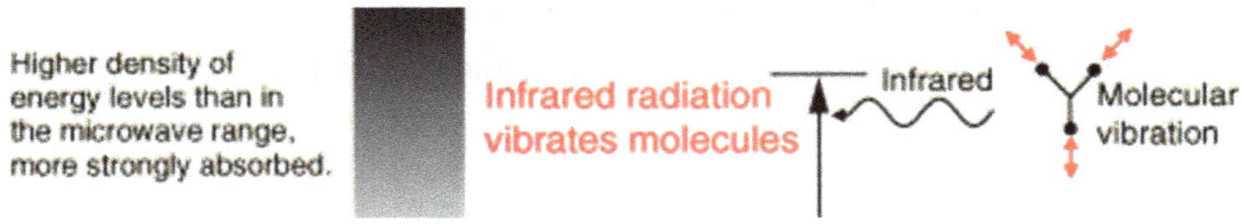

The human body is very transparent to radio waves. Microwaves, infrared, and visible light are absorbed more. UV radiation is absorbed in a thin layer of the skin. The human body becomes transparent again to electromagnetic waves with shorter wavelength, like X-Rays. It absorbs only a small fraction of the radiation, but this is enough to cause strong ionization effects (Figure 3).

Infrared cameras measure skin temperature by using the natural infrared radiation emitted by the human body (Lozano III & Hassanipour, 2019). At 37°C the human body emits heat, as shown in Figure 4. The radiation emitted by the human body is maximum at a wavelength between 9 and 10µm. The emissivity of the human body is near that of the blackbody. This emissivity was measured empirically and it is around 0.98 in the spectral band that is between 1 and 1410µm.

Infrared Technology and Infrared Cameras

Infrared technology began to be developed during the First World War. Military security then protected and made access to the technical details difficult. Measurements in the infrared region are calculated by using methods of radiometry, the science of measuring radiant energy. Radiometers absorb some of the energy from a source and convert it into another form of energy e.g., electrical, thermal or chemical energy. The conversion devices are called detectors and include radiation thermocouple, bolometer, photocell and photographic plate.

Until the 1990s, IR cameras had a low number of IR photosensitive detectors. The cameras were then cooled scanning systems and to operate them cryogenic temperatures were required. Many types of IR detectors are available nowadays. Arrays of microbolometers enable uncooled systems to be developed

Figure 3. Radiation and the human body (HyperPhysics, 2019)

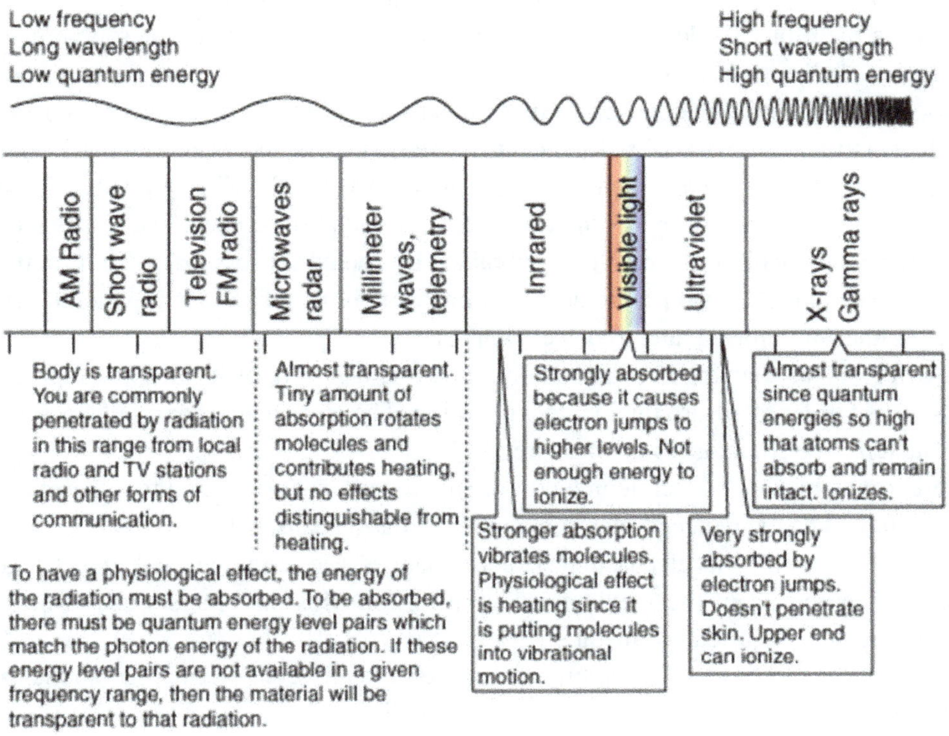

Figure 4. Typical IR detector materials and the emission of radiation from the human body (Lozano & Hassanipour, 2019)

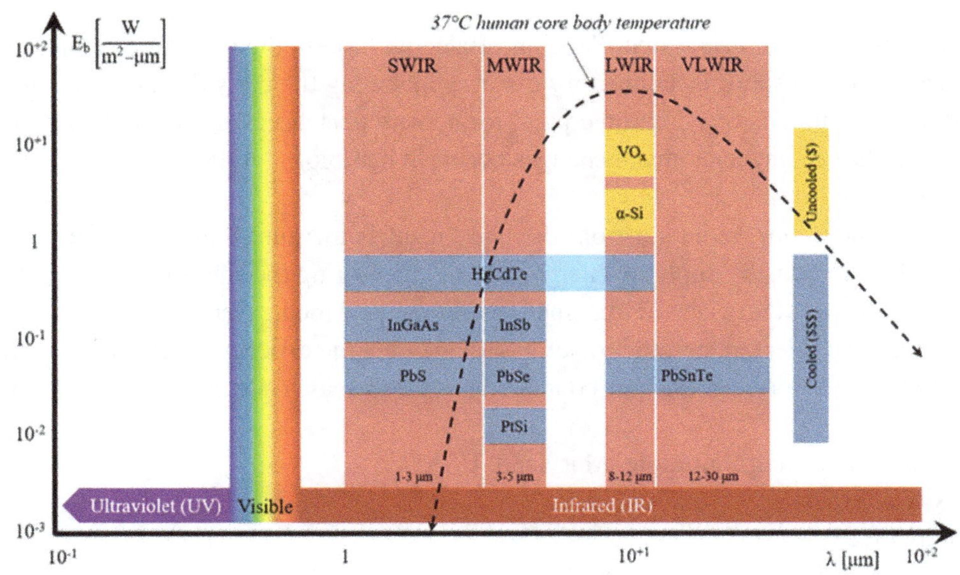

and the new systems are compact and low power. They are fabricated on top of silicon integrated circuitry and designed to measure the changes in the electrical resistance of each pixel in the array. The silicon-based circuitry is therefore an electrical and a mechanical interface for the microbolometer (Norton, Horn, Pelleggrino, & Perconti, 2008).

A microbolometer is an individual sensor that changes its electrical resistance when it is heated, including by IR radiation. It consists of a silicon chip, covered with a fine vanadium layer. These systems are very sensitive and they are able to detect changes as small as 50mK (FLIR Systems, 2004). They are compact, cheap, and consume less energy than detectors that need to be cooled. The disadvantage of using them is that they do not achieve the resolution obtained by cooled sensors made from semiconductors.

They can be used in night vision cameras (for military or civil applications), to identify fire spots, in satellites for weather monitoring, and to detect skin cancer.

Thermal detectors have an absorber and a temperature sensor or transducer. The absorber must have a high emissivity in order to absorb the incident radiation. The electrical property of the sensor must be sensitive to the temperature range to be measured.

The absorber may be a metal, semiconductor or superconductor connected to a thermal reservoir at a fixed temperature. The incidence of electromagnetic radiation causes the temperature of the absorber to increase and, consequently, its electrical resistance changes. Measurement of the electrical resistance can provide information about the incident radiation power. Most bolometers use semiconductor or superconducting materials instead of metals.

Thermal cameras have sensors that capture the emitted and reflected thermal radiations from bodies. Their optical lenses can be made of quartz, CaF2, Ge and Si.

Systems that use image converters are active systems. Systems must illuminate the target and then detect the radiation reflected. Passive systems do not emit radiation and measure the radiation emitted naturally by the target. IR cameras are passive systems.

Use of Infrared Cameras in Medical Applications

According to Diakides, Diakides, Lupo, Paul, and Balcerak (2006), there are three major areas where IR cameras can be very useful: inflammatory diseases including the early detection of cardiovascular diseases; arthritis, rheumatism and chronic pain; for neovascular diseases such as cancer. IR cameras can aid diagnoses before any anatomical changes occur; in neurology, an IR camera can detect regions where blood does not flow.

In passive thermography, radiation from the body itself is measured. In active thermography, the process is based on exciting by applying energy to it and measuring the subsequent thermal response.

The same authors state that today IR imaging is used in several medical areas such as oncology (breast and skin), vascular disorders, respiratory disorders and testing the efficacy of drugs and therapies. The following institutions in North America are conducting further research into IR Imaging and/or are using it:

- John Hopkins Hospital, Baltimore, Maryland, USA;
- University of Houston;
- University of Texas;
- NIH - National Institute of Health, Bethesda, Maryland, USA.
- And, specifically for breast cancer:
- EHH Breast Cancer and Treatment Center, Baton Rouge, LA;

- Ville Marie Oncology Research Center, Montreal, Canada.

However, note that the Ville Marie Center, which is often cited by researchers investigating breast cancer, does not have any information on breast thermography on its site: as at October, 08th, 2019 (Montreal Breast Center, 2019).

There are other countries that conduct research on the topic: China, Japan, Korea, United Kingdom, Germany, Austria, Poland and Italy. For example, in Japan there are around 1500 hospitals that use IR routinely.

Diakides et al. (2006) also say that there is a good acceptance by the medical community worldwide of IR technology. The research interests of the authors of this chapter focus on blood perfusion, breast cancer, dermatology, pain, open heart surgery, and sports medicine. They recall institutions such as the Cancer Institute Hospital (for breast cancer), University of Tokyo, Toho University and about forty other medical institutions in Japan. But currently there are no references to IR Imaging on the home pages of these institutions (Cancer Institute Hospital of JFCR, 2019; Global Cancer Control, 2019).

Faculty and student researchers at Rochester Institute of Technology, NY, USA and physicians from the Rochester Regional Health System (RRHS), developed a non-invasive process using infrared imaging to better detect cancerous tumors. The team improved an imaging option that is both comfortable for the patient and reliable (Medical Xpress, 2019). They emphasize that today the technique is more sensitive and can show more details in the image. Moreover, examinations are fast (they take about 20 min) compared to magnetic resonance imaging (MRI) which can take 45 min. Also, they suggest that further studies are needed to put this technique into practice.

Acquiring IR images is only part of the whole process. This group uses advanced computer calculations to better understand the problem under analysis. They can predict the location of tumors and their growth. These calculations give information about tumor types, location, and size which can help physicians to determine whether, how and when to make interventions. Information on the home page affirms that a highly scientific approach with advanced mathematical tools is being used.

In Toronto (CA), there is a medical service (Thermography Clinic Inc, 2019) that uses thermography to perform medical analyses, especially for breast cancer. Some patients have been attended to for up to 12 years. There is also a mobile service for companies with a large number of women employees. When companies use this service, these employees can be examined at their workplace, thereby reducing the time they need to take off work.

In the United Kingdom, EBME Services is a company that offers medical services (EBME & Clinical Engineering Articles, 2019) which uses some applications of IR techniques to analyze breast pathologies, extra-cranial vessel disease, lower extremity vessel diseases, and arthritis. But the site does not link their affirmations to the literature.

In the USA, there is a private medical service, the United Breast Cancer Foundation which has a program of breast screening (United Breast Cancer Foundation, 2019). The site lists many of the advantages of using thermography, such as:

- an abnormal infrared image is also the single most important marker of high risk for developing breast cancer;
- it is 8 times more significant than a first order family history of the disease;
- a persistent abnormal thermogram carries a 22x higher risk of future breast cancer;

- when added to a woman's regular breast health checkups, a 61% increased survival rate has been realized;
- when used as part of a multimodal approach (clinical examination + mammography + thermography) 95% of early stage cancers will be detected.

The medical service emphasizes that although thermography is also a physiological examination, it does not replace the traditional exams. Moreover, a combination of breast self-exams, physician exams, thermography, mammography and ultrasound together provide the latest detection system available

MEDICAL APPLICATIONS OF THE THERMOGRAPHY TECHNIQUES

In this section we will review the state of the art of medical thermographic applications over the past five years, especially their use as a promising technique for the early detection of breast cancer and other abnormalities of the breast. This review will consider the most important databases such as Springer Link, the IEEE Xplore Digital Library and PubMed.

Graphical analyses should be undertaken to evaluate the rate per year at which studies on such applications have been published in the period considered; what the most relevant topic was and; what different techniques were used for classification, for example.

The study of heat transfer in living tissues is of great importance, because temperature is a relevant parameter in the maintenance of life. Historically, body temperature has proven to be a good indicator of health and, since 400 BC, it has been used for clinical diagnosis (Houdas & Ring, 1982; Ring, 2007 as cited in Lahiri, Bagavathiappan, Jayakumar, & Philip, 2012).

In 1936, Hardy described the physiological role of the emission of infrared radiation by the human body and he established the importance of diagnosis based on the temperature measured by the infrared technique, which led to thermography being used in the medical sciences (Hardy & Muschenheim, 1936).

Already in 1936, Barnes demonstrated that thermograms can provide information on physical anomalies and thus be useful for diagnosing various diseases (Barnes, 1963). However, the first use of infrared thermography in medicine was reported only in 1960 due to the unavailability of quality equipment and the lack of technicians' practical knowledge (Ring, 2010). Since then, infrared thermography has shown great potential in this area and its use has been growing and is becoming widespread.

In recent years, published studies related to thermography applied to medicine have shown its versatility as a screening tool, for clinical evaluation, for surgical/postoperative support or for diagnosis in different medical areas. A search of the Pubmed.org database that includes publications related to the literature of biomedicine and papers in Life Science journals found that 373 studies had been published between January 2015 and July 2019. Figure 1 shows the number of studies involving thermography in the medical field that were published per year in this period. Not only do these studies show that thermography is being applied in different medical disciplines but that more and more institutions in the same country and in an increasing number of different countries are making use of thermography.

Studies involving thermography are related to: detecting breast cancer, diabetic neuropathy and vascular disorder; the study of thermoregulation; screening for fever, thermo-encephaloscopy (brain imaging); odontology; dermatology, diagnosing rheumatological and musculoskeletal diseases; diagnosing dry eye syndrome; treating liver disease and detecting liver metastasis; intestinal ischemia; kidney transplants; treating heart disease; making clinical evaluations in various areas of medicine; applications in gynecol-

Figure 5. Number of studies published between Jan 2015 and July 2019

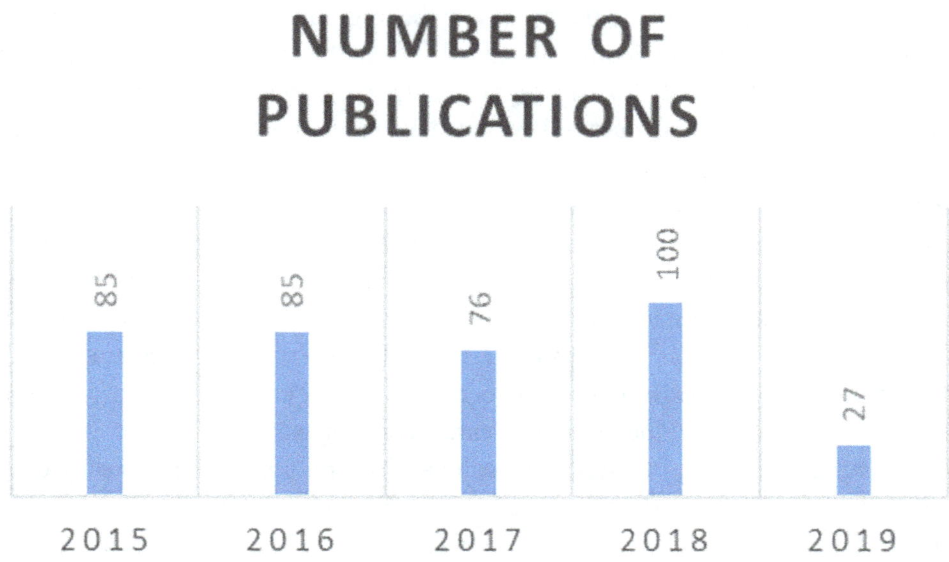

ogy and; assessing recovery from skin burns. Thermographic images have also been used in treatment with acupuncture, cryotherapy, forensic medicine, plastic surgery and assessing radiation damage in the human body (Ammer & Ring, 2006; Jung et al., 2003 as cited in Lahiri et al., 2012).

When monitoring thermoregulation processes using thermography, Lahiri, Bagavathiappan, Soumya, Jayakumar, and Philip (2015) investigated the local raising of the temperature of the cheek and ear region due to using cellular devices. The authors observed that the temperature of a device increases exponentially when it is switched off but is simultaneously receiving an electric charge. This temperature may rise even more depending on the size of the battery of the phone. The temperature of the cheek and ear peaked when the mobile phone kept in contact with these parts of the body and whenever it was being recharged and used at the same time during a phone call. Some results showed that the increase in skin temperature due to using devices exceeded the 1° C limit value, which, according to the researchers, may lead to health problems because the homeothermic system does not respond well to variations in temperature beyond this value. Thus, to reduce the increase in skin temperature, they suggested that using mobile phones during phone calls be performed in non-contact mode by using earphones, for example.

In order to prevent infectious disease pandemics quickly, effective screening techniques are required. Using neck and face thermograms, Nguyen et al. (2010) inferred that, besides being sensitive, thermography is a fast method and does not require contact with the patient's skin to monitor fever. High body temperature is one of the most common symptoms in many diseases, including infectious ones. Therefore, this method becomes a powerful tool for performing an initial screening of a certain group of people (NG, 2005). Nishiura and Kamyia (2011) used an infrared thermoscanner to screen passengers at Narita International Airport in Japan during the health crisis generated by the Influenza A (H1N1) virus. Similarly, Furuichi, Makie, Honma, Isoda, and Miyake (2015) recommended using this equipment to aid the prompt control of chikungunya and dengue.

Individuals with diabetes may be hospitalized due to vascular complications in the extremities of the body. The main causes of these complications are the decrease in blood irrigation (vascular disease) and loss of sensitivity (neuropathy). These factors lead to changes in the surface temperature of the skin and, for this reason, thermography becomes an excellent tool for diagnosing these dysfunctions. Hosaki et al. (2002) investigated peripheral circulation in a diabetic group by using thermal imaging and observed that temperature gradients, indicating abnormal flow in the affected regions, are correlated with clinical findings. Similarly, Liu et al. (2013) integrated a thermographic camera into the clinical routine for frequent examinations of patients' feet and designed a quantitative tool for analyzing thermograms. In this case, using thermography made it possible to identify the risk of ulcers or other complications based on the rise/ drop in temperature in the limbs evaluated.

Besides being used in studies involving individuals with a transplanted heart (Manginas et al., 2010), thermography may also assist in detecting early signs of atherosclerosis and thus act as an early indicator of heart attack. Research by Santos, Bianco, and Brioschi (2015) evaluated using this technique in the study of the endothelial function and correlated it with the risk of cardiovascular events. The results showed that there is a strong correspondence between thermographic findings (e.g. sympathetic hyperactivity and maximum ischemia temperature) and cardiovascular risk.

Gynecology is a field in which thermography can have several applications, mainly due to the fact that during pregnancy the internal female genitals undergo significant changes in the size, vascularity and volume of the uterus, thereby causing an increase in blood vessels and temperature of the area (Birnbaum & Kliot, 1964, as cited in Lahiri et al., 2012). Menczer and Eskin (1969) as cited in Lahiri et al. (2012) studied postpartum nipple pain, for example. They report that the temperature of patients in pain is higher compared to those without postpartum pain. This pain is usually caused by venous and lymphatic engorgement or filling of the acini with milk. These processes cause the increase in vascularization and temperature, which makes the application of thermography to detect these increases effective.

When planning plastic surgery, there is a need to be aware of the anatomy of the circulation of the tissues that will be mobilized. To this end, Nogueira, Nogueira and Ely (2015) proposed integrating infrared thermography with routine imaging for diagnosis, prognosis and/ or follow-up of a particular specialty. The results suggest that this technique has a very positive role in plastic surgery, and proves to be a practical, fast and effective method that can minimize tissue loss rates and improve the quality of surgical and postoperative results (e.g. follow-up of pressure ulcers).

Thermograms are also used in a complementary manner to assess disorders and injuries of the musculoskeletal system. Its use is related to identifying which part of the system is affected by a disease or injury or to assess the effectiveness of a treatment. Hildebrandt, Raschner, and Ammer (2010), for example, used thermography to evaluate repetitive knee strain injuries and patellar tendinopathy in skiers. A group of fifteen athletes was monitored. Of this group, seven athletes reported symptoms of local reactions in the knee and the others were asymptomatic. Symptomatic athletes presented mean temperature differences between the symptomatic knee and the contralateral knee of 1.4 ± 0.58 °C, while non-symptomatic athletes presented an average temperature variation between the two knees of 0.3 ± 0.61 °C.

The post-fracture phase of bone regeneration is characterized by an increase in metabolism and, consequently, in the temperature of local tissues. Based on this fact, Morasiewicz, Dudek, Orzechowski, Kulej, & Stepniewski (2008) evaluated the correlation of thermographic analysis with radiographic evidence. To do so, they followed the case of 18 patients undergoing osteogenic distraction treatment for bone lengthening with the Ilizarov external fixator. The results indicated a statistically significant correlation between bone regeneration and thermal indices. The mean values of the Spearman correlation coefficient for the tibia and femur were 0.925 ($p < 0.01$) and 0.724 ($p < 0.05$), respectively. Thermography has proven to be a valuable complement to traditional methods for diagnosing fractures that can be used to monitor and evaluate bone formation and remodeling at all stages of treatment.

In the area of physiotherapy, Trafarski, Róanski, Straburzynska-Lupa, & Korman (2008) used thermography to evaluate the effectiveness of the local cryotherapy procedure in patients with rheumatoid arthritis. To do so, they determined the thermal intensity during the procedure and the duration of the body's response to the stimulus. The procedure consisted of applying liquid nitrogen vapors or fresh air on the hand. A comparison of the temperature distribution on the surface of the hand was made at different times: before, immediately after and at certain intervals after applying the stimulus. The body's response to stimulation with liquid nitrate vapors lasted about 2 hours and, in the case of cold air, the cooling lasted for 90 minutes. Research has shown that thermography is a viable measurement technique for this procedure and is useful in evaluating the progress and monitoring of treatment.

In the prognostic assessment, it was observed that thermography can objectively and quantitatively distinguish variation in surface temperature in order to correlate with changes in the intensity of pain after therapeutic physiotherapy.

In Odontology, thermography may complement anatomical physical examination, as it presents physiological conditions in real time, according to temperature (Amorim et al., 2019). This technique can help to diagnose and plan the treatment of orofacial changes such as inflammatory and infectious processes in the orofacial region, postoperative follow-up and the routine evaluation of patients with temporomandibular dysfunction (TMD) (Haddad, Brioschi, Arita, 2012; Dibai-Filho, Costa, Packer, de Castro, & Rodrigues-Bigaton, 2015).

In a preliminary study using thermography as a complementary diagnosis for myogenic TMD the chewing muscle regions of 23 women were evaluated by lateral projections and clinical examination and were divided as follows: patients with and without the pathology. The authors found that the masseter and anterior temporal muscle regions had a lower temperature in the presence of myogenic TMD when compared to the control group. They also state that thermography is a useful, noninvasive, non-ionizing method that can assist in diagnosing this dysfunction (Haddad et al., 2014). Other areas of odontology are also involved in thermographic research, such as endodontics, periodontics, stomatology, oral pathology, implantology and oral surgery.

Overall, thermography is inexpensive, noninvasive, simple, painless, safe (without side effects), practical, and requires no contact or compression, and no radiation or venous access (Tan, Queck, Ng, & Ng, 2007). This technique enables the physiological responses of tissues to be detected, thereby providing functional information that is often evaluated better than anatomical characteristics (Wang et al., 2010). Good interpretation of the thermal image is fundamental for the correct diagnosis (Queiroz, 2014).

A RECENT REVIEW ON BREAST THERMOGRAPHY APPLIED TO DIAGNOSING BREAST CANCER

This topic describes the recent evolution of a thermography technique applied to diagnosing breast cancer. It includes a survey of the recent literature in this field, in the last five years.

The use of thermography as a tool for investigating breast lesions began in the 1950s when studies carried out by Ray N. Lawson found some alterations in the surface temperature of the skin of the breast due to breast cancer.

In subsequent years, several researchers published studies that recommended using thermography for breast cancer screening (Isard, Becker, Shilo, & Ostrum, 1972; Stark, & Way, 1974a; Stark, & Way, 1974b) while others rejected thermography as a screening tool (Moskowitz, Milbrath, Gartside, Ermeno, & Mandel, 1976; Nathan, Burn, & MacErlean, 1972; Moskowitz et al., 1981).

Those studies that regarded thermography favorably showed that it had potential for detecting breast cancer. However, due to the method for evaluating thermograms and inconsistencies observed in the diagnoses, this technique was not formally approved by any national authority anywhere in the world (Ng & Sudarshan, 2004). Despite these conflicting studies, in 1982, the United States Food and Drug Administration (FDA) approved the use of thermography but only as an adjunct tool to mammography.

Infrared technology has advanced significantly in the past 5 decades. In the early 1970s, thermographic cameras had a cooled detector with a resolution of approximately 100×100 and a sensitivity of approximately 0.2°C. In the nineties, new generations of thermographic cameras appeared. These IR cameras are uncooled with a 320×240 detector resolution or similar, have a temperature range of 0–500°C, sensitivity of <0°C, and 2°C accuracy. Today, an uncooled IR camera has a resolution of up to 1024×768, a temperature range of −40–2,000°C, sensitivity of <0.02°C, and 1°C accuracy (Lozano & Hassanipour, 2019).

This new IR technology coupled with machine learning techniques has allowed breast thermography to become quantitative. Several machine learning tools can be used to assess breast abnormalities in thermographic images, thus fueling a growing interest in this type of evaluation.

In this section, we undertake a systematic review of papers published from 2015 through mid-2019 that involve thermography applied to breast abnormalities. The research articles were obtained from ScienceDirect, IEEEXplore and PubMed Central databases. The keywords used were "thermography", "breast", "thermal" and "infrared" combined with the Boolean descriptor "OR". The papers were initially selected by title and then by reading the abstract so as to confirm the paper matched our criteria.

Based on these selection criteria, 59 articles that were published between 2015 and mid-2019 were identified. In this broad area, over the past five years, the average annual publication rate has been 11.8 papers. Figure 6 shows the total number of papers published annually involving breast thermography

Figure 6. Number of papers on breast thermography published annually between 2015 and mid-2019

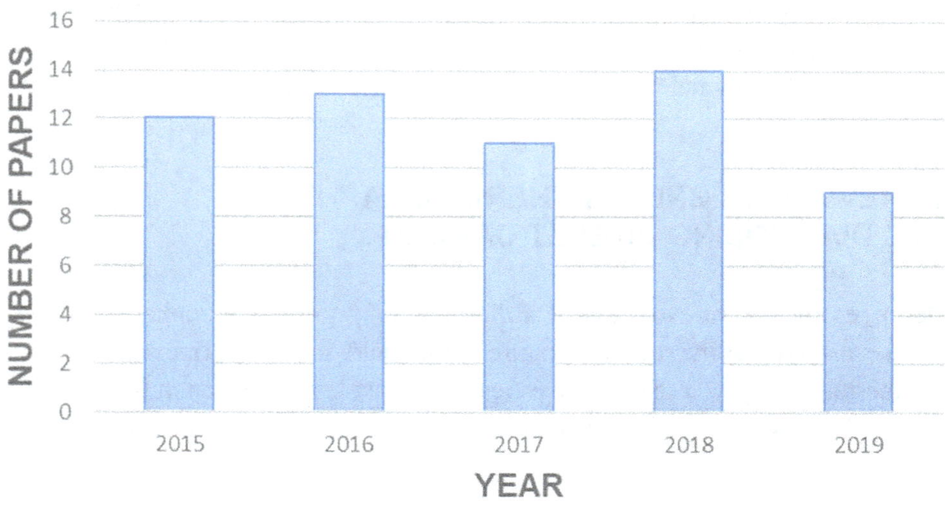

Figure 7. Main sub-areas of published papers – 2015 to mid-2019.

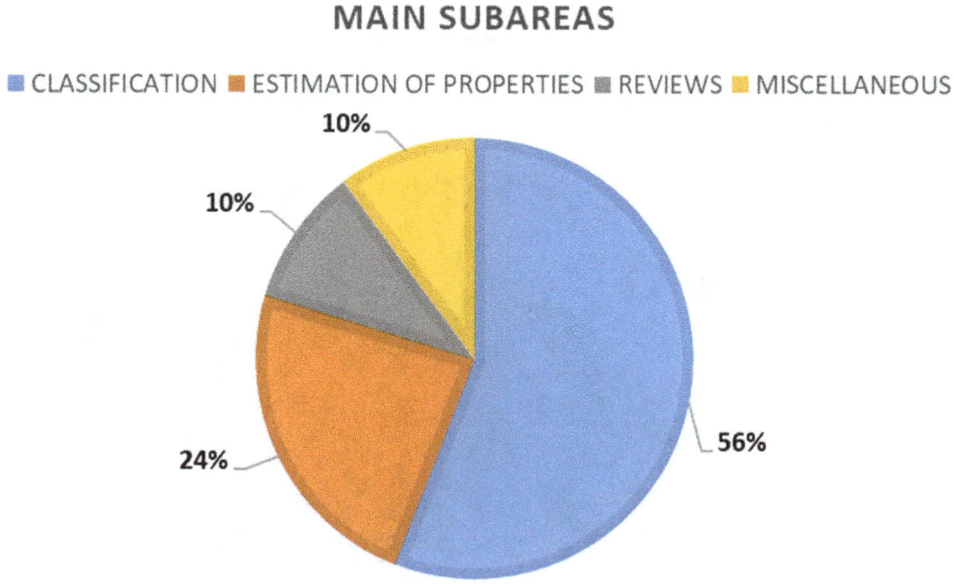

from 2015 to mid-2019, thus demonstrating a continuous interest in the subject. Papers published in this area can be further divided into sub-areas, as illustrated in Figure 7.

The main sub-areas are: Classification, Numerical modeling/Estimation of Properties and Reviews. The sub-area "Miscellaneous" shown in Figure 7 contains papers that cannot be grouped in any of the other classes.

Classification

Most of the 59 articles selected for this study focused on the classification process. In fact, fifty-five percent of all publications selected were related to classification. Many machine learning tools can be used and combined with each other to increase the efficiency of making use of the ability of thermography to identify breast abnormalities in thermograms. Furthermore, the classification process also includes some sub-steps such as segmentation and feature extraction. Many authors devote their papers to examining and refining the steps required to accomplish the task of classification. In addition, there are papers on classification which focus on comparing different trends in medical imaging.

Figure 8 is a pie chart which shows a percentage break-down of the articles placed in the category of Classification divided into four sub-areas. These are: the process of classification itself; segmentation; the extraction of features; and the comparison of thermography with other trends in medical imaging.

Segmentation

The segmentation of a medical image is the stage during which a large effort is made to delineate the structures of interest and make these stand out from the rest of the image (Bankman, 2009). The accuracy of the classification depends on the correct segmentation of the object studied (Araújo, Lima, & Souza, 2014). Around 8.33% of the papers selected for this study focused on image segmentation of the breasts.

Figure 8. Division of the category of Classification into sub-areas

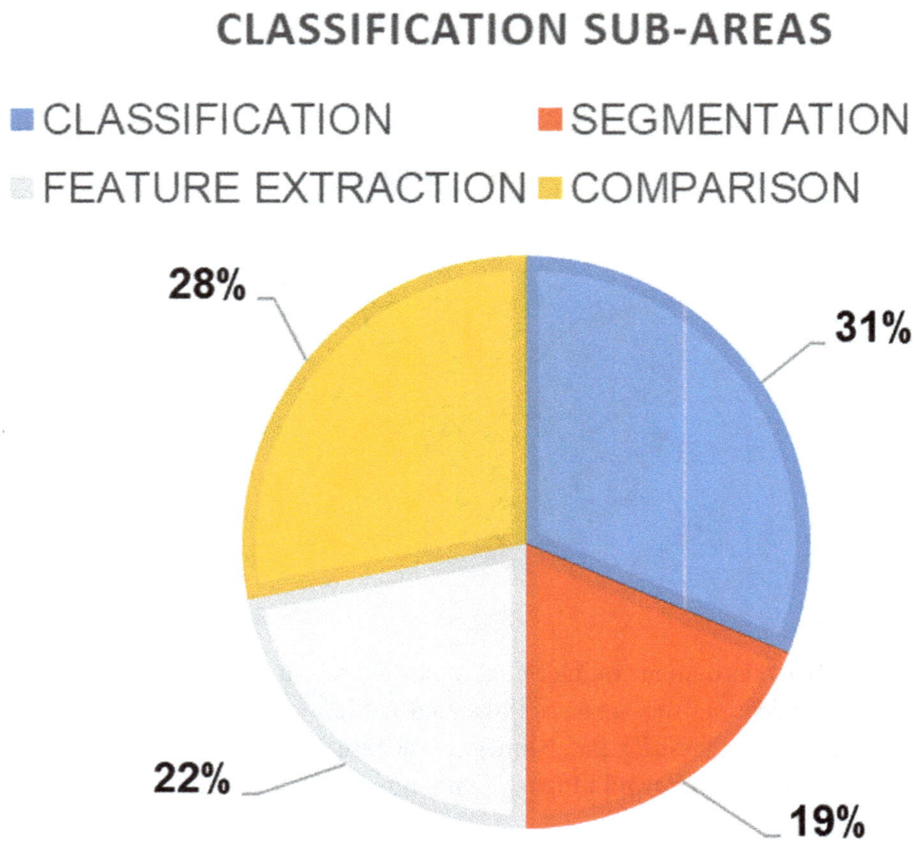

This sub-area represents 19% of the published papers placed in the category of Classification. Good segmentation can improve the task of classification and this helps diagnose breast cancer. Segmentation can be done manually or automatically. Manual segmentation is usually more accurate, but it is time-consuming, while an automated technique can be quick but inaccurate. Recently published papers have sought to improve automated breast cancer segmentation. The greatest difficulty lies in the anatomical variability of different patients' breasts and concerns the characteristics of the thermal imaging itself, which makes it difficult to detect edges in areas at the same temperature (Kermani, Samadzadehaghdam, & EtehadTavakol, 2015; Mahmoudzadeh, Montazeri, Zekri, & Sadri, 2015; Marques, Conci, Perez, Andaluz, & Mejia, 2016; Mahmoudzadeh, Zekri, Montazeri, Sadri, & Dabbagh, 2016; Garduño-Ramón, Vega-Mancilla, Morales-Henández, & Osornio-Rios, 2017; Díaz-Cortés et al., 2018)

Feature Extraction

The features extracted from the IR image are the input data that will be provided to the classifier. The main objective of feature extraction is to obtain a set of variables that can discriminate between a healthy breast and a breast with tumors or cysts. Physically, we seek to maximize the differences between the temperatures at the site of a tumor and those of the contralateral mirror image of a site that is healthy. The better these sites discriminate the problem, the better the classification results will be. Several features can be extracted from the IR image. Commonly used features are statistical measures like mean, variance, skewness, kurtosis, entropy and the histogram of each breast. Image texture also can be used as a feature. Common texture measures are run percentage, contrast, correlation, energy and homogeneity (Prabha, Suganthi, & Sujatha, 2015; Milosevic, Jankovic, & Peulic, 2015; Silva et al., 2015; Madhu, Kakileti, Venkataramani, & Jabbireddy, 2016; Sarigoz, Ertan, Topuz, Sevim, & Cihan, 2018; Kirubha, Anburajan, Venkataraman, & Menaka, 2018; Gogoi, Bhowmik, Bhattacharjee, & Ghosh, 2018). Around 22% of the papers selected for this study that were placed in the category of Classification focused on extracting features of the breast.

Classification

Data classification is the task of classifying information. This is the main step in pattern recognition techniques. In breast thermography, this step is used to determine if the patient has a healthy or an unhealthy breast. To classify a dataset into several different classes, the algorithm must be trained with a set of data with the corresponding classes. This is called a training set. Then the algorithm is tested with a different dataset from that used for training, without having prior knowledge of its property class.

Many machine learning algorithms such as Fuzzy Logic, Artificial Neural Networks, Distance Classifiers, K-NN, Decision Trees and Deep Learning techniques have been used alone or combined to classify breast abnormalities detected by thermography. This classification problem can be addressed as a binary classification (cancer and non-cancer). Recently, some papers have addressed the classification problem with more than two classes to discriminate breast pathologies (malignant, benign, cyst and healthy), which increases the complexity of the problem (Araújo et al., 2014). In this case, authors must determine a set of features that favors separating classes.

The classification problem (including its sub-steps) represents 55% of all the papers selected for our study that analyzed breast cancer detected by thermography. Although studies that evaluate segmentation and feature extraction use classification tools such as a comparison metric, this classification is not their primary focus. As to the papers that address the sub-areas of the category of Classification, the classification problem itself accounts for 31% of this category, the other sub-areas being segmentation, feature extraction and comparison.

Comparison

Thermography is considered a physiological exam, while mammography and tomography, for example, are anatomical exams. Many papers focus on comparing the results from classifying breast thermograms with those obtained for mammography or other breast screening techniques. Comparative studies between thermography, mammography, ultrasound and tomography focus on increasing the detection of cancer by adding information from different exams. Thermography alone is not suitable for detecting cancer, but the benefit derived from IR thermography is maximized when it is used as a tool to complement other conventional screening techniques (i.e., mammography, ultrasound, tomography).

Estimation of Properties/ Numerical Modeling

The breast consists of different tissues and the interaction of these different tissues inside the breast creates a non-homogeneous medium. The presence of a tumor between these tissues creates a local thermal pattern. Because IR thermography is basically a surface measurement, thermal transport between the tumor and the skin surface is a critical factor for the thermography-based detection of cancer. Some breast tumors that are small or deep may not be detectable on the surface of the skin, thus resulting in a false negative assessment. The sensitivity of thermography is relatively low for deep and small tumors (Borchartt, Conci, Lima, Resmini, & Sanchez, 2013). Therefore, the properties of a tumor, for example, size, depth, metabolic heat generation and the thermal properties of tissue, play an important role in detecting breast abnormalities by thermography (Lozano & Hassanipour, 2019).

Many authors are interested in calculating the influence of these properties on the surface temperature of the breast by designing a numerical thermal simulation. To model tissue, scientists have proposed various mathematical models to describe the behavior of this complex material. These models must consider the geometry of the breast, the size of the tumor and its location. Thermography can be used to validate simulations or as input to inverse modeling problems. The known measured temperatures are used to estimate unknown tumor properties.

This field represented 25% of all the published papers on breast thermography selected for this study.

Other Studies

10% of the articles selected do not fall into the subcategories listed above. These research papers involve studies that seek to determine medical protocols for applying thermography, creating thermographic databases, constructing phantoms for thermal breast simulation, proposing an index to estimate breast similarities and evaluating infrared thermography of the breast in the asymptomatic population (screening).

Table 1 lists the papers selected by sub-area, author's name and title.

POSSIBILITY OF USING THERMAL INFRARED IMAGES AS AN AUXILIARY TOOL TO DETECT BREAST CANCER

This topic will discuss the theoretical foundations that allow thermography to be used to validate calculated temperature profiles. Surface temperature distribution associated with the inverse heat transfer problem can be used to estimate thermophysical properties of the breast and tumors, thereby enabling thermography to be used as an auxiliary tool for detecting breast cancer.

Table 1. Papers selected that were published between 2015 and mid-2019

Authors Title of Paper Sub-area

Krawczyk, Schaefer, & Woźniak, 2015 A hybrid cost-sensitive ensemble for imbalanced breast thermogram classification CLASSIFICATION

Zadeh, Haddadnia, Ahmadinejad, & Baghdadi, 2015 Assessing the potential of thermal imaging in recognition of breast cancer CLASSIFICATION

Kirubha, Anburajan, Venkataraman, & Menaka, 2015 Comparison of PET–CT and thermography with breast biopsy in evaluation of breast cancer: a case study COMPARISON

Zore, Filipović-Zore, Stanec, Batinjan, & Matejčić, 2015 Association of clinical, histopathological and immunohistochemical prognostic factors of invasive breast tumors and thermographic findings CLASSIFICATION

Souza et al., 2015 Reference breast temperature: proposal of an equation MISCELLANEOUS

Han, Shi, Liang, Wang, & Li, 2015 A simple and efficient method for breast cancer diagnosis based on infrared thermal imaging ESTIMATION OF PROPERTIES

Prabha et al., 2015 An approach to analyze the breast tissues in infrared images using nonlinear adaptive level sets and Riesz transform features. FEATURE EXTRACTION

Kermani et al., 2015 Automatic color segmentation of breast infrared images using a gaussian mixture model SEGMENTATION

Mahmoudzadeh et al., 2015 Extended hidden Markov model for optimized segmentation of breast thermography images SEGMENTATION

Milosevic et al., 2015 Comparative analysis of breast cancer detection in mammograms and thermograms FEATURE EXTRACTION

Silva et al., 2015 Thermal signal analysis for breast cancer risk verification FEATURE EXTRACTION

Venkataramani et al., 2015 Semi-automated breast cancer tumor detection with thermographic video imaging COMPARISON

Silva et al.,2016 Hybrid analysis for indicating patients with breast cancer using temperature time series CLASSIFICATION

Rastghalam & Pourghassem, 2016 Breast cancer detection using MRF-based probable texture feature and decision-level fusion-based classification using HMM on thermography images CLASSIFICATION

Weum, Mercer, & de Weerd, 2016 Evaluation of dynamic infrared thermography as an alternative to CT angiography for perforator mapping in breast reconstruction: a clinical study COMPARISON

Prasad et al., 2016 Evaluation of efficacy of thermographic breast imaging in breast cancer: a pilot study CLASSIFICATION

Wu, Kuo, Chen, Tsai, & Wang, 2016 The association of infrared imaging findings of the breast with prognosis in breast cancer patients: an observational cohort study MISCELLANEOUS

Saniei, Setayeshi, Akbari, & Navid, 2016 Parameter estimation of breast tumour using dynamic neural network from thermal pattern ESTIMATION OF PROPERTIES

Hossain, Abdelaal, & Mohammadi, 2016 Thermogram assessment for tumor parameter estimation considering body geometry ESTIMATION OF PROPERTIES

Wahab et al., 2016 Thermal distribution analysis of three-dimensional tumor-embedded breast models with different breast density compositions ESTIMATION OF PROPERTIES

Hossain & Mohammadi, 2016 Tumor parameter estimation considering the body geometry by thermography ESTIMATION OF PROPERTIES

Amri, Pulko, & Wilkinson, 2016 Potentialities of steady-state and transient thermography in breast tumour depth detection: a numerical study ESTIMATE OF PROPERTIES

Marques et al., 2016 An approach for automatic segmentation of thermal imaging in Computer Aided Diagnosis SEGMENTATION

Mahmoudzadeh et al., 2016 Directional SUSAN image boundary detection of breast thermogram SEGMENTATION

Madhu et al., 2016 Extraction of medically interpretable features for classification of malignancy in breast thermography FEATURE EXTRACTION

Garduño-Ramón et al., 2017 Supportive Noninvasive Tool for the Diagnosis of Breast Cancer Using a Thermographic Camera as Sensor SEGMENTATION

Gourd, 2017 Breast thermography alone no substitute for mammography COMPARISON

Kandlikar et al., 2017 Infrared imaging technology for breast cancer detection – current status, protocols and new directions REVIEW

Bhowmik et al., 2017 Designing of Ground-Truth-Annotated DBT-TU-JU Breast Thermogram Database Toward Early Abnormality Prediction MISCELLANEOUS

Hatwar & Herman, 2017 Inverse method for quantitative characterization of breast tumors from surface temperature data ESTIMATION OF PROPERTIES

Rastgar-Jazi & Mohammadi, 2017 Parameters sensitivity assessment and heat source localization using infrared imaging techniques ESTIMATE OF PROPERTIES

Rahmatinia & Fahimi, 2017 Magneto-thermal modeling of biological tissues: a step toward breast cancer detection MISCELLANEOUS

Avila-Castro et al., 2017 Thorax thermographic simulator for breast pathologies MISCELLANEOUS

Ramírez-Torres et al., 2017 The role of malignant tissue on the thermal distribution of cancerous breast ESTIMATION OF PROPERTIES

de Jesus Guirro et al., 2017 Accuracy and Reliability of Infrared Thermography in Assessment of the Breasts of Women Affected by Cancer CLASSIFICATION

Araújo, Souza, Lima, & Filho, 2017 An interval prototype classifier based on a parameterized distance applied to breast thermographic images CLASSIFICATION

Díaz-Cortés et al., 2018 A multi-level thresholding method for breast thermograms analysis using dragonfly algorithm SEGMENTATION

Sarigoz et al., 2018 Role of digital infrared thermal imaging in the diagnosis of breast mass: a pilot study: diagnosis of breast mass by thermography FEATURE EXTRACTION

Kirubha et al., 2018 A case study on asymmetrical texture features comparison of breast thermogram and mammogram in normal and breast cancer subject FEATURE EXTRACTION

de Vasconcelos, dos Santos, & Lima, 2018 Analysis of methods of classification of breast thermographic images to determine their viability in the early breast cancer detection CLASSIFICATION

Gogoi et al., 2018 Singular value-based characterization and analysis of thermal patches for early breast abnormality detection FEATURE EXTRACTION

Milosevic, Jankovic, Milenkovic, & Stojanov, 2018 Early diagnosis and detection of breast cancer COMPARISON

Migowski et al., 2018 Guidelines for early detection of breast cancer in Brazil. II - New national recommendations, main evidence, and controversies COMPARISON

Mambou, Maresova, Krejcar, Selamat, & Kuca, 2018 Breast cancer detection using infrared thermal imaging and a deep learning model CLASSIFICATION

Alikhassi, Hamidpour, Firouzmand, Navid, & Eghbal, 2018 Prospective comparative study assessing role of ultrasound versus thermography in breast cancer detection COMPARISON

Neal, Flynt, Jeffries, & Helvie, 2018 Breast imaging outcomes following abnormal thermography COMPARISON

Prabha & Sujatha, 2018 Proposal of index to estimate breast similarities in thermograms using fuzzy C means and anisotropic diffusion filter based on fuzzy C means clustering MISCELLANEOUS

Espíndola, Bezerra, Santos, & Lima, 2018 Estimating breast thermophysical parameters by the use of mapping surface temperatures measured by infrared images ESTIMATION OF PROPERTIES

Zhou & Herman, 2018 Optimization of skin cooling by computational modeling for early thermographic detection of breast cancer ESTIMATION OF PROPERTIES

Yassin, Omran, El Houby, & Allam, 2018 Machine learning techniques for breast cancer computer-aided diagnosis using different image modalities: a systematic review REVIEW

Iljaž, Wrobel, Hriberšek, & Marn, 2018 Numerical modelling of skin tumor tissue with temperature-dependent properties for dynamic thermography ESTIMATION OF PROPERTIES

Raghavendra et al., 2019 Computer-aided diagnosis for the identification of breast cancer using thermogram images: a comprehensive review REVIEW

Figueiredo et al., 2019 Breast tumor localization using skin surface temperatures from a 2D anatomic model without knowledge of the thermophysical properties ESTIMATION OF PROPERTIES

Zuluaga-Gomez, Zerhouni, Al Masry, Devalland, & Varnier, 2019 A survey of breast cancer screening techniques: thermography and electrical impedance tomography COMPARISON

Lozano & Hassanipour, 2019 Infrared imaging for breast cancer detection: an objective review of foundational studies and its proper role in breast cancer screening REVIEW

Gogoi, Majumdar, Bhowmik, & Ghosh, 2019 Evaluating the efficiency of infrared breast thermography for early breast cancer risk prediction in asymptomatic population MISCELLANEOUS

Gonzalez-Hernandez et al., 2019 Technology, application and potential of dynamic breast thermography for the detection of breast cancer REVIEW

Marchena-Menéndez, Ramírez-Torres, Penta, Rodríguez-Ramos, & Merodio, 2019 Macroscopic thermal profile of heterogeneous cancerous breasts. A three-dimensional multiscale analysis ESTIMATION OF PROPERTIES

Singh & Singh, 2019 Role of image thermography in early breast cancer detection - Past, present and future REVIEW

Introduction

The first reports on using thermobiology may have been written by Hippocrates about 480 BC. After this discovery, research continued and clinical observations have proven that human body temperatures are, indeed, indicative of normal and abnormal physiological processes (Amalu, Hobbins, Head, & Elliot, 2006).

The first medical diagnosis using infrared imaging was made by Lawson (1956), when he found that the temperature of the skin over a tumor in the breast was higher than normal tissue. He also showed that the venous blood that drains the malignant tumor is often warmer than that supplied by the arterial system. After the first discoveries made by Lawson, several technological advances were made in infrared detection systems.

In 1965, Gershen-Cohen, Haberman, and Brueschke (1965) as cited in Amalu et al. (2006), introduced using infrared imaging for diagnosing cancer in the USA. Using a Barnes infrared camera, they had, in the 4,000 cancer cases analyzed, a sensitivity of 94% and a false positive rate of 6%.

Spitalier et al. (1982) as cited in Amalu et al. (2006) examined 61,000 women using thermography over a 10-year period. The authors observed that thermography detected 91% of non-palpable malignant tumors. Gautherie (1980), based on a population of 85,000 patients, showed that the sensitivity of thermography was 90%.

Thomassin (1984) conducted a study with a group of 4,000 patients, all of whom had been diagnosed as having breast cancer. In this group, the author observed 130 carcinomas with a diameter of 3 - 5 mm. Of the 130 cases, thermography detected 50% of early cancer cases, while mammography identified only 10% of cases. The accuracy of the test is similar or better than that indicated by self-exams.

In 1986, in a study by Nyirjesy et al. as cited in Amalu et al. (2006), the authors had three groups of patients: 4,716 patients who had been diagnosed as having a carcinoma; 3,305 patients with a benign tumor and 8,757 patients with healthy breasts, totaling 16,778 patients. They compared the clinical examinations, mammograms and thermographs of all these patients all of whom had been diagnosed with breast cancer. The results showed that clinical examinations had a sensitivity of 75% in detecting all tumors and 50% in tumors smaller than 1 cm. Mammography had an average sensitivity of 80% and thermography had an average sensitivity of 88% (85% in tumors smaller than 1 cm). The authors suggested that none of these techniques is sufficiently accurate to be used alone for detecting breast cancer.

According to Gautherie (1983), there is a symmetry regarding the temperature distribution in healthy breasts and this symmetry can be observed for long periods of time. Thermal variations can be associated with the menstrual cycle and with a possible pregnancy. Such physiological changes somehow affect both breasts. When the breast presents a change, this symmetry is lost and changes in temperature levels begin to occur. In the case of tumors, the changes occur due to the excessive production of nitric oxide (NO) by cancer cells. This oxide is one of those responsible for a new vascularization (angiogenesis) near the region of the tumor and the main contributory factor to vasodilation present in angiogenesis. (Miles et al., 1995).

The new vascularization raises local blood flow, causing the temperature of the tumor region to rise, thus prompting cancer cells to generate more heat than normal cells. In breast tumors, this rise in the local temperature can be observed on the surface of the breast by thermography, and the difference in temperature between healthy and carcinogenic tissue can be expressed when there is a 2 to 3°C increase in the local temperature on the surface of the skin below which the tumor is located (Harris, Greeining, & Aichroth, 1966, as cited in Hu, Gupta, Gore, & Xu, 2004). In this region, the blood perfusion rate and the generation of metabolic heat are higher than in a healthy breast (Gautherie, 1980). Thermography, therefore, is closely linked to patients' blood perfusion, thus reflecting the microcirculatory dynamics of the surface of the patient's skin. Therefore, it is a physiological test, while other forms of diagnosis, such as mammography and ultrasound, are anatomical tests (Ng & Sudarshan, 2004; Diakides, Diakides, Lupo, Paul, & Balcerak, 2006; Schaefer, Z ´Avisek, & Nakashima, 2009; EtehadTavakol, Chandran, Ng, & Kafieh, 2013; Borchartt et al., 2013).

The use of processing techniques applied to thermographic images has grown in recent decades, and thermograms have started to be processed to emphasize regions with hotspots, which are indicative of some kind of breast disease (Schaefer et al., 2009). The resulting images show that there are different distribution characteristics for different classes of image, such as malignant, benign and normal classes. These differences are often subtle and apparent only to a trained eye. Automated classification of thermograms then became of great interest to screening for breast cancer (EtehadTavakol et al., 2013).

Ng and Kee (2008) analyzed thermographic images of the breast using artificial neural networks, biostatistical methods, including linear regression and receiver operating characteristic (ROC) methods to evaluate medical diagnosis. The proposed technique presented an accuracy rate of 80.95%, with a sensitivity of 100% and 70.6% of specificity in identifying breast cancer.

Schaefer et al. (2009) analyzed thermograms of the breast to detect cancer. The authors used statistical characteristics extracted from thermograms in conjunction with a fuzzy classification system based on a diagnostic rule to quantify bilateral differences between the left and right breasts. With a data set of about 146 thermograms (29 malignant and 117 benign) they achieved a classification that was 80% accurate. Sensitivity and specificity were also around 80% accurate at detecting a malignant tumor.

Serrano, Lima, Melo, and Conci (2010) presented a study on using fractal measurements in thermal imaging for diagnosing early stage breast cancer. The methodology is based on lacunarity and machine learning techniques. The results showed that the method is able to separate normal breasts from those with some type of alteration.

Dumansky, Lyakh, Gorshkov, Gurianov, and Prihodchenko (2012) analyzed the feasibility of applying the Hurst exponent algorithm to reveal any difference between normal thermograms and those that show a malignant tumor. The results showed the proposed algorithm can be used to classify malignant tumors.

Acharya, Ng, Tan, and Sree (2012) evaluated the feasibility of using thermographic images as a potential tool for detecting breast cancer. The authors used 50 thermograms, 25 of which were normal and 25 showed malignant tumors. All images were from patients at the General Hospital of Singapore. Texture characteristics were extracted from the co-occurrence matrix. These characteristics, after being normalized, fed the SVM (Support Vector Machine) classifier in order to classify breast conditions automatically. The results showed an accuracy of 88.1%, sensitivity of 85.71% and specificity of 90.48%.

Etehad, Tavakol et al. (2013) used invariant bispectral features to detect breast cancer using thermographic images. The authors showed that higher order characteristics of the spectrum were able to differentiate between different classes, such as normal breast, malignant and benign tumors. First of all, the thermograms were converted to rectangular images of hot regions using image processing. Invariant bispectral features are extracted from random projections of the images. The results showed that thermogram images perform well at discriminating between malignant and benign cases. Malignant cases were detected with 95% accuracy in a test set of 32 cases (9 malignant, 12 benign and 11 normal).

Thermographic Images and Numerical Simulations

Thermographic images in conjunction with numerical simulations can be an auxiliary tool for detecting breast cancer (Ng & Sudarshan, 2001, 2004). According to Jiang, Zhan, and Loew (2011), numerical modeling techniques can quantify complex relationships between thermal behaviors and the physiological conditions of the breast. Therefore, it can be concluded that the geometric modeling, which is needed for computer modeling, is extremely important in the attempt to find factors that relate to a possible diagnosis of any alteration in the breast. However, few studies represent the breast with real geometries, but, instead, use simplified geometries.

When attempting a real reconstruction of the geometry of the breast, several surrogate geometries have been used by the research group (Biomechanical Engineering Group -UFPE). They were initially obtained from a semi-sphere (Bezerra, 2007), then from a phantom (Santos, 2009), and from silicone prostheses of the external breast (Viana, 2010). Then, in the search for custom geometries for each patient, silicone prostheses were used, but adapted to the individual curves obtained from thermographic images (Viana, 2016) and three-dimensional volumes of the breast obtained directly from the curves provided by each patient's thermography (Melo, Queiroz, Bezerra, & Lima, 2019). The latter are getting closer and closer to the real geometry of each patient's breasts, volume errors being negligible. Figure 9 shows examples of substitute geometries obtained by the group.

Figure 9. Substitute Geometries

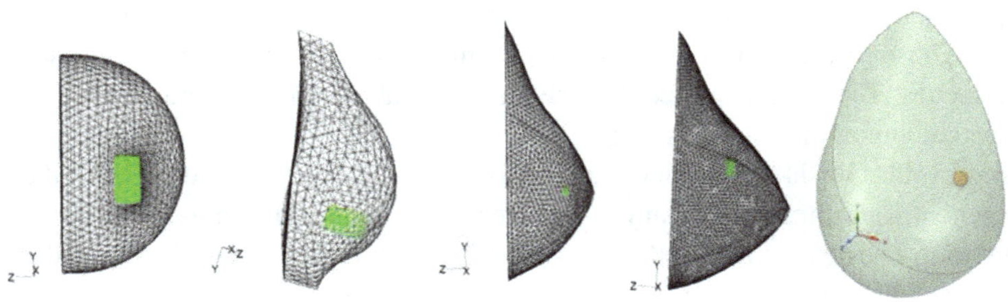

The external prostheses used are of models SG-419 and SG-420 and in sizes 1, 2, 4, 6, 8, 10 and 12, manufactured by Ortho Pauher. All prostheses were donated by the manufacturer.

Some papers that used numerical simulations in breasts are commented on below.

The first attempts to simulate breast temperatures due to the subcutaneous sources of heat were based on analytical solutions (Jiang et al., 2011). Chen et al. as cited in Jiang et al. (2011) performed two-dimensional numerical simulations showing that the temperature of the breast is very sensitive to blood perfusion rate of tissues. Since then, several studies with three-dimensional models have been conducted and are discussed below.

Osman and Afify (1984) developed a three-dimensional mathematical model to calculate the normal breast temperature distribution in a healthy breast using the Finite Element Method, in which the breast was modeled as a semi-sphere. Osman and Afify (1988) developed a mathematical model to simulate a breast that has a malignant tumor. This model takes into account the effect of the size of the tumor and its location on the production of metabolic heat. The tumor was modeled as an important which generated heat equal to the total production of metabolic heat. Based on the results obtained from the simulation, the authors state that the temperature profile of the surface of the abnormal breast may not be directly related to the presence of the tumor.

Ng and Sudarshan (2001) conducted three-dimensional numerical simulations under cold stress, incorporating the behavior of a vasomotor. They used the Finite Element Method to solve the Pennes equation in steady and transient states. To investigate the effect of cold stress, they considered skin temperature to be the same as room temperature. They reached this value after running a numerical simulation considering an ambient temperature of 21°C and obtained a temperature of 27°C on the surface of the skin. As Pennes had observed in 1948 that applying 70° alcohol to the forearm reduces the skin temperature by 4-5°C, the authors reduced the surface temperature of the breast by 6°C to run simulations. Transient solutions were obtained by the process of rewarming the breast. These were obtained for various blood perfusion rates considering a model breast that was healthy and another that had a tumor. The authors compared the results obtained numerically with thermograms of three volunteers. One of the volunteers had healthy breasts and the other two had a benign tumor in one breast. They concluded that the parameters that most influence the surface temperatures of the breast are: blood perfusion, the metabolic heat of the subcutaneous region and the heat transfer coefficient. They also concluded that numerical simulation can be used as a complementary tool, but it is far from being an independent detection tool.

Hu et al. (2004) used a model based on the Bio Heat Transfer Equation to obtain the temperature distribution in healthy breasts and breasts with malignant tumors undergoing forced convection in a wind tunnel. Numerical simulations were performed using FLUENT™ software. Breast geometry and the unstructured mesh were made in GAMBIT and the geometry of the breast was modeled as a semi-sphere. Parametric studies were conducted to verify the influence of airflow on the surface of the breast. The results showed that cooling the surface plays a very important role in determining the surface temperatures of the cancer patient.

Bezerra (2007) used thermographic images to validate the numerical calculation of temperatures in breast tissues, and compared the temperatures obtained from thermographic images with those obtained by using three-dimensional simulations, performed on a simplified model in which breast geometry was modeled by a semi-sphere. The CFD (Computational Fluid Dynamics) commercial program, FLUENT™, was used to run the numerical simulations. Due to the simplified physical model used for the breast, only the maximum surface temperatures were used for the validation.

Santos (2009) developed a computational tool to conduct parametric analyses. A parametric study was done to evaluate the influence of the position and size of a tumor on the surface temperatures of the breast. The substitute geometry used was obtained from a phantom representing a female torso and the coordinates of which were measured by a Coordinate Measuring Machine (CMM).

Zhang, He, and Zhu (2009) conducted a parametric study in which they analyzed the influence of the size and location of a tumor, room temperature and the convection coefficient on the surface temperatures of the breast. The breast was modeled by a semi-sphere and the tumor by a sphere. The Finite Element Method was used to discretize the equations and the results showed that tumors deeper than 3 cm are difficult to locate using surface temperature. The results also showed that the effects of ambient temperature on the surface temperature are very significant, while this is not the case for the heat exchange coefficient by convection.

Viana (2010) used surrogate geometries of various sizes and developed a computational tool using the Least Squares Methods to determine the substitute geometry best suited to the patient's breast. Numerical simulations were performed to validate such geometries.

Jiang et al. (2011) developed a three-dimensional model, based on thermal modeling and elastic techniques, to thoroughly characterize the thermophysical and elastic properties of tissues, to investigate their effects on the temperature field of normal and tumor-bearing breasts. The model underwent a progressive deformation due to applying the elastic model. Results indicate that elastic deformation influences surface temperatures. They also showed that surface temperatures are less sensitive to the sizes of the tumor than to its depth.

Inverse Problems in Heat Transfer

Modeling via inverse problems is an area of research that has grown considerably in recent decades. This has evolved from theoretical research topics for an important tool for practical engineering analysis. Being of a multidisciplinary nature, this type of problem combines the mathematical analysis of problems with experimental data. It is applied in several areas, such as engineering, image reconstruction, medicine, geophysics, astrophysics and other branches of science (Silva Neto & Moura Neto, 2005).

Huang and Huang (2007) applied the Levenberg-Marquardt Method to estimate thermal conductivity and volumetric heat capacity in biological tissues based on temperature measurement using the Bio Heat Transfer Equation. The accuracy of the inverse problem is analyzed using the exact simulated temperature and temperature measurements with additions of random errors. A statistical analysis is performed to obtain the 99% confidence limits for the estimated thermal properties. The results show that good estimates of thermal conductivity and volumetric heat capacity can be obtained using the Levenberg-Marquardt algorithm.

Partridge and Wrobel (2007) used the Dual Reciprocity Method (DRM) coupled with a genetic algorithm in an inverse process whereby the size and location of a skin tumor can be obtained from temperature measurements on the surface of the skin. In this case, DRM does not need internal nodes. Results are presented for tumors of different sizes and positions relative to the surface of the skin.

Ghafi, Batcha, and Raghavan (2009) predicted effective thermal conductivity in hydride metal beds for storing hydrogen. The Raghavan and Martin model was chosen for analysis as it combines simplicity with physical rigor. The expected result succeeded in predicting the thermal conductivity of particles and in determining the heat transfer rates of hydrides governing the absorption and desorption of hydrogen rates in the storage system.

In Mitra and Balaji (1992), Paruch and Majchrzak (2007), Mital (2008), Jiang et al. (2011), Agnelli, Barrea, and Turner (2011) some thermophysical and geometric parameters of tumors and the breast were estimated using the temperature distribution on the surface of the breast. This was obtained by numerical simulation which simulated an experimentally measured temperature profile.

Paruch and Majchrzak (2007) solved an inverse problem using an evolutionary algorithm, in conjunction with the multiple reciprocity boundary element (MRBEM) method in order to simultaneously estimate some thermophysical properties and geometric parameters (thermal conductivity, metabolic heat, blood perfusion, location and size) of the region of the tumor. Once again, numerically calculated surface temperatures of the breast are assumed to be experimental temperatures. Using this methodology led to satisfactory results, but in three-dimensional simulations the method was slow. The author suggested that the method presented can be used as an effective noninvasive diagnostic tool in medical practices.

Mital (2008) and Mitra and Balaji (1992) used optimization methods using genetic algorithms and neural networks to estimate the parameters, using a simplified two-dimensional model (circle) and a three-dimensional geometry (semi-sphere). These studies suggest that such studies can be undertaken using thermographic images.

It can be seen that several studies have shown that thermographic images have a great potential to be used in conjunction with heat transfer optimization problems, with a view to determining the thermophysical properties of the materials. But none of them used the temperatures obtained from infrared imaging. They only solved the inverse problems using surface temperatures obtained from numerical simulations. Some studies in which thermographic images were used to solve inverse problems are discussed below.

Bezerra et al. (2013) developed a methodology for estimating the thermophysical properties of the breast and breast tumors using thermographic images in conjunction with optimization techniques. Commercial CFD software, FLUENT™, which uses the Finite Volume Method, was used for numerical simulations and the Sequential Quadratic Programming Method (SQP) was used to solve the inverse problem.

Espíndola et al. (2018) estimated the thermophysical properties of the breast and breast tumors using mapping of the surface temperatures of the breast as measured by patient infrared imaging on top of three-dimensional volumes representing the breast. The Transfer Equation was used to calculate the temperature profiles of the breast. The Sequential Quadratic Programming method was used to estimate the thermal conductivity and blood perfusion of the breast tissue and the tumor. The results indicated that this method does not guarantee that the values obtained represent the global minimum of the objective function of the optimization problem.

Melo et al. (2019) developed a methodology based on thermographic images to obtain a reliable three-dimensional model of patients' breasts. Using this geometry, numerical simulations were run to determine temperature profiles, combined with temperatures measured by thermography, thereby allowing the physical properties of breast tissue and of breast pathologies to be measured. The model was developed using the profile curve of the breast obtained from the thermographic image and by adapting the volume of an external orthoprosthesis. The Sequential Quadratic Programming Method (SQP) was used to estimate the thermal conductivity of the glandular tissues and nodules using the maximum temperature in the region of the lesion which was measured by using the thermographic image. The results were compared with those of other authors and the values were measured by thermographic camera, thereby validating the calculations reported.

ADVANTAGES AND DISADVANTAGES OF THE THERMOGRAPHIC TECHNIQUE FOR DETECTING BREAST CANCER

In this section we will consider the main advantages of thermographic technique and how to reduce the disadvantages. In later chapters of this book, we will introduce some numerical and statistical tools commonly used in engineering to show some ways to use this type of imaging to detect disease for which scientific bases are used.

According to Norton et al. (2008), beginning in 1994, US defense agencies, focused their efforts to explore the potential of IR technology associated with image processing and its use then spread to medicine.

The issues that the authors considered important, such as challenges for acceptance by the medical community, were:

1. Standardization and quantification of clinical data;

2. Better understanding of the nature and physiology of pathologies and their "thermal signature";
3. Intensive publication of IR imaging results in journals and at conferences;
4. Characterization of the "thermal signature" by means of iterative databases;
5. Training in acquiring IR images and interpreting them.

The infrared imaging technique, proposed as an auxiliary tool in breast cancer screening, has advantages and disadvantages, which are summarized below.

Advantages:

- It does not emit ionizing radiation;
- There is no physical contact with the patient;
- It can be used as often as necessary;
- It is suitable for young women and men;
- The equipment is cheap compared to the cost of ultrasound or mammography equipment;
- The portability of the IR camera;
- It can make a physiological analysis of the breasts;
- It allows access to low-resource screening locations;
- There is no need for a doctor to acquire the images;
- It is able to show thermal asymmetries that can be classified with similar BIRADS indexes;
- It can be used to validate the profiles of the temperature of the breast, which have been calculated numerically.

Disadvantages:

- The image captures surface temperatures only;
- It may be inefficient at detecting small or very deep nodules;
- It cannot make an image-only diagnosis (a problem that is identical to other exams);
- The image needs to be segmented and classification techniques used to better understand all the physics involved;
- Numerical simulations of temperature profiles of the breast as well as techniques for estimating parameters are needed to help understand and interpret thermographic images;
- It needs a massive investment in being advertised in medical circles because the technique is still barely known in this area.

The topics are well known and discussed, but more effort is needed to make the technique come to be seen as an important complementary tool for detecting breast cancer early.

Recent academic papers on this area are listed in the Item 3 of this chapter.

Research Conducted at the Federal University of Pernambuco (UFPE) – Brazil

To support the infrared imaging technique, the authors of this chapter have synthesized satisfactorily and objectively the limitations and comments made by Diakides et al. (2006), and outlined directions that have been used by the Biomechanical Engineering Group of the Department of Mechanical Engineering of the Federal University of Pernambuco (DEMEC/ UFPE), which since 2006 has been working on developing the project registered in the Brazilian Ministry of Health under the number CEP/CCS/UFPE No. 279/05. Since then, the group has received support from the Brazilian funding agencies CAPES – the Higher Education Coordination Unit (by means of a project that lasted 5 years, funding scholarships and research and was about the cooperation between the Federal University of Pernambuco and the Universidade Federal Fluminense), and CNPq - National Council for Research and Development, by means of six projects that were included in Universal Promulgations (*Editais Universais*, in Portuguese), two of which are still in force on the present date (CNPq Projects and 425334/2016-3 and 430797/ 2018-4).

The IR images used by our research group were acquired with an FLIRS45 camera, with an uncooled microbolometer detector, 320X240 pixels. Its thermal sensibility is 0.08°C and it is ±2°C accurate. It works in a spectral range from 7.5 to 13 μm. The camera was calibrated in the range from -40° to 120°C, using a blackbody emitter, and in that interval its accuracy was ±1°C (Bezerra, 2013).

The inspection using infrared (IR) images has been performed on patients of the Mastology Outpatient Clinic of the Hospital das Clinicas of UFPE, with a view to analyzing the feasibility of using this tool as an aid in the early detection of cancer, together with conventional exams.

During the period 2006-2019, several scientific articles were produced which were published in national and international journals and congresses, in addition to which Master and Doctorate courses were successfully run under the Postgraduate Program in Mechanical Engineering of UFPE. These researchers/teachers are multipliers who irradiate knowledge in this area. Some products of our research are referred in Items 3 and 4 of this chapter.

Later chapters of this book present the results of applications of the use of breast images obtained by the IR technique. These chapters include the following: numerical simulation of temperature profiles of the breast using three-dimensional substitute geometries, customized for each patient analyzed; estimation of thermophysical parameters of breast tissues and breast pathologies; classification techniques of these pathologies using IR images; and computational frameworks that manage the use and integration of all the techniques mentioned. The results obtained can be used to reinforce and support the view that thermographic images can be used as a complementary exam in the pursuit of detecting breast cancer early.

The main objective of all the effort expended on the study and development of the topics mentioned above is to provide understanding of the thermal behavior of the breast so that, together with the thermographic images, these can provide doctors and researchers with informed data on the presence of breast anomalies. Among the objectives of computational frameworks is that they can be used by people who have no prior knowledge of numerical simulation techniques or of the classification of breast anomalies (Queiroz, 2014).

Recent Research in Organizations in Other Countries

Mention will be made in this topic of some institutions where the technique was applied or is being applied, as well as the advantages and disadvantages cited in each of these sites.

Nowadays the modalities routinely used for breast cancer screening and detection are well known. These are mammography and ultrasound, associated with the indispensable clinical examination. Digital mammography is the most used, but it is known to be inadequate at analyzing dense breasts of young patients and to be difficult to use on men. Magnetic resonance imaging has been used as well, but still has a high rate of false positives despite being well accepted by doctors for precisely locating tumors, an important fact for planning surgery.

The IR technique is based on the fact that the chemical activity of the vessels is higher in tissues next to a breast pathology than in the other normal regions of the breast. These tissues need abundant nutrients in order to maintain their growth, and send chemical components in order to keep blood vessels open and to permit the creation of new vessels (neoangiogenesis). In addition, there is local vasodilation. These facts cause the temperature to rise in the region.

At ebme.co.uk, it can be seen that medical thermography is proposed as a multipurpose tool. Among the many and possible proposals is to apply it so as to detect breast pathologies, but there is a lack of references that present scientific or clinical results. A series of clinical engineering articles is listed on the site, but none of them deals with breast thermography.

It is also stated that IR images have the facility of being statistically analyzed. And that IR images, provided they are acquired by accurate cameras, can be analyzed by doctors who can determine if there are areas of abnormal heating. This private-sector organization also states that the Food and Drug Administration (FDA) has approved the thermographic procedure for screening for breast cancer, diseases of the head and neck vessels, neuro-musculoskeletal disorders and lower extremity vascular diseases of the lower extremities.

The site claims that over the past decade the application of thermography has been controversial in the medical world, but recent technological advances have made technology an important weapon for tracking and detecting breast anomalies, as demonstrated in numerous studies (EBME & Clinical Engineering Articles, 2019).

In 2019, the FDA released a paper stating that thermography should not be considered as a screening tool to replace mammography. It is possible to observe in the greater part of the recent bibliography, that for many years, the academic community involved in research in the exams and it is not intended to replace any modality in current use. This effort has been monitored by the medical institutions mentioned in this item.

The United Breast Cancer Foundation (2019), New York / USA, includes on its website the importance of thermography as an auxiliary tool for detecting breast anomalies. It also states that ultra-sensitive cameras and sophisticated computers are currently used to analyze and produce diagnostic images of temperature changes, and cites the advantages already listed earlier in this chapter.

It also states that over 250,000 women have been included as study participants in the past 30 years worldwide. And that more than 800 articles have been published in journals. There are studies involving from 37,000 to 118,000 participants and some of these studies followed patients for up to 12 years.

The Foundation's main conclusions are that:

- An abnormal thermogram is an important marker of high risk of developing breast cancer.
- Is eight times more important than a family history;
- A persistently abnormal thermogram may carry a 22-fold increased risk of future breast cancer.
- When added to regular checkup exams, there was a 66% increase in survival rate;
- When added to traditional exams, 95% of early stage breast cancer cases can be detected.

The Rochester Institute of Technology (RIT) in New York, USA, was formed in 2008 with the mission to innovate in medical treatment, teaching and research. An alliance was made with the Rochester General Health System. Together they set about improving cancer screening and studying the benefits of using thermography for this purpose.

According to Prof. Satish Kandlikar, "Modern infrared imaging has the potential to significantly increase the accuracy of screening for breast cancer and could have broad implications for preventive medicine" (Rochester Institute of Technology, 2019).

The method proposed by Kandlikar combines IR images with an artificial intelligence system which can predict the location and size of tumors on a thermal map. The algorithms will simulate scenarios based on numerical models of thermal patterns derived from mammography and magnetic resonance exams conducted at Rochester General Hospital (EurekAlert, 2019).

PROTOCOL FOR ACQUIRING INFRARED IMAGES OF THE BREAST

The objective of this section is to present the protocol for acquiring thermographic images of the breast that the Biomechanical Engineering Group, DEMEC / UFPE drew up and has been using since 2012. Key topics include ensuring that the examination room is adequate and patients are properly prepared; describing the mechanical apparatus developed and built to capture images and that it is properly maintained. A comparison with protocols used by other researchers will be included.

The Biomechanical Engineering Group of the Federal University of Pernambuco (UFPE) drew up and began to use the protocol for acquiring thermographic images in 2012. It continues to be used today to guide the capture of infrared images of patients from the Mastology Outpatient Clinic of the Hospital das Clínicas UFPE, Recife.

Figure 10. Mechanical apparatus designed and built in DEMEC. Source: Oliveira (2012).

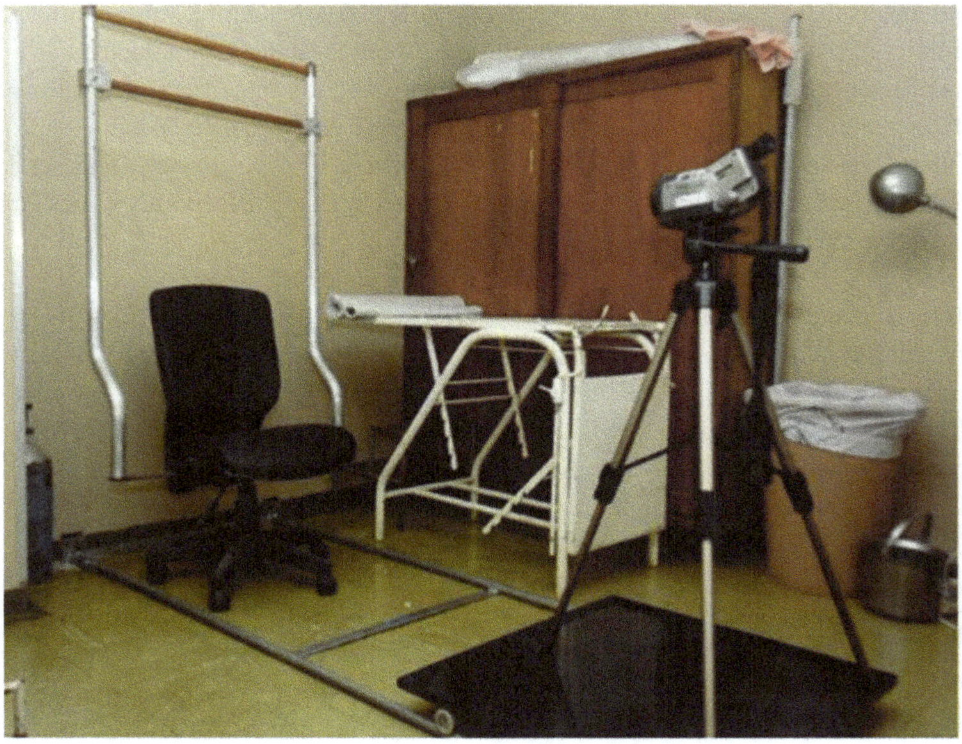

When drawing up the protocol, we bore in mind several characteristic aspects of the public health network in Brazil and the difficulties encountered by the group, such as: the room is not used exclusively to capture images; it is not possible to warn patients in advance that they will undergo this examination; and there are deficiencies in controlling the temperature and relative humidity of the room. There are three main topics that make up the protocol: ensuring the adequacy of the room; preparing the patient preparation; and acquiring images (Oliveira, 2012).

Making the Room Adequacy: Measuring approximately 3x4 meters, the exam room has a door and two windows. To control the air flow in the room, the door is opened and closed by the technical group. The windows are kept shut. The room is air conditioned by an air conditioner and a thermo-hygrometer is used to check the temperature and relative humidity. In order to standardize the acquisition of images, a mechanical apparatus has also been designed and built by the Biomechanics Group (Oliveira, 2012).

Preparing the patient: Patients are referred after consultation with the mastologist taking part in this research. Prior to the exam, the research group explains to the thermographic exam to the patient and how she should behave during the imaging. The patient needs to sign an informed consent form if she agrees to take part in the research. Upon arriving at the thermographic examination room, and due to the characteristics of being attended to at the Hospital das Clinicas UFPE, the patient has spent at least two hours without exposure to sunlight, without performing physical exercises, without eating more than a snack and some liquid and without taking a shower (Oliveira, 2012).

Oliveira (2012) also mentions that after the exam has been explained to the patient, she is asked to remove clothing from the upper part of her body, is given a disposable gown to wear and is asked to wait for approximately ten minutes, without touching her breasts, in order that they reach thermal equilibrium with the environment (process acclimatization process).

Acquisition of images: Oliveira (2012) states that the patient is asked to sit on the swivel chair of the mechanical apparatus. The height and distance of the camera from the patient's breast are adjusted. Then the parameters that are set are those of emissivity, reflected temperature, atmospheric temperature, relative humidity of the environment and the distance between the camera and the patient.

Two sets of images are collected: one set is taken that is slightly more than one meter between the patient and the camera and the other set is taken with the camera closer to patient, but with no predefined distance. The second set is for the physician who will make a qualitative analysis. This set does not require rigorous standardization. The first set of images is used by the UFPE Biomechanics Group. There are seven images in this set (Figure 11):

a) T1 - frontal image of both breasts, hands on the waist;
b) T2 - frontal image of both breasts, with hands raised and resting on the upper bar of the mechanical apparatus;
c) T2 - frontal image of both breasts with grid, raised and supported on the upper bar of the mechanical apparatus;
d) LIMD - internal lateral of the right breast;
e) LIME - internal lateral of the left breast;
f) LEMD - external lateral of the right breast;
g) LEME – external lateral of the left breast.

Figure 11. Standardized thermographic images acquired for each patient.
Source: Oliveira (2012).

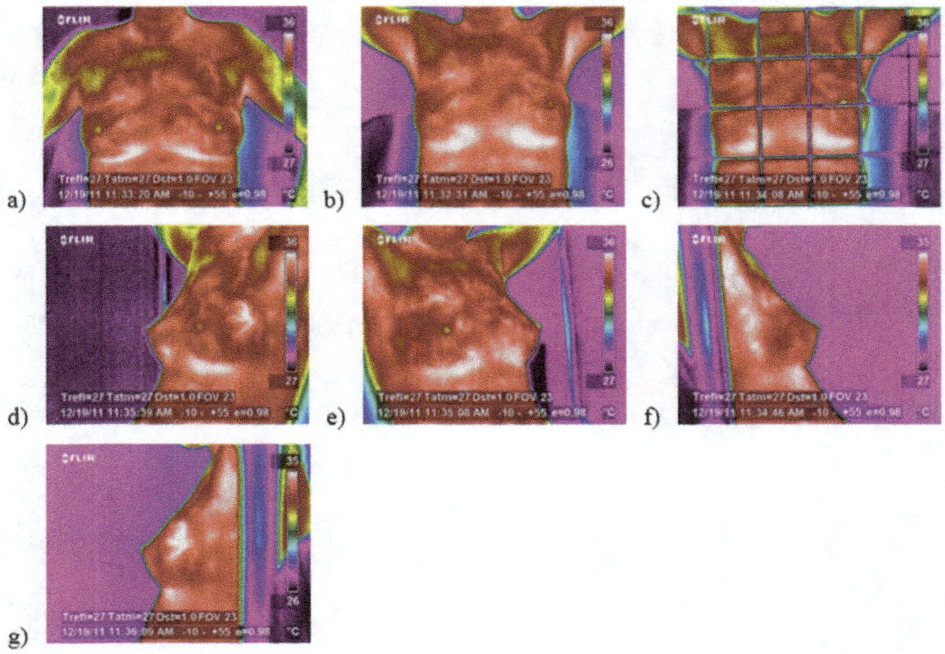

The protocols used by several research groups on the use of infrared imaging to aid the detection of breast anomalies have some differences, but there are some similar characteristics. Comments are given on some of these protocols below.

Ali et al. (2015) recommend that the patient avoids alcohol and caffeine intake, physical exercise and nicotine use for two hours prior to the exam. The room temperature should be kept between 20°C and 22°C. In the preparation step, the patient is asked to remove her necklace, earrings and any other jewelry. Then, the patient's body temperature is checked, and she is positioned between 0.8 and 1.2 meters away from the camera and with her arms resting on the bar of the mechanical apparatus. The ambient temperature, relative humidity and distance between patient and camera parameters are set into the camera. There is a 10-minute waiting period (acclimatization period) and then the first infrared (front) image is captured. Then there is a further wait of 15 minutes after which a new image is captured, also frontal.

Ramón, Mancilla, Henández, and Rios (2017) present the image acquisition protocol used for research conducted on 454 volunteer women to detect breast cancer by means of infrared images. Among the requirements of the protocol are:

a) Avoid using lotions, cosmetic creams, perfumes, deodorant or antiperspirants in the breast region.
b) Do not remove hairs from the breast area on the day of the exam.
c) Do not drink coffee and alcohol for 24 hours prior to the test.
d) Avoid smoking two hours before the exam and avoid exercise one hour before.

Figure 12. Regions with analyzed temperatures. Source: Ramón et al., 2017.

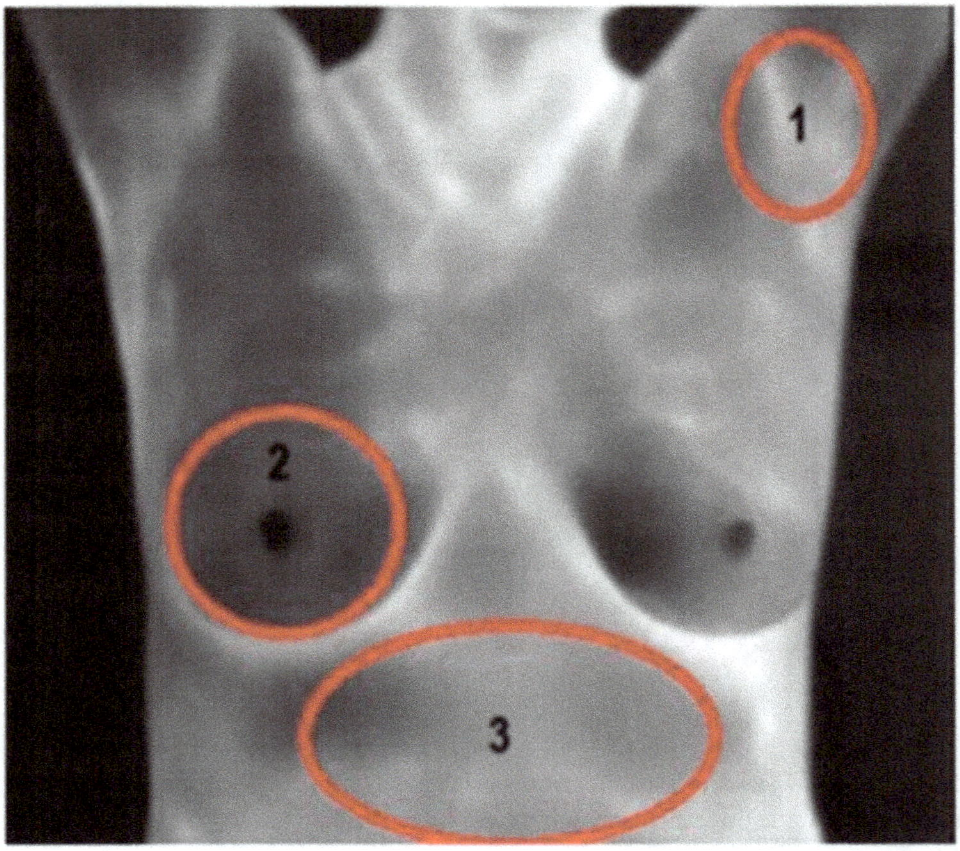

Figure 13. Temperatures taken at the points indicated. Source: Ramón et al., 2017.

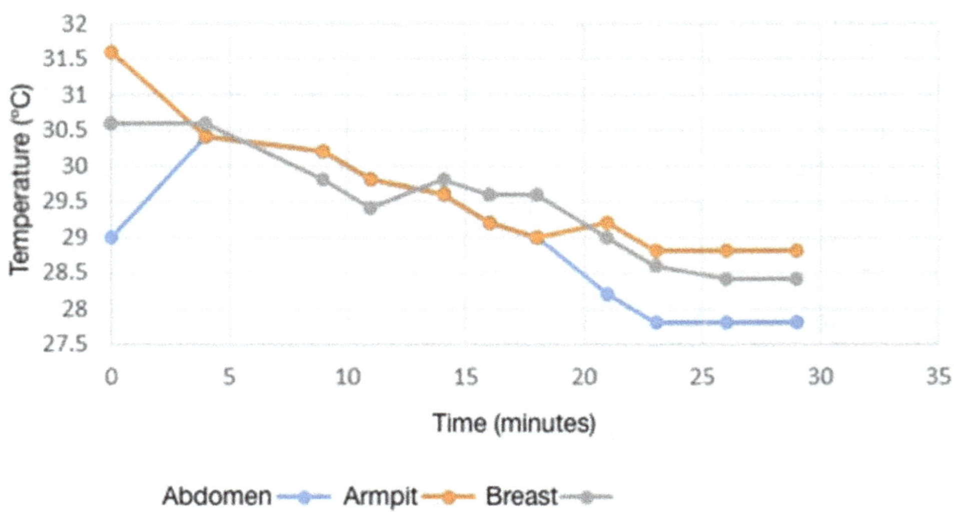

Figure 14. Thermographic images collected. Source: Ramón et al., 2017.

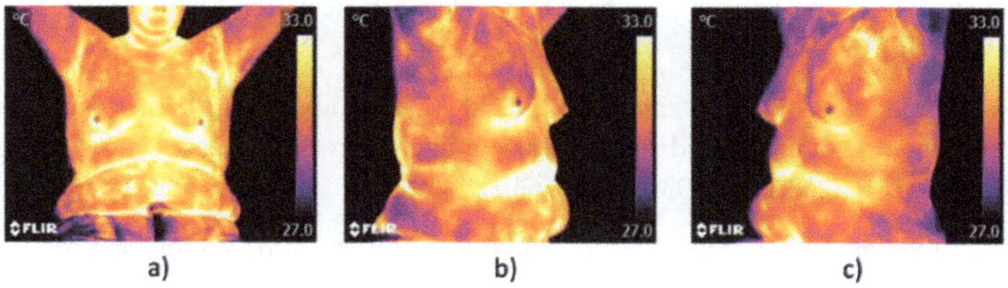

There is an analysis of three specific points (armpit, right breast and abdomen) of the patient, where surface temperature values are collected until they reach thermal equilibrium (Figure 12). The behavior observed when using this analysis indicates that it takes twenty-five minute for temperatures to be stabilized (thermal equilibrium) (Figure 13).

Three infrared images are collected: one frontal image and two semi oblique images (right and left). Images are collected in a controlled environment, the patient being 1.2 meters away from the camera (Figure 14).

Bhowmik et al. (2016) cite a list of items that the patient should avoid before the exam: long exposures to sunlight during the week prior to the exam, applying lotions or talcum on the breasts, physical activity on the day before the exam, pain medications on the day of the exam, tightly fitting clothing, smoking or drinking caffeine or alcohol before the exam, avoid contact with heavy metals and women should be at a certain period of the menstrual cycle. Initially a form with personal information and symptoms that the patient may be feeling should be completed. As for environmental control, the examination room should have neither fans nor windows. The temperature should be maintained between 20°C and 24°C by means of air conditioning cooling. Relative humidity should be checked using a thermo-hygrometer.

In the acclimatization process, the patient is asked to remove her jewelry. The patient should lie on a stretcher and then there is a 15-minute wait until the patient's body achieves thermal balance with the environment. In this period, the room remains darkened. Images should be captured in a room that is 2.5 meters long and 1.5 meters wide and that has black walls that are 1.83 meters high. The patient should be positioned at a distance of one meter from the camera. Eight images are obtained of each patient, and the views are: supine, frontal, left lateral, right lateral, left oblique, right oblique, of each breast.

REFERENCES

Acharya, U. R., Ng, E. Y. K., Tan, J. H., & Sree, S. V. (2012). Thermography based breast cancer detection using texture features and support vector machine. *Journal of Medical Systems*, *36*(3), 1503–1510. doi:10.100710916-010-9611-z PMID:20957511

Agnelli, J. P., Barrea, A. A., & Turner, C. V. (2011). Tumor location and parameter estimation by thermography. *Mathematical and Computer Modelling*, *53*(7-8), 1527–1534. doi:10.1016/j.mcm.2010.04.003

Ali, M. A. S., Sayed, G. I., Gaber, T., Hassanien, A. E., Snasel, V., & Silva, L. F. (2015). Detection of Breast Abnormalities of Thermograms based on a New Segmentation Method. *ACSIS*, *5*, 255–261. doi:10.15439/2015F318

Alikhassi, A., Hamidpour, S. F., Firouzmand, M., Navid, M., & Eghbal, M. (2018). Prospective comparative study assessing role of ultrasound versus thermography in breast cancer detection. *Breast Disease*, *37*(4), 191–196. doi:10.3233/BD-180321 PMID:30124439

Amalu, W. C., Hobbins, W. B., Head, J. F., & Elliot, R. L. (2006). Infrared imaging of the breast - an overview. *The Biomedical Engineering Handbook, 25*, 1–20.

Ammer, K., & Ring, E. F. (2006). Standard Procedures for Infrared Imaging in Medicine. In Medical Devices and Systems, The Biomedical Engineering Handbook. CRC Press.

Amorim, A. M. A. M., Barbosa, J. da S., Freitas, A. P. L. de F., Viana, J. E. F., Vieira, L. E. M., Suassuna, F. C. M., Bento, P. M., & de Melo, D. P. (2019). Termografia Infravermelha na Odontologia. *HU Revista*, *44*(1), 15–22. doi:10.34019/1982-8047.2018.v44.13943

Amri, A., Pulko, S. H., & Wilkinson, A. J. (2016). Potentialities of steady-state and transient thermography in breast tumour depth detection: A numerical study. *Computer Methods and Programs in Biomedicine*, *123*, 68–80. doi:10.1016/j.cmpb.2015.09.014 PMID:26522612

Araújo, M. C., Lima, R. C. F., & Souza, R. M. C. R. (2014). Interval symbolic feature extraction for thermography breast cancer detection. *Expert Systems with Applications*, *41*(15), 6728–6737. doi:10.1016/j.eswa.2014.04.027

Araújo, M. C., Souza, R. M. C. R., Lima, R. C. F., & Filho, T. M. S. (2017). An interval prototype classifier based on a parameterized distance applied to breast thermographic images. *Medical & Biological Engineering & Computing*, *55*(6), 873–884. doi:10.100711517-016-1565-y PMID:27629552

Avila-Castro, I. A., Hernández-Martínez, A. R., Estevez, M., Cruz, M., Esparza, R., Pérez, R., & Rodríguez, A. L. (2017). Thorax thermographic simulator for breast pathologies. *Journal of Applied Research and Technology*, *15*(2), 143–151. doi:10.1016/j.jart.2017.01.008

Bankman, I. N. (2009). *Handbook of medical imaging: Processing and analysis* (3rd ed.). Academic Press.

Barnes, R. B. (1963). Thermography of the Human body. *Science*, *140*(3569), 870–877. doi:10.1126cience.140.3569.870 PMID:13969373

Bezerra, L. A. (2007). *Uso de imagens termográficas em tumores mamários para validação de simulação computacional* (Master's thesis). Universidade Federal de Pernambuco, Recife, PE, Brazil. Retrieved from https://repositorio.ufpe.br/handle/123456789/5486

Bezerra, L. A. (2013). *Estimativa de parâmetros termofísicos da mama utilizando método inverso* (Unpublished doctoral thesis). Universidade Federal de Pernambuco, Recife, Brazil.

Bezerra, L. A., Oliveira, M. M., Rolim, T. L., Conci, A., Santos, F. G. S., Lyra, P. R. M., & Lima, R. C. F. (2013). Estimation of breast tumor thermal properties using infrared images. *Signal Processing*, *93*(10), 2851–2863. doi:10.1016/j.sigpro.2012.06.002

Bhowmik, M. K., Gogoi, U. R., Das, K., Ghosh, A. K., Bhattacharjee, D., & Majumdar, G. (2016). Standardization of Infrared Breast Thermogram Acquisition Protocols and Abnormality Analysis of Breast Thermograms. *Thermosense: Thermal Infrared Applications XXXVIII. SPIE, 9861.*

Bhowmik, M. K., Gogoi, U. R., Majumdar, G., Bhattacharjee, D., Datta, D., & Ghosh, A. K. (2017). Designing of Ground-Truth-Annotated DBT-TU-JU Breast Thermogram Database Toward Early Abnormality Prediction. *IEEE Journal of Biomedical and Health Informatics*, *22*(4), 1238–1249. doi:10.1109/JBHI.2017.2740500 PMID:28829321

Birnbaum, S. J., & Kliot, D. (1964). Thermography-obstetrical applications. *Annals of the New York Academy of Sciences*, *121*(1), 209–222. doi:10.1111/j.1749-6632.1964.tb13697.x PMID:14237513

Borchartt, T. B., Conci, A., Lima, R. C. F., Resmini, R., & Sanchez, A. (2013). Breast thermography from an image processing viewpoint: A survey. *Signal Processing*, *93*(10), 2785–2803. doi:10.1016/j.sigpro.2012.08.012

Cancer Institute Hospital of JFCR. (2019). Retrieved from https://www.jfcr.or.jp/hospital-en/

de Jesus Guirro, R. R., & Vaz, M. M. O. L. L. (2017). Accuracy and Reliability of Infrared Thermography in Assessment of the Breasts of Women Affected by Cancer. *Journal of Medical Systems*, *41*(5), 87. doi:10.100710916-017-0730-7 PMID:28405947

de Vasconcelos, J. H., dos Santos, W. P., & Lima, R. C. F. (2018). Analysis of Methods of Classification of Breast Thermographic Images to Determine their Viability in the Early Breast Cancer Detection. *IEEE Latin America Transactions*, *16*(6), 1631–1637. doi:10.1109/TLA.2018.8444159

Diakides, N., Diakides, M., Lupo, J., Paul, J., & Balcerak, R. (2006). Advances in Medical Infrared Imaging. In J. D. Bronzino (Ed.), Medical Devices and Systems, The Biomedical Engineering Handbook (3rd ed.). CRC Press. doi:10.1201/9781420003864.sec3

Díaz-Cortés, M., Ortega-Sánchez, N., Hinojosa, S., Oliva, D., Cuevas, E., Rojas, R., & Demin, A. (2018). A multi-level thresholding method for breast thermograms analysis using Dragonfly algorithm. *Infrared Physics & Technology*, *93*, 346–361. doi:10.1016/j.infrared.2018.08.007

Dibai-Filho, A. V., Costa, A. C., Packer, A. C., de Castro, E. M., & Rodrigues-Bigaton, D. (2015). Women with more severe degrees of temporomandibular disorder exhibit an increase in temperature over the temporomandibular joint. *The Saudi Dental Journal*, *27*(1), 44–49. doi:10.1016/j.sdentj.2014.10.002 PMID:25544814

Dumansky, Y., Lyakh, Y., Gorshkov, O., Gurianov, V., & Prihodchenko, V. (2012). Fractal dimensionality analysis of normal and cancerous mammary gland thermograms. *Chaos, Solitons, and Fractals*, *45*(12), 1494–1500. doi:10.1016/j.chaos.2012.07.006

EBME & Clinical Engineering Articles. (2019, October 4). Retrieved from https://www.ebme.co.uk/articles/clinical-engineering/medical-thermography

Espíndola, N. A., Bezerra, L. A., Santos, L. C., & Lima, R. C. F. (2018). Estimating Breast Thermophysical Parameters by the Use of Mapping Surface Temperatures Measured by Infrared Images. *IEEE Latin America Transactions, 16*(10).

EtehadTavakol, M., Chandran, V., Ng, E. Y. K., & Kafieh, R. (2013). Breast cancer detection from thermal images using bispectral invariant features. *International Journal of Thermal Sciences*, 1–16.

EurekAlert. (2019). Retrieved from https://www.eurekalert.org/pub_releases/2019-06/riot-iit062619.php

Figueiredo, A. A. A., do Nascimento, J. G., Malheiros, F. C., da Silva Ignacio, L. H., Fernandes, H. C., & Guimaraes, G. (2019). Breast tumor localization using skin surface temperatures from a 2D anatomic model without knowledge of the thermophysical properties. *Computer Methods and Programs in Biomedicine*, *172*, 65–77. doi:10.1016/j.cmpb.2019.02.004 PMID:30902128

Furuichi, M., Makie, T., Honma, Y., Isoda, T., & Miyake, S. (2015). Laboratory-Confirmed Dengue Fever and Chikungunya Fever Cases at the Narita Airport Quarantine Station in 2013. *Japanese Journal of Infectious Diseases*, *68*(2), 142–144. doi:10.7883/yoken.JJID.2014.242 PMID:25420667

Garduño-Ramón, M. A., Vega-Mancilla, S. G., Morales-Henández, L. A., & Osornio-Rios, R. A. (2017). Supportive Noninvasive Tool for the Diagnosis of Breast Cancer Using a Thermographic Camera as Sensor. *Sensors (Basel)*, *17*(3), 497. doi:10.339017030497 PMID:28273793

Gasiorowicz, S. (1979). Física Quântica (G. Dois, Ed.). Academic Press.

Gautherie, M. (1980). Thermopathology of breast cancer: Measurements and analysis of in vivo temperature and blood flow. *Annals of the New York Academy of Sciences*, *335*(1), 383–415. doi:10.1111/j.1749-6632.1980.tb50764.x PMID:6931533

Gautherie, M. (1983). Thermobiological assessment of benign and malignant breast diseases. *American Journal of Obstetrics and Gynecology*, *147*(8), 861–869. doi:10.1016/0002-9378(83)90236-3 PMID:6650622

Gershen-Cohen, J., Haberman, J., & Brueschke, E. (1965). Medical thermography: A summary of current status. *Radiologic Clinics of North America*, 3. PMID:5846852

Ghafir, M. F. M., Batcha, M. F. M., & Raghavan, V. R. (2009). Prediction of the thermal conductivity of metal hydrides - the inverse problem. *International Journal of Hydrogen Energy*, *34*(16), 7125–7130. doi:10.1016/j.ijhydene.2008.06.033

Global Cancer Control. (2019, October 4). Retrieved from https://www.uicc.org/membership/national-cancer-research-center-japan

Gogoi, U. R., Bhowmik, M. K., Bhattacharjee, D., & Ghosh, A. K. (2018). Singular value based characterization and analysis of thermal patches for early breast abnormality detection. *Australasian Physical & Engineering Sciences in Medicine*, *41*(4), 861–879. doi:10.100713246-018-0681-4 PMID:30171500

Gogoi, U. R., Majumdar, M., Bhowmik, M. K., & Ghosh, A. K. (2019). Evaluating the efficiency of infrared breast thermography for early breast cancer risk prediction in asymptomatic population. *Infrared Physics & Technology*, *99*, 201–211. doi:10.1016/j.infrared.2019.01.004

Gonzalez-Hernandez, J., Recinella, A. N., Kandlikar, S. G., Dabydeen, D., Medeiros, L., & Phatak, P. (2019). Technology, application and potential of dynamic breast thermography for the detection of breast cancer. *International Journal of Heat and Mass Transfer*, *131*, 558–573. doi:10.1016/j.ijheatmasstransfer.2018.11.089

Gourd, E. (2017). Breast thermography alone no substitute for mammography. *The Lancet. Oncology, 18*(12), e713. doi:10.1016/S1470-2045(17)30833-1 PMID:29103872

Haddad, D. S., Brioschi, M. L., & Arita, E. S. (2012). Thermographic and clinical correlation of myofascial trigger points in the masticatory muscles. *Dento Maxillo Facial Radiology, 41*(8), 621–629. doi:10.1259/dmfr/98504520 PMID:23166359

Haddad, D. S., Brioschi, M. L., Vardasca, R., Weber, M., Crosato, E. M., & Arita, E. S. (2014). Thermographic characterization of masticatory muscle regions in volunteers with and without myogenous temporomandibular disorder: Preliminary results. *Dento Maxillo Facial Radiology, 43*(8), 20130440. doi:10.1259/dmfr.20130440 PMID:25144605

Han, F., Shi, G., Liang, C., Wang, L., & Li, K. (2015). A simple and efficient method for breast cancer diagnosis based on infrared thermal imaging. *Cell Biochemistry and Biophysics, 71*(1), 491–498. doi:10.100712013-014-0229-5 PMID:25194831

Hardy, J. D., & Muschenheim, C. (1936). The radiation of heat from the human body. V. *The Journal of Clinical Investigation, 15*(1), 1–8. doi:10.1172/JCI100746 PMID:16694368

Harris, D. L., Greeining, W. P., & Aichroth, P. M. (1966). Infra-red in the diagnosis of a lump in the breast. *British Journal of Cancer, 20*(4), 710–721. doi:10.1038/bjc.1966.82 PMID:5964605

Hatwar, R., & Herman, C. (2017). Inverse method for quantitative characterisation of breast tumours from surface temperature data. *International Journal of Hyperthermia, 33*(7), 741–757. doi:10.1080/02656736.2017.1306758 PMID:28540793

Hildebrandt, C., Raschner, C., & Ammer, K. (2010). An overview of recent application of medical infrared thermography in sports medicine in Austria. *Sensors (Basel), 10*(5), 4700–4715. doi:10.3390100504700 PMID:22399901

Hosaki, Y., Mitsunobu, F., Ashida, K., Tsugeno, H., Okamoto, M., Nishida, N., Takata, S., Yokoi, T., Tanizaki, Y., Ochi, K., & Tsuji, T. (2002). Non-invasive study for peripheral circulation in patients with diabetes mellitus. *Annual Reports of Misasa Medical Branch, 72*, 31–37.

Hossain, S., Abdelaal, M., & Mohammadi, F. A. (2016). Thermogram Assessment for Tumor Parameter Estimation Considering Body Geometry. *Canadian Journal of Electrical and Computer Engineering, 39*(3), 219–234. doi:10.1109/CJECE.2016.2541661

Hossain, S., & Mohammadi, F. A. (2016). Tumor parameter estimation considering the body geometry by thermography. *Computers in Biology and Medicine, 76*, 80–93. doi:10.1016/j.compbiomed.2016.06.023 PMID:27416548

Houdas, Y., & Ring, E. F. J. (1982). *Human Body Temperature*. Plenum Press. doi:10.1007/978-1-4899-0345-7

Hu, L., Gupta, A., Gore, J. P., & Xu, L. X. (2004). Effect of forced convection on the skin thermal expression of breast cancer. *Journal of Biomechanical Engineering, 126*(2), 204–211. doi:10.1115/1.1688779 PMID:15179850

Huang, C., & Huang, C. (2007). An inverse problem in estimating simultaneously the effective thermal conductivity and volumetric heat capacity of biological tissue. *Applied Mathematical Modelling*, *31*(9), 1785–1797. doi:10.1016/j.apm.2006.06.002

Hudson, R. D. Jr. (1969). *Infrared System Engineering*. John Wiley and Sons Inc.

HyperPhysics. (2019). *The Interaction of Radiation with the Matter*. Department of Physics and Astronomy, Georgia State University. Retrieved from http://hyperphysics.phy-astr.gsu.edu/hbase/mod3.html

Iljaž, J., Wrobel, L. C., Hriberšek, M., & Marn, J. (2019). Numerical modelling of skin tumour tissue with temperature-dependent properties for dynamic thermography. *Computers in Biology and Medicine*, *112*, 112. doi:10.1016/j.compbiomed.2019.103367 PMID:31386971

Incropera, F. P., & Witt, D. P. (1996). Introduction to heat transfer (3rd ed.). Wiley Ed.

Isard, H. J., Becker, W., Shilo, R., & Ostrum, B. J. (1972). Breast thermography after four years and 10,000 studies. *AJR. American Journal of Roentgenology*, *115*(4), 811–821. doi:10.2214/ajr.115.4.811 PMID:5054275

Jiang, L., Zhan, W., & Loew, M. H. (2011). Modeling static and dynamic thermography of the human breast under elastic deformation. *Physics in Medicine and Biology*, *56*(1), 187–202. doi:10.1088/0031-9155/56/1/012 PMID:21149948

Kandlikar, S. G., Perez-Raya, I., Raghupathi, P. A., Gonzalez-Hernandez, J., Dabydeen, D., Medeiros, L., & Phatak, P. (2017). Infrared imaging technology for breast cancer detection – Current status, protocols and new directions. *International Journal of Heat and Mass Transfer, 108*(Part B), 2303 – 2320.

Kermani, S., Samadzadehaghdam, N., & EtehadTavakol, M. (2015). Automatic color segmentation of breast infrared images using a Gaussian mixture model. *Optik (Stuttgart)*, *126*(21), 3288–3294. doi:10.1016/j.ijleo.2015.08.007

Kirubha, A. S. P., Anburajan, M., Venkataraman, B., & Menaka, M. (2015). Comparison of PET–CT and thermography with breast biopsy in evaluation of breast cancer: A case study. *Infrared Physics & Technology*, *73*, 115–125. doi:10.1016/j.infrared.2015.09.008

Kirubha, A. S. P., Anburajan, M., Venkataraman, B., & Menaka, M. (2018). A case study on asymmetrical texture features comparison of breast thermogram and mammogram in normal and breast cancer subject. *Biocatalysis and Agricultural Biotechnology*, *15*, 390–401. doi:10.1016/j.bcab.2018.07.001

Krawczyk, B., Schaefer, G., & Woźniak, M. (2015). A hybrid cost-sensitive ensemble for imbalanced breast thermogram classification. *Artificial Intelligence in Medicine*, *65*(3), 219–227. doi:10.1016/j.artmed.2015.07.005 PMID:26319694

Lahiri, B. B., Bagavathiappan S., Jayakumar T., & Philip, J. (2012). Medical applications of infrared thermography: A review. *International Journal Infrared Physics and Technology*, 222-232.

Lahiri, B. B., Bagavathiappan, S., Soumya, C., Jayakumar, T., & Philip, J. (2015). Infrared thermography based studies on mobile phone induced heating. *Infrared Physics & Technology*, *71*, 242–251. doi:10.1016/j.infrared.2015.04.010

Lawson, R. N. (1956). Implications of surface temperatures in the diagnosis of breast cancer. *Canadian Medical Association Journal, 75*(5), 309–310. PMID:13343098

Lawson, R. N. (1957). Thermography – a new tool in the investigation of breast lesions. *Canadian Services Medical Journal, 13*, 517–524. PMID:13460932

Liu, C., Heijden, F., Klein, M. E., Baal, J. G., Bus, S. A., & Netten, J. J. (2013). Infrared dermal thermography on diabetic feet soles to predict ulcerations: A case study. *Advanced Biomedical and Clinical Systems, 11*, 8572. doi:10.1117/12.2001807

Lozano, A. III, & Hassanipour, F. (2019). Infrared imaging for breast cancer detection: An objective review of foundational studies and its proper role in breast cancer screening. *Infrared Physics & Technology, 97*, 244–257. doi:10.1016/j.infrared.2018.12.017

Madhu, H., Kakileti, S. T., Venkataramani, K., & Jabbireddy, S. (2016). *Extraction of medically interpretable features for classification of malignancy in breast thermography*. 38th Annual International Conference of the IEEE Engineering in Medicine and Biology, Orlando, FL.

Mahmoudzadeh, E., Montazeri, M. A., Zekri, M., & Sadri, S. (2015). Extended hidden Markov model for optimized segmentation of breast thermography images. *Infrared Physics & Technology, 72*, 19–28. doi:10.1016/j.infrared.2015.06.012

Mahmoudzadeh, E., Zekri, M., Montazeri, M. A., Sadri, S., & Dabbagh, S. T. (2016). Directional SUSAN image boundary detection of breast thermogram. *IET Image Processing, 10*(7), 552–560. doi:10.1049/iet-ipr.2015.0347

Mambou, S. J., Maresova, P., Krejcar, O., Selamat, A., & Kuca, K. (2018). Breast Cancer Detection Using Infrared Thermal Imaging and a Deep Learning Model. *Sensors (Basel), 18*(9), 2799. doi:10.339018092799 PMID:30149621

Manginas, A., Andreanides, E., Leontiadis, E., Sfyrakis, P., Maounis, T., Degiannis, D., Alivizatos, P., & Cokkinos, D. (2010). Right ventricular endocardial thermography in transplanted and coronary artery disease patients: First human application. *The Journal of Invasive Cardiology, 22*, 400–404. PMID:20814045

Marchena-Menéndez, J., Ramírez-Torres, A., Penta, R., Rodríguez-Ramos, R., & Merodio, J. (2019). Macroscopic thermal profile of heterogeneous cancerous breasts. A three-dimensional multiscale analysis. *International Journal of Engineering Science, 144*, 144. doi:10.1016/j.ijengsci.2019.103135

Marques, R. S., Conci, A., Perez, M. G., Andaluz, V. H., & Mejia, T. M. (2016). An approach for automatic segmentation of thermal imaging in Computer Aided Diagnosis. *IEEE Latin America Transactions, 14*(4), 1856–1865. doi:10.1109/TLA.2016.7483526

Medical Xpress. (2019). *Infrared imaging technology being developed to better detect breast cancer*. Retrieved from https://medicalxpress.com/ news/2019-06-infrared-imaging-technology-breast-cancer.html?utm_sour ce=TrendMD&utm_medium=cpc&utm_campaign=MedicalXpress_TrendMD_1

Melo, J. R. F., Queiroz, J. R. A., Bezerra, L. A., & Lima, R. C. F. (2019). Development of a three-dimensional surrogate geometry of the breast and its use in estimating the thermal conductivities of breast tissue and breast lesions based on infrared images. *International Communications in Heat and Mass Transfer*, 108.

Menczer, J., & Eskin, B. A. (1969). Evaluation of postpartum breast engorgement by thermography. *Magazine Obstetrics and Gynecology*, *33*(2), 260–263. PMID:4886952

Migowski, A., Silva, G. A. E., Dias, M. B. K., Diz, M. D. P. E., Sant'Ana, D. R., & Nadanovsky, P. (2018). Guidelines for early detection of breast cancer in Brazil. II - New national recommendations, main evidence, and controversies. *Cadernos de Saude Publica*, *34*(6). PMID:29947654

Miles, D. W., Thomsen, L. L., Happerfield, L., Bobrow, L. G., Knowles, R. G., & Moncada, S. (1995). Nitric oxide synthase activity in human breast cancer. *Journal of Cancer*, *72*(1), 41–44. doi:10.1038/bjc.1995.274 PMID:7541238

Milosevic, M., Jankovic, D., Milenkovic, A., & Stojanov, D. (2018). Early diagnosis and detection of breast cancer. *Technology and Health Care*, *26*(4), 729–759. doi:10.3233/THC-181277 PMID:30124455

Milosevic, M., Jankovic, D., & Peulic, A. (2015). Comparative analysis of breast cancer detection in mammograms and thermograms. *Biomedizinische Technik. Biomedical Engineering*, *60*(1), 49–56. doi:10.1515/bmt-2014-0047 PMID:25720034

Mital, M. (2008). Breast tumor simulation and parameters estimation using evolucionary algorithms. *Modelling and Simulation in Engineering*, *10*(1), 7–14.

Mitra, S., & Balaji, C. (1992). A neural network based estimation of tumor parameters from a breast thermogram. *Modelling and Simulation in Engineering*, *10*(1), 7–14.

Modest, M. F. (2013). *Radiative heat transfer* (3rd ed.). Academic Press. doi:10.1016/B978-0-12-386944-9.50023-6

Montreal Breast Center. (2019, October 8). Retrieved from http://www.vmmed.com

Morasiewicz, L., Dudek, K., Orzechowski, W., Kulej, M., & Stepniewski, M. (2008). Use of thermography to monitor the bone regenerate during limb lengthening - preliminary communication. *Ortop Traumatol Rehabil 2, 10*(3), 279-85.

Moskowitz, M., Fox, S. H., del Re, R. B., Milbrath, J. R., Bassett, L. W., Gold, R. H., & Shaffer, K. A. (1981). The potential value of liquid-crystal thermography in detecting significant mastopathy. *Radiology*, *140*(3), 659–662. doi:10.1148/radiology.140.3.7280232 PMID:7280232

Moskowitz, M., Milbrath, J., Gartside, P., Ermeno, A., & Mandel, D. (1976). Lack of efficiency of thermography as a screening tool for minimal and Stage I breast cancer. *Journal of Medicine*, *295*(5), 249–252. PMID:934189

Nathan, B. E., Burn, J. I., & MacErlean, D. P. (1972). Value of mammary thermography in differential diagnosis. *British Medical Journal*, *2*(5809), 316–317. doi:10.1136/bmj.2.5809.316 PMID:5022040

Neal, C. H., Flynt, K. A., Jeffries, D. O., & Helvie, M. A. (2018). Breast Imaging Outcomes following Abnormal Thermography. *Academic Radiology, 25*(3), 273–278. doi:10.1016/j.acra.2017.10.015 PMID:29275941

Ng, E. Y. (2005). Is thermal scanner losing its bite in mass screening of fever due to SARS? *Medical Physics, 32*(1), 93–97. doi:10.1118/1.1819532 PMID:15719959

Ng, E. Y. K., & Kee, E. C. (2008). Advanced integrated technique in breast cancer thermography. *Journal of Medical Engineering & Technology, 32*(2), 103–114. doi:10.1080/03091900600562040 PMID:17852648

Ng, E. Y. K., & Sudarshan, N. M. (2001). Effect of blood flow, tumor and cold stress in a female breast: A novel time-accurate computer simulation. *Proc. Instn Mech Enghs. Part H, 215*, 393–404. PMID:11521762

Ng, E. Y. K., & Sudarshan, N. M. (2004). Computer simulation in conjunction with medical thermography as an adjunct tool for early detection of breast cancer. *BMC Cancer, 4*(17), 1–6. doi:10.1186/1471-2407-4-17 PMID:15113442

Nguyen, A. V., Cohen, N. J., Lipman, H., Brown, C. M., Molinari, N. A., Jackson, W. L., Kirking, H. P., Szymanowski, T. W., Wilson, B. A., Salhi, R. R., Roberts, D. W., & Strykar, D. B. (2010). Comparison of 3 infrared thermal detection systems and self-report for mass fever screening. *Emerging Infectious Diseases, 16*(11), 1710–1717. doi:10.3201/eid1611.100703 PMID:21029528

Nishiura, H., & Kamiya, K. (2011). Fever screening during the influenza (H1N1-2009) pandemic at Narita International Airport, Japan. *BMC Infectious Diseases, 11*(1), 11–121. doi:10.1186/1471-2334-11-111 PMID:21539735

Nogueira, C. H. F. V., Nogueira, C. F., & Ely, J. B. (2015). Termografia por Infravermelho em Cirurgia Plástica – Novos Horizontes. *Pan American Journal Medical Thermology, 2*(1), 81–87.

Norton, P. R., Horn, S. B., Pelleggrino, J. G., & Perconti, P. (2008). Infrared detector and detectors arrays. In N. A. Diakides, & J. D. Bronzino (Eds.), Medical Infrared Imaging. CRC Press.

Nyirjesy, I., & Ayme, Y. (1986). *Clinical evaluation, mammography, and thermography in the diagnosis of breast carcinoma* (Vol. 1). Thermology.

Oliveira, M. M. (2012). *Desenvolvimento de protocolo e construção de um aparato mecânico para padronização da aquisição de imagens termográficas de mama* (Unpublished Master's dissertation). Universidade Federal de Pernambuco, Recife, Brazil.

Osman, M. M., & Afify, E. (1984). Thermal modeling of the normal woman's breast. *Journal of Biomechanical Engineering, 106*(2), 123–130. doi:10.1115/1.3138468 PMID:6738016

Osman, M. M., & Afify, E. (1988). Thermal modeling of the malignant woman's breast. *Journal of Biomechanical Engineering, 110*(4), 269–276. doi:10.1115/1.3108441 PMID:3205011

Partridge, P. W., & Wrobel, L. C. (2007). An inverse geometry problem for the localization of skin tumours by thermal analysis. *Engineering Analysis with Boundary Elements, 31*(10), 803–811. doi:10.1016/j.enganabound.2007.02.002

Paruch, M., & Majchrzak, E. (2007). Identification of tumor region parameters using evolutionary algorithm and multiple reciprocity boundary element method. *Engineering Applications of Artificial Intelligence*, *20*(5), 647–655. doi:10.1016/j.engappai.2006.11.003

Pellegrino, J. G., Zeibel, J., Driggers, R. G., & Perconti, P. (2008). Infrared Camera Characterization. In N. A. Diakides & J. D. Bronzino (Eds.), Medical Infrared Imaging. CRC Press.

Prabha, S., Suganthi, S. S., & Sujatha, C. M. (2015). An approach to analyze the breast tissues in infrared images using nonlinear adaptive level sets and Riesz transform features. *Technology and Health Care*, *23*(4), 429–442. doi:10.3233/THC-150915 PMID:26409908

Prabha, S., & Sujatha, C. M. (2018). Proposal of index to estimate breast similarities in thermograms using fuzzy C means and anisotropic diffusion filter based fuzzy C means clustering. *Infrared Physics & Technology*, *93*, 316–325. doi:10.1016/j.infrared.2018.08.018

Prasad, S. S., Ramachandra, L., Kumar, V., Dave, A., Mestha, L. K., & Venkatarmani, K. (2016). Evaluation of efficacy of thermographic breast imaging in breast cancer: A pilot study. *Breast Disease*, *36*(4), 143–147. doi:10.3233/BD-160236 PMID:27767959

Queiroz, K. F. F. C. (2014). *Análise da repetitividade e melhoria de segmentação semiautomática de ROIs em imagens termográficas de mama* (Unpublished bachelor's degree dissertation). Universidade Federal de Pernambuco, Recife, Brazil.

Raghavendra, U., Gudigar, A., Rao, T. N., Ciaccio, E. J., Ng, E. Y. K., & Acharya, U. R. (2019). Computer-aided diagnosis for the identification of breast cancer using thermogram images: A comprehensive review. *Infrared Physics & Technology*, *102*, 102. doi:10.1016/j.infrared.2019.103041

Rahmatinia, S., & Fahimi, B. (2017). Magneto-Thermal Modeling of Biological Tissues: A Step Toward Breast Cancer Detection. *IEEE Transactions on Magnetics*, *53*(6), 1–4. doi:10.1109/TMAG.2017.2671780

Rajmanova, P., Nudzikova, P., & Vala, D. (2015). Application and technology of thermal imaging camera in medicine. *IFAC-PapersOnLine*, *48*(4), 492–497. doi:10.1016/j.ifacol.2015.07.083

Ramírez-Torres, A., Rodríguez-Ramos, R., Sabina, F. J., García-Reimbert, C., Penta, R., Merodio, J., Guinovart-Díaz, R., Bravo-Castillero, J., Conci, A., & Preziosi, L. (2017). The role of malignant tissue on the thermal distribution of cancerous breast. *Journal of Theoretical Biology*, *426*, 152–161. doi:10.1016/j.jtbi.2017.05.031 PMID:28552555

Ramón, M. A. G., Mancilla, S. G. V., Henández, L. A. M., & Rios, R. A. O. (2017). Supportive Noninvasive Tool for the Diagnosis of Breast Cancer Using a Thermographic Camera as Sensor. *Sensors (Basel)*, *17*(3). PMID:28273793

Rastgar-Jazi, M., & Mohammadi, F. (2017). Parameters sensitivity assessment and heat source localization using infrared imaging techniques. *Biomedical Engineering Online*, *16*(1), 113. doi:10.118612938-017-0403-2 PMID:28934956

Rastghalam, R., & Pourghassem, H. (2016). Breast cancer detection using MRF-based probable texture feature and decision-level fusion-based classification using HMM on thermography images. *Pattern Recognition*, *51*, 176–186. doi:10.1016/j.patcog.2015.09.009

Ring, F. (2010). Thermal imaging today and its relevance to diabetes. *Journal of Diabetes Science and Technology*, *4*(4), 857–862. doi:10.1177/193229681000400414 PMID:20663449

Ring, F., Jung, A., & Zuber, J. (2015). *A Case Book of Infrared Imaging in Clinical Medicine*. IOP Publishing.

Rochester Institute of Technology. (2019). Retrieved from https:// www.rit.edu/news/rit-rrh-working-improve-cancer-screening

Saniei, E., Setayeshi, S., Akbari, M. E., & Navid, M. (2016). Parameter estimation of breast tumour using dynamic neural network from thermal pattern. *Journal of Advanced Research*, *7*(6), 1045–1055. doi:10.1016/j.jare.2016.05.005 PMID:27857851

Santos, E. B., Bianco, H. T., & Brioschi, M. L. (2015). Thermography in Assessing Cardiovascular Risk. *Pan American Journal Medical Thermology*, *2*(1), 23–25. doi:10.18073/2358-4696/pajmt.v2n1p23-25

Santos, L. C. (2009). *Desenvolvimento de ferramenta computacional para análise paramétrica da influência da posição e do tamanho de um tumor de mama em perfis de temperatura* (Master's thesis). Universidade Federal de Pernambuco, Recife, Brasil. Retrieved from https://repositorio.ufpe.br/handle/123456789/5021

Sarigoz, T., Ertan, T., Topuz, O., Sevim, Y., & Cihan, Y. (2018). Role of digital infrared thermal imaging in the diagnosis of breast mass: A pilot study: Diagnosis of breast mass by thermography. *Infrared Physics & Technology*, *91*, 214–219. doi:10.1016/j.infrared.2018.04.019

Saxena, A., Ng, E. Y. K., & Lim, T. S. (2019). Infrared (IR) thermography as a potential screening modality for carotid artery stenosis. *Computers in Biology and Medicine*, *113*, 113. doi:10.1016/j.compbiomed.2019.103419 PMID:31493579

Schaefer, G., Závišek, M., & Nakashima, T. (2009). Thermography based breast cancer analysis using statistical features and fuzzy classification. *Pattern Recognition*, *47*(6), 1133–1137. doi:10.1016/j.patcog.2008.08.007

Serrano, R. C., Lima, R. C. F., Melo, R. H. C., & Conci, A. (2010). Using fractal geometry to extract features of thermal images for early breast diseases. *ICGG - Proceedings of the 14th International Conference on Geometry and Graphics.*

Silva, L. F., Santos, A. A. S. M. D., Bravo, R. S., Silva, A. C., Muchaluat-Saade, D. C., & Conci, A. (2016). Hybrid analysis for indicating patients with breast cancer using temperature time series. *Computer Methods and Programs in Biomedicine*, *130*, 142–153. doi:10.1016/j.cmpb.2016.03.002 PMID:27208529

Silva, L. F., Sequeiros, G. O., Santos, M. L., Fontes, C. A., Muchaluat-Saade, D. C., & Conci, A. (2015). Thermal Signal Analysis for Breast Cancer Risk Verification. *Studies in Health Technology and Informatics*, *216*, 746–750. PMID:26262151

Silva Neto, A. J., & Moura Neto, F. D. (2005). *Problemas Inversos - Conceitos fundamentais e aplicações*. Ed. UERJ.

Singh, D., & Singh, A. K. (2019). Role of image thermography in early breast cancer detection- Past, present and future. *Computer Methods and Programs in Biomedicine*, 183. PMID:31525547

Souza, G. A., Brioschi, M. L., Vargas, J. V., Morais, K. C., Dalmaso Neto, C., & Neves, E. B. (2015). Reference breast temperature: Proposal of an equation. *Einstein (Sao Paulo, Brazil)*, *13*(4), 518–524. doi:10.1590/S1679-45082015AO3392 PMID:26761549

Spitalier, H., & Giraud, D. (1982). *Does infrared thermography truly have a role in present-day breast-cancer management?Biomedical Thermology*. Alan R. Liss.

Stark, A. M., & Way, S. (1974). The use of thermovision in the detection of early breast cancer. *Cancer*, *33*(6), 1664–1670. doi:10.1002/1097-0142(197406)33:6<1664::AID-CNCR2820330629>3.0.CO;2-7 PMID:4834161

Stark, A. M., & Way, S. (1974). The screening of well women for the early detection of breast cancer using clinical examination with thermography and mammography. *Cancer*, *33*(6), 1671–1679. doi:10.1002/1097-0142(197406)33:6<1671::AID-CNCR2820330630>3.0.CO;2-4 PMID:4834162

FLIR Systems. (2004). *ThermaCAM S45: Manual do operador*. Author.

Tan, T. Z., & Queck, C. (2007). A novel cognitive interpretation of breast cancer thermography with complementary learning fuzzy neural memory structure. *International Journal of Thermal Sciences*, *33*, 652–666. PMID:32288331

Thermography Clinic Inc. (2019). Retrieved from http:// www.thermography-mw.com

Thomassin, L. (1984). *Proceedings of the third international congress of thermology*. New York: Plenum Press.

Trafarski, A., Róanski, L., Straburzynska-Lupa, A., & Korman, P. (2008). The Quality of Diagnosis by IR Thermography as a Function of Thermal Stimulation in Chosen Medical Applications. *9th International Conference on Quantitative InfraRed Thermography*, Krakow, Poland. 10.21611/qirt.2008.03_13_17

United Breast Cancer Foundation. (2019). Retrieved from https://www.ubcf.org/your-health/breast-thermography/

Venkataramani, K., Mestha, L. K., Ramachandra, L., Prasad, S. S., Kumar, V., & Raja, P. J. (2015). Semi-automated breast cancer tumor detection with thermographic video imaging. *Conference Proceedings; ... Annual International Conference of the IEEE Engineering in Medicine and Biology Society. IEEE Engineering in Medicine and Biology Society. Conference*, 2022–2025. doi:10.1109/EMBC.2015.7318783 PMID:26736683

Viana, M. J. A. (2010). *Simulating the temperature profile in the breast using surrogate geometry obtained from an external breast prosthesis* (Master's thesis). Universidade Federal de Pernambuco, Recife, Brasil. Retrieved from https://repositorio.ufpe.br/handle/123456789/17939

Wahab, A. A., Salim, M. I., Ahamat, M. A., Manaf, N. A., Yunus, J., & Lai, K. W. (2016). Thermal distribution analysis of three-dimensional tumor-embedded breast models with different breast density compositions. *Medical & Biological Engineering & Computing*, *54*(9), 1363–1373. doi:10.100711517-015-1403-7 PMID:26463520

Wang, J., Chang, K., Chen, C., Chien, K., Tsai, Y., Wu, Y., Teng, Y., & Shih, T. T. (2010). Evaluation of the diagnostic performance of infrared imaging of the breast: A preliminary study. *Biomedical Engineering Online*, *9*(3), 1–14. doi:10.1186/1475-925X-9-3 PMID:20055999

Weum, S., Mercer, J. B., & de Weerd, L. (2016). Evaluation of dynamic infrared thermography as an alternative to CT angiography for perforator mapping in breast reconstruction: A clinical study. *BMC Medical Imaging*, *16*(1), 43. doi:10.118612880-016-0144-x PMID:27421763

Williams, K. L., Phillips, B. H., Jones, P. A., Beaman, S. A., & Fleming, P. J. (1990). Thermography in screening for breast cancer. *Journal of Epidemiology and Community Health*, *44*(2), 112–113. doi:10.1136/jech.44.2.112 PMID:2370497

Wu, L. A., Kuo, W. H., Chen, C. Y., Tsai, Y. S., & Wang, J. (2016). The association of infrared imaging findings of the breast with prognosis in breast cancer patients: An observational cohort study. *BMC Cancer*, *16*(1), 541. doi:10.118612885-016-2602-9 PMID:27464553

Yassin, N. I. R., Omran, S., El Houby, E. M. F., & Allam, H. (2018). Machine learning techniques for breast cancer computer aided diagnosis using different image modalities: A systematic review. *Computer Methods and Programs in Biomedicine*, *156*, 25–45. doi:10.1016/j.cmpb.2017.12.012 PMID:29428074

Zadeh, H. G., Haddadnia, J., Ahmadinejad, N., & Baghdadi, M. R. (2015). Assessing the Potential of Thermal Imaging in Recognition of Breast Cancer. *Asian Pacific Journal of Cancer Prevention*, *16*(18), 8619–8623. doi:10.7314/APJCP.2015.16.18.8619 PMID:26745126

Zhang, H., He, L., & Zhu, L. (2009). Critical conditions for the thermal diagnosis of the breast cancer. *3rd International Conference on Bioinformatics and Biomedical Engineering*. 10.1109/ICBBE.2009.5162563

Zhou, Y., & Herman, C. (2018). Optimization of skin cooling by computational modeling for early thermographic detection of breast cancer. *International Journal of Heat and Mass Transfer, 126*(Part B), 864 – 876.

Zore, Z., Filipović-Zore, I., Stanec, M., Batinjan, B., & Matejčić, A. (2015). Association of clinical, histopathological and immunohistochemical prognostic factors of invasive breast tumors and thermographic findings. *Infrared Physics & Technology*, *68*, 101–205. doi:10.1016/j.infrared.2014.12.009

Zuluaga-Gomez, J., Zerhouni, N., Al Masry, Z., Devalland, C., & Varnier, C. (2019). A survey of breast cancer screening techniques: Thermography and electrical impedance tomography. *Journal of Medical Engineering & Technology*, *43*(5), 305–322. doi:10.1080/03091902.2019.1664672 PMID:31545114

Chapter 8
Thermography in Biomedicine: History and Breakthrough

Iskra Alexandra Nola
https://orcid.org/0000-0002-8268-210X
School of Medicine, University of Zagreb, Croatia

Darko Kolarić
Ruđer Bošković Institute, Zagreb, Croatia

ABSTRACT

The historical details are important to understand the development and application of thermography with particular emphasis on its application in medicine, explained on breast cancer detection. Today, recommendations for breast cancer include the use of mammography as the gold standard screening method. In public health, the importance of screening women for possible breast cancer is indisputable, especially in light of the fact that the size of the cancer directly corresponds to the success of the cure. A method that will allow early detection of cancer and/or successful follow-up of postoperative or adjuvant treatment is unquestionable. Thermography as a non-invasive method is harmless and therefore enables repetition without harmful radiation to the patient, unlike mammography. These features should be sufficient to empower its application. However, its breakthrough does not proceed as expected. This chapter particularly emphasizes the importance of conducting studies in a uniform manner to enable the collected data to be comparable appropriately with the methods used so far.

INTRODUCTION

Infrared thermography, thermal imaging, infrared radiometry, infrared imaging, IR condition monitoring, (dynamic) digital infrared thermal imagining ((D)DITI) or only digital infrared imagining (DII) and thermovision are all terms used for this growing research field. In simplest terms, thermography means "picture of heat" (thermograms) and utilizes highly resolute and sensitive infrared (thermographic) cameras. Thermal imaging cameras detect radiation in the infrared range of the electromagnetic spectrum (8–14 μm) and produce images of that radiation (thermography).

DOI: 10.4018/978-1-7998-3456-4.ch008

Modern term also used for thermography is thermology. Thermology became medical science that could be used in diagnostic using highly detailed and sensitive infrared images of the human body. However, in practice is often used the term thermography.

This equipment usually has two parts, the IR camera and a standard PC or laptop computer with the respective software. This software supports thermal analysis and image presentation in numerical and graphical forms of temperature value of any part of surface inside the thermographic scan. The computer is routinely used to capture and analyze the infrared data (terms: computerized thermography, digital thermography, computerized thermal imaging, computerized infrared imaging, computed thermal imaging, digital infrared thermal imaging, digital infrared imaging, etc.). The addition of the prefix "clinical" or "diagnostic" is used for thermography in the health care field.

Thermal imaging as a diagnostic instrument or inspection tool has potential diverse applications: from thermal environmental studies to medical thermography including monitoring and follow-ups in breast thermography. In this chapter the main historical progresses in thermography development and their relation to thermography breakthrough in some of most interested area of biomedicine, especially breast cancer detection, is presented. This chapter particularly emphasizes the importance of conducting studies in a uniform manner to enable the collected data to be comparable appropriately with the methods used so far.

BACKGROUND

"Thermography should not be relied on for early detection of breast cancer." (Australian Government). And nobody says it should. At least not in scientific community that tries to facilitate breast cancer screening by using solutions that are non-invasive and easy to perform. However, this before mentioned statement of Australian government shows how things could go wrong easily. From FDA approval and classification of thermography as an adjunctive diagnostic screening procedure for the detection of breast cancer to announcement that this methodology is not reliable went barely 40-some years. Enough to "bury" the methodology?

The review of papers published in last 10 years (over 131 of them appeared at PubMed when the search included "thermography" AND "breast cancer" terms) will enlighten the story behind. After getting so many papers, narrowed search included "free full text" and "review" criteria for further work. These criteria are very important while this chapter will discuss the breakthrough of thermography into (bio) medicine and the establishment of any new methodology depends on its reliability which in science is mainly approved by review studies. This narrowed search gave 3 (three!) papers in total:

"Artificial intelligence methods for the diagnosis of breast cancer by image processing: a review" by Sadoughi et al. Breast Cancer (2018);

"Breast Cancer Detection Using Infrared Thermal Imaging and a Deep Learning Model" by Mambou et al. Sensors (2018); and

"The benefits and harms of screening for cancer with a focus on breast screening" by Brodersen Jørgensen and Gøtzsche Pol Arch Med Wewn. (2010).

Even though these articles are reviews, it is visible that two of them are from 2018 and one from 2010. Moreover, in search of 10 years, maybe in another database will results be different, but the most important was to show how small proportion of them one can find in the set of 131 papers related to the thermography and breast cancer.

The answer pop-ups by itself – there is no enough review done on the subject. In ten years, only three reviews. In addition, as it will be visible through this chapter – the main obstacle in introducing new methods, methodologies or techniques in medicine is the lack of reviews and analysis that will comprehensively present data, results and their strengths and weaknesses.

Sideward the fact that there is a lack of reviews and meta-analysis in area of scientific thermography, we must see that there is also a visible difference in approach and conclusions weather the study was conducted primarily by physicians or engineers or by interdisciplinary teams. The latter should have more credibility in presenting the benefits and/or shortcomings of chosen methodology.

The use of offered possibility from PubMed to switch the search to "Best matches for thermography and breast cancer", gave 3 more papers, but none of them were review:

"Breast thermography alone no substitute for mammography" by Gourd et al. Lancet Oncol. (2017);

"Early diagnosis and detection of breast cancer" by Milosevic et al. Technol Health Care. (2018); and

"Evolution of Imaging in Breast Cancer" by Garcia et al. Clin Obstet Gynecol. (2016).

Through this chapter, the pros and cons of thermography will be presented, in light of thermography development through history and its application in last few decades, with the emphasize on further possibilities on its progression in the field of medical application.

THERMOGRAPHY BREAKTHROUGH IN BIOMEDICNE

"Historia est magistra vitae". It is true. But, how does this proverb fits into thermography in biomedicine? The thermography breakthrough into biomedicine does not proceed as expected. Here is shown how things could get in the wrong direction if we are not willing to learn from our past. Even though the beginning was fabulous.

Historical and Physical Basis of Thermography

Hippocrates, around 480 BC, first recorded the thermobiological differences visible at human body. With putting mud on the abdomen of the patient and the change in colour when getting dry, he observed that some areas would dry first. This was thought to indicate underlying organ pathology.

Santorio, an Italian physician, made first measurements of body temperatures. He was the first one using a "thermometer" based on Galileo Galilei's "thermoscope", which reflected the changes in sensible heat. Santorio's thermomether had a scale, which the thermoscope had not. In 18th century dr Wunderlich from Leipzig, Germany, developed clinical thermometer and thus introduced thermal measurement into clinical routine.

Throughout history, several physical achievements explained the causes of this phenomenon. In 1800' William Herschel discovers invisible infrared (IR) rays, and in 1840 John Herschel receives the first infrared image. As a result of continuing testing, they found that each body at a temperature above 0° K radiates thermal energy to the environment, in proportion to the temperature at which it is heated.

However, the bodies in real life radiate very diverse. Therefore, it was important to consider the simplified laws of a body model with „ideal“ radiation and then applied it to actually occurring objects. This body model in radiation physics is "black body“. This model distinguishes itself by the fact that, of all bodies of equal temperature, it shows the largest possible emitted radiation.

This "black body" model is irreplaceable tool since the real objects we are measuring more or less deviate from the given parameter. The parameter of emittance then shows this deviation through the measure of body's capability to emit IR radiation. The black body with the highest possible emittance with the value of 1, depending also on wavelength is the referent point to point the value of emittance of the body which IR radiation we are measuring. This body will also have more or less dependence on wavelength, but also the material composition, surface roughness, temperature etc. are the factors that influence the whole process and the result of measurement.

Today, the physical laws teach us that all objects with a temperature above absolute zero (−273 K) emit infrared radiation from their surface. The Stefan-Boltzmann Law defines the relation between radiated energy and temperature by stating that the total radiation emitted by an object is directly proportional to the object's area and emissivity and the fourth power of its absolute temperature. The emissivity of human skin is extremely high (~0.98), so measurements of infrared radiation emitted by the skin can be converted directly into accurate temperature values.

Thermography Breakthrough in Biomedicine

Body temperature is crucially indicative in many medical situations. Raised temperature in body or some parts of the body present natural warning mechanism. The fact that thermography can, by non-invasive approach and without the body contact, detect this temperature rise could be useful in many diagnostic situations.

Infrared imaging as an ideal procedure to evaluate body surface temperatures becomes primarily military interest. Military research on infrared monitoring systems for nighttime troop movements in the 1950s opened a new era in thermal diagnostics. These findings first were applied in development of military thermal remote sensing devices in the early 1950' in the Korean War. These first thermographic devices were very cumbersome, and were used mainly in laboratory settings or mounted on trucks for field use.

Knowing the physical principles of infrared emission was the beginning of future thermography. Military researches added an extra value: they improved methodology. This was important to elevate research to another level: to discover why different temperature occur at different body parts. They basically initiated continued research and clinical observations that finally proved that certain temperatures of different body parts could be related to normal and abnormal physiological processes.

Professor Czerny, spectroscopist, provided us with the first human infrared image in Frankfurt in 1928, presented in his work "Über Photographie im Ultraroten". However, the medical use of infrared thermography started in 1952 in Germany, and the first medical thermographic device dates from 1953 (made by manufacturer Schwamm&Reeh). The physician Schwamm and the physicist Reeh made a single detector, infrared bolometer, for thermal measurement of specific parts of the human body surface. They made it for diagnostic purposes.

When declassified from military purposes only, in the mid-1950s, infrared imaging technology became available for medical purposes as well. In 1956th Lawson used infrared imaging in breast cancer patients and discovered higher skin temperature above cancer spot than of normal tissue. His researches also reveal that the venous blood draining the cancer is often warmer than its arterial supply. After his achievements, started thermography development and exceeds the experimental state as a diagnostic procedure being used for over 40 years as an adjunctive screening procedure in the evaluation of the breast cancer.

Liquid crystal contact (LC) thermographic device was the first one in general use, and it is interesting that this device remained in use for medical research till late 1970'. The major drawback of this device was the interference between probe and the object, which was measured. Because of the contact of the two, measurements often were incorrect.

At the end of 1960' and beginning of 1970' new palette of sensors at the area of spatial configuration were introduced, with linear and matrix thermal sensors of higher degree of integration, higher thermal sensitivity and spatial resolution. The result of this technological progress was due to developing space programs for military purposes. This progress matches the scientific discoveries on neoangiogenesis by Folkman in 1971.

Angiogenesis, the process of developing new blood vessels, refers to creation of them from preexisting vessels. Until recently, this process was perceived as the only mechanism of blood vessel creation in postnatal life. The vascular system development in embryo, vasculogenesis, begins with in situ differentiation of endothelial progenitors or angioblasts. Over the last few years, studies have shown that endothelial stem cells can be found in the adult as well where participating in creation of new blood vessel in normal and pathological states, including tumor "neoangiogenesis". The "neo" prefix refers to the fact this process is present in adults, in stages where presumably all the blood vessels should be already formed.

Folkman presented the new way of thinking about cancers. He made a new approach in which cancer, in order to survive and grow, require blood vessels, and by cutting off that blood supply, a cancer would be forced to go into remission. The researches who join his idea started to study these mechanisms and together with the results of his work unraveled the processes that regulate angiogenesis. The research on the underlying biological processes responsible for cancer spread continue but the most important result of Folkman' research is this distinction between angiogenesis and neoangiogenesis. Based on that fact, that cancer creates its own blood vessels in order to survive and grow, IR imaging become suitable for cancer detection. Namely, the process of developing new blood vessels in certain area will cause the increased temperature at specific spot, which can be "catch" by thermography.

Numerous medical centers and clinics used thermography for different diagnostic purposes. At the same time significant advances have been made in the application of sophisticated computerized image processing. Many studies pointed breast cancer as a type of cancer where thermography is useful, especially when repeated check-ups are needed. Supported by this studies and application, the Food and Drug Administration on January 29, 1982, published its approval and classification of thermography as an adjunctive diagnostic screening procedure for the detection of breast cancer.

Thermography Application

Today there are numerous areas of thermography application. Many of them are very well established. In aerospace industry for achieving safety standards or testing the materials. In automotive industry for quality control or testing the tires. In chemical industry, the most important use is measuring the temperature of chemical process without contact, or checking the levels of liquids in tanks. In electrical engineering, thermography is used for measurements of temperature distribution of smallest electronic components, which is very important in producing temperature sensors while with thermography measurements are made contactless. In glass industry, thermography detects distribution of heat through and on glass by using selected spectral filters. In metallurgy, efficiently reduce the energy consumption and can detect defects in insulation processes. In plastic industry, enable measurements necessary for defining thickness of the material. In environmental studies, thermography allows measurement of smallest temperature differences in environment, biotops, laboratories, very precisely. This is important in the area of preservation (animals, environment) and in research of biological models. In studies of environmental health, today when global temperature changes occur, thermography is present in measurement of objects radiation (loss of energy), which radically contributes to elevated environmental temperature in cities creating hot zones which affect human health. Finally, thermography is applicable in medicine as well. However, proven effectiveness of thermography in other areas has not facilitated its penetration into medicine. This application is from the beginning under the greatest pressure and scrutiny by medical professional. When it comes to human body and our health, the precaution is expected. However, biomedical thermography application, except historical background, has recently conducted many studies that show its applicability in biomedicine as well. In many areas, its strength is in detection of abnormality, but also there are areas where thermography is to be expected as one of future non-invasive diagnostic tool. The most important factor that contributes to acceptable results in thermography diagnose in medicine is use of appropriate clinical infrared imaging system.

Biomedical use of thermography through history was predominately pointed towards cancer research and detection. Until nowadays, this research presents growing area especially while thermography systems are more developed and become more accurate. As thermography detects changes in the temperature of the surface, the fact that our body is very sensitive to any change in surrounding area or inner processes, makes this methodology very suitable to reveal slightly differences in skin temperature at the spots of interest. This is possible simply by following the basic physics.

In the electromagnetic spectrum, infrared rays are found within the wavelengths of 0.75 μm to 1 mm. The infrared radiation emitted from the human skin is mainly in the 2–20 μm wavelength range, with an average peak between 9 and 10 μm. Based on the application of Plank's equation and Wein's Law, it is found that approximately 90% of emitted infrared radiation in humans is in the longer wavelengths (6–14 μm). Based on that fact it was possible to create systems capable to "catch" this radiation and to analyze them in a light of pathological changes present. The main problem in thermography use in medicine is the accuracy of obtained results. This problem is solvable by using appropriate clinical infrared imaging system.

The choice of an appropriate clinical infrared imaging system is very important and demand adequate technical aspects. Absolute, spatial, and temperature resolution along with thermal stability and adequate computerized image processing are just a few of the critical specifications. Today there are minimum equipment standards established where, from research studies, infrared physics, human anatomic and physiologic parameters are applied. The most important parameter in selection of clinical infrared imaging equipment remains the wavelength sensitivity of the infrared detector.

The object we want to investigate and the type of detection are crucial parameters in defining the area of the infrared spectrum that is base for selection of a detector. In medicine object of interest is the human body and belonging environmental conditions, so Plank's equation leads us to select a detector in the 8–12 μm range. The environment under which the examination takes place is not free from possible sources of detection errors. Imaging room environmental artifacts such as reflectance can cause errors when shorter wavelength detectors (fewer than 7 μm) are used. Consequently, the optimum infrared detector to use in imaging the body should have sensitivity in the longer wavelengths spanning the 9–10 μm range. The problems encountered with first generation infrared camera systems: incorrect detector sensitivity (shorter wavelengths), thermal drift, calibration, and analogue interface, has been solved for almost two decades ago. In the end of the 20th century occurred an expansion of models and manufacturers of IR camera, also used for medical purposes. The first IR cameras applied for medical use were noisy, instable, with fixed pattern and thermal drift.

Modern computerized infrared imaging systems, with a new technology, uncooled plane array (FPA) microbolometer IR-cameras can discriminate petty variations in thermal emissions while producing extremely high-resolution images digitally processed by sophisticated computerized analysis.

Technical factors, described previously are controllable factors, but still very differ between researchers presenting wide range of choice that could be considered as one of obstacles in relation to required uniformity for good systematic review and meta-analysis of existing data and results.

Another part of factors contributing successful use of thermography includes environmental factors. Factors that are in relation to the natural environment to which patients are exposed and thermography takes place. These factors are very important but luckily controllable (room temperature, size, humidity etc.). Even though we can control them, still the best option represents the way of thermography use where patients are invited in prearranged space. Rather than go to them with the camera. That is how many environmental factors could be seen as non-interrupting ones.

Use of thermography is also influenced by individual factors. Individual factors are important and relevant for individual assessment but also individual characteristics can affect the skin temperature (age, gender, therapy, metabolic rate, genetic, etc.) or can be the obstacle in providing best reading if they affect skin temperature by their presence/absence (cosmetics, tobacco, food consuming, etc.). Here thermography faces the problem while controlling those individual factors seems impossible. Using other instruments, which does not rely on skin temperature that can be affected by so many factors, can be perceived as more reasonable, but this is not the reason to stop develop thermography as one new, affordable tool with its niche for use.

Obviously, thermography does not provide the information on structure of the organs of interest, but indicate changes in temperature and overall condition of the tissue in relation to its pathophysiology. To see if there is a space for develop the thermography to be more uniform in use is of great value while its non-invasive feature could be valuable in early detection.

Biomedical Areas of Thermography Use and Breast Cancer

Thermography is useful, biologically inert method capable to diagnose early signs of skin temperature changes in relation to different types of diseases, especially carcinogenesis which will lead to the specific cancer in observed area.

Thermography is based on the principle that, because of metabolic activity and vascular circulation, the temperature of tissue and surrounding area in which changes are occurring is always higher than in other parts. Tumors are in need for nutrients and they increase circulation to cells by keeping open existing vessels, opening dormant and creating the new ones. The process of neoangiogenesis, accented by Guido and Smith in 1996 when they described angiogenesis factors release as the beginning of early stage of tumor cells growth, put these physiological principles as the one that allows thermography to "catch" the early signs of hypervascularity and hyperthermia.

By measuring local skin temperature thermography can detect these changes in each part of human body. If the change is visible by thermography, this is the proof of raised metabolic activity in certain area. This still does not mean that there is a tumor cells developing, while certain other processes could be the reason for elevated metabolic activity: inflammation, for example. Still, for precancerous changes, thermography could have enormous potential. If we exclude other causes, then the precancerous changes are very likely the reason.

All these facts pushed many researchers to investigate possible areas of thermography application. This resulted in researches and results of thermography application in breast cancer, arthritis, vascular and nervous system disorders, metabolic disorders, headaches, neck and back problems, etc. Somewhere in early 1990', researches of thermography use for early cancer detection get the wings and the number of studies raised in almost each before mentioned areas. This was also encouraged by more innovative approach to the thermography cameras development, and more physical and electro engineering research. When the infrared technology became available and developed (better spatial resolution for example), the more research was conducted with more significant results.

Studies showed that thyroid gland, in relation to its thermo-physical properties, if it is affected by tumor, presents significant variation in temperature. Also, skin cancer, which present uncontrolled growth of abnormal skin cells (often cause by ultraviolet radiation), is visible as the temperature difference between affected and non-affected skin area. These examples prove that, where is the raised metabolic activity, there will be notifications visible by thermography.

In all this areas studies discovered that temperature difference between suspicious spot and the healthy one tells the story about clinical change. The problem was that many of these studies did not go further and try to systematize their findings. In some area, the main obstacle was the fact that their findings were not comparable with other studies while the chosen methodology were too different. However, this was not the case with breast cancer.

Breast cancer is known from ancient times. It is described in ancient Egyptian and Greek culture as a bulging disease spread over the breast. In first and second century A.D. physicians tried to incise and cauterize the formations found in female breasts. They discovered it is in relation to the age and menstrual cycle. This was the time when Galen, well known Roman physician and philosopher of Greek origin, attributed cancer to the “black bile in the blood”, and named it as “cancer” (“crab”) while he wanted to accent the fact that there were dilated veins radiating from the affected tissue. During the middle ages, almost until 1500', the approach to surgical methods was diminished. Medieval postulates in healing preferred faith and miracles over surgery. There were some improvement in Islamic part of the world but the European populations were forced to wait progress in that area. During the Renaissance period started the golden era for revival of surgery. The theories were spreading all over and causes of breast cancer differ from infection, through family factors, environment, to the trauma and personality. In that period, the “lymph” replaced “black bile”. In 19th century, the generally accepted fact that the cancer is spread through lymph led to the radical surgery approaches, including mastectomy. The surgical principle ruled until the late 19th and early 20th century when development of radiology made changes. The urge for the detecting the early signs of disease emerged and introduction of mammography changed the approach. Mammography was introduced in early 1960' when became methodology of choice for diagnosing. This happened after technical innovations enabled higher quality images easier to interpret. Not long after, the mammography was tested as a screening tool. This was important while researchers discovered that the most important factor that contributes to better breast cancer outcome (survival) is the time of detection (particularly the size). Thus, screening for early cancer detection became the most important tool for public health efforts in general population' health preservation. Really, at the beginning, the detection of cancers was impressive and breast cancer mortality was reduced. However, for last decade or more these results seem to stagnate. To make them more accurate, the more contrast is needed in contrast-enhanced mammography, which is dangerous for patients with kidney disease, for example.

Early detection, biopsy, surgery, chemotherapy and radiation today are all the methods available in breast cancer treatment. However, parallel to development of clinical breast cancer management, public health started to be more and more important while epidemiology and statistics showed increased number of women with breast cancer in populations. The main task of public health is to prevent the disease in population. When this is not possible, public health wants to detect early signs of the disease in order to minimize the possible damage.

Early signs of breast cancer are detectable by mammography and, in some cases, genetically (when this genetic test only reveal the predisposition). Genetic tests are expensive and public health needs the methodology by which screening the population of interest is possible. Mammography, over the years, became the golden standard for breast cancer screening, but it has limitations as well. First, it radiates. Second, because of radiation, it could not be used frequently. Moreover, as we know, a tumor can grow in a few months from the small one (perceived as curable without any grave consequences) to one which will need a most comprehensive management to be treated properly.

As the mammography present possible threat to human health if the use exceed the benefits, and the breast cancer became more and more presented in population, the method that will allow more often checkups was needed. This was the main reason why many studies were performed on development of possible method for breast cancer detection. This is simple to explain: breast cancer is the most common cancer, it was the cancer with highest rate of mortality and became, after introducing mammography, the most screened cancer.

When the number of discovered breast cancers began to rise, by simple use of mammography, some physicians/researchers started to consider possible implication of X-ray film mammography more frequent and its consequences in sense of human radiation exposure. Because the main focal point in each cancer management is early detection, while uniform, defined prevention is still missing, and treatment is still very invasive, any progress in non-invasive technology that could be used for that matter became very important.

The rising number of studies that benefit thermography present the results with a visible difference between healthy tissue and cancerogenic ones. In other areas of application, thermography also showed some progress in temperature changes and differences detection that allowed researches to try to conclude what is the primary benefit of thermography use. Almost all of them agreed that thermography as additional tool/method, which allows more checkups, while is non-invasive and biologically inert, is worth to be additionally investigate. Finally, why not to try using it as follow-up tool after the treatment? It will be worthy to have a tool that could diagnose recurrence in the breast after breast-conserving therapy simply by rise in breast temperature much earlier than other diagnostic tools. Thermographic images can be a sort of individual baseline. They are thermal fingerprints and stay relatively the same through our lifetime. First image after breast-conserving therapy should be the baseline, and all future images will be compared with that one. They can be rated as well: as high or low risk. This will help the physician to decide when the next appointment with the patient will be. This will also be a good model for follow-up of the effects of intervention and therapies.

All these promising situations are the good reasons to enhance further researches. Still, we are attending the situations where thermography is more than ever under the suspicious of being deceiving, not accurate enough and problematic when it comes to the diagnosing the exact spot that represent tumor at image. Why is that so?

PROS AND CONS

During the history of breast cancer, and cancers as well, the primary outcome to be expected was the detection of cancer presence. With the development of science, medicine and public health, the humans changed their focus: the most important thing became to find it still very small so we can treat it with minimal therapy. To detect something small, in its infancy, and to be sure that is malignant is the 21st century task.

Mammography is the approved tool for breast cancer screening. It is invasive (it radiates), and present for over the 50 years. What are its characteristics? The overall sensitivity is about 79%, which means that mammography correctly identifies 79% of women who truly have breast cancer. Sensitivity is higher in 50+ women and lower in younger and those with dense breasts (National Cancer Institute). This means that there are situations when false-positive and/or false-negative findings occur. False-positive results are the results when mammogram shows there is a cancer when in fact there is no cancer in the breast. This often produce fear and anxiety in women recalled after such mammograms. After several years of mammograms, the chance of having false-positive mammograms is increased, it is about 50-60%. However, the specificity of mammography measures the non-cancer that were pronounced as non-cancer. This measure is very important for screening in the domain of public health while those are women not to be recall for additional check-ups.

Is there any need, with so high statistical data on mammography accuracy, for another diagnostic tool? As mentioned before, mammography is not harmless, and the screening plans very differ from country to country. All available data are the results of many studies conducted. The most valuable are those performed as a part of screening programs. However, which method is suitable for women with dense breasts and younger than 50 years? This question opens the niche for new tools for detection. Thermography would be suitable for younger or elder women. Thus, studies that are uniformed, focused on same age group are needed.

The tumor size is in relation to the degree of hyperthermia. The fact that hyperthermia occurs in relatively small number of physiological changes, is very attractive for further investigation: any inflammatory process is visible on thermograms and inflammatory process is also in a base of tumor as well. To do accurate thermography findings we still need follow up to be done by using methodology (such as pathohistology methods) to confirm suspicious spots at thermography image. Numerous studies confirm thermography findings as significant enough, many of them followed by pathohistology, but there are still shortcomings that does not allow us to say that thermography can be used as screening tool.

This is how study design became important and when compared to studies that promote mammography things are clear. Mammography is the subject of research for more than 50 years but with the general and governmental permission and cooperation developed into very well-designed approach. The participants are uniformed, the variety of appliances is low, and the methods of reading are more comprehensive, under the regulated education. Today, based on woman' screening history, some countries (which raised the screening for breast cancer at the higher level and have centralized system of surveillance, like Denmark for example) can divide thermograms into initial (including the very first one), and subsequent ones. Having so much well-organized data, the stratification in population, related to methodology, is matter of time. This elevate the follow-up process as well by using all the screens in predefined period, adding comprehensive results in research.

All of these things are missing in many thermography researches in the area of breast cancer. We argue that new era in thermography needs well designed studies with predefined parameters to investigate. Such circumstances will allow studies to be repeatable which will lead to comprehensive data more easily to interpret and to reach uniform conclusions. With many studies conducted in such manner, the consequent meta-analysis will give final review. Only then, the results will speak for themselves.

Tumor size is a time-dependent factor and higher tumor-size should be correlated with less frequent screening. Mammography should not be performed too frequently and thus public health needs tool that could be used many times without being harmful. Here lies the possible benefit of thermography.

Untrained Personnel and Protocol Violations

Thermography has not been widely recognized few decades ago while the technology was still in its infancy, but during 1990' and 2000', this situation changed. In addition, the skepticism resists. Why? Precautionary principle is the most important one in good public health. This is why is understandable the point of view where thermography is not welcomed (yet) in everyday clinical use. However, one can still argue that research on thermography should be continued and supported having on mind its non-invasive and harmless approach. Technology progress of thermography research gives new possibilities to increase sensitivity and technologically improved sensors and methods for pathological changes detection (such as "machine learning, "deep learning" and neuron network).

In this situation, it is to be expected that many deny and downplay the contribution of thermography to cancer (especially breast cancer) detection. Articles are mainly citing the quotes where its contribution is ranked from negative to not satisfactory. They also include recommendations from their leading public health institutions (USA FDA, New Zealand, Canada and Australia governmental and public health institutions). All of them are putting thermography into a group of devices that cannot be used for malignant diseases detection. However, the focal point is missed. The problem is not the thermography by itself (and it never was). The problem are people using these devices without proper training, trying to earn money. Total market congestion with free interpreted thermal images made a disservice with its references. Thermography must stay in the field of medical diagnostic, must include realistic assessments and very well educated, interdisciplinary teams. This will protect patients and enable proper progress in developing thermography as a valuable diagnostic tool. Nevertheless, it is strange that there is no meta-analysis of studies on thermography in medicine. Especially when we know that the simplicity of changes visible on thermal images led to unprofessional approach to thermography use. This was another critical moment in which easy detection of some diseases (Raynaud's syndrome, benign/malignant skin changes, fibromyalgia, etc.) made wrong impression that thermography could be also easily used in other much more complicated cases.

To enable thermography to be used in the process of detecting breast cancer, which is the predominant area of interest, it is necessary to design software support able to identify cause underlying the temperature anomaly at specific spots at individual patient' image. Development of algorithms for complex mathematical image analysis resulted in the possibility of generating a quality diagnosis for a range of diseases.

In scientific papers a whole set of procedures could be found, which based on numerical data from thermal image and with the use of existing algorithms (or specially designed procedures) seek the result that will be capable adequately diagnose the tumor. Results are more or less good but still far away from satisfactory ones. Machine learning, based on thermographic images and their readable parameters, including algorithms, interdependencies and statistical methods, is the future in tumor detection on thermal image. This model will "teach" the machine how to detect the exact combination of parameters, which then will be, with a certain amount of probability, declared tumor (or not).

That means that more samples of thermal images in certain field (breast cancer for example) we have, of course supported by pathohistology findings, we will have more examples on which the computer will learn. Computer will learn how to define more precisely the future individual combinations from thermal image. There are studies showing positive shift in the segment of methodology' specificity, based on "machine learning".

In the scientific and professional domain of research and use, thermography produces very good results in a whole range of biomedical use. The greatest advantage of thermography for the patient is the absence of harmful radiation, no restrictions on gender and age, the cheapest price of equipment and software, quick evaluation of results, and finally, the very short preparation time performing the procedure. All this facts speaks for themselves, but also give the reasonable base for continuing the work in the field of medical thermography use.

SOLUTIONS AND RECOMMENDATIONS

As shown in Table 1, the most visible problem in thermography studies is nonexistence of uniform approach in research. Until today, researches on mammography developed in an area with very well-defined research criteria. In thermography, research is connected to the level of technological development of thermovision (sensors with higher resolution and sensitivity). Thus, is very important to uniform other features in creating the study (such a study group, expected outcomes etc.).

Table 1. Problems in uniform use of thermography as seen by authors and proposed solutions

Breast thermography	Problem	Proposed solution
Detection	What is detectable?	Describe in particular what is going to be detected (the targeted size of tumor for example).
Screening	Screening whom? Screening what?	What/who is going to be screened (particular population, particular cancer, etc.)
Follow-ups	What/who is followed?	Define: follow-up of recovery, reoccurrence, women with suspicious thermograms, etc.
Check-ups	What/who is going to be checked?	Define: check-up of the first thermograms, the younger women, elder women…
Study design	Uniformity of the data Interdisciplinary approach	Making databases Ensuring availability of databases to other scientists Differ the results based on the chosen study Computer packages Include interdisciplinary teams

FUTURE RESEARCH DIRECTIONS

Future research on thermography application in breast cancer screening should incorporate development of specially designed computed packages for thermal image analysis. In addition, creation of atlas with representative images of tumors recognized by thermography (Figure 1) and proved by pathohistology (Figure 2) will ensure more accurate approach and validation of methodology. This will facilitate additional benefit for the use of thermography as an adjunct tool. The study design rests the most important feature. This means that uniform approach in standardized measurement and data collecting and processing, and results presentation is needed. This will enable thermography studies to be comparable with other methodologies used in the same or different studies.

Figure 1. ThermoMED (program package developed at Ruđer Bošković Institute), isothermal temperature display

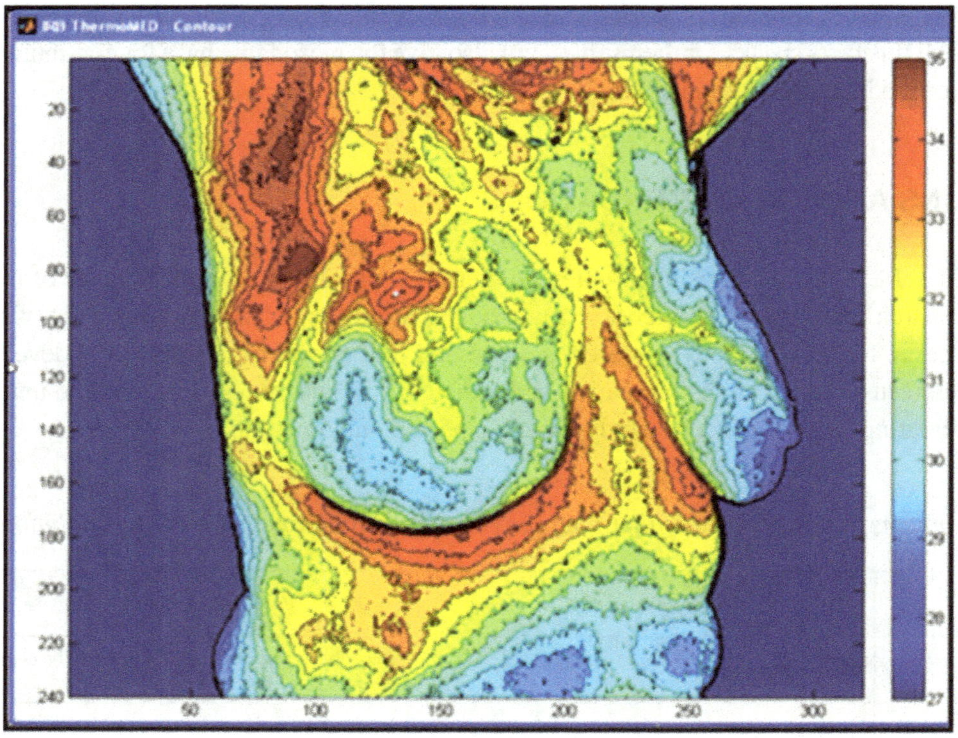

CONCLUSION

Malignant tumors are the most important findings that could be marked by using thermography. Thermal response, based on biological activity, represents the first sign that something went wrong in the area of interest. First there is a decrease in temperature (around the tumor) while it grows using existing vascularity. Then intensified blood flow is seen as hyperthermia. This is direct consequence of hypervascularity which is the result of subsequent tumor growth, when it forms own blood vessels. This are the main symptoms of area affected by tumor cells. Common knowledge on physiology of tumorous cells tells the story about how the changes that threaten human health begins. Sometimes the temperature is increased by higher metabolic rate caused by the effort of tumor to develop itself, and sometimes is caused by immunologic reaction that represent battle that body is trying to win.

Figure 2. Thermographic image patient whose tumor was proved by pathohistology. Right semi-oblique position. Right breast, in upper outer quadrant – pathological thermographic sign (also using ThermoMED program)

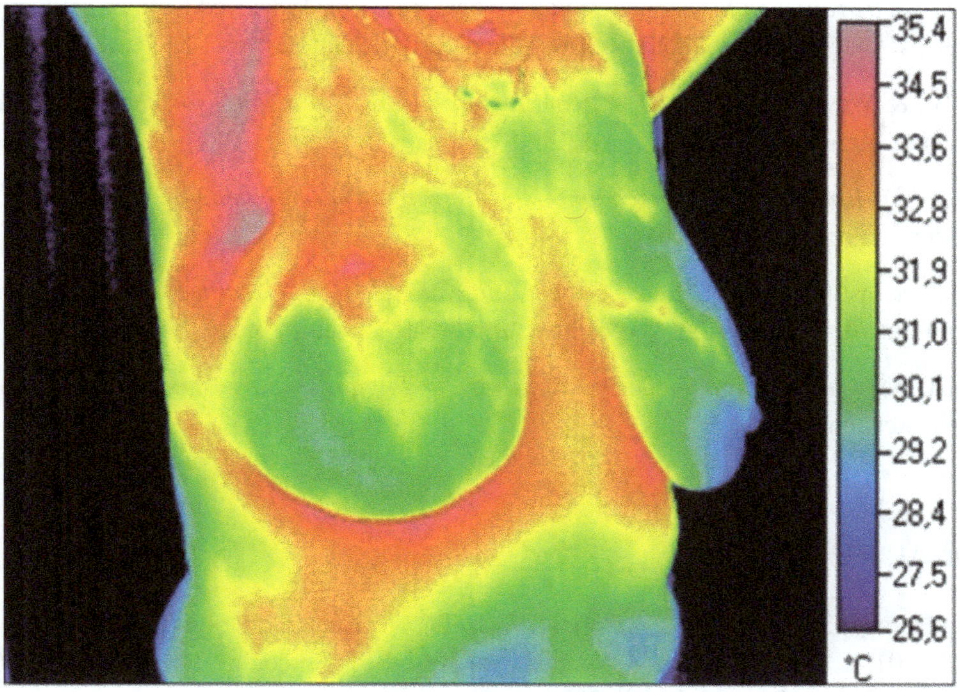

In past decade or so, technology advances in digital images and their computer-assisted analyses emerges as a possible tool for early cancer diagnosis without unnecessary irradiation. These advances are visible in better cameras, images, more accurate hot spots on images that could be easier detected and described, and the progress in this technology is promising by their possible everyday use and non-harmfulness. Proper detection of an early sign of breast cancer sets the task in front of researchers. History of breast cancer treatments, teaches us to be more open-minded. If the humans did not made discoveries in the area of anesthesia, we will still have operations with tremendous pain, without biopsy mastectomy will still rule, and without mammography, we will still be forced to the invasive surgical approach in any breast cancer type or case. Based on those principles, we argue that search for non-invasive technology that will be of help in detecting early signs of disease, and be effective in follow-up routine, must not stop. Here we see thermography as a very promising method that will bring future in our breast cancer management. In addition, all the studies performed should follow the uniform strategy, and the great contribution would make a central database for thermography findings. Meta-analysis performed on such data would eliminate declaration as the ones stated by National Cancer Institute "that no randomized trials have compared thermography to other screening modalities." (National Cancer Institute). In addition, "Small cohort studies do not suggest any additional benefit for the use of thermography as an adjunct modality." (National Cancer Institute). These statements should be perceived as the direction that thermography research must go. Appling the adequate approach to thermography search, studies, data processing and presentation of results will facilitate the real breakthrough of thermography into medicine.

REFERENCES

Australian Government, Department of Health, Therapeutic Goods Administration. (2019). *Thermography should not be relied on for early detection of breast cancer.* Retrieved from https://www.tga.gov.au/media-release/thermography-should-not-be-relied-early-detection-breast-cancer

Jorgensen, B., & Wewn, G. (2010). *The benefits and harms of screening for cancer with a focus on breast screening*. Academic Press.

Mambou. (2018). *Breast Cancer Detection Using Infrared Thermal Imaging and a Deep Learning Model.* Academic Press.

National Cancer Institute. (n.d.). *Breast Cancer Screening (PDQ®)–Health Professional Version.* Retrieved from https://www.cancer.gov/types/breast/hp/breast-screening-pdq#_543

Sadoughi. (2018). *Artificial intelligence methods for the diagnosis of breast cancer by image processing: a review.* Academic Press.

ADDITIONAL READING

Kolarić, D., Herceg, Ž., Nola, I. A., Ramljak, V., Kuliš, V., Katančić Holjevac, J., Deutsch, J. A., & Antonini, S. (2013). Thermography – A Feasible Method for Screening Breast Cancer? *Collegium Antropologicum, 37*(2), 583–588. PMID:23941007

Poljak-Blaži, M., Kolarić, D., Jaganjac, M., Žarković, K., Skala, K., & Žarković, N. (2009). Specific thermographic changes during Walker 256 carcinoma development: Differential infrared imaging of tumour, inflammation and haematoma. *Cancer Detection and Prevention, 32*(5/6), 431–436. doi:10.1016/j.cdp.2009.01.002 PMID:19232842

KEY TERMS AND DEFINITIONS

Machine Learning: Study of algorithms and statistical models that computers use to perform tasks for which they do not have instructions. Instead, they rely on patterns and they use acquired data to make predictions or decisions. This is one of the steps of artificial intelligence.

Precautionary Principle: Relates to promotion and protection of human health where any features, actions or methodology, if potentially harmful or not safety for individual and/or population health, is perceived as threat that must be addressed in favor of prevention.

Public Health: Science that focuses on disease prevention, prolonging life and promoting human health through public health interventions and actions, which include informing and educating society and individuals, and treatments and methods that uniformly protect them.

Screening: Strategy that aims to reduce the risk of disease in individual or population by checking them for undesirable factors or features that contribute to individual or population susceptibility to disease development.

Thermal Imaging: Represent the process of converting the IR radiation (heat) into visible images that present spatial distribution of temperature differences.

Thermography in Biomedicine: Any thermal monitoring made on living organisms in order to study, heal, or protect them.

Chapter 9
Imaging Techniques for Breast Cancer Diagnosis

Debasray Saha
Institute of Applied Medicines and Research, Ghaziabad, India

Neeraj Vaishnav
University of Rajasthan, India

Abhimanyu Kumar Jha
https://orcid.org/0000-0002-6798-2825
Institute of Applied Medicines and Research, Ghaziabad, India

ABSTRACT

Breast cancer is the most typical variety of cancer in women worldwide. Mammography is the "gold standard" for the analysis of the breast from an imaging perspective. Altogether, the techniques used within the management of cancer in all stages are multiple biomedical imaging. Imaging as a very important part of cancer clinical protocols can offer a range of knowledge regarding morphology, structure, metabolism, and functions. Supported by relevant literature, this text provides an outline of the previous and new modalities employed in the sector of breast imaging. Any progress in technology can result in increased imaging speed to satisfy physiological processes necessities. One of the problems within the designation of breast cancer is sensitivity limitation. To overcome this limitation, complementary imaging examinations are used that historically include screening, ultrasound, MRI, etc.

INTRODUCTION

Breast cancer is that the most ordinarily occurring cancer in women and therefore the second most typical cancer overall. There were over two million new cases in 2018. The highest twenty-five countries with the best rates of breast cancer in 2018 are given within Table 1 below (Bray F et al., 2019). BC ranks first among the cancers diagnosed in women between 20 and 59 years of age (Siegel R et al., 2012). During the past thirty years, BC mortality in Chinese females has followed a gradual upward trend, creating it

DOI: 10.4018/978-1-7998-3456-4.ch009

the fifth most typical explanation for cancer death in females (Jia M et al., 2011). BC is also a massive financial load and source of pain in patients' daily lives (Diaby V et al., 2015). The clinical outcome of BC is vastly variable, starting from complete characteristic to a time span of ten years post-surgical treatment, because of the heterogeneous cluster of tumors conferred with BC (Colombo PE et al., 2011; Pracella D et al., 2013). When breast cancer has grown to the point where physical signs and symptoms appear, the patient feels a breast lump (usually painless) (Iorio MV et al., 2011). Other shows embrace tenderness, skin irritation or dimpling, and nipple discharge or pain, scaliness, ulceration, or retraction. Breast pain typically because of benign conditions and not usually the primary symptom of breast carcinoma (Iorio MV et al., 2011).

Biomedical imaging techniques, one in all the most pillars of comprehensive cancer care, has several benefits as well as real time observation, accessibility while not tissue destruction, least or no invasiveness and would possibly operate over wide ranges of sometime and size scales involved in biological and pathological processes. Time scales go from milliseconds for super molecule binding and chemical reactions to years for diseases like cancer.

The recent role of imaging in cancer management is shown in Figure 1 and depends on screening and symptomatic unhealthiness management.

The upcoming role of imaging in cancer management is shown in Figure 2 and is bothered with pre-symptomatic, minimally invasive and targeted medical aid. Early diagnosing has been the most important think about the decrease of mortality and cancer management prices.

PRIMARY EVALUATION & STAGES

History

A thorough patient history is necessary for the physician to recognize danger factors for breast cancer. Some risk actors are well recognized, and others designate possible increased risk (Van Ongeval Ch et al.,2007, Newcomb PA et al.,2002, Weiss LK et al.,2002, Key TJ et al.,2003, Barton MB et al.,1999) (Tables 2 & 3).

STAGES

Stage 0

Stage 0 is that the earliest carcinoma stage conjointly referred to as malignant neoplastic disease in situ. At stage 0, the breast mass is noninvasive, and there's no sign that the neoplasm cells have unfold to different components of the breast or different components of the body. Often, stage 0 is taken into account a malignant tumor condition that generally needs shut observation, however not treatment.

Stage 0 carcinoma is troublesome to find. There might not be a lump which will be felt throughout a self-contemplation, and there are also no different symptoms. However, breast self-exams and routine screening are invariably necessary and may usually cause early diagnosing, once the cancer is most treatable. Stage zero sickness is most frequently found inadvertently throughout a breast diagnostic test for an additional reason, like to examine an unrelated breast lump.

Table 1. The top 25 countries with the highest rates of breast cancer in 2018.

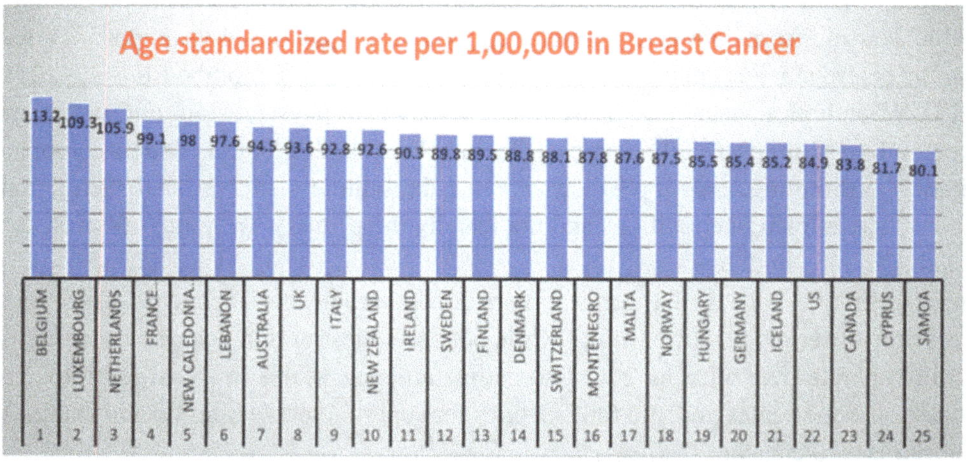

*Age-standardized rates are used in the tables. This is a summary measure of the rate of disease that a population would have if it had a standard age structure. Standardization is necessary when comparing populations that differ with respect to age because age has a powerful influence on the risk of dying from cancer.
*Reference from 1

Figure 1. The recent role of imaging in cancer management.

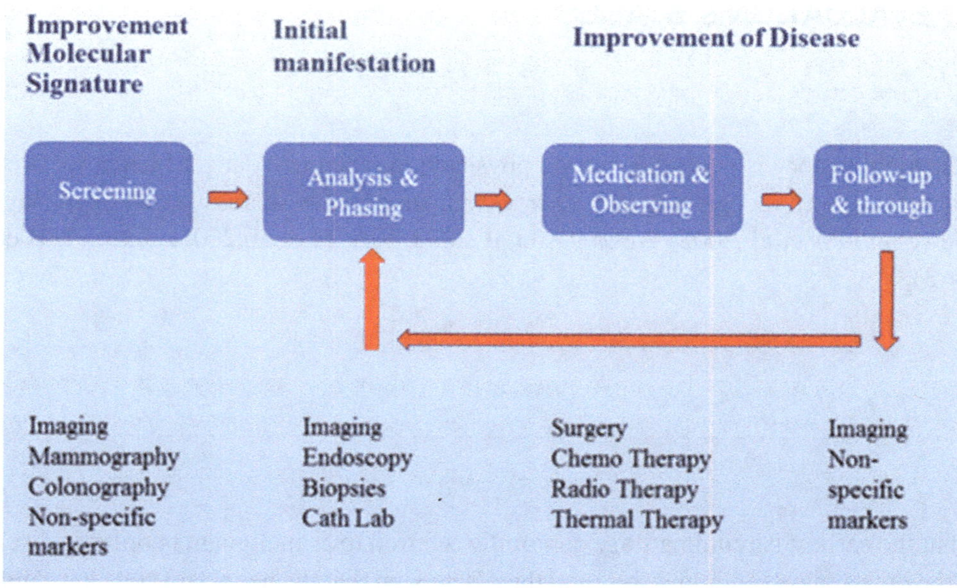

There are two classes of stage 0 breast cancer:

Ductal carcinoma in situ (DCIS) happens once carcinoma cells develop within the breast ducts. Now days, stage zero DCIS is actualiy diagnosed additional actually because additional women's are having routine roentgenogram screenings. DCIS will become invasive, therefore early treatment will be necessary.

Figure 2. The upcoming role of imaging in cancer management.

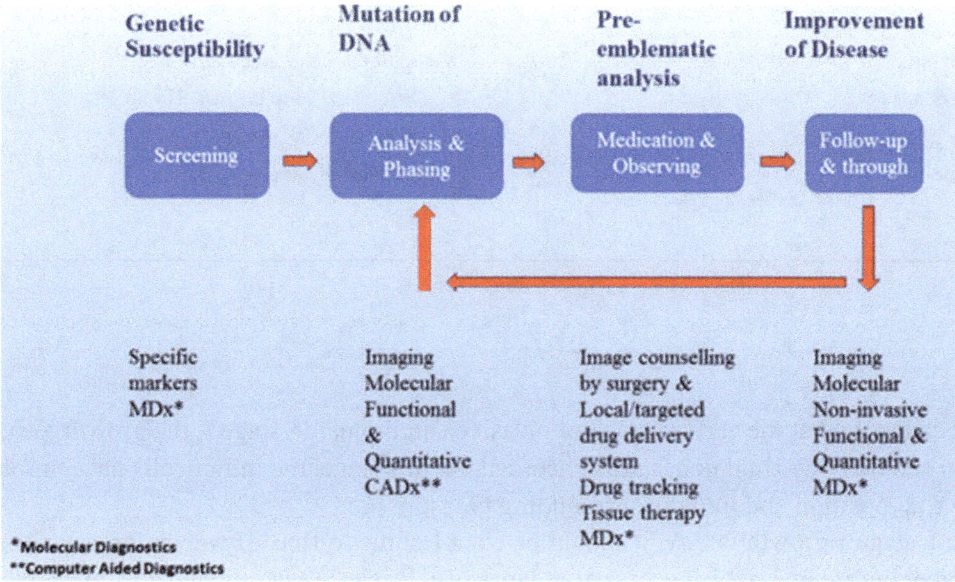

Table 2. Risk circumstances for Breast Cancer (BC)

Risk Circumstances Cannot Change	Risk Circumstances Can Change
• Getting older (after age 50)	• Taking hormones (Certain oral contraceptives (birth management pills) even have been found to boost breast cancer risk).
• Having dense breasts (Dense breasts have a lot of connective tissue than adipose tissue, which may typically create it laborious to visualize tumors on a mammogram).	• Drinking alcohol (increases with the a lot of alcohol she drinks).
• Reproductive history (Early menstrual periods before age twelve and beginning menopause after age fifty five expose women to hormones longer, raising their risk of obtaining carcinoma).	• Not being physically active (not physically active have a enhanced risk of obtaining breast cancer).
• Genetic mutations (Inherited changes (mutations) to bound genes, like BRCA1 and BRCA2).	• Being overweight or obese after menopause (i. e., BMI >= 30 kg per m^2).
• Family history of breast cancer (Having a first-degree male relative with breast cancer also raises a woman's risk).	• Reproductive history (Having the primary pregnancy when age thirty, not breastfeeding)
• Previous medication via radiation therapy(Women who had radiation to the chest or breasts like for medication of Hodgkin's lymphoma ,earlier age 30).	

Lobular carcinoma in situ (LCIS) happens once abnormal cells develop within the lobules. These cells don't seem to be cancerous and this condition seldom becomes invasive cancer. However, girls World Health Organization develop LCIS is also at improved risk for increasing breast cancer within the future. for girls World Health Organization develop LCIS, the danger of obtaining associate invasive cancer is 20% to 25% over fifteen years once the initial diagnosing.

Table 3. Compatible history with palpable breast masses in women.

Compatible History with Palpable Breast Masses in Women .	
• Breast lump characteristics	• Redness or fever
• Current medication	• Nipple discharge and inversion
• Duration of mass	• Change relative to menstrual cycle
• Breastfeeding history	• Current lactation status
• Number of baby	• Age at menopause
• Pain or swelling	• Smoking

Stage I

This breast cancer is that the earliest stage of invasive carcinoma. In stage I, the growth measures up to a pair of cm and no body fluid nodes are concerned. At this stage, the tumor cells have unfolded on the far side the first position and into the surrounding breast tissue.

Because a stage I growth is tiny, it should be troublesome to find. However, breast self-exams and schedule screening are invariably necessary and may usually cause early diagnosing, once the carcinoma is most treatable.

Stage I carcinoma is split into 2 categories:

Stage IA (Stage1A): The neoplasm measures 2 cm or smaller (about the dimensions of a pea or shelled peanut) and has not spread outside the breast.

Stage IB (Stage1B): little clusters of cancer cells measurement no over two millimeters, are found within the lymph nodes, and either there's no tumor within the breast, or the tumor is minor, determinant 2 cm or less.

The survival rate for stage IA breast cancer could also be slightly over for stage IB. However, all ladies with stage I carcinoma are thought-about to own a decent prognosis.

At stage I, TNM designations facilitate express the level of the unwellness. for instance, there could or might not be cancer cells within the humor nodes, and also the size of the growth could vary from 1 cm to 2 cm. most ordinarily, stage I breast cancer is delineate as:

- T: T1, T2, T3 or T4, looking on the dimensions and extent of the first growth
- N0: typically, cancer has not unfolded to the lymph nodes.
- M0: The unwellness has not unfold to different sites within the body.

Stage II

Also indicated to as invasive breast cancer, the tumor during this stage measures between 2 cm to 5 cm, or the carcinoma has unfolded to the lymph nodes(fig:4) underneath the arm on a similar aspect because the breast cancer. Second Stage of breast cancer indicates a rather a lot of advanced type of the unwellness. At this stage, the cancer cells have spread-out on the far side the primary location and into the surrounding breast tissue, and therefore the growth is larger than in stage I unwellness. However, stage II means that the carcinoma has not unfold to a far off a part of the body.

At stage II, a growth is also detected throughout a breast self- examination as a tough lump at intervals the breast. Breast self-exams and schedule screening are regularly essential and may characteristically cause early diagnosing, once the carcinoma is most treatable.

Stage II breast cancer is split into 2 categories:

Stage IIA (Stage 2A): one among the subsequent is true:

- There isn't any growth at intervals the breast, however cancer has unfolded to the axillary (underarm) lymph nodes, or
- The enlargement within the breast is a pair of cm or minor and cancer has unfold to the axillaris lymph nodes, or
- The growth within the breast measures 2 cm to 5 cm however cancer has not unfold to the axillaris lymph nodes.

Stage IIB (Stage 2B): one among the subsequent is true:

- The growth measures 2 cm to 5 cm and cancer has unfold to the axillary lymph nodes, or
- The growth is larger than five cm however cancer has not unfolded to the axillary lymph nodes.

The survival rate for stage IIA breast cancer is also slightly more than for stage IIB. However, all women with stage II breast cancer are thought-about to possess a decent prognosis.

At stage II, TNM designations facilitate describe the extent of the malady. most typically, stage II breast cancer is represented as:

- T: T1, T2, T3 or T4, counting on the scale and extent of the first growth
- N1: Cancer has unfolded to the lymph nodes.
- M0: The unwellness has not unfold to different sites within the body.

Stage III

Also called regionally advanced breast cancer, the growth during this stage of breast cancer is quite 2 inches in length across and therefore the cancer is intensive within the underarm lymph nodes or has unfold to different lymph nodes or tissues close to the breast. Stage III breast cancer could be a lot of advanced type of persistent breast cancer. At this stage, the cancer cells have sometimes not unfolded to a lot of distant sites within the body, however they're present in many axillary (underarm) lymph nodes. The growth may additionally be quite massive at this stage, probably extending to the chest wall or the skin of the breast.

Stage III breast cancer is split into 3 categories:

Stage IIIA (Stage 3A): one among the subsequent is true:

- ◦ No growth is originating within the breast; however, cancer is existing in axillary lymph nodes that are connected to either different or different structures, or cancer is also found within the lymph nodes close to the sternum,
- ◦ The growth is a pair of cm or smaller. Cancer has unfolded to axillary lymph nodes that are connected to every different or different structures, or cancer could have spread to liquid body substance nodes close to the sternum,
- ◦ The growth is 2 cm to 4 cm in size. Cancer has unfolded to axillary lymph nodes that are connected to every different or to different structures, or cancer could have unfolded to liquid body substance nodes close to the sternum,
- ◦ The growth is larger than 5 cm. Cancer has unfold to axillary lymph nodes which will be connected to every different or to different structures, or cancer could have unfolded to lymph nodes close to the sternum.

Stage IIIB (Stage 3B): The growth is also any size, and therefore the cancer:

- ◦ Has unfold to the chest wall and skin of the breast, and
- ◦ May have unfold to axillary lymph nodes which will be connected to every different or to different structures, or cancer could have unfolded to lymph nodes close to the sternum.
- ◦ Cancer that has unfold to the skin of the breast is inflammatory carcinoma.

Stage IIIC (Stage 3C):

There is also no sign of cancer within the breast or the growth is also any size and should have unfold to the chest wall and skin of the breast.

- Cancer cells are present in lymph nodes on top of or below the clavicle.
- Cancer cells could have unfolded to axillary lymph nodes or lymph nodes close to the sternum.
- Cancer that has unfold to the skin of the breast is inflammatory carcinoma.

Stage IIIC carcinoma is also operable or inoperable:

- Operable stage IIIC: The cancer is found in ten or a lot of axillary lymph nodes, or is in lymph nodes below the clavicle, or is in axillary lymph nodes and lymph nodes close to the sternum.
- Inoperable stage IIIC: The cancer has unfolded to the lymph nodes on top of the clavicle.

The endurance rate for stage IIIA breast cancer is also slightly more than for stage 3B, and therefore the endurance rate for stage IIIB is also slightly more than for stage IIIC. However, all women diagnosed with stage III carcinoma have many promising treatment choices.

At stage III, TNM designations facilitate express the extent of the unwellness. Higher numbers indicate a lot of intensive unwellness. most typically, stage III carcinoma is represented as:

- T: T1, T2, T3 or T4, counting on the scale and/or extent of the first growth
- N1: Cancer has unfolded to the lymph nodes.
- M0: The unwellness has not unfold to different sites within the body.

Figure 3. The symmetrically of Breast Lymph Nodes.

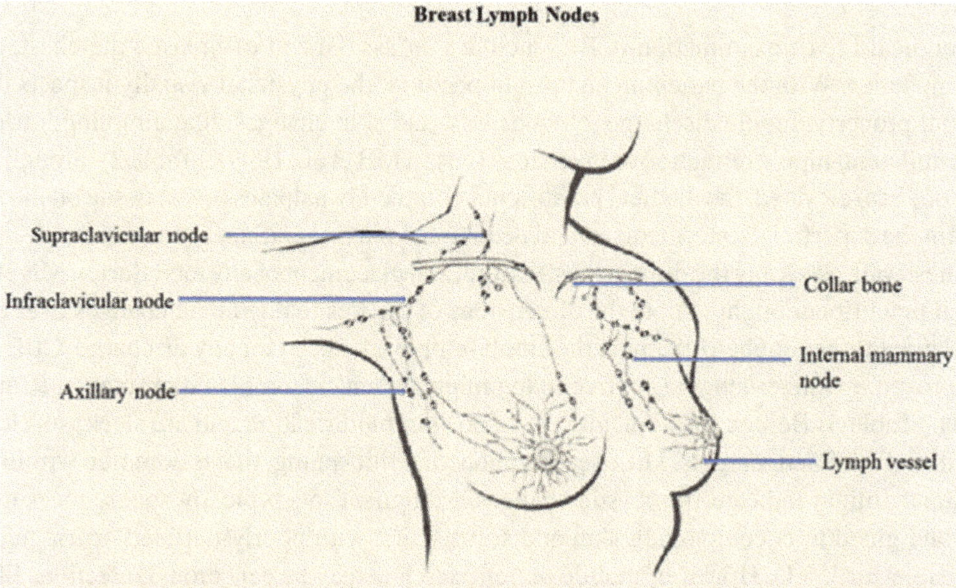

Stage IV

Also called metastatic breast cancer, the cancer during this stage has unfold on the far side the breast, underarm and internal exocrine gland body fluid nodes to different elements of the body regarding or distant from the breast. The cancer has unfolded elsewhere within the body. The affected areas may include the bones, brain, lungs or liver and more than one part of the body may be involved.

At stage IV, TNM designations facilitate define the extent of the unwellness. Higher numbers indicate additional in depth unwellness. Most ordinarily, stage IV carcinoma is represented as:

- T: T1, T2, T3 or T4, depending on the size and extent of the prime tumor.
- N1: Cancer has unfolded to the body fluid nodes,
- M1: The unwellness has unfold to different sites within the body.

Also called metastatic carcinoma, the cancer during this stage has unfold on the far side the breast, underarm and internal duct gland lymph nodes to different elements of the body with reference to or distant from the breast. The cancer has unfolded elsewhere within the body. The affected areas could embody the bones, brain, lungs or liver and over one a body part is also concerned.

At stage IV, TNM designations facilitate describe the extent of the unwellness. Higher numbers indicate additional intensive unwellness. most typically, stage IV breast cancer is delineated as (see Figure 3):

- T: T1, T2, T3 or T4, looking on the dimensions and extent of the first growth.
- N1: Cancer has unfolded to the lymph nodes
- M1: The unwellness has unfold to different sites within the body

Physical Investigation

Complete clinical breast examination (CBE) includes an assessment of breasts, the chest, axilla, and regional lymphatics. With the patient in an upright position, the physician visually inspects the breasts, noting spatial property, nipple discharge, obvious lots, and skin changes, like dimpling, inflammation, rashes, and unilateral nipple retraction or inversion (Barton MB et al., 1999). (Table 2) through the patient supine and one arm elevated, the medical practitioner completely palpates breast tissue on the raised-arm aspect within the superficial, intermediate, and deep tissue planes; axillary fossa, supraclavicular space, neck, and chest wall, assessing the dimensions, texture, and placement of any lots (Barton MB et al.,1999). The medical practitioner ought to note the dimensions of the lots to document changes over time. Next, the medical practitioner ought to examine the areola-nipple advanced for any discharge. CBE sensitivity may be improved by longer length (i.e. five to ten minutes) and accumulated exactness. (Campbell HS et al., 1991). (Table 3) Benign lots typically cause no skin modification and are sleek, soft to firm, and mobile, with well-defined margins. Diffuse, rhombohedral thickening, that is common within the higher outer quadrants, might indicate fibrocystic changes. Malignant lots typically square measure onerous, immobile, and glued to encompassing skin and soft tis-sue, with poorly outlined or irregular margins (Campbell HS et al.,1991). However, mobile or nonfixed lots may be cancerous. Infections like mastitis (a painful infection of the breast tissue) and cellulitis (affected skin appears swollen and redness) tend to be erythroderma, tender, and consider the bit.

IMAGING PLATFORM'S FOR BREAST CANCER (BC)

This section presents a review of a variety of modalities used for breast cancer detection.

Mammography

Mammography is that the commonest technique of breast imaging. It uses low-dose amplitude-X-rays to appear at the human breast. Cancerous plenty and calcium deposits seem brighter on the roentgenogram. This methodology is nice for detective work Ductal cancer in-situ (DCIS) and calcifications. Currently, mammography is the gold customary methodology to observe early stage carcinoma before the lesions become clinically palpable. enhancements over the last decade within the quality of performance and therefore the reporting of mammography studies ar the foremost necessary advances in breast imaging (Leichter et al., 2000). diagnostic technique has helped to decrease the morbidity by 25%-30% in screened ladies in comparison with an impact cluster when five to seven years (Kerlikowske et al., 1995). irregular trials of mammographic screening have provided robust proof that early identification and treatment of carcinoma reduces carcinoma mortality (Nyström et al., 2002). In addition to its quality in tele mammography, digital mammography is also additional correct than ancient mammography. Studies examination the ways are current. Studies comparing the methods are underway.

Potential new techniques embrace three-dimensional imaging, lower-dose radiation, twin energy subtraction, contrast-enhancement imaging and computer-assisted diagnosis (Hrung JM et al., 1999).

A standardized BI-RADS mammography report ought to embrace the reason(s) for doing the examination, the determined composition of the breast tissue, a description of the mammographic findings using the standardized lexicon, and a final estimation with supervision recommendation (Farewell VT et al., 1978).

Conventional Mammography (Diagnostic mammography)

Traditional mammograms produce diagnostic pictures by applying a low-dose X-ray system to look at breasts. Mammograms are accustomed monitor the breasts and assist within the early detection and diagnosing of breast diseases in ladies. X-rays are the foremost usually used variety of medical imaging.

Diagnostic mammography can help physicians decide whether a lesion is potentially cruel, and it also screens for occult dis-ease in surrounding tissue. Diagnostic mammography is employed to research suspicious breast changes like a breast lump, breast pain, an uncommon skin looks and nipple thickening or nipple discharge (Baines CJ et al., 1997). It is also used to evaluate uncharacteristic findings on a screening mammogram. Supplementary images will be made of alternative angles or specialize in areas of concern at advanced magnification.

Screening Mammography

Screening mammography is employed to find breast changes in women who haven't any signs or symptoms or noticeable breast irregularities. The goal is to find cancer before any clinical signs are visible (S. Prasad N et al., 2007). This sometimes needs a minimum of two mammograms from entirely dissimilar angles of each breast.

Digital Mammography

Digital mammography replaces ancient X-ray film with a digital chip to record pictures of the breast. This method, additionally referred to as full-field digital mammography, makes it attainable for the pictures of the breast to be viewed on a laptop monitor or written on a special film just like ancient mammograms. In digital tomosynthesis mammography, the essential mammography technique has been changed to amass 3D views of the breast (Wu T et al., 2003).

The advantages of digital mammograms embrace quicker image acquisition times, fewer total exposures and less patient discomfort. Breast health screenings that use digital mammograms are proved to find breast cancers higher than standard mammograms in 3 teams of women: those younger than fifty, those with dense breasts and people that are pre-menopausal.

3-D Mammography

3D Tomosynthesis Mammography is the latest exam to be added to our advanced array of technology. This revolutionary process allows your physician to better distinguish masses or tissues that might be cancerous. In traditional mammography, the details of the breast are viewed in one flat image. 3D mammography allows the breast to be viewed in a series of layers, allowing the radiologist to more accurately interpret the images.

The use of 3D mammography has proven to significantly reduce false positive callbacks and to be more accurate in detecting breast cancers early.

Breast Ultrasound

Ultrasonography is the most significant adjunctive imaging modality for breast cancer diagnosis. Over the years, it has also undergone significant improvements that have extended its utility for breast imaging. The traditional role of ultrasonography was to differentiate cysts from solid masses (Kopans DB et al., 1986; Joensuu H et al., 1994).

The diagnostic yield of mammography with an automated whole breast ultrasound (AWBU), for women with dense breasts and/or at elevated risk of breast cancer, is better (Kelly KM et al., 2010). A study by Kelly et al (Kelly KM et al., 2010) showed that 87% of cancer detections added by AWBU were found in the 68% of studies in women with dense/very dense breasts.

Advancements in ultrasound technology include 3D ultrasound, Automated ultrasound, Doppler Ultrasound, and Sonoelastography.

3D Ultrasound

Systematic three-dimensional (3D) ultrasound is utilized, shape, orientation, borders, and other clinically discriminating signs of malignancy can be evaluated offline without the patient being present of the breast. This method has been widely used and described for 3D ultra-sound scanning. Further, discretionary slicing permits modernization of scan planes in any orientation of the nonheritable size. Useful original 3D information should help in assessing the duct network and the relationship of a mass or lesion to the ducts, and should better demonstrate the vascularity associated with neoplasms (Fornage BD et al., 2000).

One approach to 3D ultrasound is to acquire a series of 2D ultrasound images covering the volume of interest, and build a 3D voxel-based Cartesian volume (or 3D grid) by placing each of these images in its correct location in the volume. A system for breast ultrasound scanning has been implemented and evaluated, using linear translation of an ultrasound transducer in small incremental steps covering the breast immersed in water (Riis C et al., 2005). However, in breast ultrasound scanning, the method suffers from some limitations; a majority of breast cancers are located in the upper quadrant of the breast, adjacent to the lymphatic complex in the axilla area.

A technique for systematic 3D scanning of the uncompressed breast has been developed, and is presently being subjected to evaluation and optimization. Examination is performed with the patient lying prone on an examination bed, with the uncompressed breast immersed in a water-filled cup (Riis C et al., 2005).

Automated Breast Ultrasound (ABUS)

Automated breast ultrasound (ABUS) makes waves as a new supplemental screening method for the dense breast population. ABUS's increased sensitivity about 97 percent when used in conjunction with mammography demonstrates this technology can be a beneficial screening tool for those women within the dense breast population, this dramatically decreases in women with dense breasts, falling to as low as 48 percent (Dave Fornell et al.,2017). However, because it is a relatively new technology there are certain areas that will need to be addressed as more companies decide to develop systems, and as use and technology continues to increase. In 2016, Giger and colleagues in a very reader study launched to assess and compare radiologists' performance within the recognition of carcinoma exploitation diagnostic technique alone versus diagnostic technique with ABUS (Giger et al., 2016).

The application of ABUS in India is limited due to its high cost, and its need to be used along with mammogram as it does not show calcifications (Giger et al., 2016).

Doppler Ultrasound

During a breast ultrasound investigation, the sonographer or medical practitioner accomplishment the check might use Doppler techniques to assess blood movement or deficiency of flow in any breast mass. With the development of ever more sensitive color doppler and power Doppler ultrasound machines the ability to detect flow in solid masses and even to differentiate that flow also has added another level of sophistication to ultrasound analysis of breast masses. Color doppler does not discriminate completely between benign and malignant masses; the presence of signals in a lesion that is otherwise thought to be benign should prompt a biopsy while the absence of signals in an indeterminate lesion is reassuring. Therefore, color doppler is now widely established as a useful addition to breast imaging and dynamic features of ultrasound that are useful in breast diagnosis (Makes D et al., 2005).

Sonoelastography

Sonelastography is a new imagistic method helpful in the diagnosis of breast cancer. Usually, breast cancer is more durable than the adjacent traditional tissue and this property constitutes the premise for elastography.

The basis of sonoelastography is that the tissue compression produces strain at intervals the tissue which the strain is variable looking on tissue stiffness. Determining the tissue strain we are able to estimate tissue hardness which can be helpful for differentiating malignant from benign masses. The tissue snap distribution is regenerate in a image referred to as elastogram, the size ranged from red (for elements with greatest strain) to blue (for those with no strain). (Jumuga et al., 2009).

It supplements and increases the diagnostic accuracy of conventional ultrasound, particularly of BI-RADS 3-4 lesions; further reducing unnecessary biopsies or subsequence reevaluation (Scaperrotta G et al., 2008).

Breast Thermography

Currently, breast thermograms are widely used for the correct detection of carcinoma (breast Cancer) (Ng EYK., 2009; Ring EFJ et al., 2000). Thermography could be a promising screening tool as a result of its ready to diagnose carcinoma a minimum of 10 years earlier. However, each analysis and interpretation of thermograms depends on analysts.

Thermography relies on the principle that metabolism and vas proliferation in each pre-cancerous tissue and also the space encompassing a developing carcinoma is sort of forever over in traditional breast tissue. Developing tumors increase circulation to their cells by enlarging existing blood vessels and making new ones in a very method referred to as vascularization (S. Prasad N et al., 2007).

This method often leads to a rise in regional surface temperatures of the breast. Diagnostic procedure uses ultra-sensitive infrared cameras and PCs to get high-resolution diagnostic images of those temperature variations (Mital M et al., 2007).

Magnetic Resonance Imaging (MRI)

Breast MRI is a widely used imaging modality for the early detection of breast cancer (Schnall MD et al., 2001). Initial results counsel that MRI will dramatically improve the yield of screening bound at-risk populations. resonance imaging (MRI) could be a non-invasive, typically painless medical check that helps physicians diagnose and treat medical conditions. MRI doesn't use radiation (x-rays). MRI of the breast offers valuable info regarding breast conditions that can't be obtained by different imaging modalities, like mammography or ultrasound.

MRI of the breast isn't a re-placement for diagnostic technique or ultrasound imaging however rather a supplemental tool for notice and staging breast cancer and different breast irregularities (Tofts PS et al., 1995).

Application of state-of-the-art imaging modalities, namely MRI, magnetic resonance spectroscopy (MRS), nuclear imaging, and optical imaging, for precise identification of human breast tumors and their use in monitoring chemotherapeutic responses has been discussed (Basilion JP et al.,2001). MRI helps in investigating vascular changes associated with neoangiogenic (Leach MO et al., 2001).

MRI is highly sensitive (85 to 100 percent), it lacks specificity (47 to 67 percent). MRI is inferior to diagnostic technique in notice in place cancers and cancers smaller than three millimeters, and it offer no price profit over excisional diagnostic assay for substantiating malignancy (Tofts PS et al.,1995; Muller et al.,1997). Research suggests two potential roles for MRI in breast mass diagnosis: evaluating patients with silicone breast implants and assessing patients in whom evaluation by ultrasonography and mammography is problematic (Herborn CU et al., 2002).

Technetium Sestamibi Scan (Scintimammography)

Scintimammography is additionally called nuclear medicine breast imaging, Breast Specific Gamma Imaging (BSGI) and Molecular Breast Imaging (MBI). Scintimammography may be a form of breast imaging take a look at that's accustomed discover cancer cells within the breasts of some women who have had abnormal mammograms, or for those that have dense breast tissue, post-operative connective tissue or breast implants. (Liberman et al., 2003) A compound known as technetium sestamibi has been studied to help detect breast cancer. This test is market-ed under the trade name Miraluma. The scintimammography imaging technique uses an isotope to examine lesions of the breast. during this procedure, a little quantity of the radioactive substance is injected into associate degree arm vein.

A high-resolution breast-specific gamma camera was used to evaluate the occult breast cancer in women at high risk of breast cancer (Brem RF et al., 2005). The authors originate that high-resolution breast-specific scintimammography was ready to discover tiny (< one cm), mammographically occult, nonpalpable lesions not otherwise detected by diagnostic technique or physical examination in women with exaggerated risk for breast cancer. The joint use of diagnostic technique and 99mTc-methoxy isobutyl isonitrile (MIBI) scintimammography to scale back the quantity of biopsies needed in patients with suspected carcinoma has been considered. (Prats E et al.,1999). The total number of biopsies performed was reduced by 34%. In scintimammography with Tc99m compounds, the value of planar Tc99m sestamibi scanning for auxiliary lymph node evaluation was presented (Massardo T et al., 2005). Their work confirmed that non-tomographic Tc99m sestamibi scintimammography had a very low detection rate for auxiliary lymph node involvement and may not be suitable for clinical assessment of breast cancer. The sensitivity and specificity of Breast-Specific Gamma Imaging (BSGI) for the finding of carcinoma (breast cancer) by mistreatment pathologic results because the reference normal make up my mind (Brem RF et al., 2008). BSGI showed high sensitivity (96.4%) and moderate specificity (59.5%) in the detection of breast cancers (Sree et al., 2011).

Several limitations in there through this process, first one, scintimammography is not a primary breast cancer screening tool and second, it is not a replacement for mammography or ultrasound. Nuclear medicine procedures can be time-consuming. However, the image resolution of nuclear medicine images may not be as high as that of mammography or MRI. An irregularity detected on scintimammography is also tough to search out mistreatment different imaging exams. This will build it tough to perform a diagnostic assay.

Positron Emission Tomography (PET)

Positron emission tomography (PET) is a nuclear medicine imaging technique which is used to produce three dimensional images. It detects a pair of γ rays, which are emitted from the radionuclide that is introduced into the human body. A tiny amount of radioactive substance is injected into an arm vein. This substance gives off small amount of radiation that is detected by a special PET scanner to form an image. The most commonly used substance in this test is fluorodeoxyglucose (FDG), which is a type of sugar. It is an effective means of predicting response to neoadjuvant chemotherapy in patients with breast cancer (Koga S et al., 2007).

PET used to complement mammography is known as positron emission mammography (PEM), and it has been reported that PEM may not be adversely affected by breast density, hormone replacement therapy, and menopausal status of the patient (Schilling K et al., 2008).

PET is being used to detect metastatic disease (cancer spread) and has been successful in that role. The PET scan is not currently used for primary breast cancer detection because it does not reliably detect tumors smaller than 5–10 mm, but research is being done to improve the accuracy of this test (S. Prasad N et al., 2007).

Optical Imaging (OI)

The optical molecular imaging modality uses exogenous fluorescent probes as additional contrast agents that target molecules relevant to breast cancer (A.Godavarty et al., 2004). The use of fluorescent probes has a potential in early breast cancer detection but the effectiveness of fluorescence imaging relies on the functions of the probes (D. Asanuma et al., 2015). Molecular distinction probes on specific neoplasm receptors or neoplasm associated enzymes also are below development.

Diffuse Optical Tomography (DOT)

Diffuse optical tomography (DOT) was introduced the early 1990s. DOT uses near-infrared light transmission and intrinsic breast tissue contrast for the detection and characterization of abnormal tissue (S. R. Arridge et al., 1995). It is sensitive, cost-effective, and does not involve any ionizing radiation, and has a high sensitivity due to the rich optical absorption contrast. Owing to the relatively low absorption of hemoglobin, water and lipid at wavelengths of 650–1000 nm, near-infrared (NIR) light can transmit through several centimeters of biological tissue with an adequate signal-to-noise ratio for breast tomographic imaging (H. Dehghani et al., 2009). Furthermore, in this spectral range, oxy-hemoglobin and deoxy-hemoglobin and lipids predominantly affect the absorptive properties of the breast tissue. There is a difference in total hemoglobin concentration levels between benign and malignant breast lesions, so it was a useful indicator for distinguishing between benign and malignant breast lesions (Q. Zhu et al., 2005). By combining images reconstructed by DOT at various wavelengths, concentrations of oxy-and deoxy hemoglobin and water can be determined to reveal tumors from background tissue (V. Quaresma et al., 1998).

NIR Optical Tomography

NIR optical imaging of the breast has a limited resolution due to light scattering effects it can give spectral information (H. Dehghani et al., 2003) that permits functional measurements associated with hemoglobin concentration and oxygenation, water concentration, lipid content, and wavelength dependence of tissue scattering.

Near-infrared (NIR) Optical Tomography

Near-infrared (NIR) optical tomography is associate degree imaging method with high blood-based distinction. This is due to the fact that hemoglobin absorbs visible wavelength light up to the near infrared region (Fass L. et al., 2008). There is a window of opportunity in the near infrared because water absorbs the far infrared wavelengths.

Non-invasive (NIR) Optical Tomography

Non-invasive NIR tomographic imaging has been used in organs like the breast because they can be trans illuminated externally.

A little modification in property creates an awfully enormous image distinction. The high distinction of NIR optical picturing is principally thanks to exaggerated light-weight attenuation by hemoprotein relative to water in parenchymal tissue and therefore the distinct spectral variations between the aerated and deoxygenated circumstances of hemoprotein (Fass L. et al., 2008).

Although, NIR diffuse optical tomography can distinguish cysts and solid masses (X. Gu et al., 2004).

Computed Tomography (CT)

A CT scan (also referred to as a CAT scan, or computed axial tomography scan) is associate degree X-ray technique that offers doctors info regarding the body's internal organs in 2-dimensional slices, or cross-sections. Right now, CT scans don't seem to be used habitually to judge the breast. If you have got an oversized carcinoma, your doctor might order a CT scan to assess whether or not or not the cancer has moved into the chest partition.

Generally, CT scans wouldn't be needed if, have an early-stage breast cancer. If symptoms or other findings suggest that the cancer could be more advanced, however, may need to have CT scans of the head, chest, and/or abdomen. If advanced breast cancer is found, doctor may order more CT scans during treatment to see whether or not the cancer is responding. After treatment, CT scans is also used if there's reason to suppose the carcinoma has unfolded or recurred outside the breast.

Spiral CT

It is useful for elucidating problems in the diagnosis of breast lesions. Its advantages consist in the speed of the method, comfort for the patient, absence of movement artefacts, easy standardization and wide applicability.

Dynamic Contrast-Enhanced CT

Dynamic contrast-enhanced CT of the breast has been originate to be actual for the recognition of intraductal extension of breast malignant neoplastic disease and is assumed to be helpful within the operative assessment of indications of breast-conserving surgery (Yamamoto A et al., 2006). The lesions appear attenuating compared with fatty background, and they show early enhancement on arterial phase on dynamic contrast-enhanced CT. CT is usually not the first modality to be used in imaging breast cancer, but it may be used as an adjuvant for monitoring spread. Although it involves some exposure to radiation, it should be considered in patients in whom MRI is contraindicated.

Three-Dimensional (3D) Helical CT

Three-dimensional (3D) helical CT can provide good in-formation about the spread of breast cancer and could be an alternative to 3D MRI for preoperative examination of breast cancer (Yamamoto A. et al., 2006).

In Vitro High-Resolution Helical CT

In vitro high-resolution helical CT can depict the internal structure of small nodes. Morphologic changes detected on helical CT help distinguish benign from malignant nodes (S. Prasad N et al., 2007). Tumours appear as dense lesions on CT and usually shows early contrast enhancement similar to that seen with dynamic MRI.

Electrical Impedance-Based Imaging

Our body tissues offer impedance to the flow of electric current. Studies have shown that cancerous breast tissues have lower impedance when compared to normal tissues. Electrical impedance tomography (EIT) and electrical impedance scanning (EIS) or electrical impedance mapping (EIM) are the two types of electrical impedance-based imaging techniques available.

Electrical Impedance Tomography (EIT) / Electrical Impedance Mapping (EIM)

In EIT, 2D or 3D images area unit reassembled from an oversized range of ohmic resistance values that area unit captured by putting electrodes round the breast surface in an exceedingly circular fashion. However, a planar electrode array is used and there is no need for complicated reconstruction algorithms which are used for EIT or EIM.

Electrical Impedance Scanning (EIS)

The electrical impedance scanner (EIS) model TS2000 (Mirabel Medical Systems, Austin, TX) demonstrated clinical effectiveness and received US Food and Drug Administration approval for use as an adjunct to MMG. EIS maps electrical impedance (capacitance and conductivity) of breast tissue and produces a real-time gray-scale "image" of differences in impedance measured over a broad range of frequencies. In an electrical impedance image, the nipple is a bright, white area because of its high concentration of ductal tissue that has lower electrical impedance than the surrounding more fatty tissue of the breast. The surrounding normal breast tissue is displayed in varying shades of gray (Scholz B et al., 2000; Piperno G et al., 1990; Glickman YA et al., 2002).

There is evidence that EIS does not simply detect distortions of electrical fields due to a localized cancer, but also reflects more widespread electrical changes in the breast (Dickhaut M et al.,1996).Studies measuring electrical impedance of the breast suggest that what is being measured is primarily related to generalized, premalignant, tissue-proliferative changes (Dickhaut M et al.,1996).In this regard, measurements on the nipple are a particularly sensitive indicator of ductal epithelial changes in the breast as a whole (Piperno G et al.,2002). These findings suggest that EIS has the potential to identify women at a high risk of having breast cancer, in the absence of a specific lesion that can be localized.

CONCLUSION

Current breast imaging modalities play a vital role in assisting clinicians in the primary screening of cancer, in the diagnosis and characterization of lesions, staging and restaging, treatment selection and treatment progress monitoring and in determining cancer recurrence. In this literature shows that the only radiological technique that has had significant impact on the diagnosis, staging and patient follow-up in the case of screening asymptomatic breasts for cancer is low-dose mammography. Based on current understanding and results from ongoing research, it appears that high-resolution, high-contrast, anatomical x-ray imaging either in 2-D (mammography) or with added depth information will be the primary screening modality in the next decade. However, MRI and ultrasound will have an increasingly important role for imaging high risk patients and for imaging women with dense breasts. With increasing field strength and improved homogeneity, MRS is likely to add value to dynamic contrast enhanced MRI studies. Contrast-enhanced x-ray imaging, scintimammography with dedicated cameras, dedicated SPECT, and dedicated PET offer great potential as diagnostic evaluation tools and for clinical management.

At present x-ray mammography is the most commonly used breast-imaging technique and is thus the "gold standard" in the evaluation of the breast from an imaging perspective.

Moreover, the use of computer-aided diagnosis techniques has been widely advocated for the improvement of cancer detection efficiency and for reducing the inter-observer variability that is associated with the subjective human interpretation of the images obtained. In summary, ongoing research and recent advances indicate that the prospects of substantial improvements in early detection, accurate diagnosis, and improved monitoring of therapeutic response of breast cancer are highly promising.

Conflict of Interest Statement

The authors declare that the research was conducted in the absence of any commercial or financial relationships that could be construed as a potential conflict of interest.

ACKNOWLEDGMENT

The authors acknowledge the help provided by the Department of Biotechnology, Faculty of Life Sciences, Institute of Applied Medicines and Research, Ghaziabad, Uttar Pradesh, India.

REFERENCES

22Kopans, D. B. (1986). What is a useful adjunct to mammography? Radiology, 161(2), 560–561. doi:10.1148/radiology.161.2.3532197 PubMed doi:10.1148/radiology.161.2.3532197 PMID:3532197

Amalu, W. C., Hobbins, W. B., Head, J. F., & Elliott, R. L. (2006). Infrared imaging of the breast - an overview. In Biomedical Engineering Handbook. CRC Press.

Ammer, K., & Ring, E. F. J. (2006). Standard procedures for infrared imaging in medicine. In Biomedical Engineering Handbook. CRC Press.

Arridge. (2011). Methods in diffuse optical imaging. *Philos Trans A Math Phys Eng Sci., 369*(1955), 4558-76.

Asanuma, D., Sakabe, M., Kamiya, M., Yamamoto, K., Hiratake, J., Ogawa, M., Kosaka, N., Choyke, P. L., Nagano, T., Kobayashi, H., & Urano, Y. (2015). Sensitive beta-galactosidase-targeting fluorescence probe for visualizing small peritoneal metastatic tumours in vivo. Nature Communications, 6(1), 6463. doi:10.1038/ncomms7463 PubMed doi:10.1038/ncomms7463 PMID:25765713

Baines, C. J., & Miller, A. B. (1997). Mammography versus clinical examination of the breasts. Journal of the National Cancer Institute. Monographs, 1997(22), 125–129. doi:10.1093/jncimono/1997.22.125 PubMed doi:10.1093/jncimono/1997.22.125 PMID:9709288

Barton, M. B., Harris, R., & Fletcher, S. W. (1999). The rational clinical examination. Does this patient have breast cancer? The screening clinical breast examination: Should it be done? How? Journal of the American Medical Association, 282(13), 1270–1280. doi:10.1001/jama.282.13.1270 PubMed doi:10.1001/jama.282.13.1270 PMID:10517431

Basilion, J. P. (2001). Current and future technologies for breast cancer imaging. Breast Cancer Research, 3(1), 14–16. doi:10.1186/bcr264 PubMed doi:10.1186/bcr264 PMID:11300100

Bray, F., Ferlay, J., Soerjomataram, I., Siegel, R. L., Torre, L. A., & Jemal, A. (2019, April 15). (in press). Global Cancer Statistics 2018: GLOBOCAN estimates of incidence and mortality worldwide for 36 cancers in 185 countries. CA: a Cancer Journal for Clinicians, 144(8), 1941–1953. 10.1002/ijc.31937 PubMed PMID:30207593

Brem, R. F., Floerke, A. C., Rapelyea, J. A., Teal, C., Kelly, T., & Mathur, V. (2008). Breast-specific gamma imaging as an adjunct imaging modality for the diagnosis of breast cancer. Radiology, 247(3), 651–657. doi:10.1148/radiol.2473061678 PubMed doi:10.1148/radiol.2473061678 PMID:18487533

Brem, R. F., Rapelyea, J. A., Zisman, G., Mohtashemi, K., Raub, J., Teal, C. B., Majewski, S., & Welch, B. L. (2005). Occult breast cancer: Scintimammography with high-resolution breast-specific gamma camera in women at high risk for breast cancer. Radiology, 237(1), 274–280. doi:10.1148/radiol.2371040758 PubMed doi:10.1148/radiol.2371040758 PMID:16126919

Campbell, H. S., Fletcher, S. W., Pilgrim, C. A., Morgan, T. M., & Lin, S. (1991). Improving physicians' and nurses' clinical breast examination: A randomized controlled trial. American Journal of Preventive Medicine, 7(1), 1–8. doi:10.1016/S0749-3797(18)30957-7 PubMed doi:10.1016/S0749-3797(18)30957-7 PMID:1867894

Colombo, P. E., Milanezi, F., Weigelt, B., & Reis-Filho, J. S. (2011). Microarrays in the 2010s: The contribution of microarray-based gene expression profiling to breast cancer classification, prognostication and prediction. Breast Cancer Research, 13(3), 212. doi:10.1186/bcr2890 PubMed doi:10.1186/bcr2890 PMID:21787441

Dehghani, H., Pogue, P. W., Poplack, S. P., & Paulsen, K. D. (2003). Multiwavelength three-dimensional near-infrared tomography of the breast: Initial simulation, phantom, and clinical results. Applied Optics, 42(1), 135–145. doi:10.1364/AO.42.000135 PubMed doi:10.1364/AO.42.000135 PMID:12518832

Dehghani, Srinivasan, Pogue, & Gibson. (2009). Numerical modelling and image reconstruction in diffuse optical tomography. *Philos Trans A Math Phys Eng Sci, 367*(1900), 3073-93.

Diaby, V., Tawk, R., Sanogo, V., Xiao, H., & Montero, A. J. (2015). A review of systematic reviews of the cost-effectiveness of hormone therapy, chemotherapy, and targeted therapy for breast cancer. Breast Cancer Research and Treatment, 151(1), 27–40. doi:10.1007/s10549-015-3383-6 PubMed doi:10.100710549-015-3383-6 PMID:25893588

Dickhaut, M., Schreer, I., & Frischbier, H. J. (1996). The value of BBE in the assessment of breast lesions. In Electropotentials in the Clinical Assessment of Breast Neoplasia. New York, NY: Springer-Verlag.

Farewell, V. T., Bulbrook, R. D., & Hayward, J. L. (1978). Risk factors in breast cancer: A prospective study in the island of Gnernsy, in early diagnosis of Breast cancer. New York: E. Grandmann and L. Beck Gustav Fisher Verlag Stuttgart, 1978, 43–51.

Fass, L. (2008). Imaging and cancer: A review. Molecular Oncology, 2(2), 115–152. doi:10.1016/j.molonc.2008.04.001 PubMed doi:10.1016/j.molonc.2008.04.001 PMID:19383333

Fornage, B. D. (2000). Recent advances in breast sonography. JBR-BTR; Organe de la Societe Royale Belge de Radiologie (SRBR), 83(2), 75–80. PubMed PMID:10859903

Fornell, D. (2017). *New Technology and Clinical Data in Breast Imaging, ITN, "Breast Imaging" website channel*. https://www.itnonline.com/article/new-technology-and-clinical-data-breast-imaging

Giger, M., Inciardi, M., Edwards, A., Papaioannou, J., Drukker, K., Jiang, Y., Brem, R., & Brown, J. (2016). Automated Breast Ultrasound in Breast Cancer Screening of Women with Dense Breasts: Reader Study of Mammography-Negative and Mammography-Positive Cancers. AJR. American Journal of Roentgenology, 206(6), 1–10. doi:10.2214/AJR.15.15367 PubMed doi:10.2214/AJR.15.15367 PMID:27043979

Glickman, Y.A., Filo, O., & Nachaliel, U. (2002). Novel EIS postprocessing algorithm for breast cancer diagnosis. *IEEE Trans Med Imag, 21*(710).

Godavarty, A., Thompson, A. B., Roy, R., Gurfinkel, M., Eppstein, M. J., Zhang, C., & Sevick-Muraca, E. M. (2004, May-June). Diagnostic imaging of breast cancer using fluorescence-enhanced optical tomography: Phantom studies. Journal of Biomedical Optics, 9(3), 488–496. doi:10.1117/1.1691027 PubMed doi:10.1117/1.1691027 PMID:15189086

Gu, X., Zhang, Q., Bartlett, M., Schutz, L., Fajardo, L. L., & Jiang, H. (2004). Differentiation of cysts from solid tumors in the breast with diffuse optical tomography. Academic Radiology, 11(1), 2094–2107. doi:10.1016/S1076-6332(03)00562-2 PubMed doi:10.1016/S1076-6332(03)00562-2 PMID:14746402

Herborn, C. U., Marincek, B., Erfmann, D., Meuli-Simmen, C., Wedler, V., Bode-Lesniewska, B., & Kubik-Huch, R. A. (2002). Breast augmentation and reconstructive surgery: MR imaging of implant rupture and malignancy. European Radiology, 12(9), 2198–2206. doi:10.1007/s00330-002-1362-x PubMed doi:10.100700330-002-1362-x PMID:12195470

Hrung, J. M., Sonnad, S. S., Schwartz, J. S., & Langlotz, C. P. (1999). Accuracy of MR imaging in the work-up of suspicious breast lesions: A diagnostic meta-analysis. Academic Radiology, 6(7), 387–397. doi:10.1016/S1076-6332(99)80189-5 PubMed doi:10.1016/S1076-6332(99)80189-5 PMID:10410164

Iorio, M. V., Casalini, P., Piovan, C., Braccioli, L., & Tagliabue, E. (2011). Breast cancer and microRNAs: Therapeutic impact. The Breast, 20, S63–S70. doi:10.1016/S0960-9776(11)70297-1 PubMed doi:10.1016/S0960-9776(11)70297-1 PMID:22015296

Jia, M., Zheng, R., Zhang, S., Zeng, H., Zou, X., & Chen, W. (2015). Female breast cancer incidence and mortality in 2011, China. Journal of Thoracic Disease, 7, 1221–1226. PubMed PMID:26380738

Joensuu, H., Asola, R., Holli, K., Kumpulainen, E., Nikkanen, V., & Parvinen, L. M. (1994). Delayed diagnosis and large size of breast cancer after a flase negative mammogram. European Journal of Cancer (Oxford, England), 30(9), 1299–1302. doi:10.1016/0959-8049(94)90177-5 doi:10.1016/0959-8049(94)90177-5

Jumuga, C., Macota, G., & Stoian, I. (2009). The role of sonoelastography for the diagnosis of breast cancer. *Gineco.ro, 5*, 258-262.

Kelly, K. M., Dean, J., Comulada, W. S., & Lee, S. J. (2010). Breast cancer detection using automated whole breast ultrasound and mammography in radiographically dense breasts. European Radiology, 20(3), 734–742. doi:10.1007/s00330-009-1588-y PubMed doi:10.100700330-009-1588-y PMID:19727744

Kerlikowske, K., Grady, D., Rubin, S. M., Sandrock, C., & Ernster, V. L. (1995). Efficacy of screening mammography. A meta-analysis. Journal of the American Medical Association, 273(2), 149–154. doi:10.1001/jama.1995.03520260071035 PubMed doi:10.1001/jama.1995.03520260071035 PMID:7799496

Key, T. J., Appleby, P. N., Reeves, G. K., Roddam, A., Dorgan, J. F., Longcope, C., ... (2003). Body mass index, serum sex hormones, and breast cancer risk in postmenopausal women. Journal of the National Cancer Institute, 95(16), 1218–1226. doi:10.1093/jnci/djg022 PubMed doi:10.1093/jnci/djg022 PMID:12928347

Koga, S., Nakano, S., Honma, Y., & Ogasawara, N. (2007, June 28). FDG-PET (positron emission tomography) in the detection of primary breast cancer and lymph nodes involvement [Japanese]. Japanese Journal of Clinical Medicine, 65(Suppl 6), 379–384. PubMed PMID:17682181

Leach, M. O. (2001). Application of magnetic resonance imaging to angiogenesis in breast cancer. Breast Cancer Research, 3(1), 22–27. doi:10.1186/bcr266 PubMed doi:10.1186/bcr266 PMID:11300102

Leichter, I., Buchbinder, S., Bamberger, P., Novak, B., Fields, S., & Lederman, R. (2000). Quantitative characterization of mass lesions on digitized mammograms for computer-assisted diagnosis. Investigative Radiology, 35(6), 366–372. doi:10.1097/00004424-200006000-00005 PubMed doi:10.1097/00004424-200006000-00005 PMID:10853611

Liberman, M., Sampalis, F., Mulder, D. S., & Sampalis, J. S. (2003). Breast Cancer Diagnosis by Scintimammography: A Meta-analysis and Review of the Literature. *Breast Cancer Research and Treatment, 80*(1), 115–126. doi:10.1023/A:1024417331304

Makes D Department of Radiology. (2005). Faculty of Medicine, University of Indonesia Ciptomangunkusumo General Hospital. Jakarta Biomed Imaging Interv J, 1(1), e6–e1.

Massardo, T., Alonso, O., Llamas-Ollier, A., Kabasakal, L., Ravishankar, U., Morales, R., Delgado, L., & Padhy, A. K. (2005). Planar Tc99m—sestamibi scintimammography should be considered cautiously in the axillary evaluation of breast cancer protocols: Results of an international multicenter trial. BMC Nuclear Medicine, 5(1), 4. doi:10.1186/1471-2385-5-4 PubMed doi:10.1186/1471-2385-5-4 PMID:16048648

Mital, M., & Scott, E. P. (2007, February). Thermal detection of embedded tumors using infrared imaging. Journal of Biomechanical Engineering, 129(1), 33–39. doi:10.1115/1.2401181 PubMed doi:10.1115/1.2401181 PMID:17227096

Müller-Schimpfle, M., Ohmenhäuser, K., Sand, J., Stoll, P., & Claussen, C. D. (1997). Dynamic 3D – MR mammography: Is there a benefit of sophisticated evaluation of enhancement curves for clinical routine? Journal of Magnetic Resonance Imaging, 7(1), 236–240. doi:10.1002/jmri.1880070137 PubMed doi:10.1002/jmri.1880070137 PMID:9039622

Newcomb, P. A., Titus-Ernstoff, L., Egan, K. M., Trentham-Dietz, A., Baron, J. A., Storer, B. E., ... (2002). Postmenopausal estrogen and progestin use in relation to breast cancer risk. Cancer Epidemiology, Biomarkers & Prevention, 11, 593–600. PubMed PMID:12101105

Ng, E. Y. K., & Sudharsan, N. M. (2004). Numerical modeling in conjunction with thermography as an adjunct tool for breast tumour detection. BMC Cancer, 4, 1–26. doi:10.1186/1471-2407-4-17 doi:10.1186/1471-2407-4-17

Ng, E. Y. K. (2009). A review of thermography as promising non-invasive detection modality for breast tumour. International Journal of Thermal Sciences, 48(5), 849–859. doi:10.1016/j.ijthermalsci.2008.06.015 doi:10.1016/j.ijthermalsci.2008.06.015

Nyström, L., Andersson, I., Bjurstam, N., Frisell, J., Nordenskjöld, B., & Rutqvist, L. E. (2002). Long-term effects of mammography screening: Updated overview of the Swedish randomised trials. Lancet, 359(9310), 909–919. doi:10.1016/S0140-6736(02)08020-0 PubMed doi:10.1016/S0140-6736(02)08020-0 PMID:11918907

Piperno, G., & Lenington, S. (2002). Breast electrical impedance and estrogen use in postmenopausal women. *Maturitas, 41*(17).

Piperno, G., Frei, E.H., & Moshitzky, M. (1990). Breast cancer screening by impedance measurements. *Front Med Biol Eng, 2*(111).

Pracella, D., Bonin, S., Barbazza, R., Sapino, A., Castellano, I., Sulfaro, S., & Stanta, G. (2013). Are breast cancer molecular classes predictive of survival in patients with long follow-up? Disease Markers, 35, 595–605. doi:10.1155/2013/347073 PubMed doi:10.1155/2013/347073 PMID:24288429

Prasad, S. N., & Houserkova, D. (2007). The Role of Various Modalities in Breast Imaging. Biomed Pap Med., 151(2), 209–218. doi:10.5507/bp.2007.036 doi:10.5507/bp.2007.036

Prats, E., Aisa, F., Abós, M. D., Villavieja, L., García-López, F., Asenjo, M. J., Razola, P., & Banzo, J. (1999). Mammography and 99mTc-MIBI scintimammography in suspected breast cancer. Journal of Nuclear Medicine, 40, 296–301. PubMed PMID:10025838

Qi, H., Kuruganti, P. T., & Snyder, W. E. (2006). Detecting breast cancer from thermal infrared images by asymmetry analysis. In Biomedical Engineering Handbook. CRC Press.

Quaresma, V., Matcher, S. J., & Ferrari, M. (1998, January). Identification and quantification of intrinsic optical contrast for near-infrared mammography. Photochemistry and Photobiology, 67(1), 4–14. doi:10.1111/j.1751-1097.1998.tb05159.x PubMed doi:10.1111/j.1751-1097.1998.tb05159.x PMID:9477760

Riis, C., Lernevall, A., Sorensen, F. B., & Nygaard, H. (2005). 3D Ultrasound-Based Evaluation of Lesions in the Uncompressed Breast. In E. Ueno, T. Shiina, M. Kubota, & K. Sawai (Eds.), Research and Development in Breast Ultrasound. Springer. doi:10.1007/4-431-27008-6_22 doi:10.1007/4-431-27008-6_22

Ring, E. F. J., & Ammer, K. (2000). The technique of infrared imaging in medicine. Thermology Int., 10, 7–14.

Scaperrotta, G., Ferranti, C., Costa, C., Mariani, L., Marchesini, M., Suman, L., Folini, C., & Bergonzi, S. (2008). Role of sonoelastography in non-palpable breast lesions. European Radiology, 18(11), 2381–2389. doi:10.1007/s00330-008-1032-8 PubMed doi:10.100700330-008-1032-8 PMID:18523780

Schilling, K., Narayanan, D., & Kalinyak, J.E. (2008). Effect of breast density, menopausal status, and hormone use in high resolution positron emission mammography. *Radiol Soc North Am.*, VB31–04.

Schnall, M. D. (2001). Application of magnetic resonance imaging to early detection of breast cancer. Breast Cancer Research, 3(1), 17–21. doi:10.1186/bcr265 PubMed doi:10.1186/bcr265 PMID:11300101

Scholz, B., & Anderson, R. (2000). On electrical impedance scanning: Principles and simulations. *Electromedica, 68*(35).

Siegel, R., Naishadham, D., & Jemal, A. (2012). Cancer statistics, 2012. CA: a Cancer Journal for Clinicians, 62(1), 10–29. doi:10.3322/caac.20138 PubMed doi:10.3322/caac.20138 PMID:22237781

Sree, S. V., Ng, E. Y., Acharya, R. U., & Faust, O. (2011). Breast imaging: A survey. *World Journal of Clinical Oncology, 2*(4), 171–178. doi:10.5306/wjco. v2.i4.171

Tofts, P. S., Berkowitz, B., & Schnall, M. D. (1995). Quantitative analysis of dynamic Gd – DTPA enhancement in breast tumours using a perme-ability model. Magnetic Resonance Imaging, 33, 564–568. PubMed PMID:7776889

Tofts, P. S., Berkowitz, B., & Schnall, M. D. (1995). Quantitative analysis of dynamic Gd – DTPA enhancement in breast tumours using a permeability model. Magnetic Resonance Imaging, 33, 564–568. PubMed PMID:7776889

Van Ongeval, Ch. (2007, May-June). Department of Radiology, KULeuven, UZ Gasthuisberg, Leuven, Belgium. Digital mammography for screen-ing and diagnosis of breast cancer: An overview. JBR-BTR; Organe de la Societe Royale Belge de Radiologie (SRBR), 90(3), 163–166.

Weiss, L. K., Burkman, R. T., Cushing-Haugen, K. L., Voigt, L. F., Simon, M. S., Daling, J. R., ... (2002). Hormone replacement therapy regimens and breast cancer risk (1). Obstetrics and Gynecology, 100, 1148–1158. PubMed PMID:12468157

Wiecek, B., Wiecek, M., Strakowski, R., Jakubowska, T., & Ng, E. Y. K. (2010). Wavelet-based thermal image classification for breast screening and other medical applications. In E. Y. K. Ng, R. U. Acharya, & J. S. Suri (Eds.), Performance Evaluation Techniques in Multi-modality Breast Cancer Screening, Diagnosis and Treatment. American Scientific Publishers.

Wu, T., Stewart, A., Stanton, M., McCauley, T., Phillips, W., Kopans, D. B., Moore, R. H., Eberhard, J. W., Opsahl-Ong, B., Niklason, L., & Williams, M. B. (2003). Tomographic mammography using a limited number of low-dose cone-beam projection images. Medical Physics, 30(3), 365–380. doi:10.1118/1.1543934 PubMed doi:10.1118/1.1543934 PMID:12674237

Yamamoto, A., Fukushima, H., Okamura, R., Nakamura, Y., Morimoto, T., Urata, Y., Mukaihara, S., & Hayakawa, K. (2006). Dynamic helical CT mam-mography of breast cancer. Radiation Medicine, 24(1), 35–40. doi:10.1007/BF02489987 PubMed doi:10.1007/BF02489987 PMID:16715660

Zhu, Q., Cronin, E. B., Currier, A. A., Vine, H. S., Huang, M., Chen, N., & Xu, C. (2005, October). Benign versus malignant breast masses: Optical differentiation with US-guided optical imaging reconstruction. Radiology, 237(1), 57–66. doi:10.1148/radiol.2371041236 PubMed doi:10.1148/radiol.2371041236 PMID:16183924

Chapter 10
Applications of the Use of Infrared Breast Images:
Segmentation and Classification of Breast Abnormalities

Marcus Costa de Araújo
https://orcid.org/0000-0002-1818-5686
Universidade Federal de Pernambuco, Brazil

Kamila Fernanda F. da Cunha Queiroz
https://orcid.org/0000-0003-4257-5155
Federal Institute of Rio Grande do Norte, Brazil

Renata Maria Cardoso Rodrigues de Souza
https://orcid.org/0000-0002-2849-1273
Universidade Federal de Pernambuco, Brazil

Rita de Cássia Fernandes de Lima
DEMEC, Federal University of Pernambuco, Brazil

ABSTRACT

Applications that have already been developed on using infrared (IR) imaging are proposed for a better understanding of breast cancer analysis. The first part of this chapter presents the use of interval data to classify breast abnormalities. Authors have been adapting machine learning techniques to work with interval variables that can handle the intrinsic variation of data. The second part evaluates segmentation techniques applied to breast IR images. Many authors use automatic image segmentation techniques that must consider the natural anatomical variation between people. Manual segmentation techniques can be used to minimize the problem of anatomical variations. The main purpose of such techniques is to seek to avoid the errors due to the natural asymmetry of the human body. A process that uses ellipsoidal elements to represent each breast has been chosen. The manual technique is more precise and can correct possible failures presented in the automatic method. Validation of each segmentation type was also included by using Jaccard, DICE, False Positive, and False Negative methods.

DOI: 10.4018/978-1-7998-3456-4.ch010

STATISTICAL CLASSIFICATION OF BREAST ABNORMALITIES USING INFRARED (IR) IMAGES: INTERVAL CLASSIFIERS

This topic uses interval data to classify breast abnormalities. Many authors have been adapting some machine learning techniques to work with interval variables. These kinds of variable can handle the intrinsic variation of data. In breast thermography, the use of interval data along with machine learning techniques can lead to results offering new possibilities for their use.

The IR images were acquired at the Outpatient Clinic of Mastology of the Clinical Hospital of the Federal University of Pernambuco (HC/UFPE). The project was registered in the Brazilian Health Ministry (CEP/CCS/UFPE nº 279/05) after being approved by the Ethics Committee of UFPE.

Symbolic Data

In classical data modeling, each variable is represented by a single value, which makes the analysis of complex problems involving large data sets restrictive. In contrast, a symbolic variable can represent values which are multivalued, categorical, interval, frequency histograms and subsets and functions of different semantics, such as frequency, probabilistic, and possibilistic semantics.

Symbolic objects are defined for the purpose of reducing the volume and complexity of the original data by providing a new description of such data. According to Gowda and Diday (1992), symbolic objects are an extension of classical data. In conventional databases, objects are "individualized" whereas in symbolic databases they can be "united" by means of relationships. They therefore represent a group of data that is more complex than conventional data.

This chapter focuses on using symbolic objects of an interval nature.

Symbolic Interval Objects

Let Γ be a set of symbolic objects and let $\dot{y}_i$ be an individual belonging to Γ. Let $\dot{y}_{i1}, \dot{y}_{i2}, \ldots, \dot{y}_{i3}$ be a set of *p* symbolic variables that describe the object $\dot{y}_i$. A symbolic interval object $\dot{y}_i$ is one where the variables assume values within an interval (Schnepper & Stadtherr, 1996)., i.e.,

$$\dot{y}_{ij} = \left[a_{ij}, b_{ij}\right] \subset R; a_{ij} \leq b_{ij}; a_{ij}, b_{ij} \in R; j = 1, \ldots, p$$

According to Silva and Brito (2006), the use of interval data is justified for two different situations:

1. Let there be a dataset Ω ,, which has been aggregated to a base that uses certain criteria. Each element of Ω is described by real variables $\boldsymbol{x}_j$, $\boldsymbol{j} = 1, \ldots, \boldsymbol{p}$, and the interval variables $\dot{\boldsymbol{y}}_j$ represent the variability of $\boldsymbol{x}_j$ in each group of data.
2. Each interval variable $\dot{\boldsymbol{y}}_j$ represents a set of possible values within the uncertainty of measurement of the real variable $\boldsymbol{x}_j$.

Thus, a source of interval data can naturally arise from the description of specific technical data.

Conceptually, IR imaging provides a temperature matrix of a surface. Thus, an IR image of the breast provides the distribution of temperatures over the surface of the breast. If breast temperatures are considered to have an interval-like behavior, we can represent the breasts in the IR image as a group of temperatures, rather than representing them by classical data such as average, maximum or minimum temperatures. By analyzing the temperature data of a breast as an interval of temperatures rather than single values, the intrinsic variability in the data can be taken into account.

In a thermographic image, an interval can be defined based on the temperatures contained in a region of interest by $\dot{y} = [T_{min}, T_{max}]$ where T_{min}, called the *infimum* (Inf), represents the minimum temperature obtained over the region of interest and T_{max}, called the *supremum* (Sup), represents the maximum temperature obtained over the same region of interest, i.e., they represent the lower and upper limits of the temperature interval, respectively.

Classification Based on Symbolic Data

This section will consider two approaches to using interval data to classify breast pathologies in thermographic images:

- The first approach is underpinned by the use of continuous variables derived from interval dissimilarity measures. Several dissimilarity measures were defined by Diday and Noirhomme-Fraiture (2008). Thus, the information contained in temperature intervals can be translated into classical data and conventional classifiers can be used for the task of classification (Araújo, Lima, & Souza, 2014).
- The second form of doing so is to describe the breast by means of interval variables and using interval classifiers to distinguish between malignant and nonmalignant nodules. Several authors have generalized the concept of conventional classifiers (classical data) for use with interval variables (Araújo, Souza, Lima, & Silva Filho, 2017).

Approach 1: Measurement of dissimilarity between intervals.

From the temperature matrices corresponding to the breast regions in the thermogram, which were obtained after segmenting the thermographic image, we can define an interval variable for each breast as being $\dot{y}_{LB} = [T_{min\,LB}, T_{max\,LB}]$ and $\dot{y}_{RB} = [T_{min\,RB}, T_{max\,RB}]$,where LB and RB stand for the left breast and the right breast, respectively.

From the temperature intervals for each breast, continuous variables are obtained, based on measures of dissimilarity between intervals, which will be used for the classification process. These continuous characteristics are based on the components of position (D1) and of content (D2) defined in the Gowda-Diday dissimilarity measure for intervals. (Billard & Diday, 2006).

Let there be a set Γ of interval observations $\dot{y}_i$, with $i = 1, \cdots, m$ observations at p variables, denoted by

$$\dot{y}_i = \left(\dot{y}_{i1}, \dot{y}_{i2}, \ldots, \dot{y}_{ip}\right) \quad (1)$$

The Gowda-Diday dissimilarity measure between two interval variables $\dot{y}_{RB} = [a_{RB}, b_{RB}]$ and $\dot{y}_{LB} = [a_{LB}, b_{LB}]$ belonging to an interval observation $\dot{y}_i$ is given by

$$D(\dot{y}_{RB}, \dot{y}_{LB}) = \sum_{r=1}^{3} D_r(\dot{Y}_{RB}, \dot{Y}_{LB}) \tag{2}$$

In Equation 2, D is formed by the sum of three components (D_1, D_2, D_3), where D_1 represents the position component, D_2 represents the content component, and D_3 represents the relative position between the intervals $\dot{y}_{RB}$ and $\dot{y}_{LB}$.

Components D_1, D_2 and D_3 are defined as:

$$D_1(\dot{y}_{RB}, \dot{y}_{LB}) = \frac{\left||b_{RB} - a_{RB}| - |b_{LB} - a_{LB}|\right|}{K} \tag{3}$$

where K corresponds to the junction of the intervals, i.e.

$$K = \left|\max(b_{MD}, b_{ME}) - min(a_{MD}, a_{ME})\right|$$

$$D_2(\dot{y}_{RB}, \dot{y}_{LB}) = \frac{(|b_{RB} - a_{RB}| + |b_{LB} - a_{LB}| - 2I)}{K} \tag{4}$$

where I is the length of the intersection between the intervals $\dot{y}_{RB}$ and $\dot{y}_{LB}$, given by:

$$I = \left|\max(a_{MD}, a_{ME}) - \min(b_{MD}, b_{ME})\right|$$

When there is no overlap between the intervals, $I = 0$ is assumed and finally

$$D_3(\dot{y}_{RB}, \dot{y}_{LB}) = \frac{|a_{RB} - a_{LB}|}{|\dot{y}_u|} \tag{5}$$

where $|\dot{y}_u|$ corresponds to the total length covered by the variable under analysis, considering all instances $|\dot{y}_u|$ i.e.,

$$|\dot{y}_u| = \max b_i - \min a_i \ . \tag{6}$$

Figure 1. Graphical representation of the temperature intervals for the right and left breasts of the same patient.

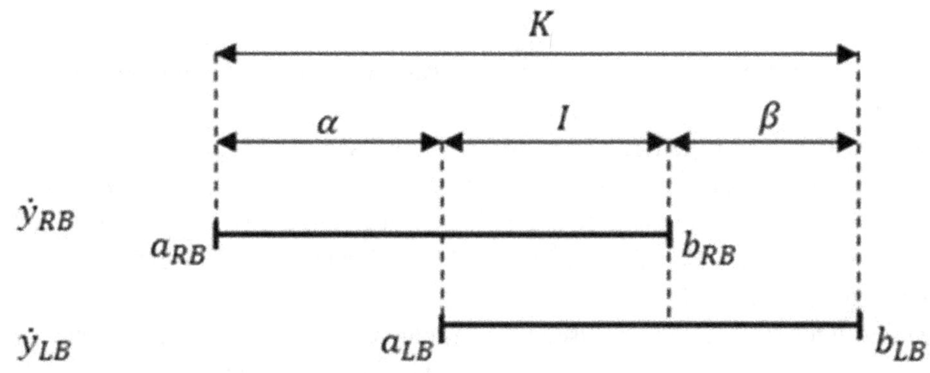

The graphical representation of two intervals $\dot{y}_{RB}$ and $\dot{y}_{LB}$ representing temperature data for the right and left breasts of the same patient, respectively, can be displayed as shown in Figure 1. Thus we can define the length of $\dot{y}_{RB}$ as

$$\left|\dot{y}_{RB}\right| = \left|b_{RB} - a_{LB}\right| = \alpha + I$$

where I represents the length of the intersection between the intervals; and $\alpha = \left|a_{LB} - a_{RB}\right|$. Similarly, the length of $\dot{y}_{LB}$ can be written as

$$\left|\dot{y}_{LB}\right| = \left|b_{LB} - a_{LB}\right| = \beta + I$$

where $\beta = \left|b_{LB} - b_{RB}\right|$.

Therefore, from Equations (4.7) and (4.8) the components D_1 and D_2 of the Gowda-Diday dissimilarity measure can be defined as:

$$D_1\left(\dot{y}_{RB}, \dot{y}_{LB}\right) = \frac{\left\|b_{RB} - a_{RB}\right| - \left|b_{LB} - a_{LB}\right\|}{K} = \frac{\left(\alpha - I\right) - \left(\beta + I\right)}{K} = \frac{\alpha - \beta}{K} \tag{7}$$

$$D_2\left(\dot{y}_{RB}, \dot{y}_{LB}\right) = \frac{\left(\left|b_{RB} - a_{RB}\right| + \left|b_{LB} - a_{LB}\right| - 2I\right)}{K} \tag{8}$$

$$= \frac{\left(\alpha + I\right) + \left(\beta + I\right) - 2I}{K} = \frac{\alpha + \beta}{K}$$

$$D_3\left(\dot{y}_{RB},\dot{y}_{LB}\right)=\frac{\left|a_{RB}-a_{LB}\right|}{\left|\dot{y}_u\right|}=\frac{\alpha}{\left|\dot{y}_u\right|} \tag{9}$$

These classical variables, obtained from the interval representation of temperature, can be used to classify breast pathologies.

Araújo et al. (2014) based their study on measures of dissimilarity between breast temperature intervals so as to classify the pathologies observed in thermographic images as "Malignant", "Benign" and "Cyst". The authors evaluated feature extraction by different classifiers, and obtained a sensitivity to the malignant tumor of 85.7% and specificity to the malignant tumor of 86.5%.

Approach 2: Interval Classifier.

In this section, interval variables are used as the input vector for a classifier. Interval classifiers represent a generalization of the classical classifiers. Diday and Noirhomme-Fraiture (2008) generalized the concept of classification by means of classical data to interval data using different classical classifiers available from the literature. Souza, Carvalho and Tenório (2004) extended the concept of the Mahalanobis distance to interval data, thus letting this interval distance be used in a minimum distance interval classifier. Araújo et al. (2017) applied a minimum interval-to-interval classifier based on a class-weighted Mahalanobis distance.

Classifier of minimum distance for intervals

The minimum distance classifier attributes an unknown pattern $\boldsymbol{x}$ to a class $\boldsymbol{\acute{E}}_i, \boldsymbol{i}=1,\ldots,\boldsymbol{C}$, based on minimizing a proximity function defined between the projection of the pattern itself and the projection of a representative $\boldsymbol{u}_i$ of class $\boldsymbol{\acute{E}}_i$, known as the prototype of the class, in the space of characteristics. This method has the advantage of being independent of the distribution of the individuals of each class (Hastie, Tibshirani, & Friedman, 2009).

The minimum distance classifier for intervals works in the same way as the minimum distance classifier for classic data. Let $\Gamma=\dot{y}_1,\ldots,\dot{y}_m$, a group of m symbolic objects described by p interval variables. Each object $\dot{\boldsymbol{y}}_i\left(\boldsymbol{i}=1,\ldots,\boldsymbol{m}\right)$ is represented as a vector of intervals $\dot{\boldsymbol{y}}_i=\left(\left[\boldsymbol{a}_{i1},\boldsymbol{b}_{i1}\right],\ldots,\left[\boldsymbol{a}_{ip},\boldsymbol{b}_{ip}\right]\right)^T$. Let P be a partition of Γ in K classes $C_1,\ldots,C_K$, where each class $\boldsymbol{C}_k\left(\boldsymbol{k}=1,\ldots,\boldsymbol{K}\right)$ has a prototype $\boldsymbol{L}_k$ which is also represented as a vector of intervals $\dot{g}_k=\left(\left[\alpha_{k1},\beta_{k1}\right),\ldots,\left[\alpha_{kp},\beta_{kp}\right]\right)^T$, where $\dot{\boldsymbol{g}}_k$ corresponds to the vector of means of the intervals of $\boldsymbol{C}_k$.

For $\boldsymbol{j}=1\ldots,\boldsymbol{p}$:

$$\left[\alpha_{kj}=\frac{\sum_{i\in C_k}a_{ij}}{n_k},\beta_{kj}=\frac{\sum_{i\in C_k}b_{ij}}{n_k}\right]$$

where $\boldsymbol{n}_k$ represents the number of elements in class $\boldsymbol{C}_k$.

The minimum distance classifier allocates an object $\dot{\boldsymbol{v}}_i$ to class $\boldsymbol{C}_k$ if

$$d^{\lambda}\left(\dot{v}_i,\dot{g}_k\right)\leq d^{\lambda}\left(\dot{v}_i,\dot{g}_r\right)\forall r,r=1,\ldots,K.$$

where the function $d''(\dot{v}_i, \dot{g}_k)$ represents a distance between intervals.

Distance Measures for Intervals

Ichino-Yaguchi dissimilarity measure

The Ichino-Yaguchi dissimilarity measure between two intervals $\dot{y}_{ij}$ and $\dot{y}_{ik}, j \neq k$, belonging to the interval variable $\dot{y}_i$, can be defined as (Billard & Diday, 2006):

$$\phi_i(\dot{y}_{ij}, \dot{y}_{ik}) = |\dot{y}_{ij} \oplus \dot{y}_{ik}| - |\dot{y}_{ij} \otimes \dot{y}_{ik}| + \gamma(2|\dot{y}_{ij} \otimes \dot{y}_{ik}| - |\dot{y}_{ij}| - |\dot{y}_{ik}|)$$

where $|A|$ corresponds to the length of the interval $A = [a, b]$, i.e., $|A| = b - a$, and $|A| = b - a$, and $0 \leq \lambda \leq 0.5$ represents a predetermined constant; and the sum and product interval operators are defined as:

$$\dot{y}_{ij} \oplus \dot{y}_{ik} = [a_{ij} + a_{ik}, b_{ij} + b_{ik}]$$

$$\dot{y}_{ij} \otimes \dot{y}_{ik} = [(a_{ij}a_{ik}, a_{ij}b_{ik}, b_{ij}a_{ik}, b_{ij}b_{ik}), (a_{ij}a_{ik}, a_{ij}b_{ik}, b_{ij}a_{ik}, b_{ij}b_{ik})]$$

Minkowsky's (weighted) generalized distance

Minkowsky's (weighted) generalized distance between two interval observations $\dot{y}_L$ and $\dot{y}_R$ is defined as (Billard & Diday, 2006):

$$d(\dot{y}_L, \dot{y}_R) = \left\{ \sum_{j=1}^{p} w_j^* [\phi(\dot{y}_{Lj}, \dot{y}_{Rj})]^q \right\}^{1/q} \quad (10)$$

where $\phi(\dot{y}_{Lj}, \dot{y}_{Rj})$ corresponds to the Ichino–Yaguchi dissimilarity measure between two interval variables $\dot{y}_{Lj}$ and $\dot{y}_{RJ}$; $W_j^* = 1/|\dot{y}_j|$ is a weight function associated with the variable *j* and is defined as in Eq. 6; *q* is called the Minkowsky order of distance. For $q = 1$ the distance corresponds to a City-Block distance for intervals; for $q = 2$, Minkowsky's distance corresponds to a normalized Euclidean distance for intervals.

Standard Hausdorf Distance

The standard Hausdorf distance between two interval variables $\dot{y}_{Lj}$ and $\dot{y}_{Rj}$ is given by (Billard & Diday, 2006):

$$\phi_j(\dot{y}_{Lj}, \dot{y}_{Rj}) = (|a_{Lj} - a_{Rj}|, |b_{Lj} - b_{Rj}|) \quad (11)$$

Class-Weighted Mahalanobis Distance

Let an interval object, represented by the interval vector $\dot{\boldsymbol{v}}_i$ and $\boldsymbol{v}_{iI} = \left(\boldsymbol{a}_{i1},...,\boldsymbol{a}_{ip}\right)^T$ and $\boldsymbol{v}_{iS} = \left(\boldsymbol{b}_{i1},...,\boldsymbol{b}_{ip}\right)^T$, be two vectors containing the values of Inf and Sup of $\dot{\boldsymbol{v}}_i$, respectively; and let $g_{kI} = \left(\alpha_{i1}, \ . \ . \ . \ ,\alpha_{ip}\right)^T$ and $g_{kS} = \left(\alpha_{i1}, \ . \ . \ . \ ,\alpha_{ip}\right)^T$ be two vectors containing the values of Inf and Sup of prototype $\dot{\boldsymbol{g}}_k$, respectively.

Souza et al. (2004) defined the Mahalanobis distance $'\left(\dot{\boldsymbol{v}}_i, \dot{\boldsymbol{g}}_k\right)$ between two interval observations $\dot{\boldsymbol{v}}_i$ and $\dot{\boldsymbol{g}}_k$ as:

$$\delta\left(\dot{v}_i,\dot{g}_k\right) = d\left(v_{iI}, g_{kI}\right) + d\left(v_{iS}, g_{kS}\right) \tag{12}$$

where

$$d\left(v_{iI}, g_{kI}\right) = \left(v_{iI} - gkI\right)^T S_I^{-1}\left(v_{iI} - g_{kI}\right) \tag{13}$$

represents the Mahalanobis distance between the Inf, vectors $\boldsymbol{v}_{iI}$ and $\boldsymbol{g}_{kI}$, and $\boldsymbol{S}_I$ corresponds to the covariance matrix for the values of Inf; and

$$\boldsymbol{d}\left(\boldsymbol{v}_{iS}, \boldsymbol{g}_{kS}\right) = \left(\boldsymbol{v}_{iS} - \boldsymbol{g}_{kS}\right)^T \boldsymbol{S}_S^{-1}\left(\boldsymbol{v}_{iS} - \boldsymbol{g}_{kS}\right) \tag{14}$$

represents the Mahalanobis distance between the Sup vectors $\boldsymbol{v}_{iS}$ and $\boldsymbol{g}_{kS}$. And $\boldsymbol{S}_S$ corresponds to the covariance matrix for the values of Sup.

From this point on, Araújo et al. (2017) defined the parameterized Mahalanobis distance by means of a common covariance matrix between Inf and Sup, parameterized for each class. Where λ_k is the control parameter of class $\boldsymbol{C}_K$, $\lambda_k \in \left[0,1\right], \left(k=1, \ . \ . \ . \ , K\right)$. A parameterized Mahalanobis distance between two interval vectors $\dot{\boldsymbol{v}}_i$ and $\dot{\boldsymbol{g}}_k$ can be defined as follows:

$$d^{\lambda}\left(\dot{v}_i, \dot{g}_k\right) = \left(v_{iI} - g_{kI}\right)^T S_k^{-1}\left(\lambda_k\right)\left(v_{iI} - g_{kI}\right) + \left(v_{iS} - g_{kS}\right)^T S_k^{-1}\left(\lambda_k\right)\left(v_{iS} - g_{kS}\right) \tag{15}$$

where $S_k\left(\lambda_k\right)\left(K = 1,...,K\right)$ represents a parameterized covariance matrix for class $\boldsymbol{C}_k$ that is defined based on a control parameter $\lambda_k \in \left[0,1\right]$. This parameter measures the degree of relevance between the limits of the intervals, i.e., between the Inf and Sup values, when the matrix of parameterized covariances of the class is calculated.

The parameterized covariance matrix of class $\boldsymbol{C}_k$ is given by

Table 1. Synthesis of the results obtained by Araújo et al. (2017).

Distance	Error	Sens. Malignant	Spec. Malignant	Spec. Benign	Spec. Benign	Sens Cyst	Spec. Cyst
Hausdorf	0.2	0.79	0.92	0.79	0.9	0.82	0.88
Minkowsky City-Block (q=1)	0.78	0.57	0.31	0.16	0.55	0	1
Minkowsky Euclidian (q=2);	0.8	0.5	0.33	0.16	0.55	0	0.94
Ichino-Yaguchi, $(\gamma = 0.2)$	0.66	1	0.11	0.16	0.97	0	1
Mahalanobis parameterized, $(\lambda_1 = 0.4; \lambda_2 = 0.4; \lambda_3 = 0)$	0.16	0.93	0.86	0.84	0.94	0.76	0.97

Note: Sens. = Sensitivity and Spec. = Specificity.

$$S_k\left(\lambda_k\right) = \frac{\left(1-\lambda_k\right)S_{kI} + \lambda_k S_{kS}}{\left(1-\lambda_k\right)n_k + \lambda_k n} \tag{16}$$

where $\boldsymbol{S_{kI}}$ and $\boldsymbol{S_{kS}}$ correspond to covariance matrices for the values of Inf and Sup of class $\boldsymbol{C_k}$, respectively; and λ_k represents the parameter of class $\boldsymbol{C_k}$.

Araújo et al. (2017) compared these different classifiers of minimum distance for intervals with a view to classifying breast pathologies in a database containing thermographies of 50 patients. The authors arrived at the results listed in Table 1. Regarding the Malignant Class, note that Table 1 shows that the classifier, based on the Ichino-Yamaguchi dissimilarity measures, obtained 100% sensitivity but presented great losses for the other classes and a high specificity value for this Malignant Class. The parameterized Mahalanobis classifier obtained a sensitivity of 93% combined with a specificity of 86% for the Malignant Class, with an overall error rate of only 16%, which shows that the classifier presented a great improvement in the results when compared to the other classifiers.

The results showed that interval temperature data can be used to represent thermographic images as they encompass the intrinsic variability of each temperature point in the thermogram. Thus, the task of classifying breast abnormalities by thermography may benefit from the use of interval variables. An approach based on a binary "cancer" and "non-cancer" analysis may benefit from the higher sensitivities found for the Malignant Class. This tool may be of great value for screening and/or early detection of cancer, especially in the analysis of thermograms of people living in locations far from large urban centers and in places with difficult access to health services.

COMPARISON AND VALIDATION OF TECHNIQUES FOR SEGMENTATION OF IR BREAST IMAGES

In this item, we will present applications that have already been developed on using IR imaging as a proposal for a better understanding of breast cancer. It will be shown how such applications can be used as a basis for enhancing the use of breast thermographic imaging as a user-friendly and inexpensive tool for the early detection of breast cancer. We also seek to show that IR imaging can be used to validate calculated temperature profiles and to classify breast abnormalities.

This topic evaluates segmentation techniques applied to breast thermographic images. Some classifiers that will be presented are based on contralateral breast comparisons. Many authors use automatic image segmentation techniques that must take into account the natural anatomical variation between people.

Manual segmentation techniques can also be used to minimize the problem of anatomical variation. The main purpose of such techniques is to seek to avoid the errors that may arise due to the natural asymmetry of the human body and this is done by turning these techniques into tools. A process that uses ellipsoidal elements to represent each breast has been chosen. The ellipses were adjusted to each patient by manually changing their diameters. The matrix containing the temperature values measured by the IR image was used instead of using colored pixels.

The quality of the results of each type of segmentation: automatic or manual, will be assessed by using the resulting image of the breast. Validation of each segmentation type will also be included, for example, by using Jaccard, DICE, False Positive, and False Negative methods.

This topic evaluates segmentation techniques applied to breast thermographic images. Some classifiers presented in Item 1 of this chapter are based on contralateral breast comparisons. An automatic method of processing and analyzing breast thermograms will be presented. The proposal includes: an automatic digital image segmenter, certain individual features and classification methods. The features will be those that best differentiate the individuals who comprise the sample, and among the classification methods, the ones with the best results will be selected.

The second technique presented for the segmentation is the manual one, which is more precise and can correct possible failures presented in the automatic method.

The quality of the results of each type of segmentation: automatic or manual, will be assessed by using the resulting breast image. Validation of each segmentation type will also be included, such as Jaccard, DICE, False Positive, and False Negative methods.

Digital Processing of the Thermographic Image

The digital thermographic image can be defined by a two-dimensional function f (x,y) of the light intensity associated with a temperature matrix **T** (x,y), where x and y are (flat) spatial coordinates and each element of **T** (x,y) represents the temperature of the point (x,y) (Gonzalez, Woods, & Eddins, 2004).

This image is represented by an indexed image, or pseudo-color, which has two components: a temperature matrix and a color map. Therefore, the thermogram is the representation of values of the temperature matrix as pointers to the color map. In this case, the colors of each pixel will depend on the color map applied and on the lower and upper temperature limits defined by the scale of the thermogram, as can be seen in Figure 2 (Queiroz, 2014).

Thus, as each pixel represents the temperature value defined by the **T** matrix, these values remain constant regardless of changing the color map or the temperature scale, thereby making it feasible to deal with the images based on the temperature values instead of the intensity of the *pixels*.

Segmentation of Thermographic Images

The analysis of images involves the automatic measurement of the objects within an image and their assignment to certain classes (Dougherty, 2009). Frequently, it is necessary to identify and isolate the objects of interest, this stage of image processing being called segmentation. The type of segmentation chosen and its correct implementation are fundamental for pattern recognition and influence the performance of automatic decision methods.

Several segmentation techniques can be applied to medical images, thus presenting different performances depending on the type of image and the structure under analysis. One can segment microcalcifications in mammograms or even the breast region in thermograms (Luz, 2007 as cited in Queiroz, 2014). However, what makes the segmentation of thermograms difficult is the absence of clear temperature limits in some places and their misshapen structures.

In order to extract the region of interest (ROI), both automatic and manual segmentation can be used

Figure 2. Thermographic images with different temperature limits.

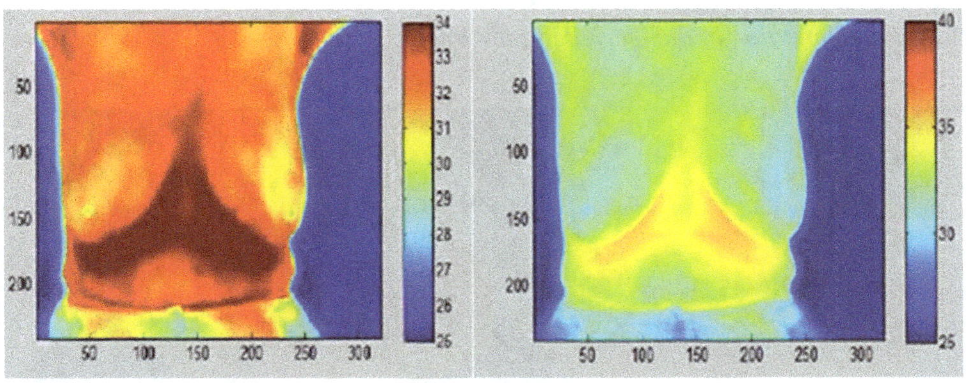

to support the diagnosis of breast cancer. Automatic segmentation without human intervention is often faster and more suitable for quick analysis. Usually, the option for manual segmentation arises from the need to reduce the segmentation errors that may arise automatically due to the natural asymmetry between the breasts and to the anatomical variations between different people. In addition, it can be easily used by a health professional to better define the area of interest (Araújo, 2014; Queiroz, 2014).

Manual Segmentation of the Breasts

The first step in segmenting a breast thermogram is to separate the breast region from the rest of the image. In this case, the **T**-temperature matrix of the thermographic image is reconstructed as a digital image using Matlab®, and assigning a color to each temperature value. Segmentation is performed on this image.

The process developed for the manual segmentation of the breast in the thermogram is to select the ROI from ellipsoidal elements, manually generated using Matlab®, over the **T**-temperature matrix. After selecting the ROI, the rest of the image is disregarded. The result of this segmentation is represented by two independent temperature matrices, MR and ML, which correspond to the right and left breast temperature matrices, respectively (Figure 3). In Figure 3, the thermographic image is manually rotated to match the ellipse axis with the orientation of the breast to be segmented.

Automatic Segmentation of the Breasts

In automatic segmentation, temperature matrices needed to be treated as grayscale images, with lighter shades indicating higher temperatures. Since temperatures are accurate to two decimal places, the 8-bit (256 shades of gray) representation was not sufficient, so 16-bit images (65536 shades of gray) had to be used. The images have been equalized for easy viewing. The process described in this chapter is detailed in Dourado Neto (2014).

The segmentation of the temperature matrix began with separating the region of the patient's body from the colder background. This was done by identifying the threshold value in the histogram that separates the two regions. Then, the regions immediately below the armpits were identified and a straight line with an angle of 60° to the horizontal defined two upper regions that were excluded, as was the region above the neck. Figure 4 presents the result of this process.

Figure 3. Breast segmentation in the thermographic image.

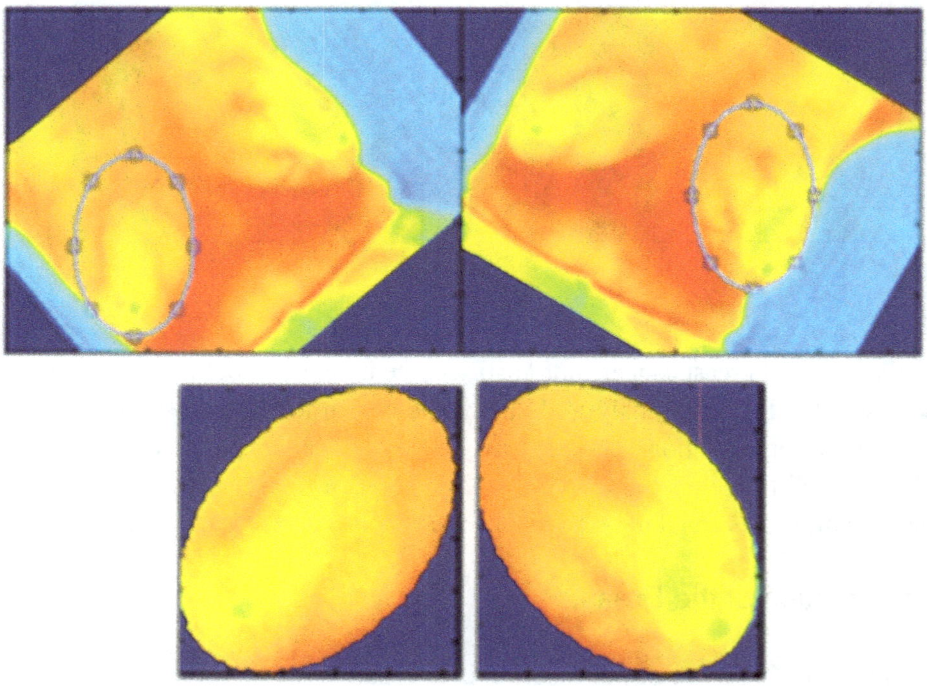

The step of removing the lower border is the most critical of the segmentation. Despite being a lighter region characterized by a high temperature, the step is a difficult one due to patients having different biotypes. The method for selecting borders begins in the central region and continues downward to each external region, excluding each pixel and its entire line below if this:

- has a value greater than or equal to $maxlin_{e - (1/}max)$, where *maxline* is the $_{\text{maximum}}$ value of the vertical line to which the pixel belongs and *max* is the global maximum value;
- has already had its most central neighbor excluded.

The result of excluding the lower border and its lower region is shown in Figure 5. In cases where the contrast of the image is very low, identifying the lower border is problematic and may result in a large loss of the ROI.

The last stage of segmentation is to remove possible residual upper lateral regions, by defining straight lines from the outer point of average height and forming 60° with the horizontal. The final segmented image of Figure 6B is displayed in grayscale corresponding to the first equalization so as to make the comparison with the original image more natural (Figure 6A).

Figure 4. Segmentation after determining the upper and lower limits and removing the residual upper lateral regions.

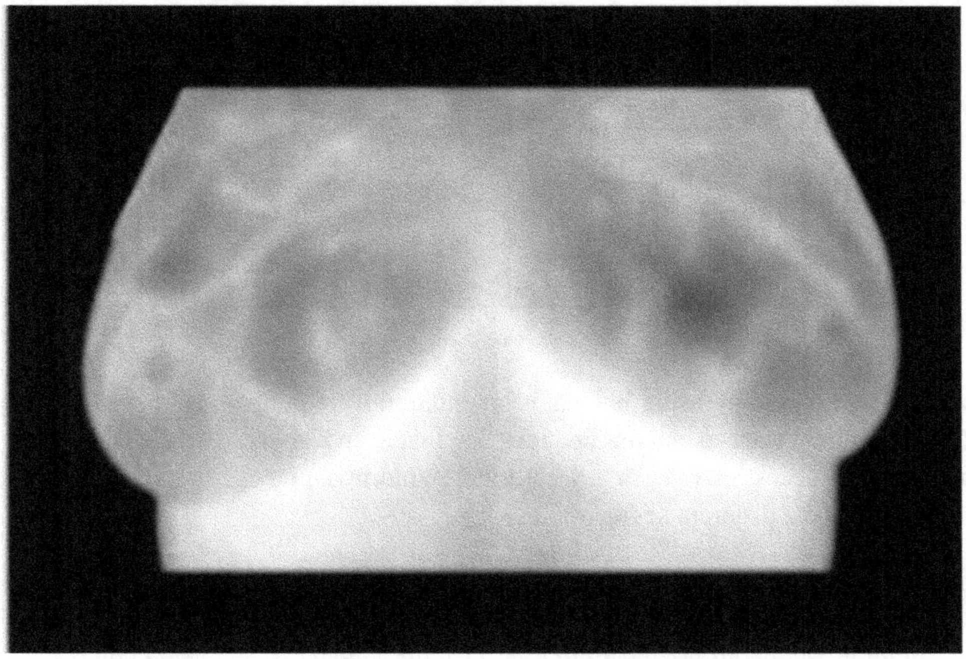

Validation of the Automatic Segmentation

As important as the segmentation methods themselves are the validation techniques. Validation should both assess the accuracy and limitations of the algorithm and make it clear whether the method can be applied. In the area of medical image processing, full validation of a method is a necessary step when it is intended to apply it to the medical routine.

To validate a method, ground truth images must be obtained that will enable the efficiency of the proposed automatic segmentation to be measured. Due to the absence of ground truth of thermographic

Figure 5. Image after removal of the border and lower region.

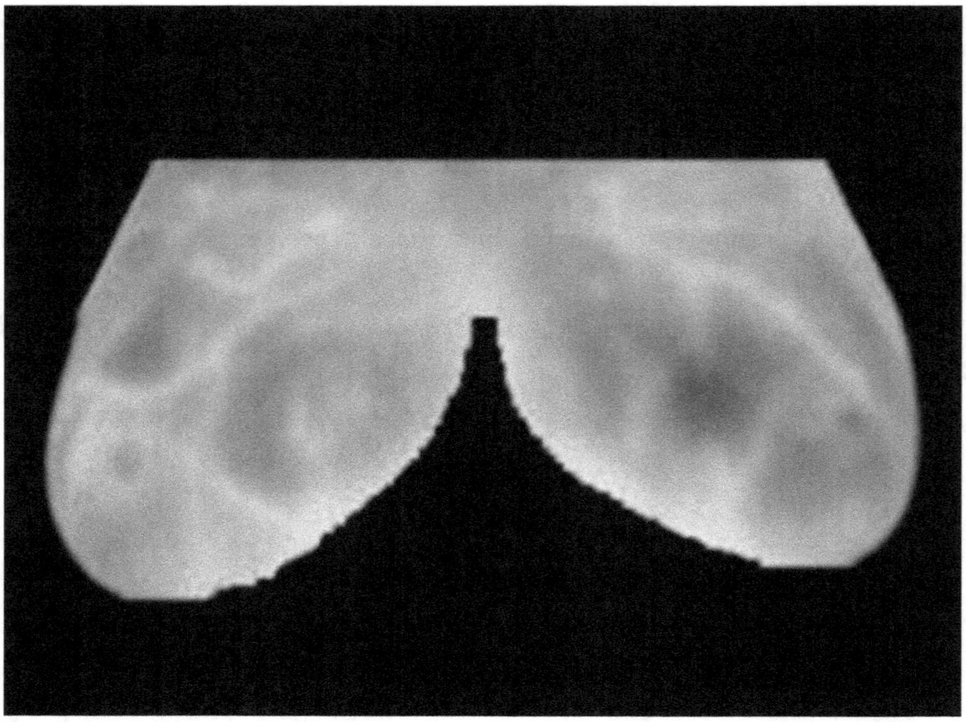

images, the results obtained by using manual segmentation were adopted as the standard (Figure 7a) (Araújo, 2014). It is important to emphasize, however, that even if more than one manual segmentation is used, this does not necessarily reach a definitive ground truth, due to the variations that there are between the results of the different segmentations.

Figure 6. Result of the automatic segmentation. A. Original image; B. Segmented image.

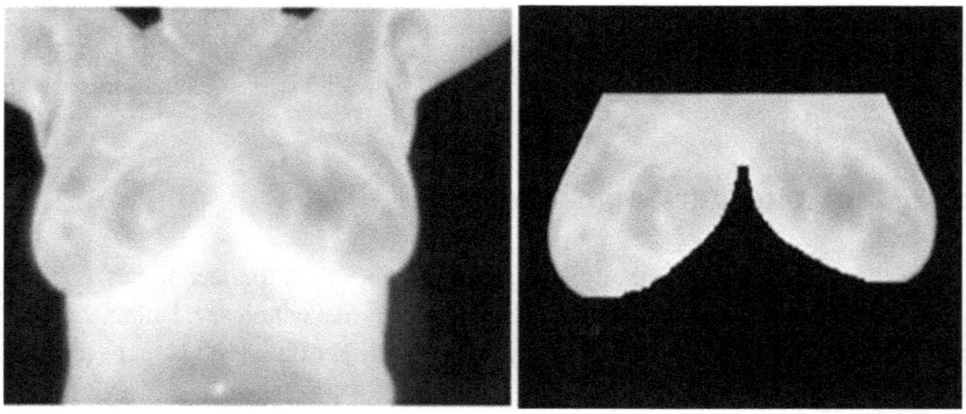

Thus, the objective of the validation method was to show that the results of automatic segmentation (Figure 7b) are within the variability between the different manual segmentations, for which the measurements of accuracy used are the Jaccard index, the Dice index, False Positive, False Negative and the similarity between the areas of the segmented regions. Table 2 presents the formulae for these metrics.

Accuracy is related to how close the result of automatic segmentation is to what can be considered the demarcation of the ground truth. This is measured by comparing each pixel of the segmentation to its ground truth counterpart.

The False Positive (FP) Rate indicates the number of pixels that are segmented as a Region of Interest (ROI) but that were not selected in the ground truth. The False Negative (FN) Rate indicates the number of pixels that were detected at the bottom of the segmented image but which are part of the ROI in the ground truth.

The Jaccard and Dice indices represent the similarity of segmentation between the automatically segmented image and the ground truth generated by manual segmentation. The closer the results are to one (1), they show that the segmentation is similar to its ground truth; results that tend to zero are those that have significant differences between automated segmentation and the corresponding gold image (Lemaître & Yong, 2010; Xie & Bovik, 2013).

Figure 7. Superimposed final images of (a) manual segmentation and (b) automatic segmentation over the thermographic image

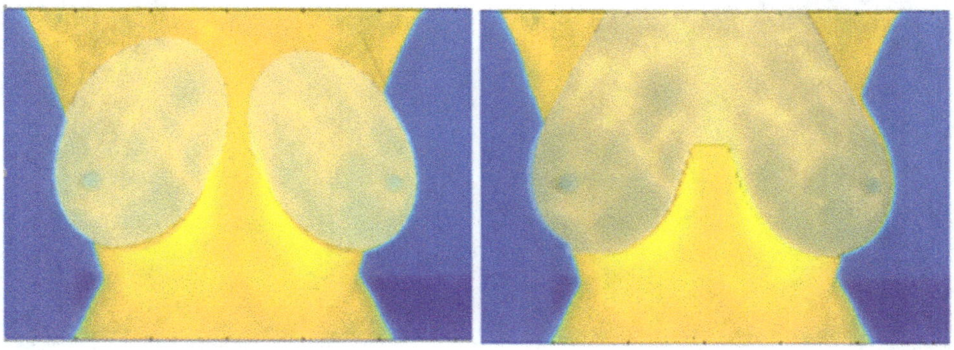

The database for validating automatic segmentation consisted of 70 thermographic images of breasts of different sizes, and these represented the maximum heterogeneity found in patients, thus enabling the scope for applying the technique to be widened.

The validation methodology was applied to both the final result of the automatic segmentation described above (Segmentation I) and to the result that it obtained in the step before excluding the lower border (Segmentation II), but by altering the lower cutoff limit (Figure 8).

The result of evaluating the segmentation methods is presented in Table 2. The experimental result shows that, among the metrics evaluated, the Dice index presented the best value (0.6988±0.1326) for the segmented images of the left breast. False positive and negative rates must be close to zero. This did not occur in Segmentation II, the false negative rate of which had a high value for the segmentation of the left breast, which indicates that it is not selecting the ROI correctly.

Table 2. Equations for the metrics of segmentation

Metrics	Equations
Jaccard Index (JI)	$JI(G,S)=\dfrac{\lvert G\cap S\rvert}{\lvert G\cup S\rvert}$
Dice Index (DI)	$DI(G,S)=\dfrac{2\lvert G\cap S\rvert}{\lvert G\rvert+\lvert S\rvert}=\dfrac{2\times J(G,S)}{1+J(G,S)}$
False Positive (FP)	$FP(G,S)=\dfrac{\lvert S\rvert-\lvert G\cap S\rvert}{\lvert G\rvert}$
False Negative (FN)	$FN(G,S)=\dfrac{\lvert G\rvert-\lvert G\cap S\rvert}{\lvert G\rvert}$

Figure 8. Automatic Segmentation with an altered lower cut-off limit.

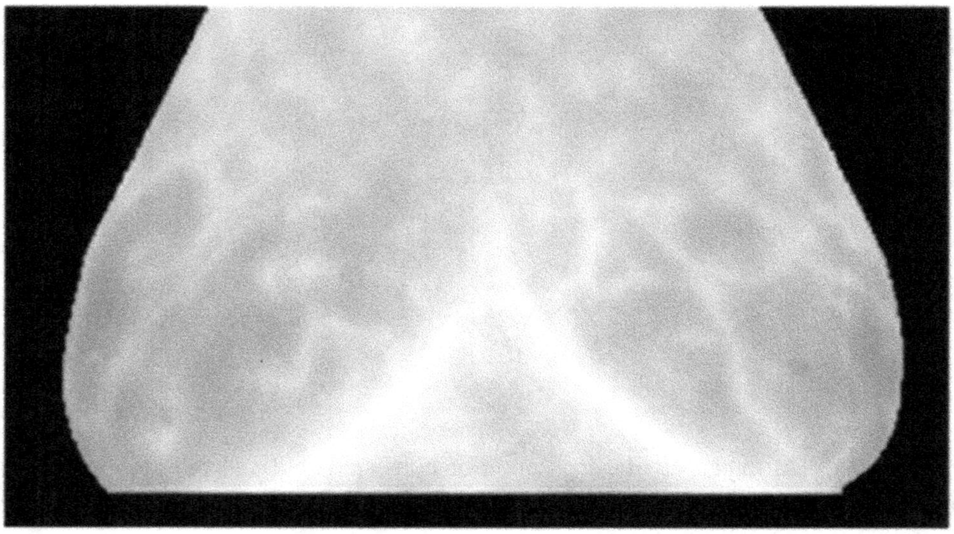

Table 2. Evaluation metrics of automatic segmentation and its variation in relation to the ground truth

Evaluation metrics	Segmentation I		Segmentation II	
	ME	MD	ME	MD
Jaccard	0.5517±0.1470	0.5209±0.1061	0.5429±0.1493	0.4700±0.1117
DICE	0.6988±0.1326	0.6783±0.0979	0.6828±0.1417	0.6314±0.1079
FP	0.3782±0.541	0.3217±0.3551	0.4214±0.3620	0.3980±0.5507
FN	0.1882±0.1849	0.1317±0.1628	230.9083±1.930.5	0.1379±0.1448

The method used in Segmentation I presented the best performance, obtaining better values in all metrics than those obtained in Segmentation II.

In order to aid in the graphic visualization of the validation process, the images of automatic segmentation (Segmentation I) and ground truth were superimposed, the nipple being taken as a reference (Figure 9). The green region represents the right breast/left breast of the ground truth and the blue region represents the right breast/left breast obtained from automatic segmentation.

The average total area shows a large difference between measurements. In particular, automatic segmentation measurements are larger than manual ones. The average difference between the areas was 2,277.0±1,939.3 pixels for the left breast and 4,033.3±1,971.3 pixels for the right breast.

The result of superimposing the final images shows coincident regions or not, between the result of automatic segmentation and ground truth, represented here by manual segmentation. In Figure 9, the darker green region represents the areas that were segmented by both methods. Thus, considering manual segmentation as ground truth, everything that was not selected by this method and was in automatic segmentation was considered a false positive.

Figure 9. Overlay of the automatic segmentation on the ground truth (light green color) of the right and left breasts, respectively.

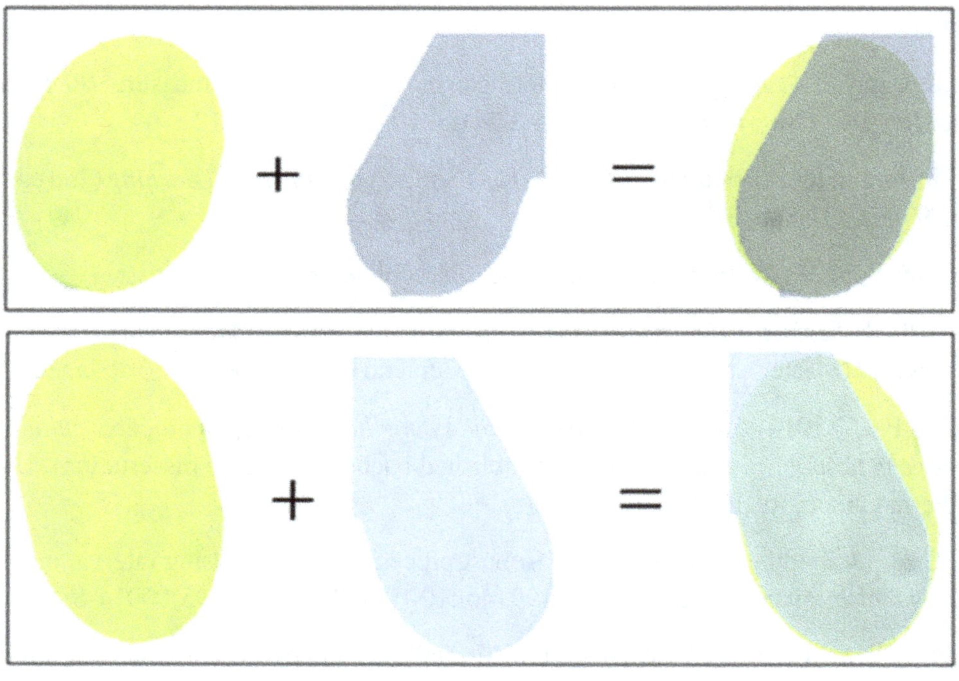

REFERENCES

Araújo, M. C. (2014). *Uso de imagens termográficas para classificação de anormalidades de mama baseado em variáveis simbólicas intervalares* (Doctoral thesis). Universidade Federal de Pernambuco, Recife, Brazil.

Araújo, M. C., Lima, R. C. F., & Souza, R. M. C. R. (2014). Interval symbolic feature extraction for thermography breast cancer detection. *Expert Systems with Applications*, *41*(15), 6728–6737. doi:10.1016/j.eswa.2014.04.027

Araújo, M. C., Souza, R. M. C. R., Lima, R. C. F., & Silva Filho, T. M. (2017). An interval prototype classifier based on a parameterized distance applied to breast thermographic images. *Medical & Biological Engineering & Computing*, *55*(6), 873–884. doi:10.100711517-016-1565-y PMID:27629552

Billard, L., & Diday, E. (2006). *Symbolic Data Analysis: Conceptual Statistics and Data Mining*. John Wiley and Sons. doi:10.1002/9780470090183

Diday, E., & Noirhomme-Fraiture, M. (2008). *Symbolic Data Analysis and the SODAS Software*. John Wiley and Sons.

Dougherty, G. (2009). *Digital Image Processing for Medical Applications*. Cambridge University Press. doi:10.1017/CBO9780511609657

Dourado Neto, H. M. (2014). *Segmentação e análise automáticas de termogramas : um método auxiliar na detecção do câncer de mama um método auxiliar na detecção do câncer de mama* (Master's thesis). Universidade Federal de Pernambuco, Recife, PE, Brazil.

Gonzalez, R. C., Woods, R. E., & Eddins, E. L. (2004). *Digital Image Processing Using Matlab*. Pearson Prentice Hall.

Gowda, K., & Diday, E. (1992). Symbolic clustering using a new similarity measure. *IEEE Transactions on Systems, Man, and Cybernetics*, *22*(2), 368–378. doi:10.1109/21.148412

Hastie, T., Tibshirani, R., & Friedman, J. (2009). *The Elements of Statistical Learning* (2nd ed.). Springer. doi:10.1007/978-0-387-84858-7

Lemaître, G., & Yong, E. W. (n.d.). Evaluation measures for segmentation. *Matrix, 1*.

Luz, L. M. S. (2007). *Segmentação em ultra-sonografia de mama com operadores morfológicos associados à função gaussiana* (Master's thesis). Universidade Federal do Rio de Janeiro, Rio de Janeiro, RJ, Brazil.

Queiroz, K. F. F. C. (2014). *Análise da repetitividade e melhoria de segmentação semiautomática de ROIs em imagens termográficas de mama* (Unpublished bachelor's degree dissertation). Universidade Federal de Pernambuco, Recife, Brazil.

Schnepper, C. A., & Stadtherr, M. A. (1996). Robust process simulation using interval methods. *Computers & Chemical Engineering*, *20*(2), 187–199. doi:10.1016/0098-1354(95)00014-S

Silva, A. P. D., & Brito, P. (2006). Linear discriminant analysis for interval data. *Computational Statistics*, *21*(2), 289–308. doi:10.100700180-006-0264-9

Souza, R. M. C. R., Carvalho, F. A. T., & Tenorio, C. P. (2004). Dynamic cluster methods for interval data based on Mahalanobis distances. *Proceedings of the meeting of the international federation of classification societies (ifcs). Classification, Clustering, and Data Mining Applications*, 351–360. 10.1007/978-3-642-17103-1_34

Xie, F., & Bovik, A. C. (2013). Automatic segmentation of dermoscopy images using. *Pattern Recognition*, *46*(3), 1012–1019. doi:10.1016/j.patcog.2012.08.012

Chapter 11
Developing and Using Computational Frameworks to Conduct Numerical Analysis and Calculate Temperature Profiles and to Classify Breast Abnormalities

Kamila Fernanda F. da C. Queiroz
https://orcid.org/0000-0003-4257-5155
Federal Institute of Rio Grande do Norte, Brazil

Marcus Costa de Araújo
https://orcid.org/0000-0002-1818-5686
Universidade Federal de Pernambuco, Brazil

Nadja Accioly Espíndola
https://orcid.org/0000-0003-1080-2173
Universidade Federal de Pernambuco, Brazil

Ladjane C. Santos
Federal Institute of Sergipe, Brazil

Francisco G. S. Santos
Universidade Federal de Pernambuco, Brazil

Rita de Cássia Fernandes de Lima
DEMEC, Federal University of Pernambuco, Brazil

ABSTRACT

In this chapter, computational tools that have been designed to analyze and classify infrared (IR) images will be presented. The function of such tools is to interconnect in a user-friendly way the algorithms that are used to map temperatures and to classify some breast pathologies. One of these performs texture mapping using IR breast images to relate temperatures measured to the points over the substitute tridimensional geometry mesh. Another computer-aided diagnosis (CAD) tool was adapted so that it could be used to evaluate individual patients. This methodology will be used when the computational framework approach for classification is described. Finally, graphical interfaces and their functionalities will be presented and explained. Some case studies will be presented in order to verify whether or not the computational classification framework is effective.

DOI: 10.4018/978-1-7998-3456-4.ch011

INTRODUCTION

In this chapter, computational tools which have been designed to analyze and classify infrared (IR) images will be presented. The function of such tools is to interconnect in a user-friendly way the algorithms that are used to map temperatures and to classify some breast pathologies.

One of these performs texture mapping, using IR breast images to relate temperatures measured to the points over the substitute tridimensional geometry mesh.

Another Computer-Aided Diagnosis (CAD) tool developed was adapted so that it could be used to evaluate individual patients. This methodology will be used when the computational framework approach for classification is described.

Finally, graphical interfaces and their functionalities will be presented and explained. Some case studies will be presented in order to verify whether or not the computational classification framework is effective.

COMPUTATIONAL FRAMEWORK TO AID THE DETECTION OF BREAST CANCER

Medical breast images obtained by different types of exam provide a high degree of relevant information to the specialist performing the analysis (Borchartt, 2013). Technological advances in areas such as computer science, computer graphics and engineering have enabled Computer-Aided Diagnosis (CAD) systems to be developed. Their function is to process images by using predefined algorithms in order to provide medical specialists with information that will speed up and/ or improve diagnosis (Cotrim, Silva, & Bezerra, 2007).

CAD systems are considered important tools which assist the medical diagnosis of breast cancer. The intention behind using them is to improve the consistency of the interpretation of the images by considering how the CAD responds to them. This answer, which may be useful when diagnosing a disease is partly based on the subjectivity of a visual analysis. Thus, double reading - by an expert physician and a computer - can significantly improve the efficiency of diagnosis (Furuie, Gutierrez, Bertozzo, & Yamagutti, 1999 as cited in Cotrim et al., 2007).

Due to the limitations of the human visual system and of physicians' experience of interpreting thermographic images, some CAD systems are being developed to improve the detection of breast abnormalities. These systems can also be used to investigate the viability of using the thermography technique as a screening exam. In other words, temperature values can be used both to analyze normal patients (without any breast abnormality) and patients who have a malignant tumor, a benign tumor or a cyst.

Typically, CAD systems are associated with graphical interfaces to facilitate how users interpret the results. One of the main advantages of creating a graphical user interface (GUI) is to make the program developed accessible to medical practitioners who do not understand programming language (Kapoor, Prasad, & Patni, 2012). By incorporating CAD systems, these human-computer interfaces may have great potential for diagnosing breast abnormalities that thermograms have identified.

Motivated by the need for a screening tool that can aid the diagnosis of breast cancer, a graphical interface was developed that lets the researcher or the mastologist evaluate a breast abnormality easily and quickly when thermographic images are used.

The results obtained came from the CAD systems, developed by Araujo (2014) and Dourado Neto (2014), based on thermographic images of the database of the system. The images used for this study were of the frontal type in which the patients were positioned with their hands raised and supported by the wooden bar of the mechanical apparatus. The tests were performed with a computer which uses the Windows 10 operating system, Intel Core i3 - 3217U (1.80 GHz), 4 GB of RAM and 64-bit Operating System.

Based on the sample that comprises the database, three different groups (the training group, the validation group and the test group) were defined for both classifiers, namely a Support Vector Machine (SVM) and Mahalanobis. The training group was formed from those that showed the characteristics of the thermographic images of the database and the algorithm was learned from this group.

The validation group was formed from patients who had been placed in diagnostic classes and this group was used to verify the generalization of the algorithm in order to adjust the classification parameters. After the program had completed the learning process, the test group was used to evaluate whether the parameters that had been set work well for any sample.

The adapted CAD systems were associated with a GUI created on the Matlab® platform. The intention was to make the process more automated. Using an interface allows the operator to use different techniques without prior knowledge of the software programming language. Figure 1 shows the GUI that was developed. It was called ANALISE IR_MAMA and has two menus (**File** and **Help**) and four panels (**Patient Information**, **Segmentation**, **Results** and **Statistics**).

Figure 1. The GUI called ANALISE IR_MAMA

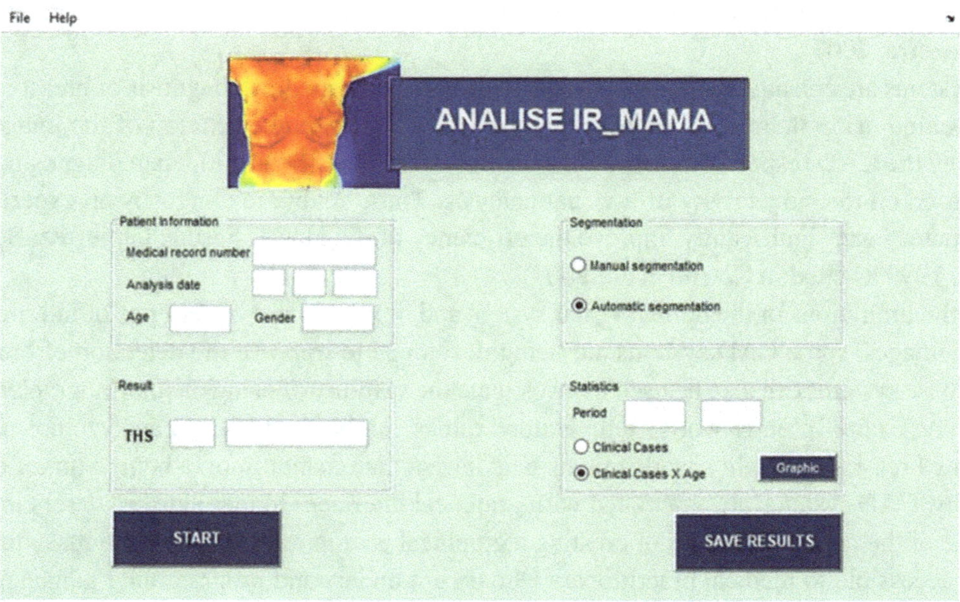

In the **File** menu the user has the option to open the IR image using the FLIR Quick Report program and he/ she can export the temperature matrix in a .csv format, or exit the interface. The **Help** menu gives a short explanation of the interface and its functionalities.

In the **Patient Information** panel, the doctor/ researcher can insert the patient's data, such as medical record number, age and gender (male/ female). The data are then stored in a .txt file so that they can be used subsequently in the Statistics panel.

In the **Segmentation** panel, the user can choose between two types of breast segmentation (semi-automatic or automatic) which are associated internally to the classifiers related to each type of segmentation.

The **Statistical** panel serves for the statistical analysis of the data recorded in a given period. For example, if the user wishes to know the number of clinical cases (normal patients, patients with malignant tumors, patients with benign tumors or patients with cysts) in 2015, the user must type 2015 2015 in the Period fields and when the button **Clinical Cases** is pressed a pie-chart with the results will appear. Similarly, if the user wishes to know the distribution of clinical cases and the age of the patients, he/she should select the **Clinical Cases × Age** button and histograms will appear for each class.

In order to standardize the results, a new THS (Thermal Statistical Index) index was defined which is based on IR images and the statistical classifiers that indicate that there may be breast pathologies. The purpose of this index is similar to that of BI-RADS (Breast Image Reporting and Data System), which is used in mammography and ultrasound exams. Table 1 shows the values set for the THS and what these indicate.

Table 1. THS Classification

Classification	Evaluation
THS 0	Non-Cancer
THS 1	Normal
THS 2	Cyst
THS 3	Benign Tumor
THS 4	Malignant Tumor

The THS 0 index was included so as to evaluate binary cases: Cancer and Non- Cancer. In this case, the patient who presents THS 0 (Non-Cancer) may have a cyst, a benign tumor or the patient may not have abnormalities. The binary class Cancer will be represented by the index THS 4 (Malignant Tumor).

For multiclass analysis, the THS index may have any of the evaluation categories 1 to 4, in accordance with the increase in the classification of the risk of malignancy.

The result associated with the THS is displayed in the **Result** panel. In the first space (Classification) a number between 0 and 4 will appear, referring to the index, and the evaluation will appear in the second space, in accordance with Table 1 above.

Finally, the classification is started when the **Start** button is selected. When the **Save Results** button is selected, the thermographic image of each patient will be saved as well as their data: medical records, diagnosis and date of IR analysis. This is intended to make the process more automated. The interface enables the operator who has no prior knowledge of software programming language to use different techniques.

Case Study

In this topic, some applications of the graphical user interface called ANALISE IR_MAMA are presented. A case study was made of a patient whose results were considered normal. The patient was 52 years old and she was diagnosed after undergoing clinical examination, ultrasonography and mammography. Her mammogram examination indicated BI-RADS 1, which means there are no abnormalities present in her breasts.

Figure 2 shows the IR image chosen for analysis (Figure 2A), the results of the semiautomatic segmentation (Figure 2B) and of the automatic segmentation (Figure 2C). Note that in the automatic

Figure 2. (A) Thermographic image of Patient 1 (B) Semiautomatic segmentation (C) Automatic segmentation.

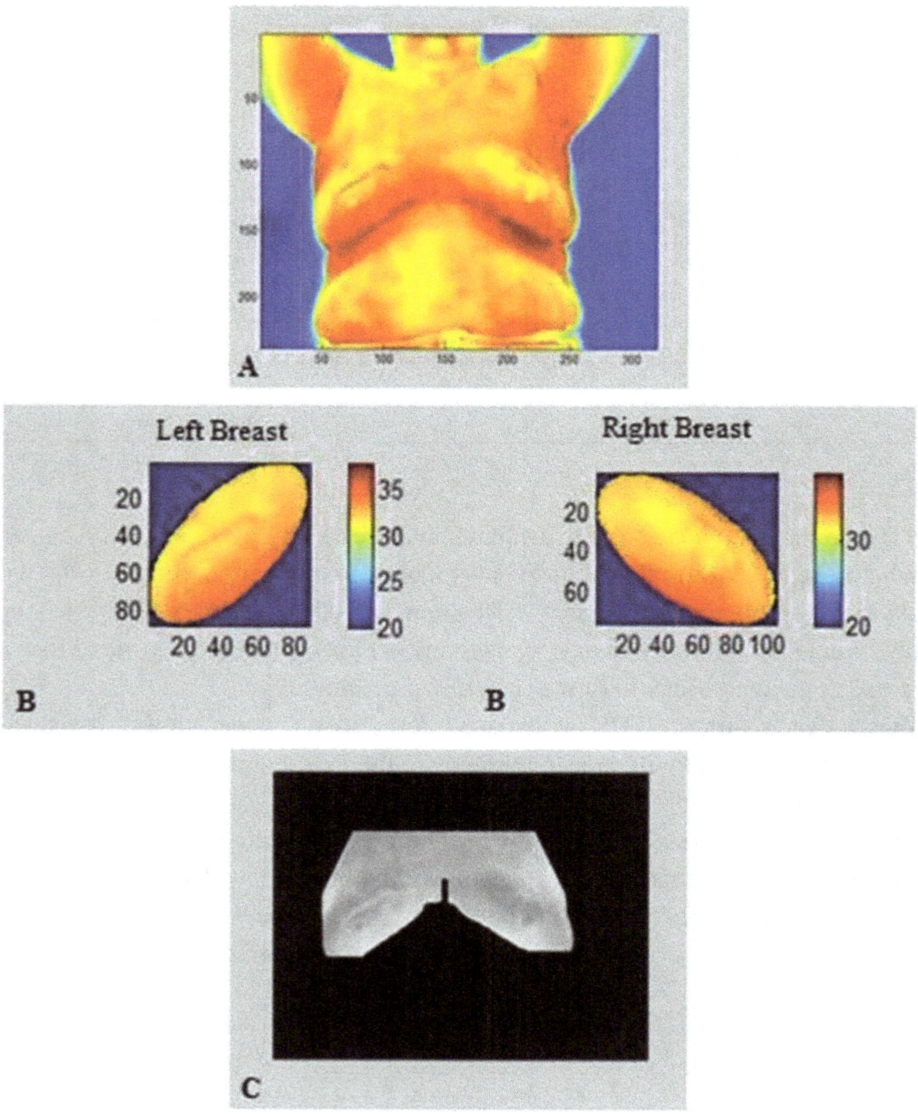

segmentation there was a small loss of the breast regions, a fact that does not occur in the semiautomatic segmentation.

The stage of manually selecting each breast lasted 58.8 seconds for the semi-automatic segmentation, whereas automatic segmentation lasted for 4.67 seconds, which is approximately 13 times less than for manual selection. Because it provides results rapidly and displays them in the most direct way, the SVM classifier can be used for fast screening of patients, thus separating the at risk and non-risk groups.

Figure 3 shows how the final SVM classification decision was displayed in the **Result** panel. The result provided by the software is a true negative because the patient was classified as not having a malignant tumor and in fact she does not. Figure 4 shows the result obtained using the adjusted Mahalanobis classifier to minimize the effects of the Normal Class variability.

Figure 3. Result for Patient 1 using the SVM classifier.

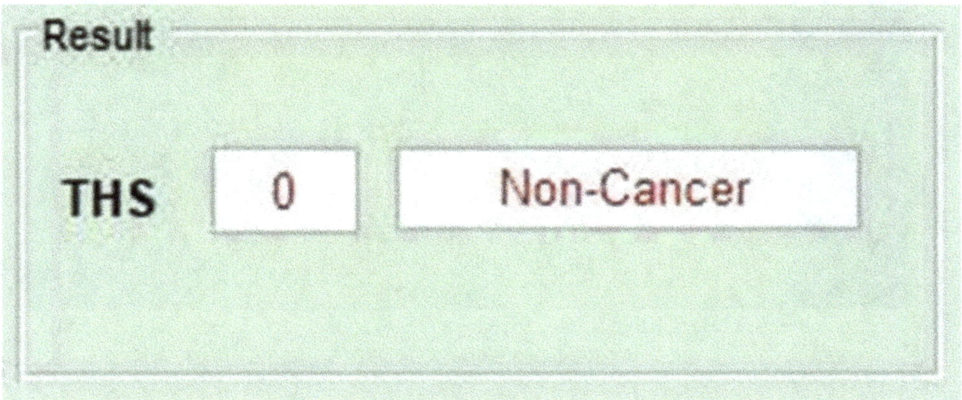

The thermographic image, with information about the patient and the result obtained by a certain classification process, was saved in *png* format when the **Save Result** button was clicked. This image can be printed and attached to the patient's medical record along with the other exams. Figure 5 shows the thermogram that was saved with regard to Patient 1.

Figure 4. Result for Patient 1 using the Mahalanobis classifier with minimization of the Normal Class.

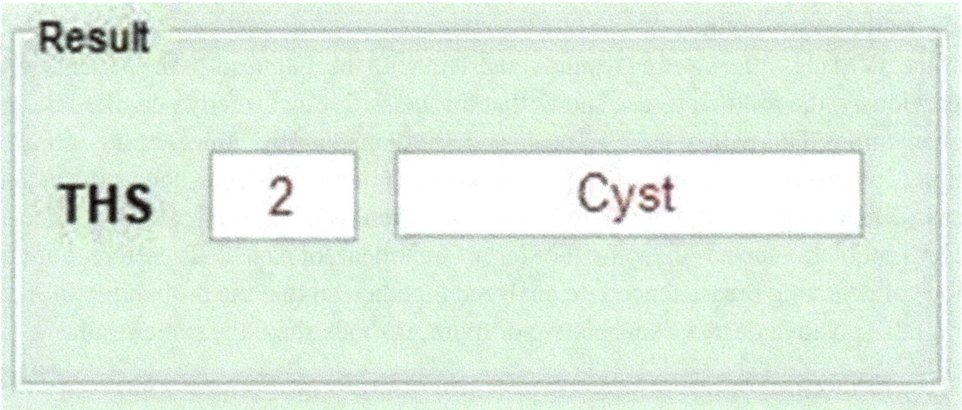

Figure 5. Image saved from Patient#1 with the result given by the SVM classifier.

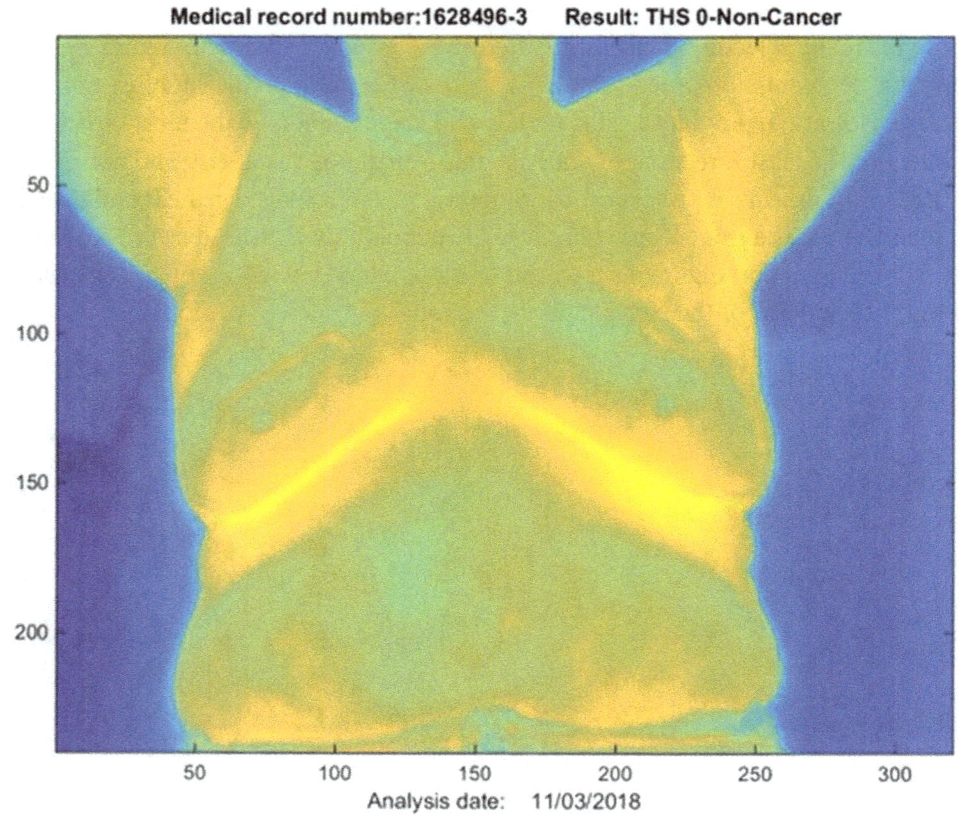

Next, a 35 year-old patient who has a malignant tumor, an invasive ductal carcinoma, was examined. Figure 6 shows the results of the segmentation of the ROIs (Regions of Interest) of the digital thermographic image. Once again, the automatic segmentation (Figure 6C) had problems detecting the lower borders of the breasts, but this did not influence extracting the ROI. The automatic segmentation process lasted 1.63s and the semiautomatic segmentation 45.39s.

The result provided by the software, using both classifiers, was a true positive (Figure 7), because the patient was classified as having a malignant tumor and in fact she does.

The same procedure was performed for the analysis of patients with cysts and with benign tumors. Table 2 presents the results found.

Whereas the SVM classifier showed results consistent with the diagnosis of the patients who had been examined previously, the following case shows that this classifier incorrectly classified the patient who had a malignant tumor. This patient is 57 years old and was diagnosed by clinical exams, ultrasonography, mammography and biopsy as having an invasive ductal carcinoma. Figure 8 shows the result obtained.

In this case, a false negative was generated. This error should be analyzed carefully since it can result in more serious problems such as delaying the start of treatment for cancer. Therefore, both this and the other methods of detecting breast cancer are analyzed together, so that the probability of having a false negative or a false positive decreases when two or more methods show the same result.

Figure 6. Segmentation of Patient #2's images: (A) Thermographic image (B) Result of the semiautomatic segmentation (C) Result of the automatic segmentation.

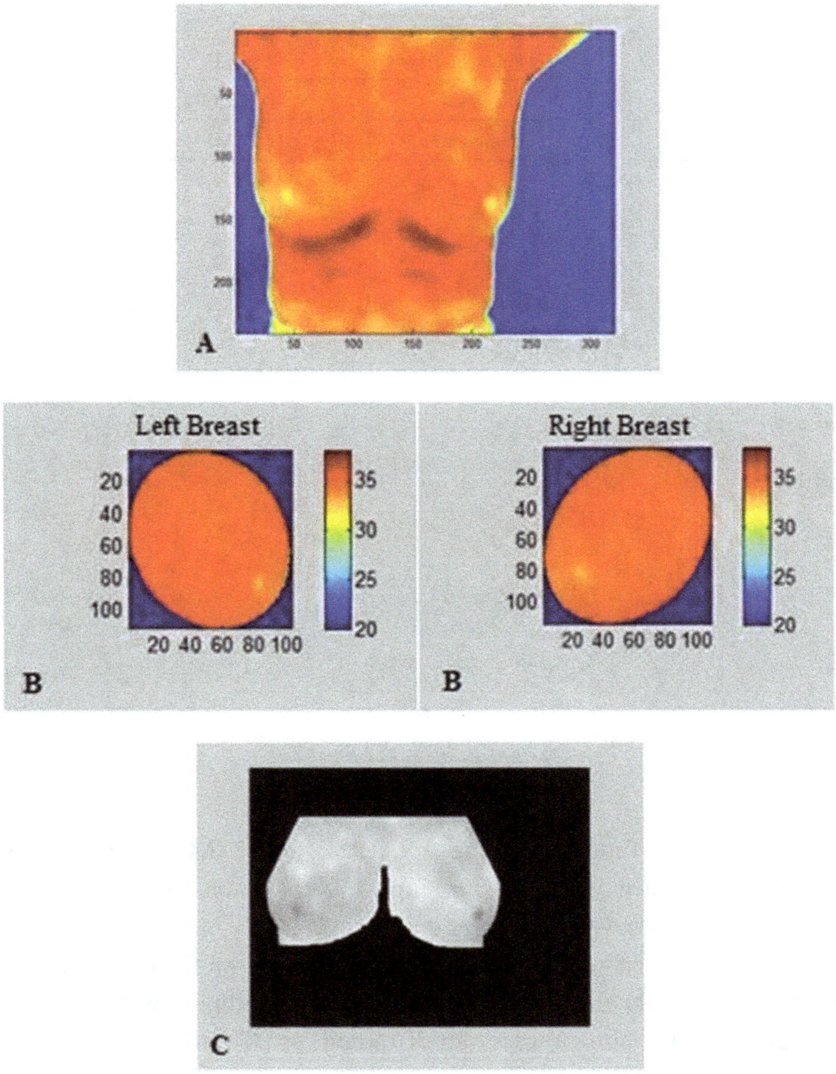

Figure 7. Result for Patient #2 using the SVM classifier and the Mahalanobis classifier with minimization of the Normal Class.

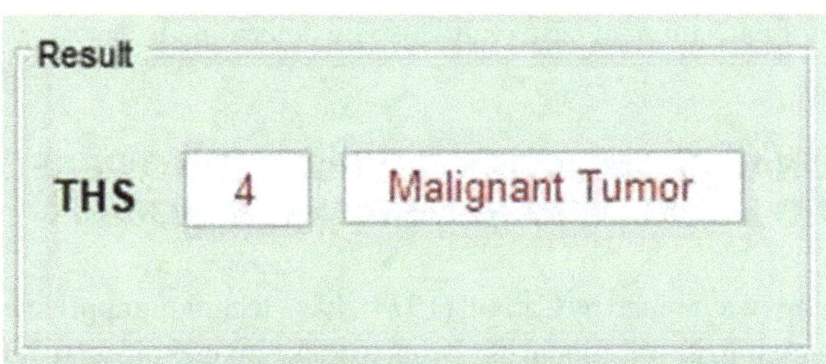

Table 2. Results obtained for the classification of the patients analyzed.

Patients	Age	Diagnostic	SVM/Binary	Mahalanobis
Patient 1	52	Normal	THS 0	THS 2
Patient 2	35	Malignant Tumor	THS 4	THS 4
Patient 3	38	Cyst	THS 0	THS 4
Patient 4	42	Benign Tumor	THS 0	THS 1

Figure 8. Result using the SVM classifier.

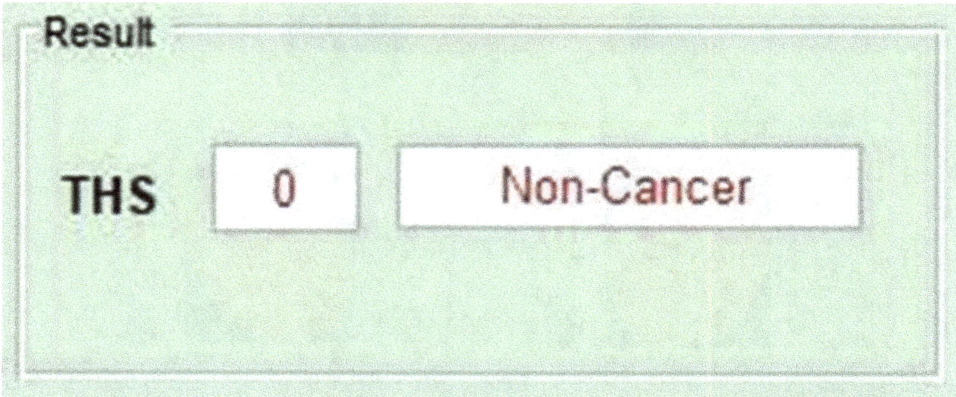

Statistical Panel

In order to assess the available functions of the ANALISE IR_MAMA software using the **Statistics** panel, some fictional data about the patients were input and the results were saved. These data include a period from 2015 to 2019 and several different diagnoses.

The first option, **Clinical Cases,** generated a pie chart that shows the quantitative results, as a percentage of the whole graph, of the diagnoses recorded in the period previously defined. Figure 9A and Figure 9B show respectively the clinical cases for 2015 and for 2015 to 2019.

The second option, **Clinical Cases × Age,** presents histograms that relate the frequency of a certain age group for each clinical case. Figure 10A and Figure 10B respectively show the histograms for 2015 and for 2015 to 2019.

From the analysis performed with the first and second option of the **Statistics** panel, an estimate could be made of the class that showed the greatest recurrence in a given period and the age group which had the highest prevalence for each clinical case could also be determined.

THE COMPUTATIONAL FRAMEWORK DEVELOPED TO PERFORM TEXTURE MAPPING USING INFRARED BREAST IMAGES

The term 'texture mapping' was coined by Catmul (1974). It is a technique applied in the areas of computer graphics and image processing, its traditional use being to make images closer to reality (Heckbert, 1986).

Figure 9. Examples of pie-charts for the distribution of clinical cases. (A) Period: 2015. (B) Period: 2015-2019.

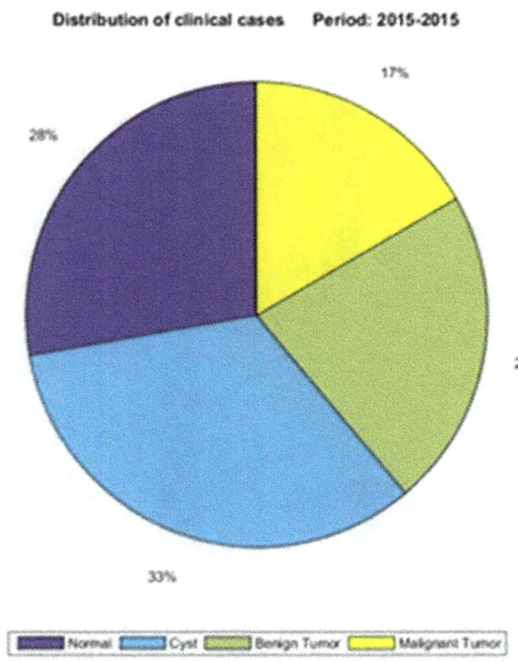

(A)

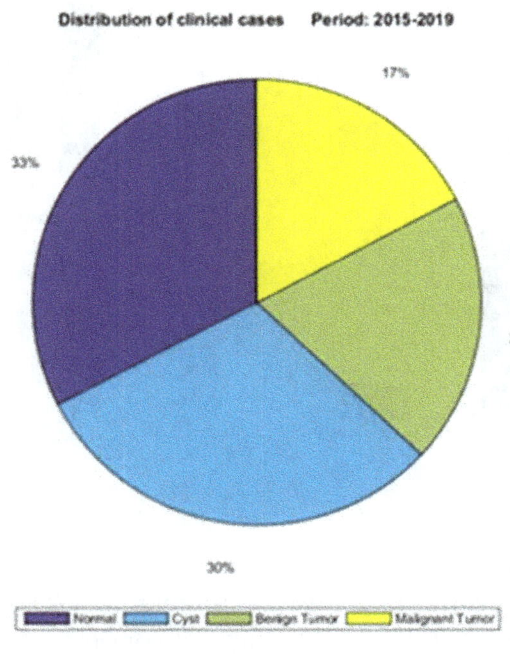

(B)

Figure 10. Examples of the Histograms Age × Frequency of each clinical case. (A) Period: 2015. (B) Period: 2015-2019.

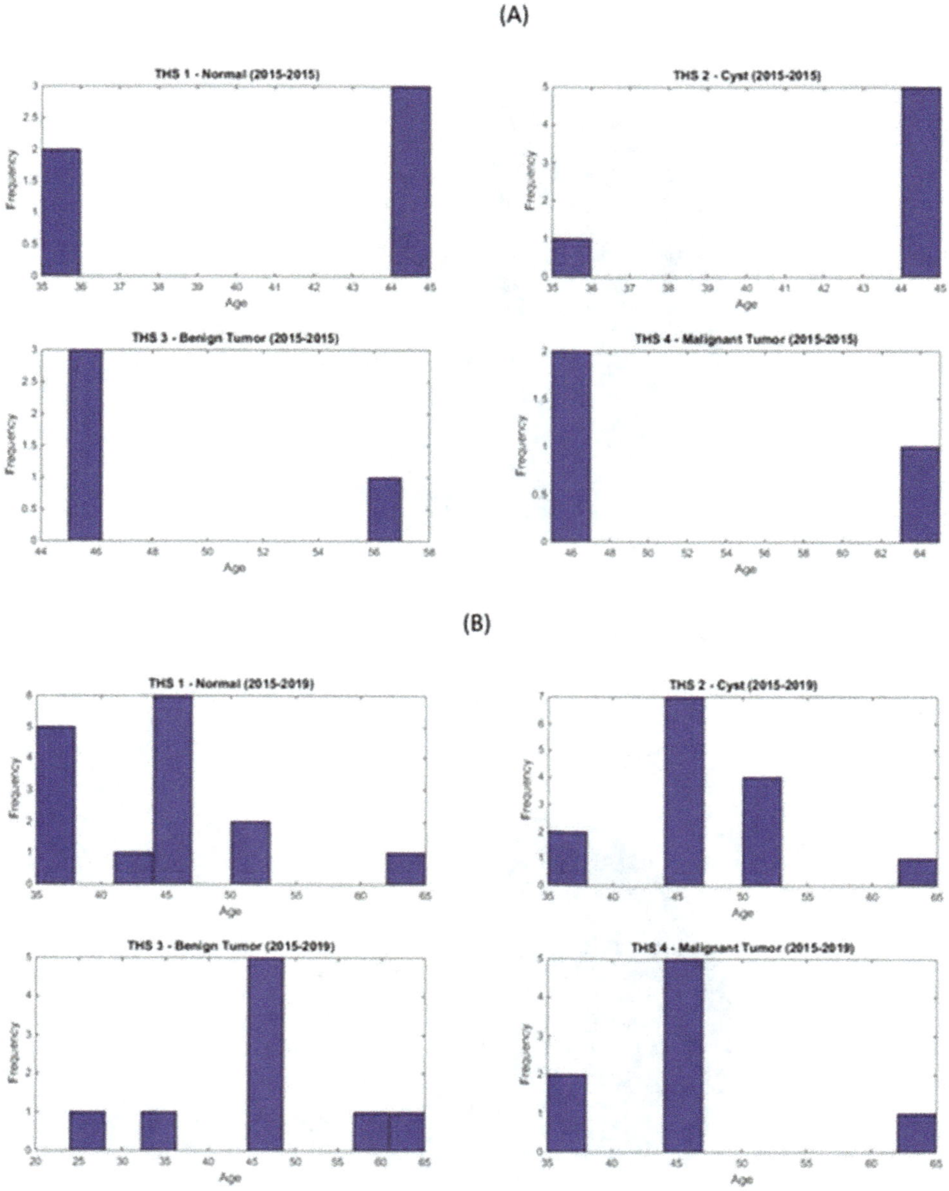

Texture mapping, performed by the software framework developed by the Biomechanics Group of the UFPE Mechanical Engineering Department, consists of transforming a 2D geometry into a 3D geometry. Specifically, 2D geometry is thermographic imaging and 3D geometry is the surrogate breast geometry of each patient analyzed (Espíndola, Bezerra, Santos, & Lima, 2018). The construction of surrogate geometry is based on the curves of each patient's breast and the size and location of the tumor, which are inserted with information obtained from the respective patient's ultrasound examination (Melo, 2019).

To transform 2D geometry into 3D geometry, it is necessary to take the coordinates of the surrogate surface (x, y, z) and then to disregard one of the coordinates, thereby obtaining a plane. Then the plane coordinates are transformed into thermography coordinates (x_t,y_t) using specific equations. Since the thermography coordinates (x_t,y_t), obtained by the transformation, do not result in whole pixels, mapping approximation and interpolation techniques are used (Santos, 2009; Espíndola et al., 2018).

The framework called "Evaluation of Breast Thermal Models - EBTM" was developed to analyze the influence of the depth of the tumor on the surface temperature of the breast, among other features. EBTM also maps the temperature values obtained by infrared images of the geometries of the breasts used in the numerical simulations. This procedure allows the temperatures obtained by infrared images to be used to validate the computational model and the physical model. Figure 11 shows the initial screen of the software.

Figure 11. First frame of EBTM framework

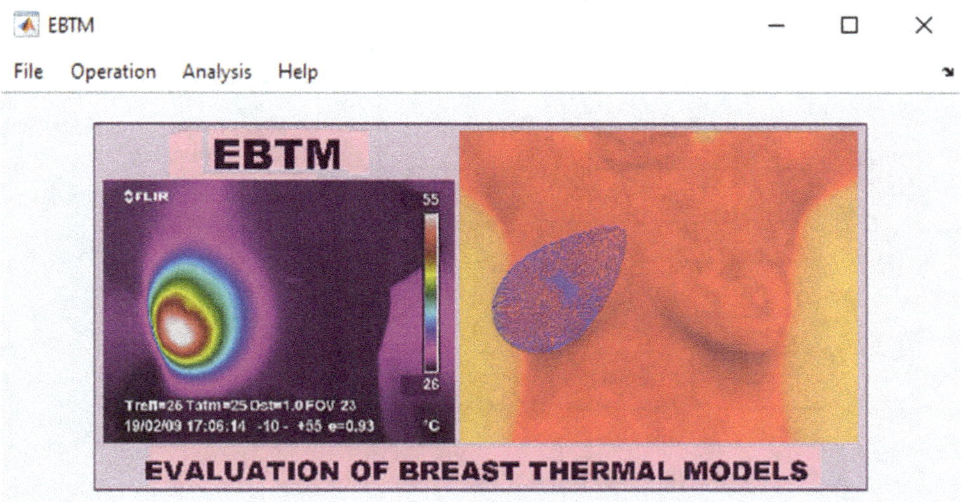

The framework allows the data analysis generated by independent software programs to be integrated. This software infrastructure connects various tools, as can be seen in Figure 12, and prepares the data that will be used for the three-dimensional simulation of temperature profiles. This software consists of modules that enable an analysis to be made of the results that are obtained by comparing the infrared images with the calculated profiles of the temperature of the breast.

The graphical interface was developed in order to automate the entire process of performing all calculations, analysis and finally presenting the results.

EBTM consists of four menus: File, Operation, Analysis, and Help. Each menu is subdivided into submenus. The Operation menu consists of the Mapping submenu which is divided into Approximation and Interpolation (Figure 13).

The Operation menu allows a parametric analysis to be conducted using the PARAMETRIC submenu. Finally the Help menu has explanations of the entire infrastructure (Figure 14).

Figure 12. Flowchart of the framework

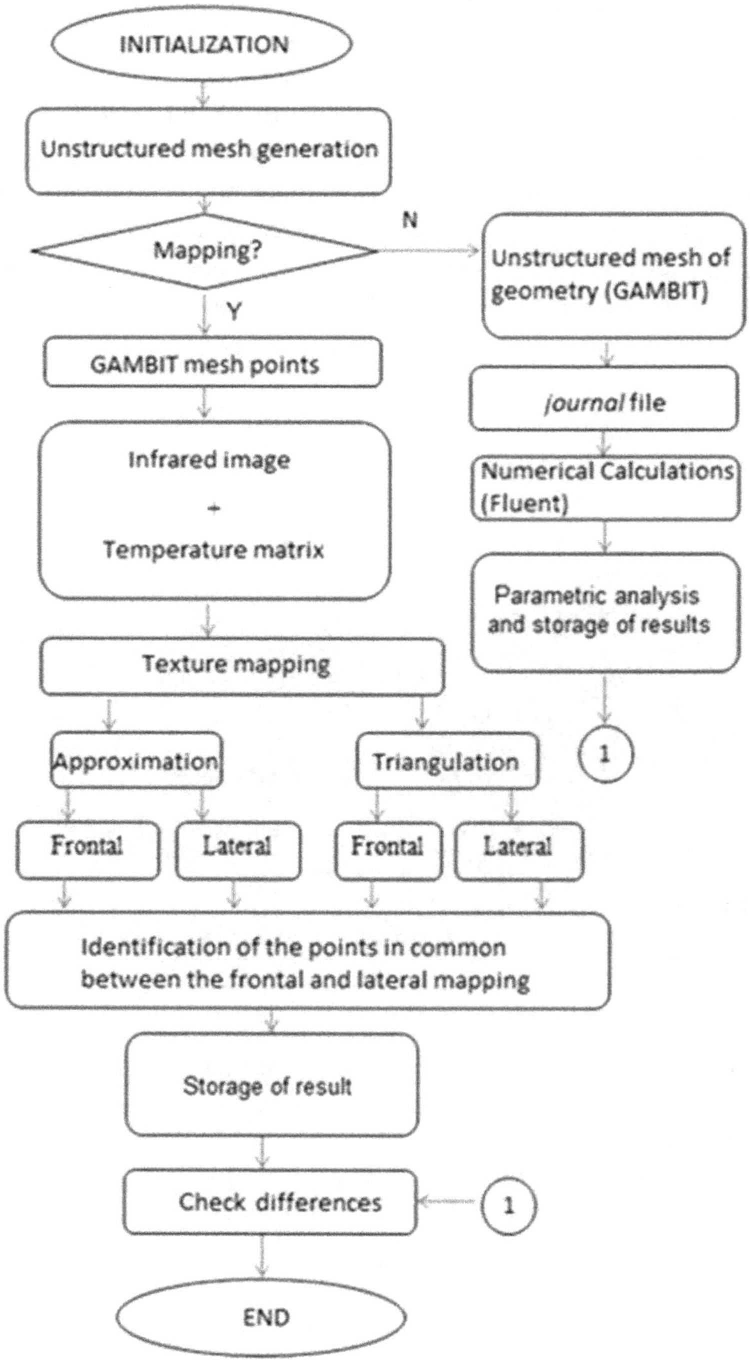

Initially, the framework imports two files: the thermographic image and the file with all the nodes of the substitute geometry mesh. Then the temperature matrix of the respective image is generated. Frontal (Figure 15) and lateral (Figure 16) mapping are carried out using this temperature matrix and the file with the nodes of the substitute geometry mesh.

The text files generated by the frontal and lateral mapping associate a temperature value to each node of the surface of the mesh of the substitute geometry of the breast using rounding techniques. Files thus

Figure 13. Framework menus

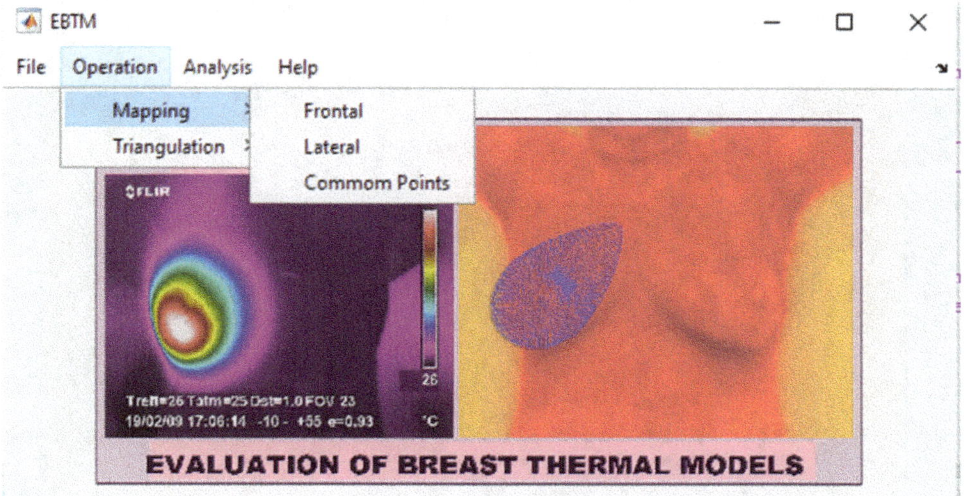

Figure 14. PARAMETRIC Submenu.

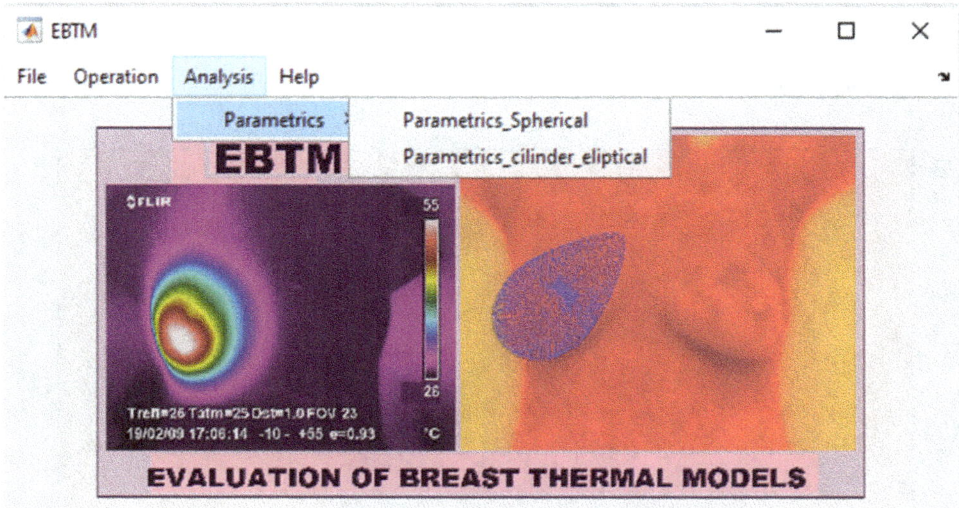

generated are used to obtain the points in common between the frontal and lateral mappings (where the temperatures are compared).

In the "Triangulation" step, a new frontal and/ or lateral mapping can be performed using interpolation techniques.

The "Parametrics" option, developed by the MATLAB platform, makes estimates of the location and size of the tumor by making numerical calculations.

Figure 15. Frontal Mapping

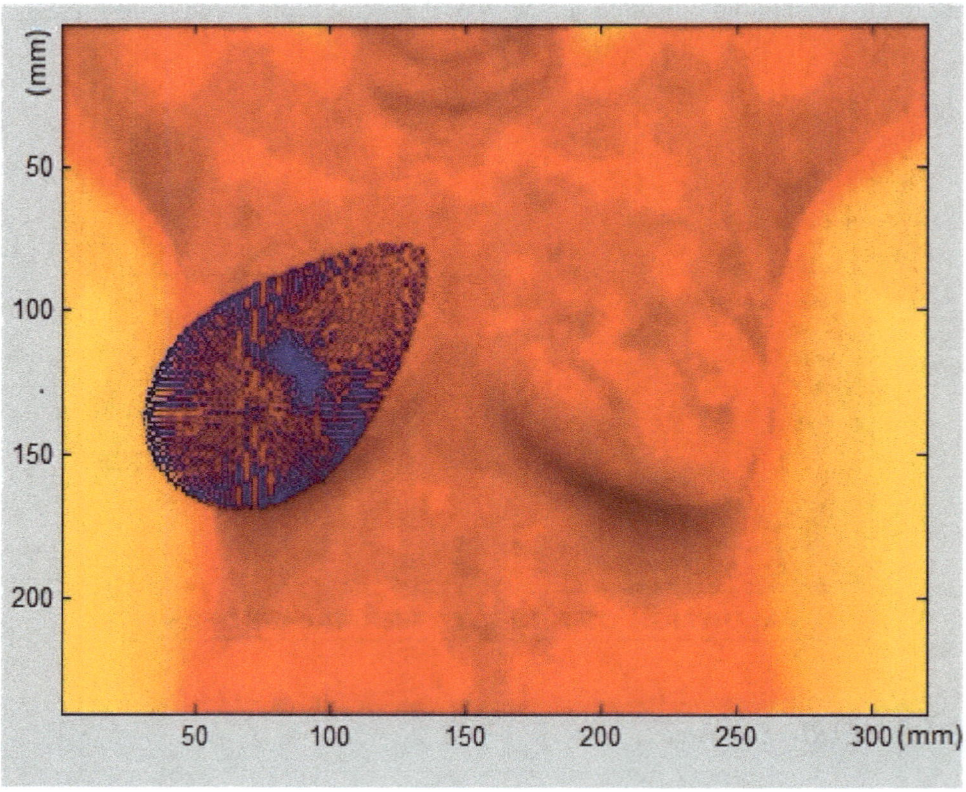

Figure 16. Lateral mapping

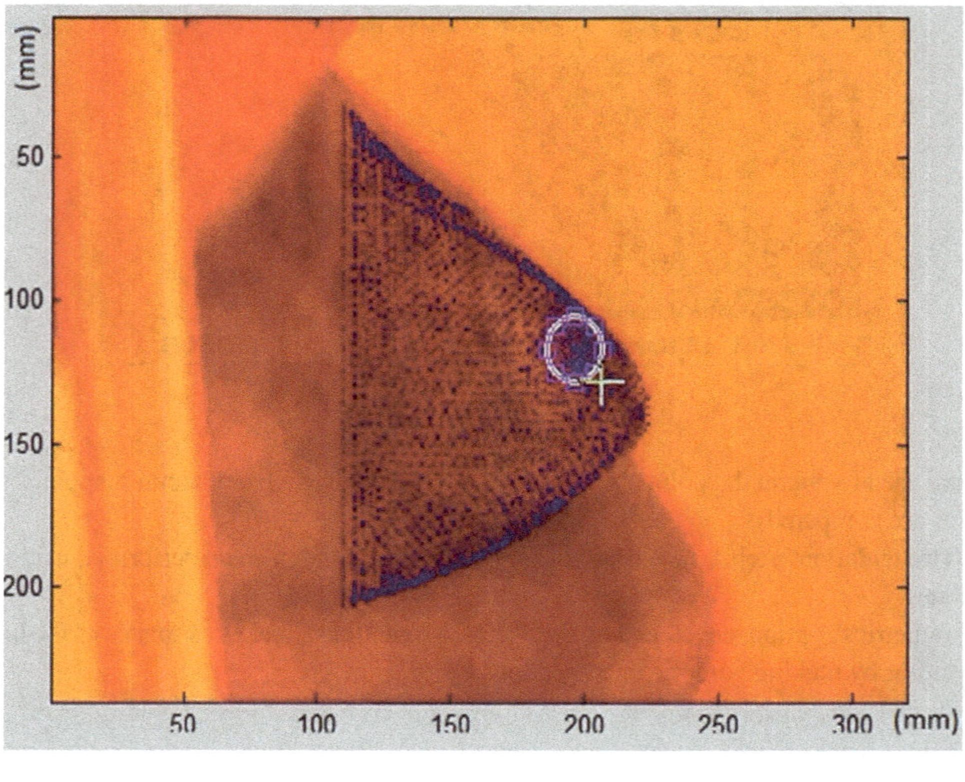

The software infrastructure can compare the calculated maximum temperature with the mapped maximum temperature, which is located on the surface of the breast in the likely region of the tumor. In order to estimate the location and size of the tumor, the framework is coupled with the PARAMETRICA software (Santos, 2009).

Validation of the software

One of the EBTM tests was to use infrared images obtained from a phantom of a female torso. The phantom breast was filled with silicone and a lamp (7W), the lamp serving as a source of heat. The surrogate geometry of the phantom was determined from coordinates obtained by using a machine that measures coordinates (Bezerra, 2013).

In the infrastructure the infrared image was converted into a temperature matrix, followed by mapping. Figure 17 presents the frontal mapping performed by the software infrastructure. Such points with their temperatures will be stored by the EBTM in a text file. The maximum temperature of the tumor region obtained by frontal mapping was 56.76°C.

The difference between the maximum calculated temperature and the maximum mapped temperature was 0.68°C.

Figure 17. Frontal mapping of the phantom.

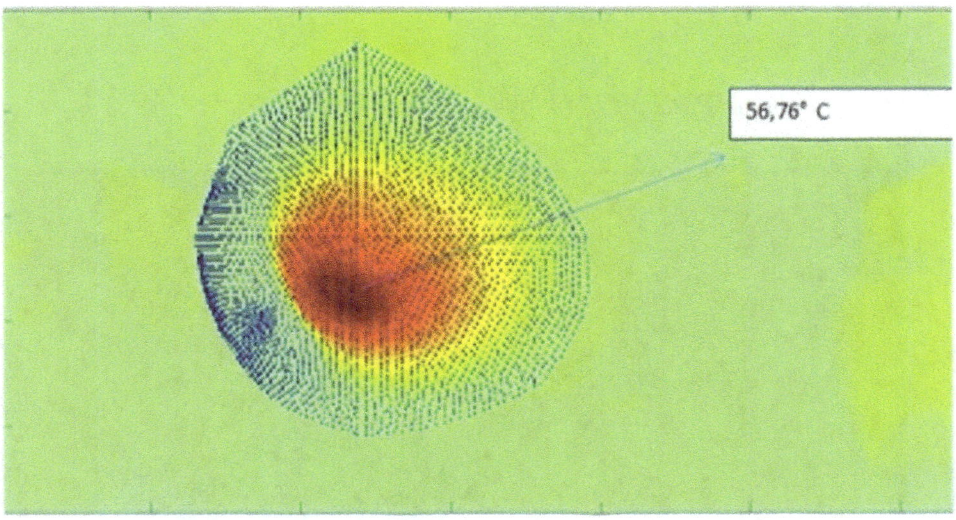

Lateral mapping was performed by EBTM and can be seen in Figure 18. The maximum temperature obtained was 54.41° C.

Analysis of an IR Image of Patient #18443694 Using the EBTM Framework

The analysis of a 49 year-old patient is presented below. She has symmetrical breasts and her adipose tissue was predominant over the glandular one. This patient has a malignant lump in the left breast that was diagnosed by clinical examination, and ultrasound and mammography exams. This tumor was located in the upper outer quadrant and its dimensions were 1.7 cm x 0.8 cm and it was located 1.6 cm below the surface of the patient's skin.

Figure 18. Lateral mapping of the phantom

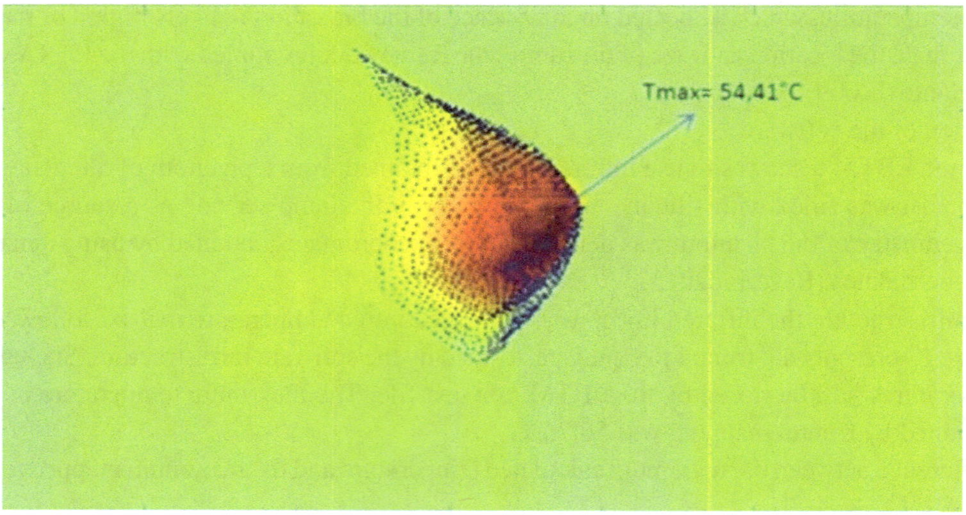

Frontal mapping was conducted using the infrastructure of the software. The result is shown in Figure 19.

Figure 19. Frontal mapping of Patient #18443694.

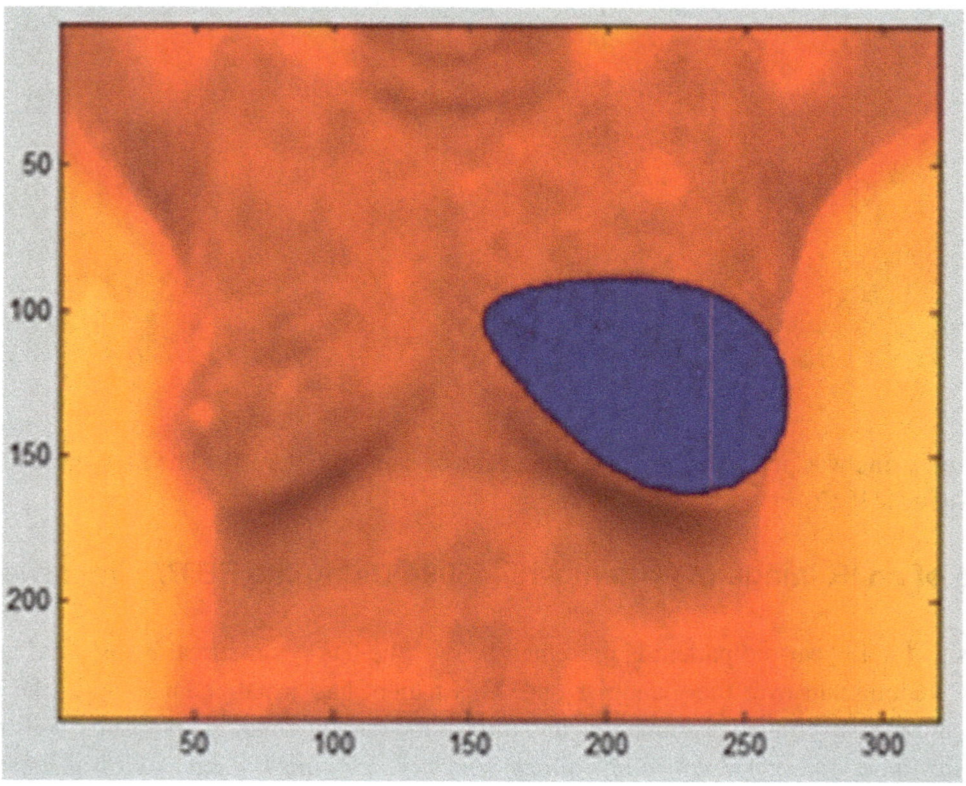

Then, a parametric analysis was performed using the EBTM software. The breast nodule was considered to be a cylinder with an ellipsoidal base. A correlation between the thermal conductivity of the breast and the patient's age (Bezerra, Oliveira, Rolim, Lyra, Lima, Conci, & Santos, 2013), was used to calculate this parameter. For this patient, its value was 0.4672 W/m°C.

Using this value, the difference between the maximum simulated temperature and maximum mapped temperature was equal to 1.56°C.

Figure 20 shows the results of the parametric analysis where for each height considered, one temperature (maximum, medium, minimum) was calculated. The results were satisfactory because the increase in the size of the tumor showed there was an increase in the maximum temperature calculated.

Figure 20. Parametric analysis of Patient #18443694.

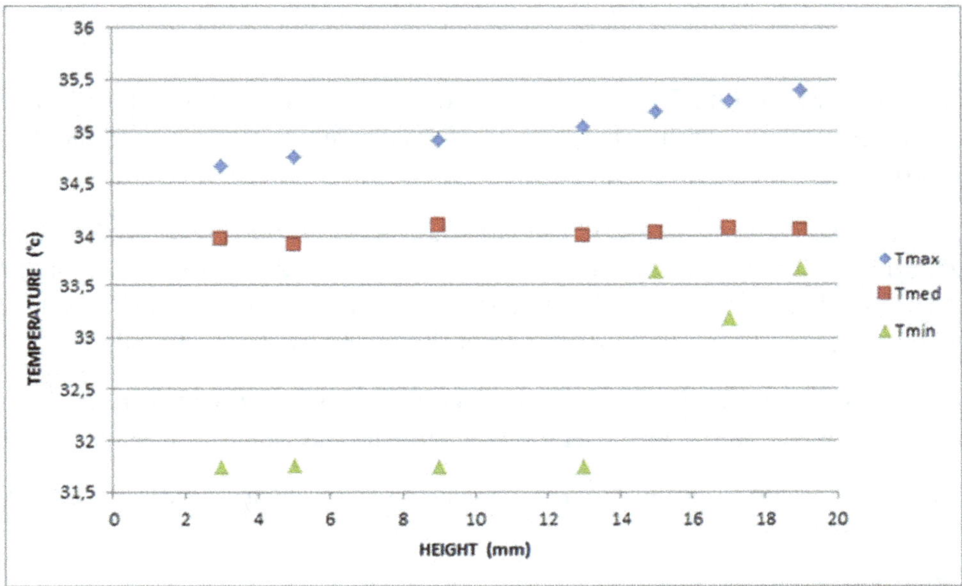

Table 3 shows the mapped temperature and the calculated temperature and the differences between them. These differences varied between 0.41°C % and 4.19°C. The differences between the maximum temperatures and the mean temperatures confirmed that the node is closer to the side of the breast.

Table 3. Differences between the mapped temperature and the simulated temperature for a 1.7 cm tumor from Patient #18443694.

	Simulated	Mapped	Difference(%)
TMAX (°C)	35.29	35.14	0.43
TMED (°C)	33.95	34.09	0.41
TMIN (°C)	31.75	33.14	4.19

The EBTM framework presented in this paper allowed breast anomalies to be analyzed using infrared images. The software used texture mapping techniques to associate all values that were measured by the infrared image with the points located on a volume that represents the geometry of the breast. To validate the entire EBTM process, the phantom that represented a woman's breast geometry was used. The software infrastructure allowed all operations to be performed easily and without the need for the user to be familiar with the operation of the routines included in the platform.

REFERENCES

Araújo, M. C. (2014). *Uso de imagens termográficas para classificação de anormalidades de mama baseado em variáveis simbólicas intervalares* [Use of thermographic images to classify breast abnormalities based on symbolic interval intervals] (Doctoral thesis). Universidade Federal de Pernambuco, Recife, Brazil.

Bezerra, L., Oliveira, M., Rolim, T., Lyra, P., Lima, R., Conci, A., & Santos, F. (2013). Estimation of breast tumor properties using infrared images. *Signal Processing*, *93*(10), 2851–2863. doi:10.1016/j.sigpro.2012.06.002

Bezerra, L. A. (2013). Estimativa de parâmetros termofísicos da mama e de distúrbios mamários a partir de termografia por infravermelho utilizando técnicas de otimização [Estimation of thermophysical parameters of the breast and maternal disturbances from infrared thermography using otimization techniques] (Doctoral thesis). Universidade Federal de Pernambuco, Recife, Brazil.

Borchartt, T. B. (2013). *Análise De Imagens Termográficas Para a Classificação De Alterações Na Mama* (Doctoral thesis). Universidade Federal Fluminense, Rio de Janeiro, RJ, Brasil.

Catmul, E. A. (1974). Subdivision algorithm for computer display of curved surfaces. Univ. Utah Computer Sci Dept, 74–133.

Cotrim, D. S., Silva, A. M., & Bezerra, E. A. (2007). Infra-estrutura de informática para sistemas de apoio ao diagnóstico aplicada a servidores pacs [Infrastructure of computing for support systems or diagnosis applied to servers pacs]. *III-SIIM*, 1-4.

Dourado Neto, H. M. (2014). *Segmentação e análise automáticas de termogramas: um método auxiliar na detecção do câncer de mama um método auxiliar na detecção do câncer de mama* [Automatic segmentation and analysis of thermograms: an auxiliary method for detecting breast cancer, an auxiliary method for detecting breast cancer] (Dissertação de mestrado). Universidade Federal de Pernambuco, Recife, PE, Brasil.

Espíndola, N. A., Bezerra, L. A., Santos, L. C., & Lima. R. C. F. (2018). Estimating Breast Thermophysical Parameters by the Use of Mapping Surface Temperatures Measured by Infrared Images. *IEEE Latin America Transactions, 16*(10).

Furuie, S., Gutierrez, M., Bertozzo, N., Figueriedo, J. C. B., & Yamaguti, M. (1999). Archiving and Retrieving Long-Term Cineangiographic Images in a PACS. *Computers in Cardiology*, 142–144. doi:10.1109/CIC.1999.826001

Heckbert, P. (1986). Survey of texture mapping. *IEEE Computer Graphics and Applications*, *6*(11), 56–67. doi:10.1109/MCG.1986.276672

Kapoor, P., Prasad, S. V., & Patni, S. (2012). Image Segmentation and Asymmetry Analysis of Breast Thermograms for Tumor Detection. *International Journal of Computers and Applications*, *50*(9), 40–45. doi:10.5120/7803-0932

Melo, J. F. R. (2019). *Metodologia para desenvolvimento de geometria tridimensional de mama e seu uso na estimativa de parâmetros usando imagens termográficas* [Methodology for the development of three-dimensional geometry of the breast and its use in estimating parameters using thermographic images] (Master's thesis). Universidade Federal de Pernambuco, Recife, PE, Brazil.

Santos, L. C. (2009). *Desenvolvimento de ferramenta computacional para análise paramétrica da influência da posição e do tamanho do tumor da mama e perfis de temperatura* [Development of computational hardware for parametric analysis of the influence of the position and size of the breast and temperature profiles] (Master's thesis). Universidade Federal de Pernambuco, Recife, PE, Brazil.

Chapter 12
Applications of the Use of Infrared Breast Images:
Numerical Calculations of Temperature Profile and Estimates of Thermophysical Properties

Luciete Alves Bezerra
https://orcid.org/0000-0002-5363-7545
Federal University of Pernambuco, Brazil

João Roberto Ferreira de Melo
Federal University of Pernambuco, Brazil

Paulo Roberto Maciel Lyra
DEMEC, Federal University of Pernambuco, Brazil

Rita de Cássia Fernandes de Lima
DEMEC, Federal University of Pernambuco, Brazil

ABSTRACT

In this chapter, procedures for and applications of using infrared (IR) imaging that have been developed will be presented and proposed means by which a better detailed understanding of breast cancer can be reached. It will be shown how such applications can be used as a basis for enhancing the use of breast thermographic imaging as a user-friendly and inexpensive tool for the early detection of breast cancer. The authors intend to show that IR imaging can also be used to validate temperature profiles that have been calculated and to classify breast abnormalities as set out in previous chapters. IR images can also be used to estimate thermophysical properties of the breast, and discussion of how this is done is included. The IR images were acquired at the Outpatients Clinic of Mastology of the Hospital das Clínicas of the Federal University of Pernambuco (HC/UFPE). The research project was registered in the Brazilian Health Ministry (CEP/CCS/UFPE nº 279/05) after being approved by the Ethics Committee of UFPE.

DOI: 10.4018/978-1-7998-3456-4.ch012

INTRODUCTION

In this chapter, procedures for and applications of using infrared (IR) imaging that have been developed will be presented and proposed means by which a better detailed understanding of breast cancer can be reached. It will be shown how such applications can be used as a basis for enhancing the use of breast thermographic imaging as a user-friendly and inexpensive tool for the early detection of breast cancer. We intend also to show that IR imaging can also be used to validate temperature profiles that have been calculated and to classify breast abnormalities, as set out in previous chapters.

IR images can also be used to estimate thermophysical properties of the breast and discussion of how this is done is included.

The IR images were acquired at the Outpatients Clinic of Mastology of the *Hospital das Clínicas* of the Federal University of Pernambuco (HC/UFPE). The research project was registered in the Brazilian Health Ministry (CEP/CCS/UFPE nº 279/05) after being approved by the Ethics Committee of UFPE.

More and more early women are being diagnosed with some alteration in the breast. Mammography, despite being a highly sensitive test, does not provide reliable results when the breast tissue is very dense, with a predominance of glandular tissue. Therefore, its sensitivity is directly related to the patient's age. For this reason, and because mammography uses ionizing radiation, mammography is therefore considered a risk factor for breast cancer (El-Bastawissi, White, Mandelson, & Taplin, 2001, 2010). Therefore, mammography is not indicated for very young women, it being recommended only for women over 40 years old (Udesc, 2007). On the other hand, thermography can play an important role in early diagnosis for young patients with dense breasts (Schaefer, Z ´Avisek, & Nakashima, 2009; Acharya, Ng, Tan, & Sree (2012); Lahiri, Bagavathiappan, Jayakumar, & Philip, 2012; EtehadTavakol, Chandran, Ng, & Kafieh, 2013). According to these authors, the technique in conjunction with clinical examination shows sensitivity for detecting breast cancer, close to that of mammography, for women under 40 years of age.

IR images can also be used to validate three-dimensional, numerical simulations. The aim of such simulations is to achieve a better understanding of breast abnormalities. According to Ng and Sudarshan (2001) and Ng and Sudarshan (2004), numerical simulations in conjunction with thermography can be used as an auxiliary tool for mammography in the detection of breast cancer, in addition to which these simulations reduce the false positives of thermography in the diagnosis of cancer. To build a more realistic model for the breast, reliable values of thermophysical properties are needed for the various types of breast tissues and the various disorders of the breast. Finding values for such properties is therefore the biggest limitation of precise numerical simulation in living tissues. To overcome this difficulty, it is proposed to use thermographic images in conjunction with an inverse method coupled to a numerical simulator to make a first estimate of the real thermophysical properties of the breast and of nodules of the breast, using a simplified breast model, which initially was considered to consist of a homogeneous medium.

Several authors such as: Mitra and Balaji (1992), Paruch and Majchrzak (2007), Mital (2008), Jiang, Zhan, and Loew (2011), Agnelli, Barrea, and Turner (2011) estimated the thermophysical properties of tumors using temperatures obtained from numerical simulations with an additional random error. In this chapter, temperatures obtained from the IR images of each patient will be used, thus improving understanding, and the estimate of thermophysical properties will then be customized for each patient analyzed. These images have great potential as an auxiliary tool in detecting breast cancer.

MATHEMATICAL MODEL

In 1948, Harry H. Pennes presented the first quantitative relationship that described heat transfer in human tissues and included the metabolic and blood flow effects on tissue temperature (PENNES, 1948; CHARNY, 1992; WISSLER, 1998). This model, which represents the temporal and spatial distribution of temperature in living systems, is known as the Bioheat Transfer Equation (BHTE). Since it was first published, this equation has been widely used to analyze various types of heat transfer phenomena in living tissues (Ng & Sudarshan, 2001; Gonzàlez, 2007).

The BHTE is the heat diffusion equation, with a specific volumetric heat generation terms: one due to blood perfusion, Q_p, another due to metabolic heat, Q_m, in addition to the volumetric generation of heat due to external sources, Q. This equation was obtained by using the total energy balance considering storage, internal energy, heat conduction and the local generation of heat. To obtain it, chemical, physical, nuclear and electrical effects were disregarded. The temperature field is described for a homogeneous biological medium for each tissue, which is isotropic and has constant thermophysical properties (ρ, c, k_t) (Bezerra, Oliveira, Rolim, Conci, Santos, Lyra, & Lima, 2013). Considering only one tissue, this gives,

$$\rho_t c_t \frac{\partial T_t}{\partial t} = \nabla.\left(k_t \nabla T_t\right) + Q_P + Q_m + Q \tag{1}$$

where, k_t is the thermal conductivity of the tissue; ρ_t is the specific mass of the tissue; c_t is its specific heat; T_t is its local temperature; and t is the time variable. In Eq. 1, Q was not considered, due to the non-existence of external heat sources.

The source of heat due to blood perfusion can be modeled by Q_p (Diller, 1982):

$$Q_P = \omega \rho_b c_b \left(T_a - T_v\right) \tag{2}$$

where ω is the blood perfusion rate of the tissue ((m^3/s) of blood per m^3 of tissue); ρ_b is the specific mass of the blood; c_b is the specific heat of the blood; T_a is the temperature of the arterial blood entering the tissue; and T_v is the temperature of the venous blood leaving the tissue.

Pennes' main contribution (1948) was to model the rate of heat transfer between blood and tissue that is proportional to the product of the volumetric perfusion rate and the difference between the temperature of arterial blood and the temperature of local tissue (Wissler, 1998).

To justify this theory, it is assumed that the temperature of the blood entering the capillary region is equal to the temperature of the arterial blood T_a, and that the temperature of the blood that leaves it, is the temperature of the venous blood, T_v. This can be considered equal to the local temperature T_t of the tissue (Charny, 1992). Therefore, the term source of heat due to blood perfusion, becomes:

$$Q_P = \omega \rho_b c_b \left(T_a - T_t\right) \tag{3}$$

The blood perfusion rate, ω, is specific for each tissue. This rate is a major factor in the local transport of heat and one of the factors responsible for increasing the temperature of the region in which the tumor is located.

The model chosen will be used in the study of breast disorders, whether these are benign, malignant or cysts.

According to Gautherie (1980), Osman & Afify (1988), Mitra & Balaji (1992), Ng & Sudarshan (2001b), the duplication time (or doubling time) of the tumor size and the metabolic rate are related because of the hyperbolic function:

$$Q_m \tau = C \tag{4}$$

where, C is a constant equal to 3.27 x 10^6 W day/m^3 and τ is the time necessary for the tumor to double its volume. The diameter of the tumor D (m) is related to τ, by the expression:

$$D = 0.01e^{[0.002134\ (\tau - 50)]} \tag{5}$$

where, τ must be expressed in days.

The last two equations are used to calculate the metabolic heat, for each patient, using the information acquired from her ultrasound exams. For nodules with a diameter less than 1 cm, the metabolic heat considered is 65,400 (W/m^3) (Ng & Sudarshan, 2001b). The metabolic heat of the breast is considered to be 450 W/m^3.

To solve Equation (1), the following boundary and initial conditions were imposed:

- Dirichlet boundary condition was imposed on the chest wall, which represents a prescribed temperature $\underline{T_0}$ over this region:

$$T = \underline{T_0} \tag{6}$$

- Cauchy or Robin boundary condition, also known as the mixed boundary condition, was imposed on the external surface of the breast, where heat transfer by convection occurs to the environment.

$$-k_t \frac{\partial T_t}{\partial \eta} = h\left(T_t - T_\infty\right) \tag{7}$$

In this equation, η is the normal unit vector, T is the ambient temperature and h is the coefficient of heat transfer by convection, for which the value of 13.5 W/m^2°C was adopted. This value takes into account a combination of the effects of convection, radiation and the evaporation of sweat (Ng & Sudarshan, 2001b).

Finally, the initial condition is expressed by:

$$T = \underline{T_0} \tag{8}$$

where the initial breast temperature $\underline{T_0}$ was considered equal to 37°C.

The thermophysical properties adopted for the analyses in this chapter are described in Table 1.

Table 1. Thermophysical properties of the breast.

Tissue	k (W/m°C)	ρ (kg/m³)	c (J/kg°C)	ω (s⁻¹)
Glandular	0.48	1,080	3,000	0.00018
Malignant Tumor	0.48	1,080	3,500	0.009
Fibroadenoma	0.48	1,080	3,500	0.0018
Blood	---	1,060	4,200	---

Source: (Bezerra, Ribeiro, Lyra, & Lima, 2020)

NUMERICAL CALCULATION

The software used for numerical simulations in this study was FLUENT™. This CFD (Computational Fluid Dynamics) program uses a technique based on the Finite Volume Method to convert the governing equations into algebraic equations that can be solved numerically. This technique consists of integrating the governing equations on each of the control volumes that make up the discretization of the domain, thus providing discrete equations that keep each property in the control volume. This method is intrinsically linked to the concept of flow balance between regions, or adjacent volumes (Fortuna, 2000).

The net amount of any quantity φ (mass or energy), which crosses the boundaries of the control volume per unit of time, is calculated by the integration on these boundaries, of the difference between the flows that enter and those that leave the control volume. These flows are basically of two types: convective and diffusive.

- Convective flows: they are due to the speed of the fluid. These types of flows have the general form $\rho\varphi\vec{v}$, where ρ is a term of specific mass, $\vec{v}$ is the velocity of fluid vector and φ is the property being transported (Fortuna, 2000).
- Diffusive flows: they are caused by the φ gradients. These types of flows have the general form $\Gamma_\varphi \nabla_\varphi$, in which Γ_φ is the diffusion coefficient, which is not necessarily constant, and φ is the property being diffused (Fortuna, 2000; Maliska, 1995).

In the case of a generic property φ and considering the convective and diffusive flows, in addition to possible generation and/or internal consumption, the problem can be solved considering the conservation of φ: a) net entry of φ into V; b) net production of φ in V; c) rate of time variation of φ in V.

The net entry of φ into V is determined from the balance, or difference, between the convective and diffusive flows of φ that enter and that leave V. The net amount of φ that enters the control volume, per unit of time, is given by integrating this balance on the boundaries of V as shown in Eq. (9). Net production, which is the difference between the generation and the consumption of φ within V, is represented in the equation by the term source.

In general, we can express a conservation law that is resolved in CFD programs as follows:

$$\frac{\partial p\phi}{\partial t} + \nabla.(p\phi\vec{v}) = \nabla.\Gamma_{\phi}\nabla\phi + S_{\phi} \tag{9}$$

where, the first term of the equation represents the storage rate, the term $(\nabla.(\rho\varphi\ \vec{v}))$ is the convective flow, the term $(\nabla.\Gamma_{\varphi}\nabla_{\varphi})$ is the diffusive flow and S_{φ} is the source term or sink.

As to the problem to be addressed in this study, the energy equation is obtained by making $\varphi = T$ and $\Gamma_{\varphi} = \frac{k}{c}$. The term source is responsible for accommodating all those terms that do not fit into the form represented by Eq. (9). In this study, there is no influence of convective flows, since these are due to the velocity of the fluid, which in this case is zero, as the medium is at rest. Thus, this equation can be rewritten as follows:

$$p\frac{\partial T}{\partial t} = \nabla.\frac{k}{c}\nabla T + S \tag{10}$$

where, S is the term source of heat generation. In Equation (10), which represents the physical model of this paper, the source term is given by the terms Q_m and Q_p.

As to the stationary regime, the equation written in integral form and using the divergence theorem, the discretization of the governing equation (Eq. 10) can be represented by Equation (11) for an arbitrary control volume (or cell) V, of the computational domain.

$$\oint_V \frac{k}{c}\nabla T.d\vec{A} + \int_V S dV = 0 \tag{11}$$

where $\vec{A}$ is the area vector and S is the source term per volume unit. Figure 1 shows an example of a section of the domain discretized using triangular cells. The discretization for each cell is given by Equation (12) (Fluent, 2005).

$$\sum_{f}^{N_{faces}} \frac{k}{c}(\nabla T)_n \vec{A}_f + SV = 0 \tag{12}$$

where, N_{faces} is the number of faces that surround the cell, $\vec{A}_f$ is the vector that represents the area of the face, ΔT is the temperature gradient on the face f and S is the average value of S in V.

Figure 1. Control volume to illustrate the discretization of the diffusion equation of a scalar
Source: (Fluent, 2005).

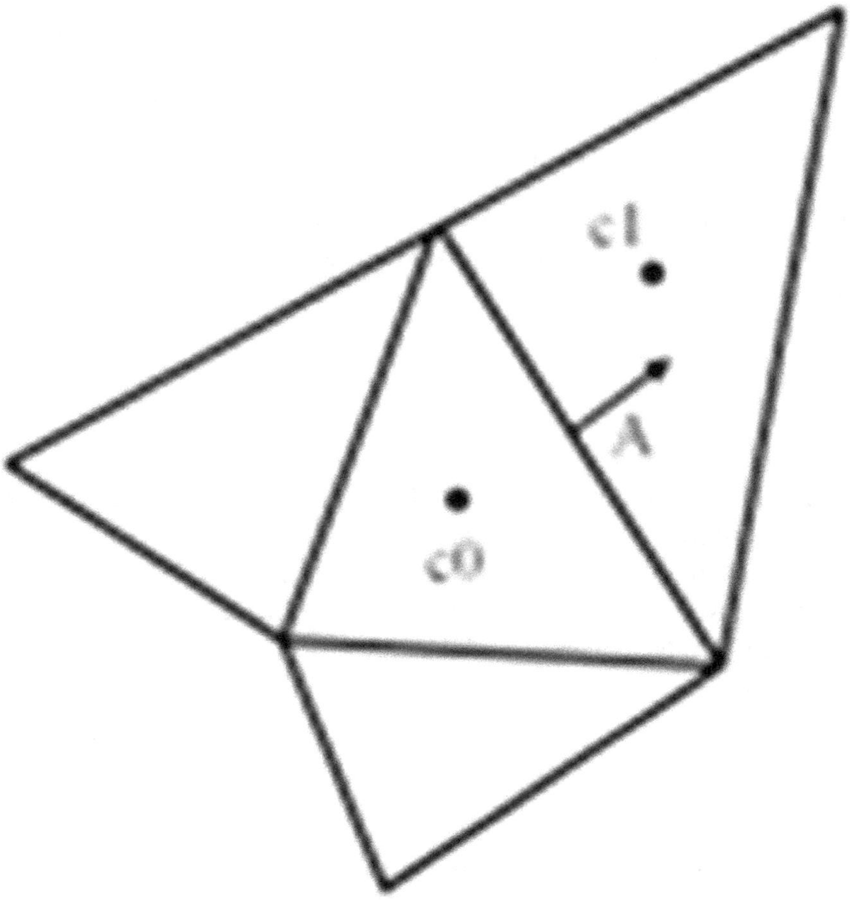

The mathematical equations solved by FLUENT™ assume the general form of Equation (12) which can be applied in cases of two or three dimensions with structured or unstructured meshes consisting of polyhedral elements. In the standard mode of the software, the discrete value of *T* is stored in the center of the cell (c0 and c1) as shown in Figure 1 (Fluent, 2005).

INVERSE PROBLEM

Modeling via inverse problems is an area of research that has grown considerably in recent decades. These problems evolved from theoretical research themes into becoming an important practical engineering analysis tool. As it is multidisciplinary in nature, this type of problem unites the mathematical analysis of problems to experimental data, and is applied in several areas, such as: engineering, reconstructing images, medicine, geophysics, astrophysics and other branches of science (Silva Neto & Moura Neto, 2005).

Inverse heat transfer problems (IHTP) can be classified according to the heat transfer process, such as: conduction, convection, radiation, conduction and radiation, conduction and convection, and phase change. They can also be classified as to the type of cause to be determined: an inverse problem of heat transfer of boundary condition, of thermophysical properties, of initial condition, of source term and of geometry.

Researchers such as Liu & Ozisik (1995), Kim, Jung, Kim, & Lee (2003), Romero-Méndez et al. (2009) have investigated the use of inverse methods to estimate thermophysical properties in heat conduction problems. Numerical and experimental methods have been developed to predict thermal conductivity, in addition to studies that were performed to estimate thermal conductivity from experimental temperatures (Liu & Ozisik, 1995; Char, Chang, Tai, 2008; Chang & Chang, 2009; Sundberg & Hellstrom, 2009). According to Kim et al. (2003), most of the methods used to estimate this property in IHTP problems use iterative optimization techniques, in which the thermal conductivity is found by minimizing the residue between the calculated temperature and the experimental temperature at specific points of the medium (Chang & Chang, 2009).

Huang and Huang (2007) applied the Levenberg-Marquardt Method to estimate the thermal conductivity and the volumetric heat capacity in biological tissues based on temperature measurement, using the Bioheat Transfer Equation. The accuracy of the inverse problem is analyzed using the exact simulated temperature and temperature measurements with additions of random errors. A statistical analysis is performed to obtain the 99% confidence limits for the thermal properties estimated. The results show that good estimates of thermal conductivity and volumetric heat capacity can be obtained using the Levenberg-Marquardt algorithm.

Partridge and Wrobel (2007) used the Dual Reciprocity Method (DRM) coupled with a genetic algorithm, in an inverse process by which the size and the location of a skin tumor can be obtained from temperature measurements on the surface of the skin. In this case, the DRM does not need internal nodules. The results are presented for tumors of different sizes and positions in relation to the surface of the skin.

Paruch and Majchrzak (2007) solved an inverse problem using an evolutionary algorithm in conjunction with the Multiple Reciprocity Boundary Element Method (MRBEM) in order to simultaneously estimate some thermophysical properties and geometric parameters (thermal conductivity, metabolic heat, blood perfusion, location and size) of the tumor region. Once again, numerically calculated breast surface temperatures are assumed as if they were experimental temperatures. Using this methodology presented satisfactory results. However, in three-dimensional simulations the method proved to be slow. The author suggested that the method presented can be used as an effective tool for non-invasive diagnosis in medical practices.

A very comprehensive definition of the reverse method is presented by (Engl, Hanke, & Neubauer, 1996):

To solve an inverse problem is to determine unknown causes based on the desired or observed effects.

Thus, in this study, the objective is to minimize the difference between the experimental temperatures, obtained from IR images, and those calculated numerically. The objective function F(**x**), (Eq. 13), represents the norm of the residuals between the calculated temperature, T_{cal}, and the temperature measured experimentally by the thermography, T_{exp}. The numerical values for T_{cal}, were obtained from a numerical solution of the Bioheat Transfer Equation, using the Finite Volume Method.

Now, **x** is considered to be the vector of design variables, where i = 1, ..., I and I is the total number of experimental measures. The vector **x** = [k, ω] represents the set of unknown parameters, i.e. values that will be defined by using the optimization process (Bezerra, Oliveira, Araújo, Viana, Santos, Santos, Rolim, Lyra, Lima, Borschartt, Resmini, Conci, 2013b; Bezerra, et al., 2013, 2020).

The formulation of the optimization problem to be solved can be described mathematically by the following expression:

$$\min_{\mathrm{x}} \mathrm{F}(\mathbf{x}) = \sum_{\mathrm{i}=1}^{\mathrm{I}} \left[\mathrm{T}_{\mathrm{cal}_\mathrm{i}}(\mathbf{x}) - \mathrm{T}_{\mathrm{exp}_\mathrm{i}} \right]^2 \tag{13}$$

subject to

$$k^L \le k \le k^U$$

$$\omega^L \le \omega \le \omega^U$$

where, k^L, k^U and ω^L, ω^U are the lower and upper limit restrictions for thermal conductivity and blood perfusion, respectively.

To minimize the objective function, the SQP (Sequential Quadratic Programming) method is used (Yang, Deng, Yu, & Luo (2009); Teles & Gomes, 2010). In this method, quadratic subproblems (QP) are solved at each iteration, and it is based on the quasi-Newton approximation of the Hessian of the Lagrangian and in a search direction, with a quadratic objective function and linear constraints (Nocedal & Wright, 2006). A code was developed on the Matlab® platform that makes use of its *fmincon function* of the optimization Toolbox™. The flowchart illustrated in Figure 2 outlines the process. A tolerance of 10^{-6} was adopted for its convergence.

In order to assess the influence of the parameters on the temperature distribution on the surface of the breast, a sensitivity analysis was performed for each case studied. This analysis is very important in order to make an assessment of which parameters can be estimated, and which parameters are the most important in the process (Blackwell, 1989).The sensitivity of the parameter to be determined must be large enough to ensure that the model responds to minor disturbances of these parameters.

The numerical approximation by finite differences was used to analyze the sensitivity coefficients. The Finite Difference Method (FDM) is a method that is easy to implement, but of high computational cost, which is directly proportional to the number of design variables. The method consists of disturbing each design variable x_i independently, with a relatively small value. Using the FDM, a first order (advanced) approach to the first derivative is given by:

$$\frac{\partial T}{\partial x_i} \approx \frac{\Delta T}{\Delta x_i} = \frac{T(x_i + \Delta x_i) - T(x_i)}{\Delta x_i}. \tag{14}$$

According to Blackwell (1989), if estimating the parameters is simultaneous, the sensitivity coefficients must be linearly independent and must also be large enough to determine the estimate successfully.

Figure 2. Flowchart of the optimization method.
Source: (Bezerra et al., 2013).

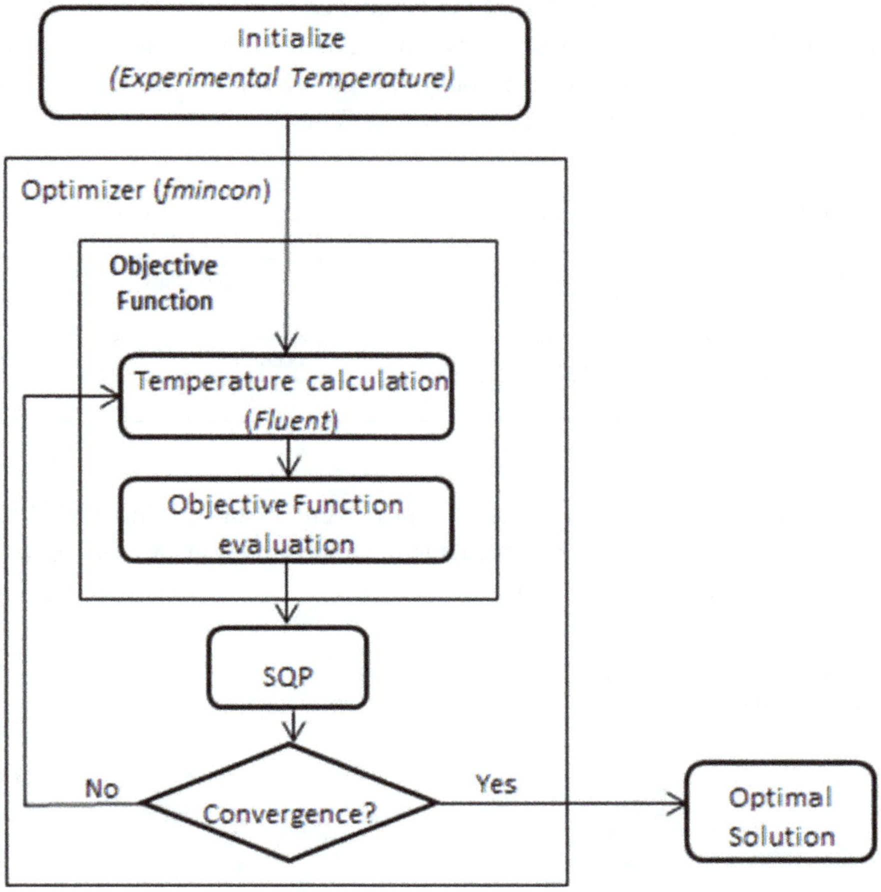

EXPERIMENTAL VALIDATION OF THE METHODOLOGY

To validate the methodology used to estimate the parameters, an experiment was carried out that uses a PVC phantom of the female torso. In this experiment, a 7 W incandescent lamp was inserted into the right breast of the phantom and this was filled with industrial silicone (Araújo, Bezerra, Santos, Rolim, Santos, Lyra, & Lima, 2008). A coordinate measuring machine (CMM) of the mobile bridge type, model CRYSTA547, manufactured by MITUTOYO, belonging to the Measurement of Coordinates Laboratory of the Department of Mechanical Engineering at UFPE, was used to obtain the coordinates of the points on the surface of the breast of the phantom. This machine has a calibration certificate issued by a laboratory belonging to the Brazilian Calibration Network (Santos, 2009).

Using the coordinates cited, it was possible to generate the real geometry of the phantom breast. The lamp was modeled as a cylinder with a radius of 1 cm and a height of 3 cm. The filament of the lamp was modeled as a cylinder with a radius of 3 mm and a height of 1.5 cm.

The geometry generated was used to conduct the numerical calculation of the temperature profiles. The boundary conditions involved were: heat exchange by convection between the surface of the breast and the environment at 25.4°C; the thoracic region was considered to have a prescribed temperature of 37.2°C.

The volumetric rate of heat generation of the lamp is equal to 1.65 x 10^7 W/m^3 (equivalent to its power of 7 W). The lamp was considered as a cylinder full of air and the material used in the filament was tungsten. For the breast filling, the thermophysical properties of silicone rubber were considered. The thermophysical properties considered are shown in Table 2.

Table 2. Thermophysical properties of the materials in the phantom experiment.

Material	k (W/m°C)	ρ (kg/m³)	c (J/kg°C)
Silicone rubber	0.21	970	65.68
Air	0.0242	1,006.43	1.225
Tungsten	174	19,250	132

The geometry and the unstructured tetrahedral mesh were obtained using the GAMBIT preprocessor. Figure 3 shows the geometry and the unstructured tetrahedral mesh adopted for the phantom. It has 6,006 nodes, 32,888 elements and 66,726 faces.

Figure 3. Unstructured mesh used for the phantom.
Source: (Bezerra et al., 2013).

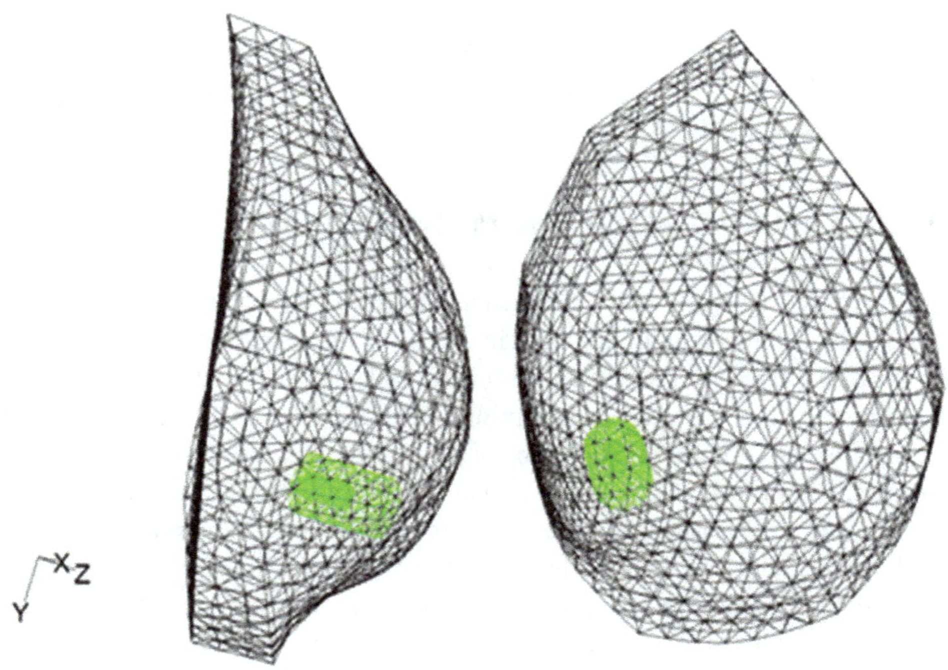

Figure 4a shows the thermogram of the front surface of the phantom. This image was taken when the steady state was reached after the lamp was turned on. The information printed on the image is generated directly by the thermographic camera. On the image, regions of interest, such as lines and boxes, can be selected. Some other parameters such as maximum and minimum temperature are shown. The maximum temperature measured over the region where the lamp is located is 47.1°C. Figure 4b shows the temperature distribution on the surface of the breast. The maximum temperature obtained using numerical simulation was also 47.1°C.

As the phantom breast was filled with only one material, it was considered a simple model to validate the methodology due to the fact that the breast model consists of a homogeneous and isotropic medium, quite unlike a real human breast. In addition, the positioning of the lamp was known.

Figure 4. a) Thermogram of phantom breast; b) Distribution of the temperature calculated on the surface of the breast.

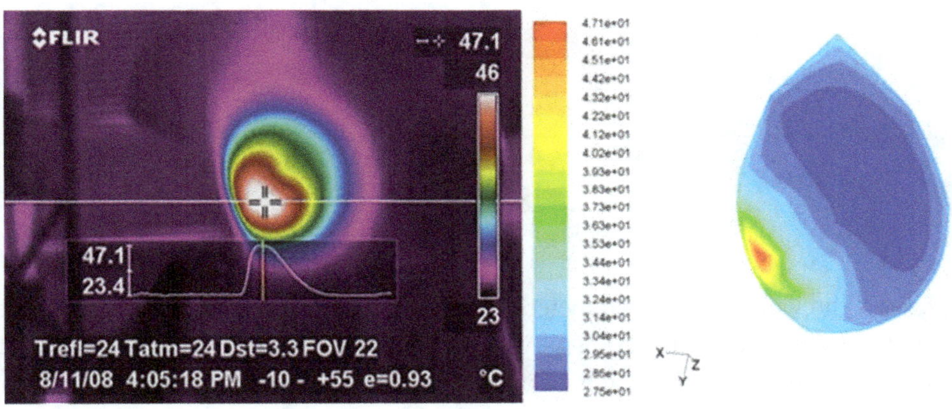

For a better understanding of the thermal behavior of the breast, a sensitivity analysis was performed, which is shown in Figure 5. This analysis showed that the sensitivity coefficients of the thermal conductivities of silicone and tungsten are linearly dependent. This implies that it is not possible to estimate both properties simultaneously. However, as the sensitivity coefficients of the conductivity of silicone and of air are not linearly dependent, they can be estimated simultaneously. The sensitivity coefficients for the thermal conductivities are practically zero up to the position of 0.06 m. In this position, these sensitivity coefficients start to vary, due to the presence of the lamp in this region.

Table 3. Thermophysical parameters of the phantom.

Design variables (W/m°C)	Actual	Estimated	Error
$k_{Silicone}$	0.21	0.2127	1.28%
k_{Air}	0.0242	0.0241	0.41%
$k_{Tungsten}$	174	174.0372	0.021%

Figure 5. Sensitivity analysis for the phantom.

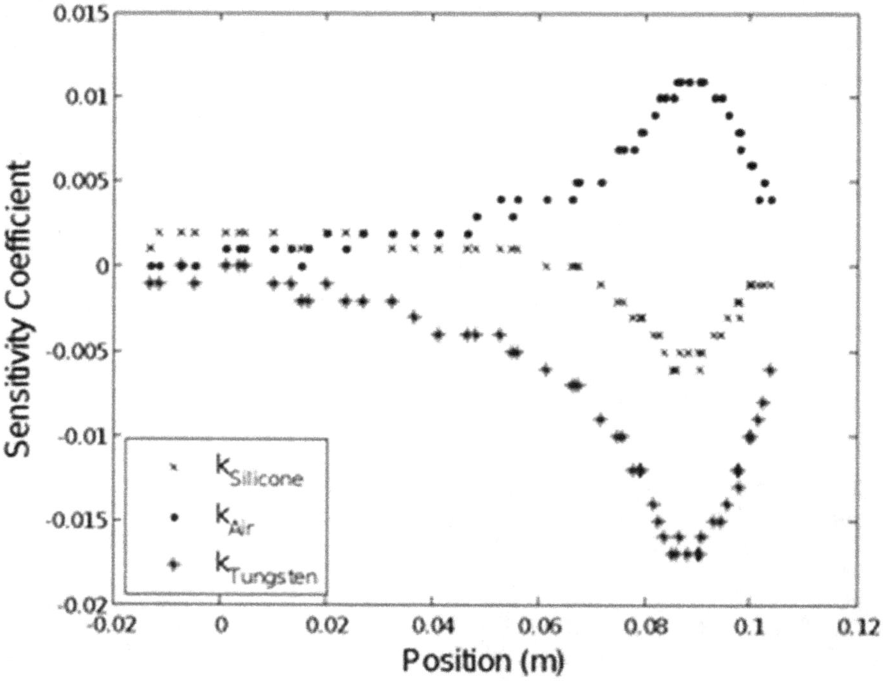

Table 3 presents the values of the parameters found in the literature and those that were estimated, using the methodology described in Section 4. A very small error was obtained for all parameters. After analyzing this, it is concluded that the estimates of thermophysical properties reached satisfactory values using the maximum temperature measured by infrared images. The maximum error was 1.28%, indicating that this procedure can be used to estimate the thermophysical properties of the breast.

CONSTRUCTION OF BREAST SURROGATE TRIDIMENSIONAL GEOMETRIES BASED ON IR IMAGES

In this topic, the methodology developed to construct a customized three-dimensional breast geometry will be presented. The model in discussion was built based on curves extracted from the patient's thermograms. The frontal and the profile breast curves were extracted using the SpaceClaim software. These curves are necessary to generate the 3D model of the breast. Then, the geometric modeling itself will be tackled by presenting the volume generated. This volume will be presented and will then be used for numerical calculations by Ansys software. Finally, some case studies will be presented for patients with malignant and benign neoplasia and the temperatures obtained by numerical simulations will be compared with previous studies by other authors.

Figure 6. The profile curve of a patient obtained by using SpaceClaim®
Source: (Melo et al., 2019).

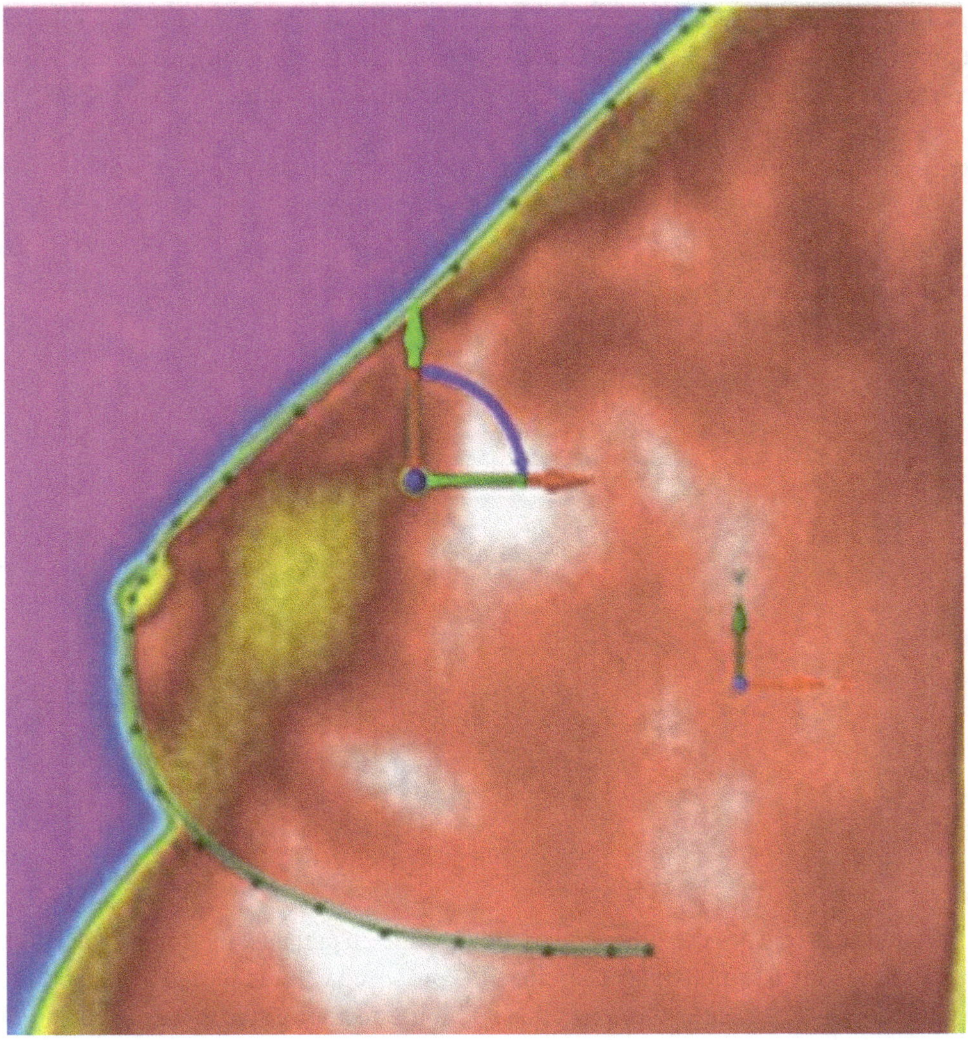

Generation of Substitute Geometry Obtained by using IR images

The use of the SpaceClaim® software, with its ability to adjust the curve, allowed the individual characteristics of the breast profile of each patient, presented in their lateral thermographic images, to be extracted. Section by section, the curve can be constructed by allocating the points in the limit region of the breast, thereby providing a more rigorous adjustment of the profile, exemplified in Figure 6. Once generated, the next step is to scale it to the actual size of the breast. It is important to note that even though this is a manual procedure, the volumes generated with the technique showed satisfactory results, thus making it viable for the proposed objective (Melo, Queiroz, Bezerra, & Lima, 2019).

Adjustment of the personalized volume based on a breast prosthesis

The posterior part of the breast in contact with the chest wall also plays an essential role in characterizing its geometry. To date, there is no one defined standard for forming such a surface. This region has already been represented by circles and ellipses. Among the forms adopted, Viana (2010) used breast implants of the trade name Ortho Pauher, series SG-419, sizes 01, 04, 08, 09 and 12, to configure the region. Figure 7 exemplifies one of the parts used.

Figure 7. Ortho Pauher breast prosthesis
Source: *https://www.orthopauher.com/2014/produtofinal.asp?pid=245&language=pt*

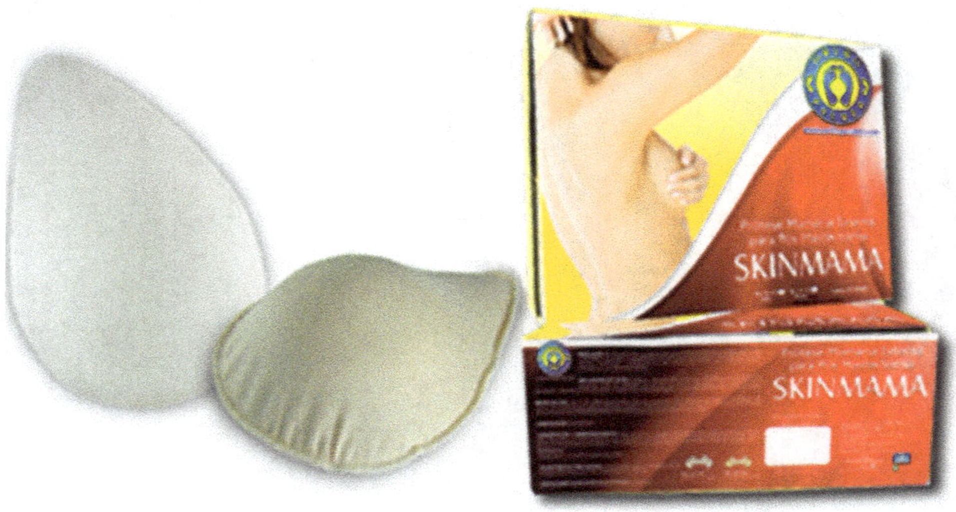

Due to the good suitability to the silhouette of mastectomized patients, the commercial prostheses are good references for geometric modeling. Therefore, the proposed volume started to adopt this configuration to constitute its posterior region. The fact that its limits are not formed by easily constructed curves often requires the use of more specific measurement techniques, as was the case for Viana (2010) who used a Coordinate Measuring Machine from the Laboratory for Measuring Coordinates of the Mechanical Engineering Department of the Federal University of Pernambuco (DEMEC/UFPE).

Analyzing the specimens and their plastic packaging, which are called cradles, the possibility was found of constructing the plane by using the spline tool to interconnect the ends of its horizontal and vertical axes. The proposed technique is illustrated in Figure 8. As the prosthesis has a practically perfect fit with its plastic wrapping (cradle), its measurements can be obtained directly from such wrapping, which is not flexible and thus can be more easily measured by the machine mentioned above (Melo et al., 2019).

Figure 8. Technique used to construct the drop shape.
Source: (Melo et al., 2019).

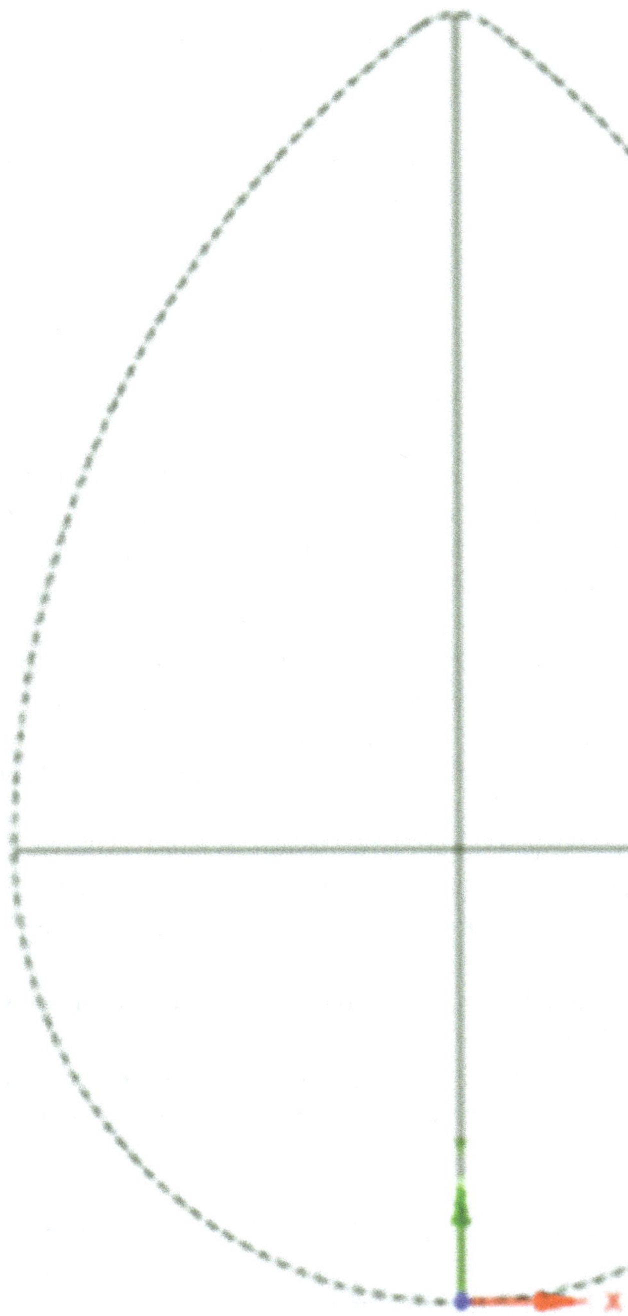

With the aid of a scalimeter on the scale of 1:1 of the trademark Trident and of a pair of set squares – one being a scalene and the other an isosceles – the measurements of the axes of all the prostheses were obtained. Table 4 summarizes the values found.

Table 4. Measurements of the axes of the external prostheses.

No. of the prosthesis	Smaller axis (mm)	Larger axis (mm)
01	107	150
04	124	174
08	151	212
09	158	222
12	167	235

Source: (Melo et al., 2019).

The values contained in the aforementioned table let the chest wall of each of the available prostheses be constructed, as shown in Figure 9.

On analyzing the formats obtained, it was found that their dimensions are related by means of a factor of proportion. As the intention is to build a more reliable model for the anatomy of the breast, it was observed that any of the surfaces could be used to generate the volume, as long as its measurements are rectified according to each patient. Due to the lack of clear boundaries in the upper region of the breast, the vertical axis is corrected proportionally to the adjustment of the horizontal axis. The entire development of the case studies of this paper was based on Prosthesis #4.

The frontal thermographic image of the patient, who was positioned behind a 75 mm metal grid, was used to construct the posterior surface. In order to obtain the correct dimension, a horizontal line (MH) needs to be inserted in the image, which must pass through the nipple, with extremities at the limiting points of the breast. This step is illustrated in Figures 10 (a) and 10 (b).

With the rear wall dimensioned, the profile curve obtained in Figure 6 can be adapted to the extremities of the vertical axis.

Finally, in order to generate the desired volume, a second curve was included, in the horizontal plane. To do so, it was decided to choose a semi-ellipse, the smaller axis of which is the same size as the line (MH). Figures 11 (a) and 11 (b) illustrate the two existing alternatives, in which (Option II) presented a minor volumetric error, that was validated in the results.

The profile curve of the breast and Curve II, considering only the frontal segment, provide the creation of the basis of the geometry, explained in Figure 12a, which was sufficient to generate the final volume. Finally, the nodule was inserted according to the information contained in the ultrasound exams, which in addition to providing its dimensions, locates it in relation to the nipple and its distance from the skin (Fig. 12b).

Validation of the substitute geometry constructed using a breast prosthesis

In order to validate the geometric model proposed in this study, it was decided to compare the actual volume of an object with the shape closest to that of a patient's breast with its computationally generated volume. Among the options, the external prosthesis mentioned in the methodology and its plastic wrapping, or cradle, proved to be suitable for this.

Figure 9. Construction of the flat surfaces of breast prosthesis
Source: (Melo et al., 2019).

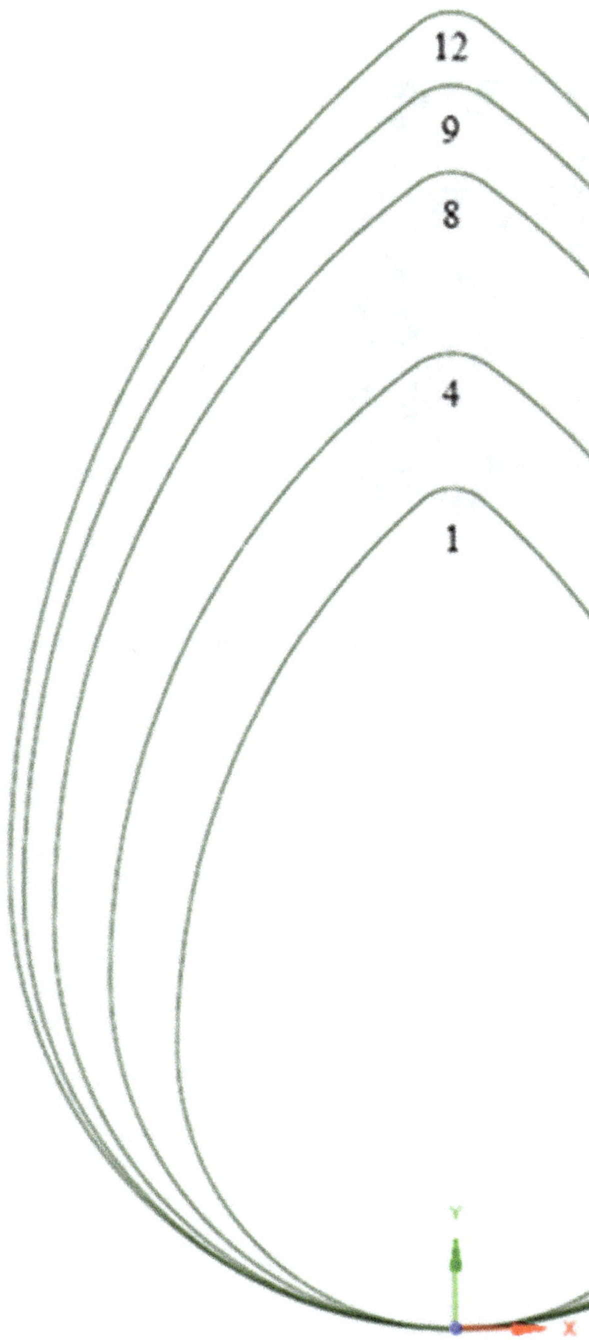

Figure 10. Technique for dimensioning the substitute geometry. (a) Front image of the patient located behind a metal grid with the straight line (MH) for dimensioning. (b) Adjustment of the thoracic base with the measurement of the straight line (MH)
Source: (Melo et al., 2019).

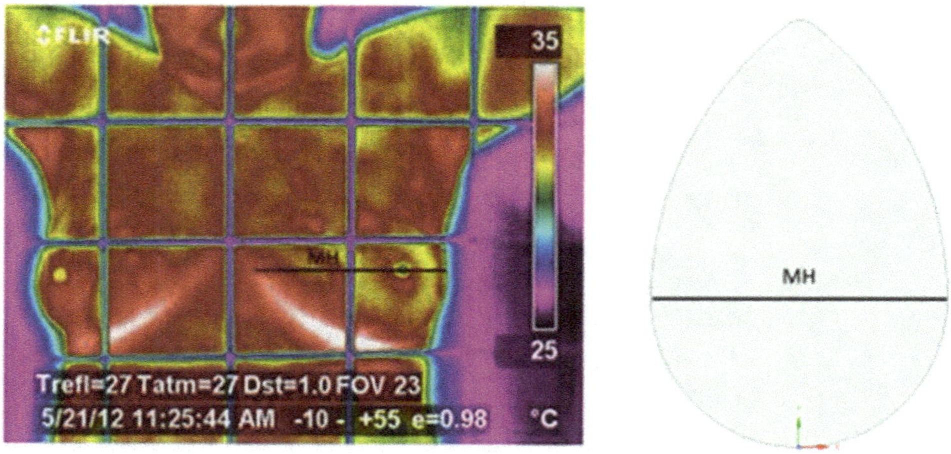

Figure 11. Alternatives available for the second curve. (a) Isometric view (b) Top view Source: (Melo et al., 2019).

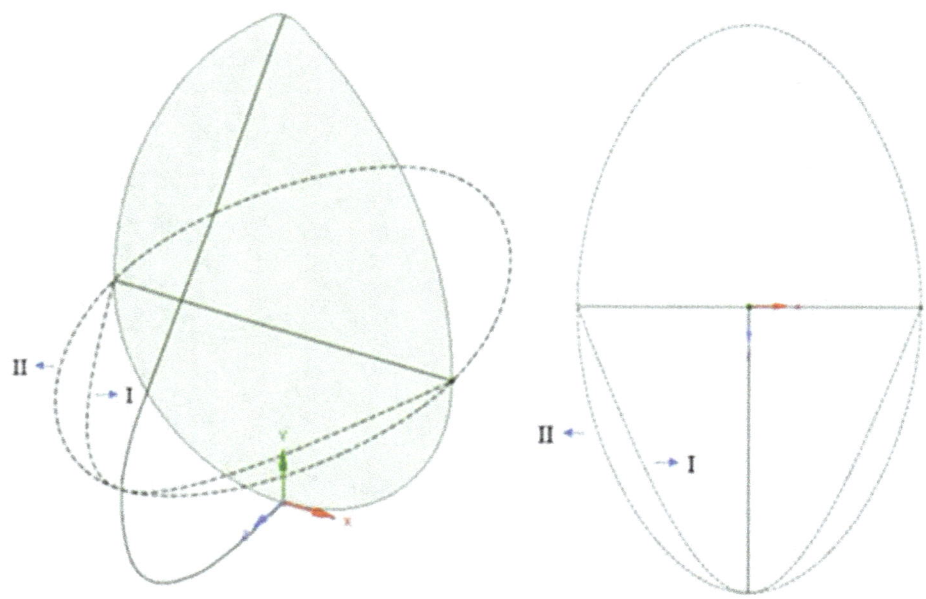

In order to measure its volume in a simplified way, it was decided to fill the cradle of the prosthesis with water, thus providing a good approximation of the real value. With the aid of a scale, a total water mass of approximately 0.404 kg was obtained, which could be converted to a unit of volume according to the volumetric density (ρ) of this fluid equal to 997 kg/m^3.

Figure 12. Basis of the substitute geometry of the breast (a). Geometry is constituted from glandular and tumor tissue (b).
Source: (Melo et al., 2019).

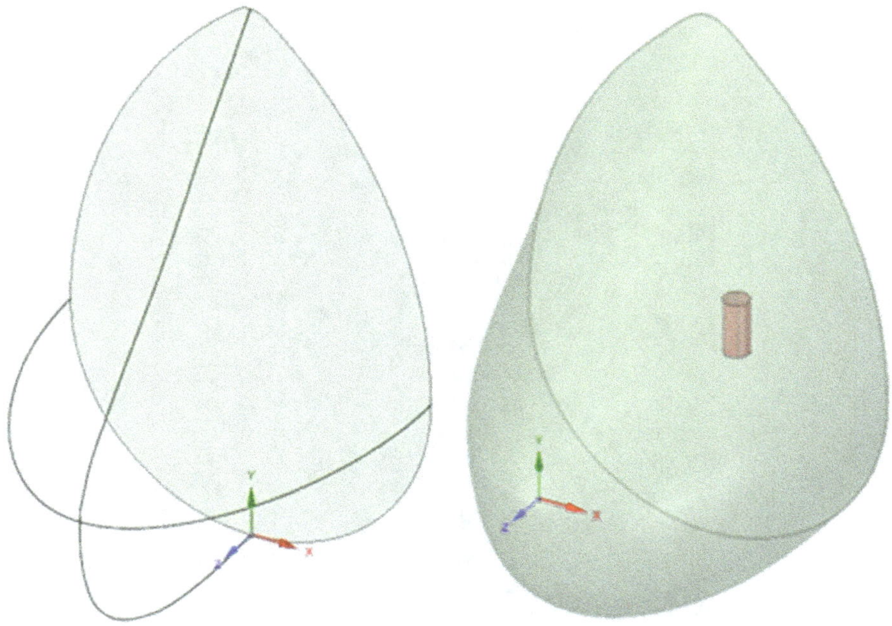

Using the plastic wrapping, due to its verisimilitude with the part and the greater facility for capturing the basic images of the model, the second step turned to the computational development of its volume. The profile curve was extracted from the cradle of the part, Figure 13, which supported the construction of the preliminary three-dimensional geometry.

After making the geometry adjustment using the horizontal measurement of the surface (MH), equal to 105 mm, the profile curve was adapted to the point of correcting the preliminary geometry, as illustrated in Figure 14 (a). In this way, the final volume was obtained and is shown in Figure 14 (b).

To assess the results, Table 5 shows how the volumes compare with each other: the real one with that of its computational three-dimensional geometry. A volumetric error of approximately 0.17% was observed, which legitimizes the proposed geometric technique.

Cases Studied

In this section, some case studies will be presented, using the geometric modeling developed for different breast pathologies.

Figure 13. Profile curve of the cradle of the prosthesis
Source: (Melo et al., 2019).

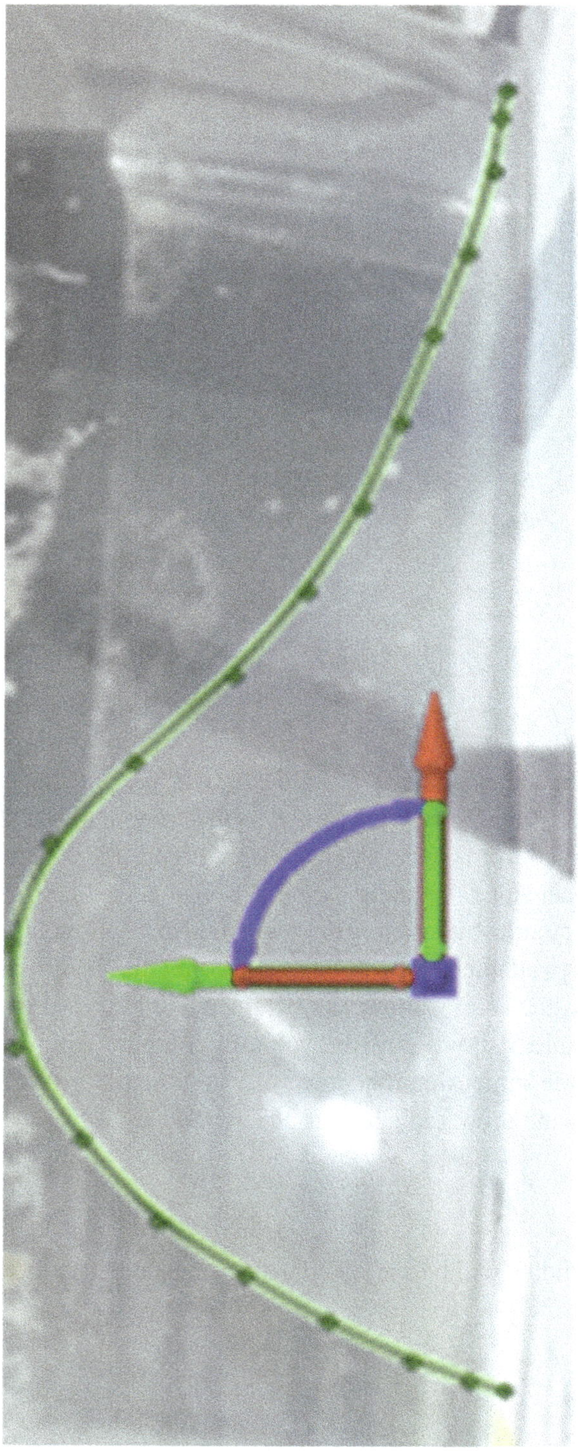

Figure 14. Geometry of the prosthesis cradle. (a) Preliminary (b) Final
Source: (Melo et al., 2019).

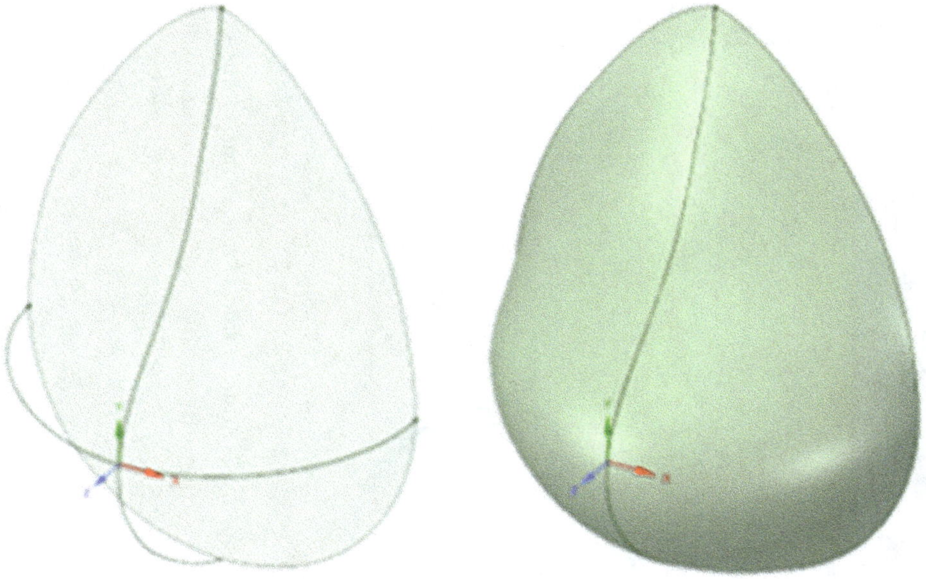

Table 5. Comparison of the computational volume with the real volume of the prosthesis

Object of study	Volume (dm^3)
Prosthesis	0.3992
Geometry	0.3985

Source: (Melo et al., 2019).

Figure 15. Thermographic images of Patient # 1301345-4. (a) Front (b) Profile

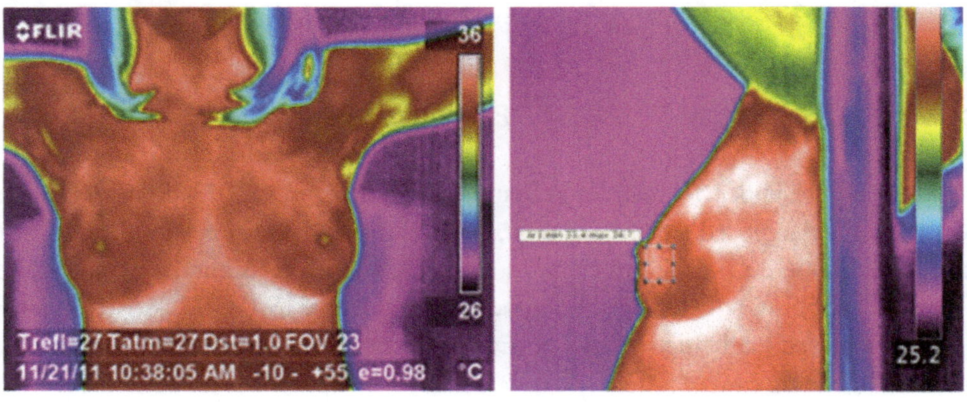

Figure 16. Extraction of the profile curve of Patient #1301345-4.
Source: (Melo et al., 2019).

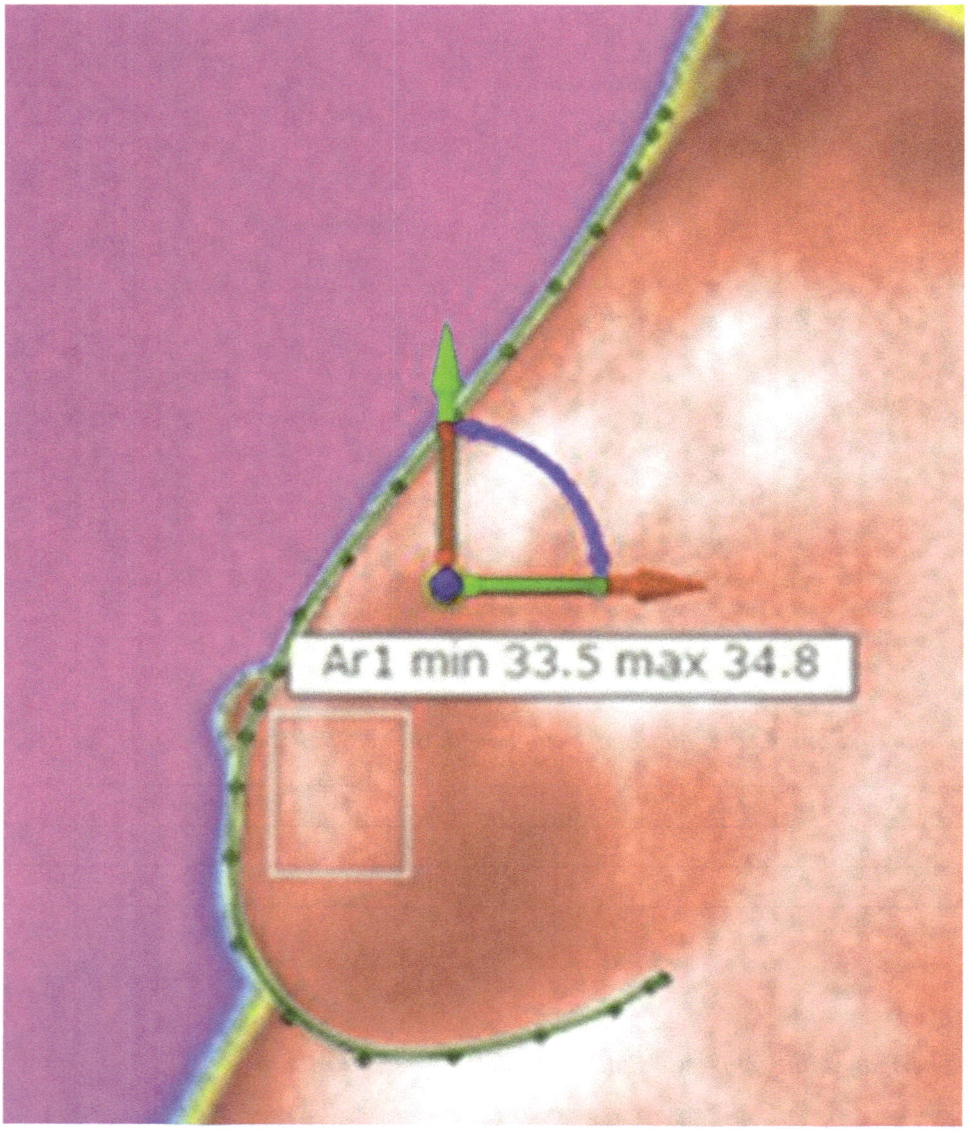

Patient of Medical Record #1301345-4 - Benign Case

The first case studied presents a 34-year-old patient (Medical Record #1301345-4). Her mammography and ultrasound exams diagnosed a fibroadenoma, a benign neoplasm, in her left breast located in the lower external quadrant (LEQ). The tumor has a spherical shape of 13 mm in diameter and is 6 mm from the skin surface. For it, a metabolic heat generation rate equal to 18,907.76 W/m^3 was calculated, according to the proposed mathematical model (Eq.4). Figures 15 (a) and 15 (b) illustrate the patient's thermographic images.

Figure 17. Geometric model of Patient # 1301345-4.
Source: (Melo et al., 2019).

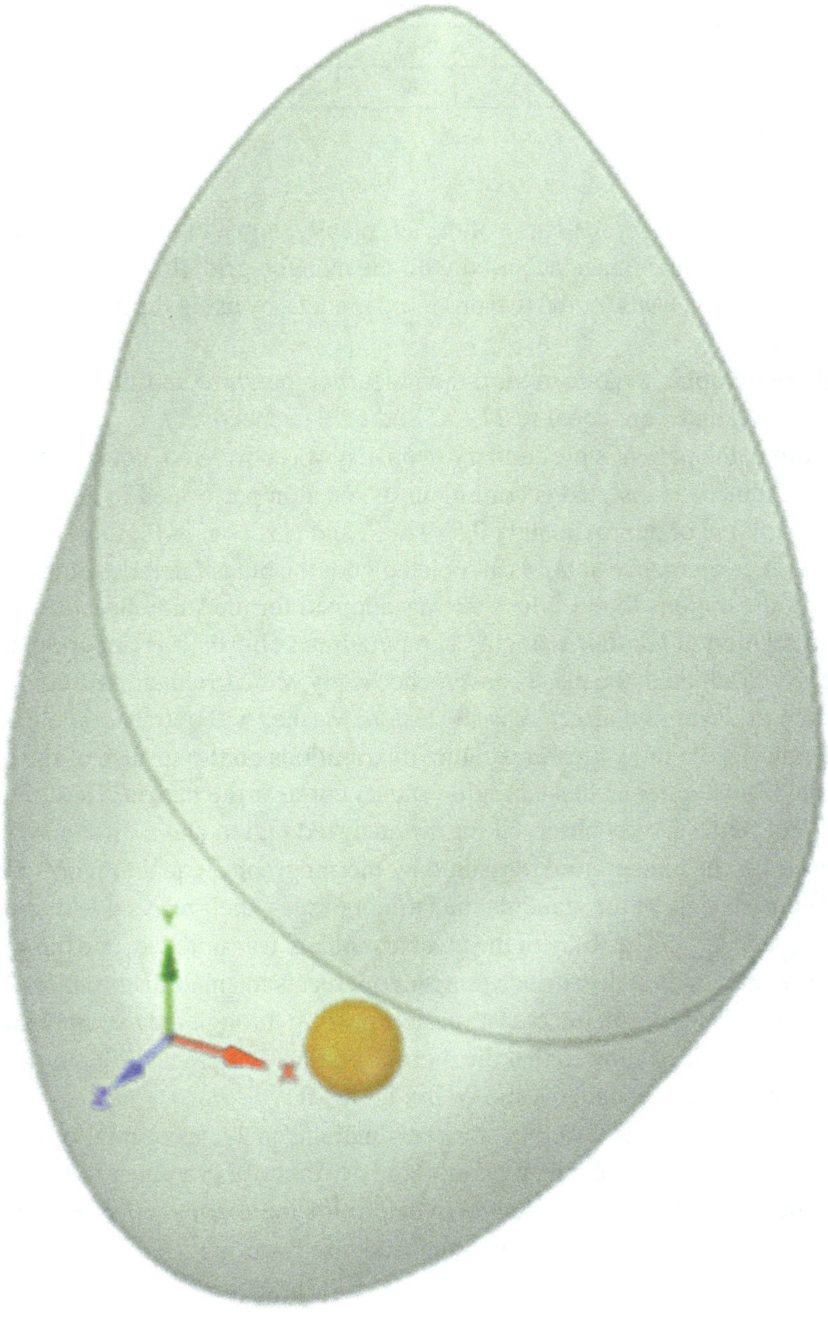

Table 6. Convergence of the mesh of Patient #1301345-4

Mesh	No. of nodes	Maximum Temperature (°C)
1	113420	35.05
2	242449	35.65
3	361107	35.66

Source: (Melo et al., 2019).

Based on Figure 15 (b), the profile curve of the left breast, shown in Figure 16, could be constructed. Later, using the thermographic image acquired with the metallic grid, the preliminary geometry of this breast could be adjusted, the basis for the two proposed models, by using the measurement of the straight MH equal to 114 mm.

During the thermographic examination, the ambient temperature and the relative humidity of the local air were measured and were equal to 27.4°C and 62%, respectively.

Using the MH line, the patient's preliminary geometry was corrected, obtaining her final geometry. Subsequently, the nodule was inserted according to its location performed by the ultrasound examination, resulting in a volume of approximately 0.549 dm^3, and is shown in Figure 17.

Initially, the mesh convergence analysis associated with the breast/ nodule set was presented, shown in Table 6. Among the options found, Mesh #2 was adopted for the study because it presents a difference of 0.01°C in relation to #3, thus reducing computational efforts. It is important to emphasize that regardless of the model adopted, the mesh convergence study was carried out in relation to the maximum surface temperature in the region affected by the lesion. Meshes with tetrahedral elements were used.

Figures 18 (a) and 18 (b) show the temperature distributions on the surface of the breast affected by the presence of the lesion, where a heated region stands out near the patient's left nipple. A maximum temperature (T_{max}) of 35.65°C was observed for the analyzed region and a difference of approximately 0.14% was obtained for the temperature measured by thermography, equal to 35.60°C.

As the model consists only of the glandular and tumor tissues, their respective thermal conductivities were named as k_{mama} and k_{tumor}. The study of the inverse problem was initiated, and the sensitivity analysis was conducted. It was found that the surface temperature reacts to small disturbances of the parameters referred to. Taking a vertical line on the breast surface, passing through the maximum temperature point (Figure 19), the result obtained showed that the thermal conductivities can be estimated simultaneously because they are linearly independent, as shown in Figure 20.

Thus, the thermal conductivities were estimated simultaneously, according to the results presented in Table 7. Comparing the results obtained by this study with those presented in Bezerra (2013), it was observed that the new volume made it possible to determine the thermal conductivity of the nodule of this patient, a fact that had not been possible in the study by Bezerra (2013).

Figure 18. Calculated temperature profile (°C) of the geometric model of Patient #1301345-4 (a) Front view (b) Profile view.
Source: (Melo et al., 2019).

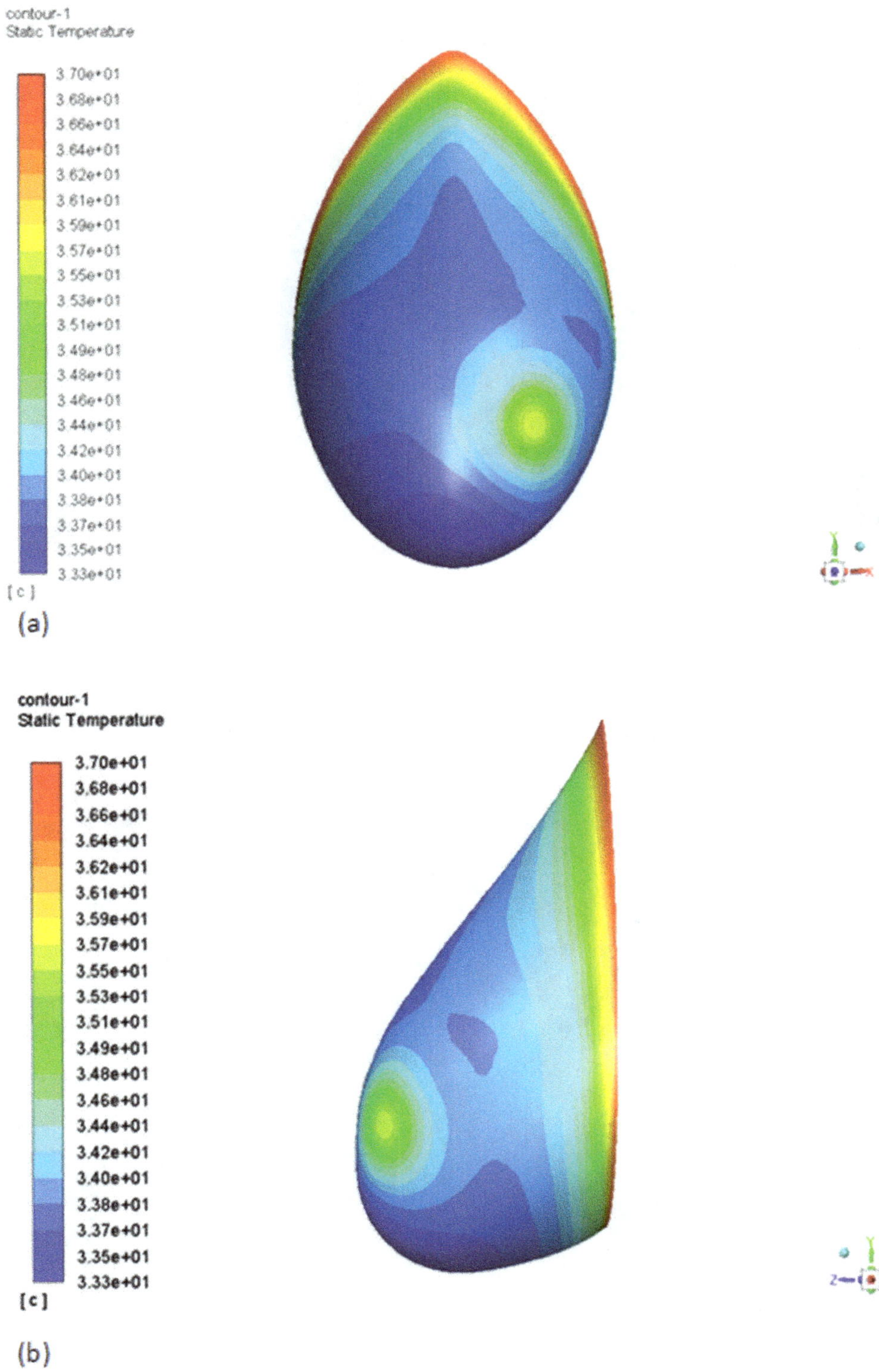

Figure 19. Vertical line used for sensitivity analysis of Patient #1301345-4.
Source: (Melo et al., 2019).

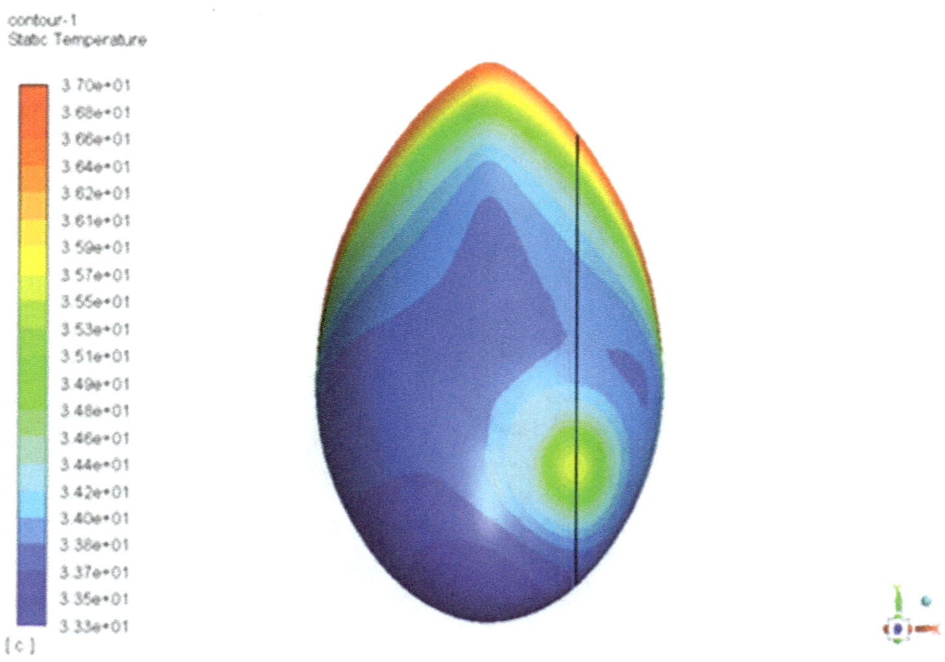

Figure 20. Sensitivity curves of the thermal conductivities of Patient #1301345-4
Source: (Melo et al., 2019).

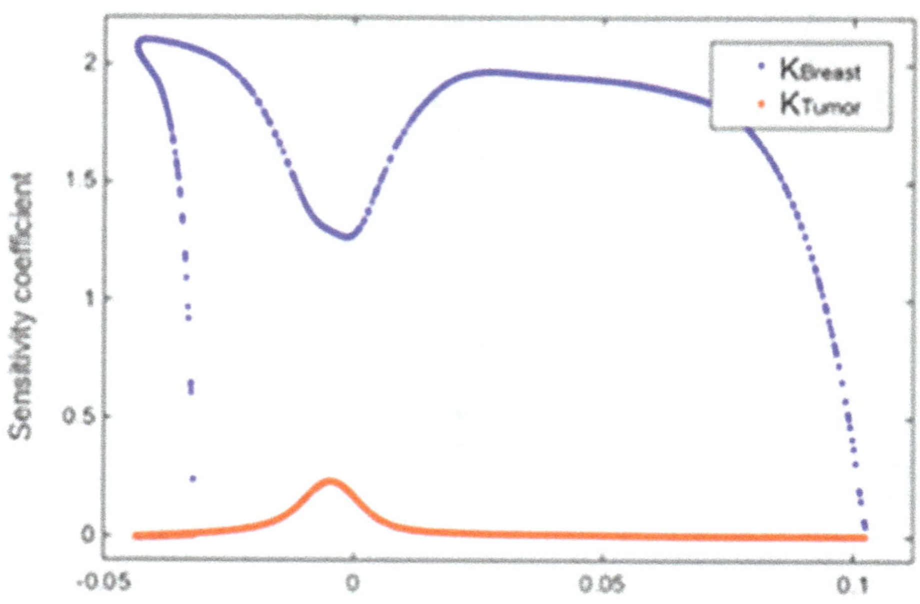

Table 7. Estimate of the thermal conductivities of Patient #1301345-4

Parameter	Reference (Table 3)	Bezerra (2013)		This study	
		Estimate	Percentage Difference	Estimate	Percentage Difference
k_{mama} ($W.m^{-1}.K^{-1}$)	0.48	0.4846	0.95%	0.4581	4.56%
k_{tumor} ($W.m^{-1}.K^{-1}$)	0.48	No results	-	0.4772	0.58%

Source: (Melo et al., 2019).

Patient of Medical Record #1844369-4 - Malignant Case

The second patient analyzed is a 49-year-old woman (Medical Record #1844369-4), who was diagnosed with a solid nodule in the left breast. This pathology was classified as BI-RADS V according to her mammography and ultrasound exams, and the result for cancer after the biopsy exam was positive. The dimensions of the lesion are 17 mm x 8 mm and it is 16 mm deep in the skin, located in the upper outer quadrant. Its geometry was approximated by a cylinder and the rate of metabolic heat generation was calculated (Eq. 4) resulting in a value equal to 25,848 W/m^3. Figures 21 (a) and 21 (b) show the thermographic images for this case.

Figure 21. Thermographic images of Patient #1844369-4. (a) Front (b) Profile

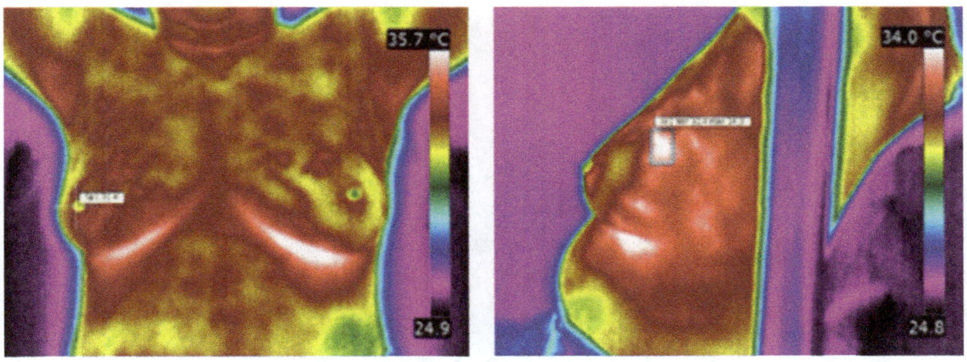

Due to her age, the liposubstitution of her breast parenchyma is more advanced than that of the previous patient. Shown in Figure 23, the geometry has a volume of approximately 0.765 dm^3. The mesh convergence analysis appears in Table 8. From the results shown, the variation of 0.01°C between Meshes #3 and #4 indicates that the first should be chosen in order to mitigate the computational effort.

Figures 23 (a) and 23 (b) show the calculated surface temperature profile of this breast, using Mesh #3. From the result obtained, the heating caused by the malignant tumor in the upper outer quadrant is noticed, the maximum local temperature, T_{max}, being 35.46°C. Comparing this with the value measured by the thermographic camera, of 35.27°C, a difference of 0.53% was verified.

Figure 22. Geometry consisting of glandular and tumor tissue.
Source: (Melo et al., 2019).

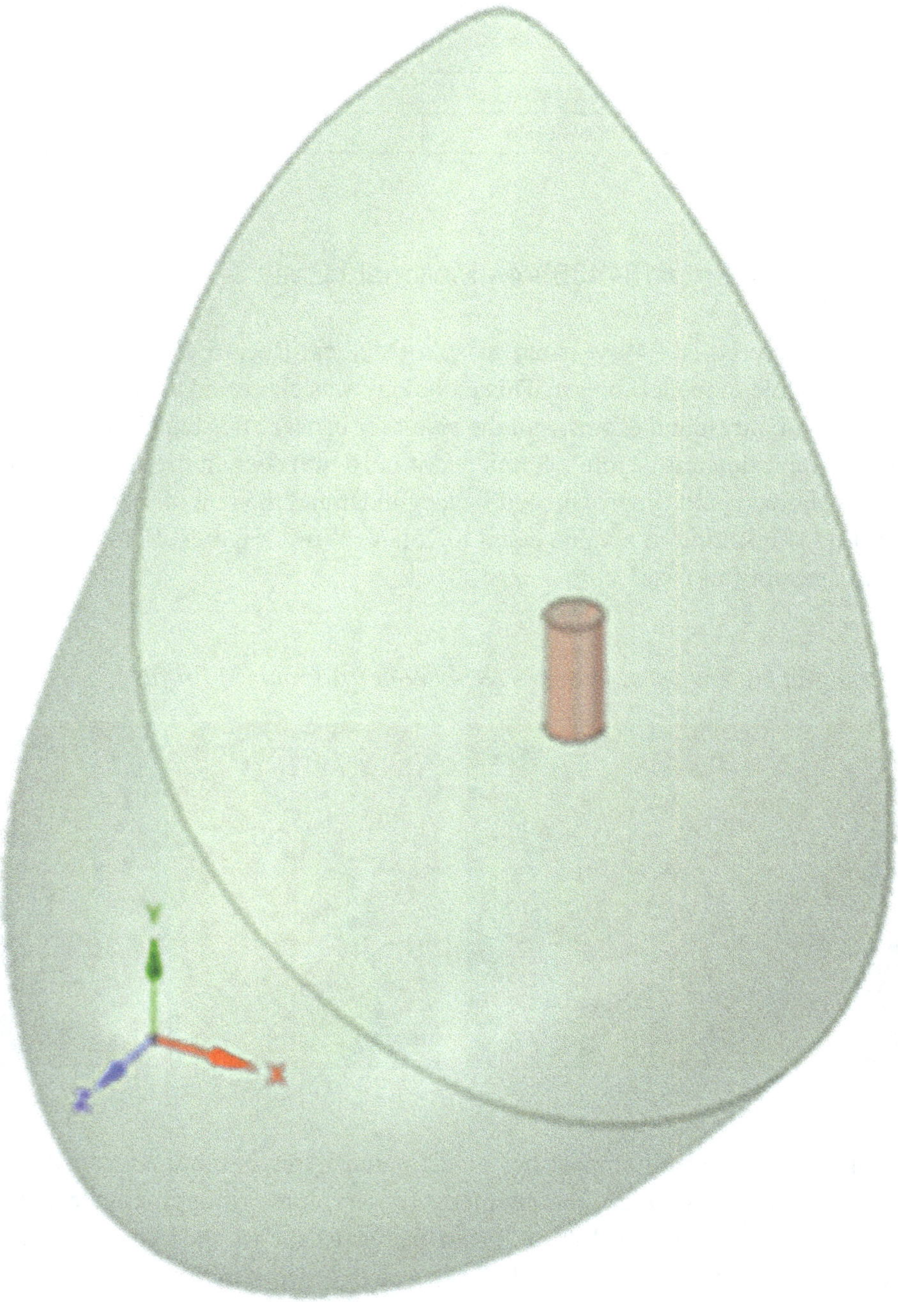

To analyze the influence of the thermal conductivities of the breast tissue and the tumor on the surface temperature profile of the breast, the associated sensitivity coefficients were also analyzed. In an identical way to the previous case, a vertical curve was used passing through the point of maximum surface temperature, as illustrated in Figure 24. Figure 25 presents the results for the sensitivity coefficients of the thermal conductivities.

Table 8. Convergence of the mesh of Patient #1844369-4

Mesh	No. of nodules	Maximum Temperature (°C)
1	240,296	35.37
2	338,357	35.43
3	459,084	35.46
4	560,079	35.47

Source: (Melo et al., 2019).

The result of the sensitivity analysis indicates that thermal conductivities can be estimated simultaneously, due to their linear independence. After solving the proposed inverse problem, the results obtained are shown in Table 9. Observing the estimates of each case, it is noticed that as the patient ages, the average thermal conductivity of the breast becomes lower. This characteristic occurs due to the substitution of glandular tissue with adipose tissue. Regarding the tumor, both results identified values above those found for benign changes.

In addition to the two cases presented here in detail, properties were estimated for seven other patients.

Table 10 presents a summary of the results of the estimated properties for such patients, as well as the sizes and types of breast nodules, and the age of the patients.

DEVELOPMENT OF AN EMPIRICAL CORRELATION BETWEEN THE PATIENT'S AGE AND THE THERMAL CONDUCTIVITY OF THE BREAST

An empirical correlation between the patient's age and the thermal conductivity of the breast was proposed to obtain a first estimate of the patient's thermal conductivity according to her age. The degree of breast tissue replacement with age is very often reported on mammograms and is done by using visual inspection, there being no correlation whatsoever in the literature that allows an objective assessment of the substitution referred to.

In Figure 26, it can be verified that the points that represent the estimated thermal conductivity are around the regression line, with the exception of the point corresponding to the age of 90 years, due to the fact of it being considered that the breast of a 90-year-old patient consisted entirely of fat. Nevertheless, the linear regression model can reliably predict a value for the thermal conductivity of the breast, since the value of the determination coefficient r^2 is 0.83083.

Using data of the first seven patients from Table 10, the regression line was determined (Equation 15):

$$k_B = 0.63702 - 0.0041124 \, . I_{years} \quad (15)$$

where, I_{years} is the patient's age in years and k_B is obtained in W/m oC. Patients # 8 and # 9 were added later and will be used to evaluate the linear regression obtained.

Figure 23. Calculated temperature profile (°C) of the geometric model of Patient #1844369-4. (a) Front view (b) Profile view.
Source: (Melo et al., 2019).

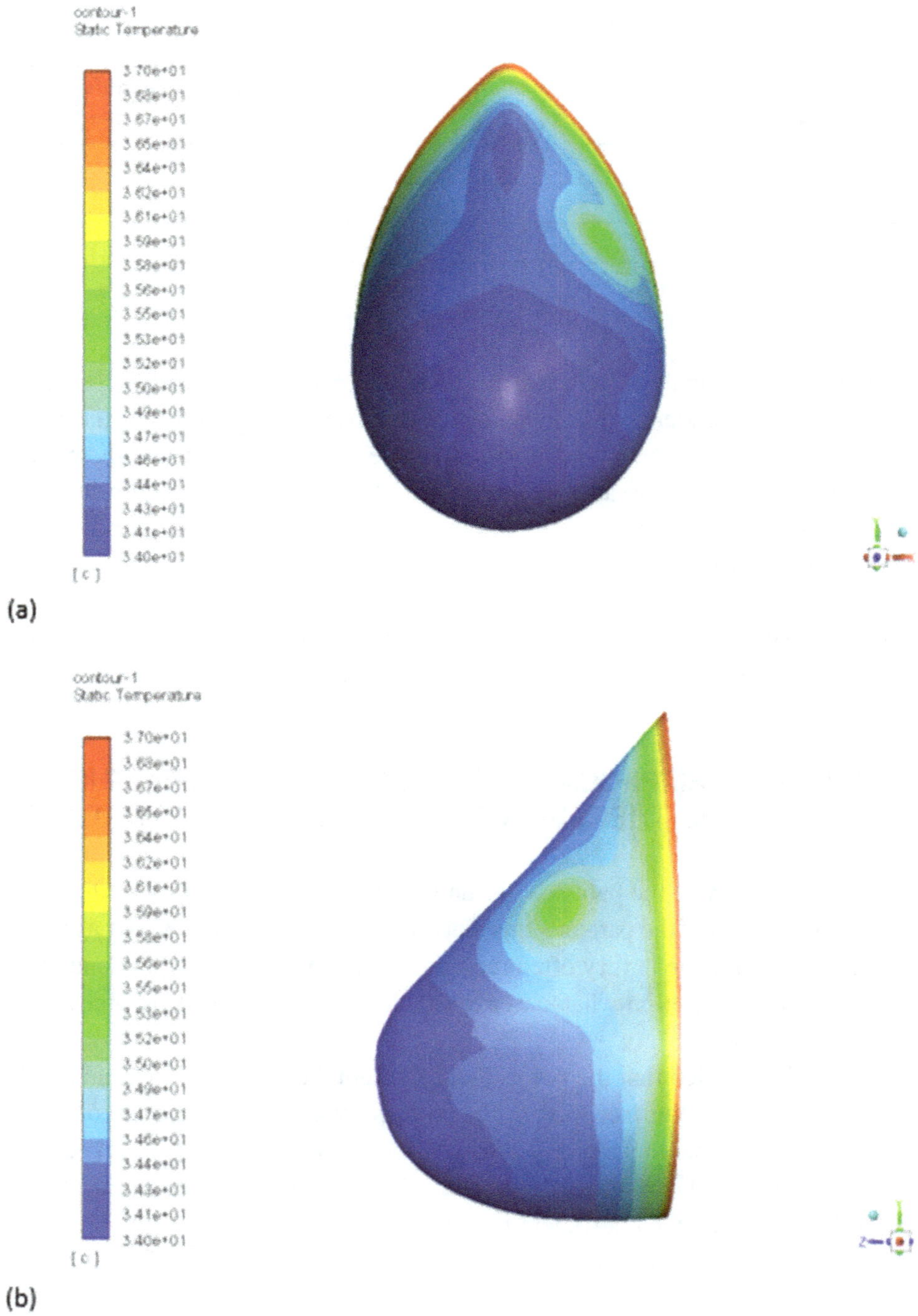

Figure 24. Vertical line used for sensitivity analysis of Patient # 1844369-4
Source: (Melo et al., 2019).

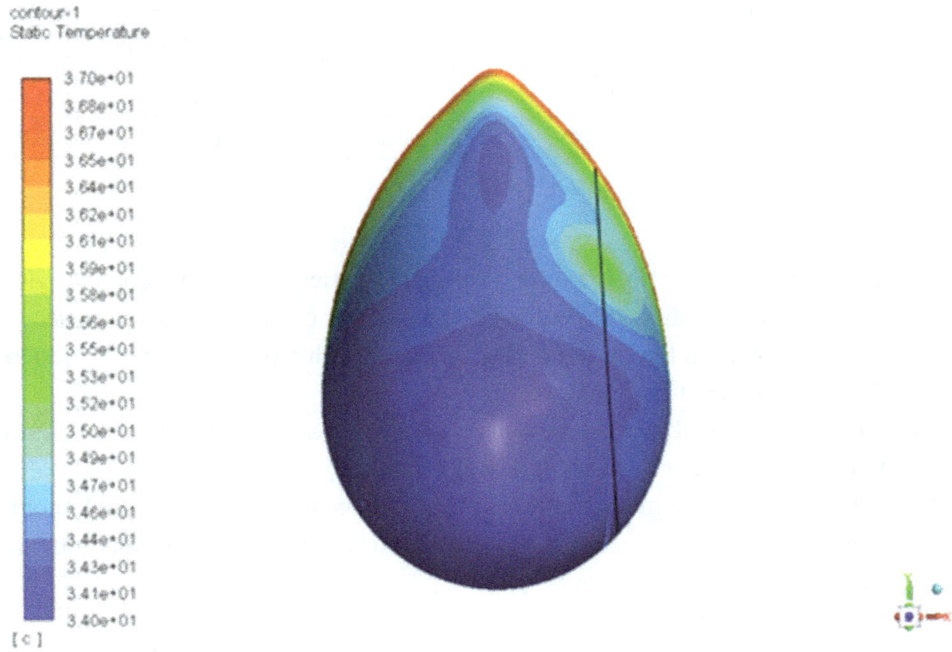

Figure 25. Sensitivity curve of the thermal conductivities of Patient #1844369-4
Source: (Melo et al., 2019).

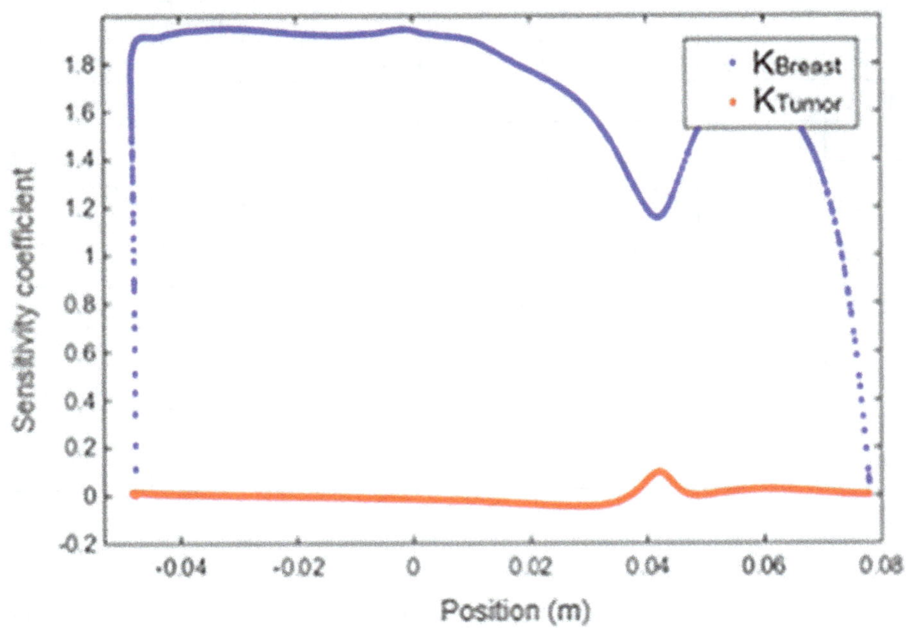

Table 9. Estimate of the thermal conductivities of Patient #1844369-4.

Parameter	Reference (Table 3)	Bezerra (2013)		Presente trabalho	
		Estimate	Percentage Difference	Estimate	Percentage Difference
k_{mama} ($W.m^{-1}.K^{-1}$)	0.48	0.4672	2.67%	0.4169	13.15%
k_{tumor} ($W.m^{-1}.K^{-1}$)	0.48	0.6143	27.98%	0.5932	19.08%

Source: (Melo et al., 2019).

Using the empirical correlation (Eq.15) for a 34-year-old patient, a thermal conductivity of 0.4972 W/m°C was obtained. Figure 27 shows the temperature profiles calculated for the patient when what were used were the value found in the literature, the estimated value of the thermal conductivity of the breast and that calculated by the empirical correlation.

The empirical correlation (Eq. 15) was assessed for four new patients who were outside the group of patients adopted to obtain the linear regression model (Table 11).

In the table, T (IR) is the maximum temperature obtained from the IR image in the tumor region; T_{Cor} is the maximum temperature calculated using k_B - empirical correlation; T_{Ref} is the maximum temperature calculated using k_B - [Ng (2001); Gautherie [43]].

Source: (Bezerra et al., 2020).

A 43-year-old patient with fibroadenoma located in the lower external quadrant of the right breast was analyzed. The ultrasound data were used for numerical simulation. The dimensions of the nodules were 3.7 cm × 0.8 cm × 3.4 cm and were located 1 cm from the skin surface, close to the nipple.

Table 10. Estimates of the thermophysical properties of the patients under study.

	Age	Anomaly	Size (cm)	Design variables			
				k_B (W/m°C)	k_T(W/m°C)	ω_B (s^{-1})	ω_T (s^{-1})
Patient #1	49	Malignant	1.7 × 0.8	0.467	0.614	0.000177	0.00915
Patient #1	49	Cyst	2.7 × 1.6	0.459	0.274	—	—
Patient #2	54	Malignant	2.8 × 2.2 & 2.8 × 1.6	0.422	0.497	0.00013	0.0062
Patient #3	27	Benign	2.3 × 1.5	0.483	0.500	0.000196	0.0023
Patient #4	34	Benign	1.3	0.485	—	0.000191	—
Patient #5	55	Benign	0.5 × 0.3 & 0.7 × 0.4	0.463	—	0.000137	—
Patient #6	69	Benign	2.1 × 1.7 × 1.0	0.375	—	0.000135	—
Patient #7	32	Benign	0.6 × 0.4	0.481	—	0.000176	—
Patient #8	43	Benign	3.7 x 0.8 x 3.4	0.453	—	—	—
Patient #9	46	Benign	1.3 & 1.1	0.431	—	—	—

Source: (Bezerra et al., 2020)

Using the empirical correlation (Eq. (15), the thermal conductivity of the calculated breast was 0.4602 W/m °C. Fig. 28 shows the temperature profiles calculated for the patient when using three different values for thermal conductivity: the one found in the literature, the value estimated by the inverse method in this study and the value calculated by the new empirical correlation In this figure, the region (- 0.014 to 0.078 m) is the region where the tumor is located. The maximum temperature obtained by the numerical solution, using the values of the thermal conductivity of the breast, calculated by the empirical correlation, was 34.48°C. The maximum temperature measured by thermography was 34.42°C, showing a difference of 0.06° C between those values.

Figure 26. Linear regression line between the thermal conductivity of the patients' breasts and age.
Source: (Bezerra et al., 2020).

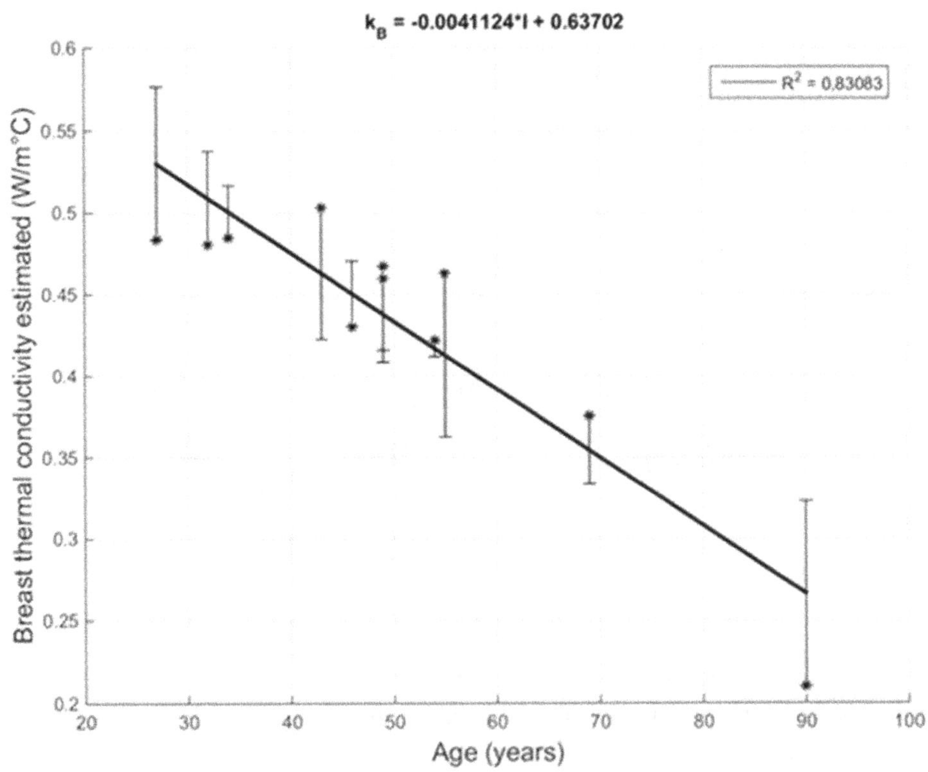

CONCLUSION

Reliable thermophysical properties for different breast tissues and nodules are not easily found. Due to this fact, the use of optimization methods in estimating these properties is an interesting approach. The main objective of using the methodology presented in this chapter is to estimate the thermophysical properties of the breast and mammary nodules, based on infrared (IR) or thermographic images of patients of the Outpatients Clinic of Mastology of the Hospital das Clínicas of the Federal University of Pernambuco (HC/UFPE), Brazil.

Figure 27. Temperature profiles calculated using three different values: the value found in the literature (Ng (2001); Gautherie (1980)); the value estimated by this paper and the value calculated by the empirical correlation for Patient #1301345-4
Source: (Bezerra et al., 2020).

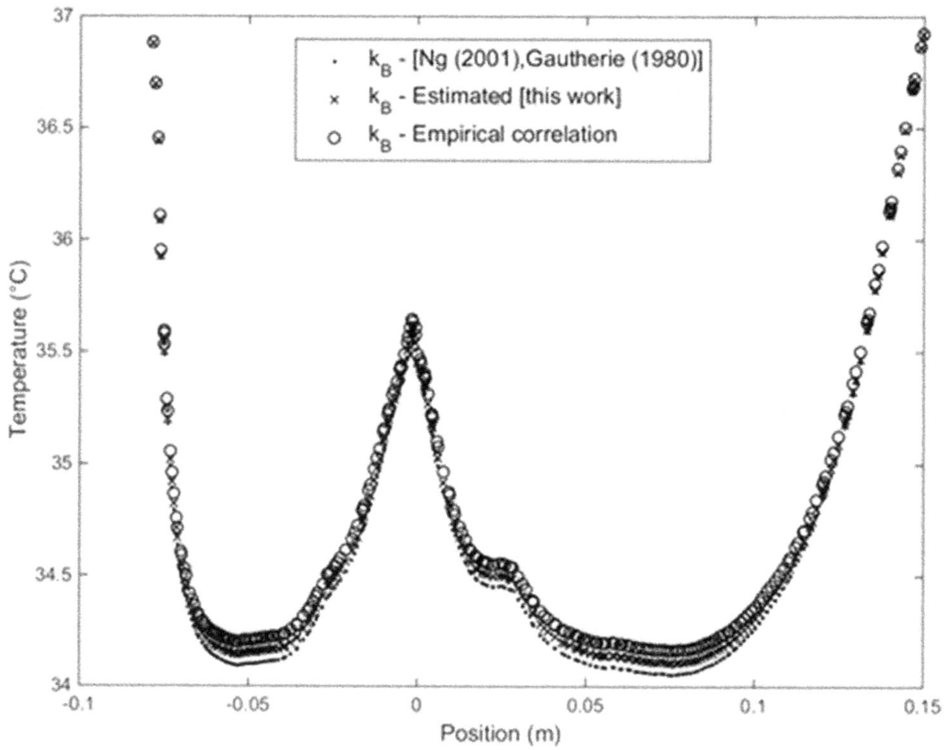

In this chapter, a new methodology was also presented for the construction of a personalized breast substitute geometry for each patient based on their thermographic images. Even though it was extracted manually, the profile curve of the female breast proved to be a viable alternative to approximate the mammary geometry to the real anatomy of the organ, given that the volumetric validation demonstrated a good approximation between the object used and its constructed three-dimensional geometry.

Table 11. Evaluation of the empirical correlation for the thermal conductivity of the breast.

	Age	Anomaly	Size (cm)	k_B(Eq.(15)	$T_{(IR)}$ (°C)	T_{Cor} (°C)	T_{Ref} (°C)
Patient #8	43	Benign	3.7 x 0.8 x 3.4	0.4602	34.42	34.48	34.94
Patient #9	46	Benign	1.3 & 1.1	0.4479	34.47	34.51	34.53
Patient #10	42	Malignant	4.0 x 2.8 x 1.0	0.4677	34.9	35.08	35.19
Patient #11	58	Benign	0.8 x 0.3	0.4008	34.49	34.52	34.71
Patient #11	58	Benign	0.7 x 0.4 & 0.7 x 0.3	0.4008	34.89	34.88	35.07

Figure 28. Temperature profiles were calculated using three different values: the value found in the literature (Ng (2001); Gautherie, 1980)); the one estimated by this study and the one calculated by the empirical correlation for Patient #08 (Table 11).
Source: (Bezerra et al., 2020).

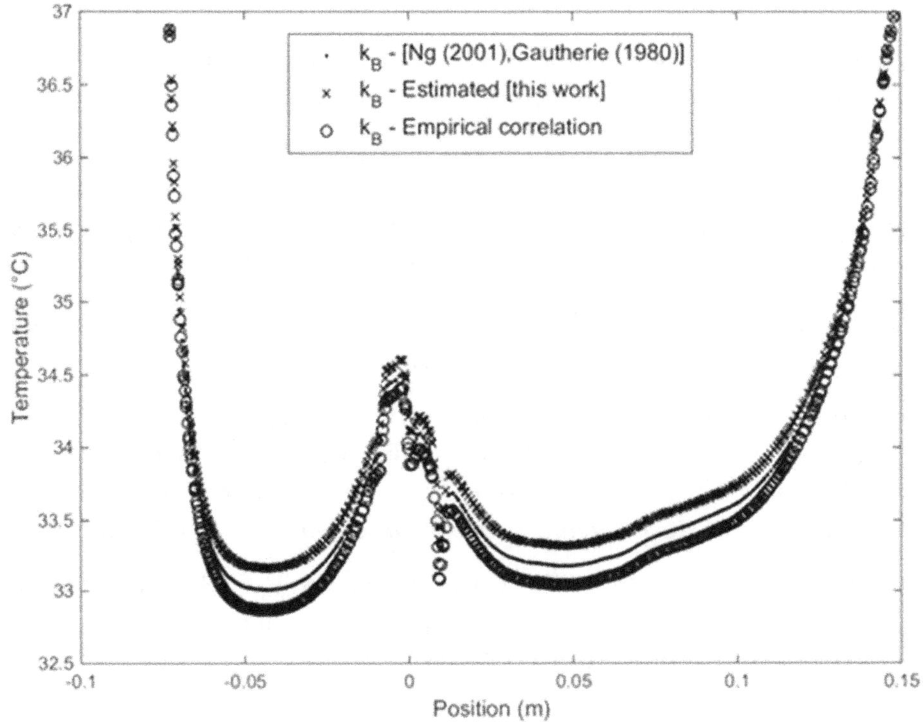

With the new developed geometry, breast temperature profiles were calculated. The cases presented here are a first attempt to estimate thermophysical properties using the SQP optimization method. The results showed that it is possible to determine these parameters satisfactorily despite use being made of the maximum temperature of the thermography, located on the skin surface, approximately over the tumor region.

Using some of the patients previously analyzed by Bezerra (2013) and varying only the geometric modeling, this study was able to estimate the thermal conductivities of their breasts and nodules, demonstrating that geometry can be an influential factor in the numerical simulations of breast temperature profiles.

The results of the estimates of the thermophysical parameters showed a smaller relative error for the youngest patient when compared with the values obtained in the literature. It is believed that this fact may be related to the amount of fat in the breast given that glandular tissue is substituted with adipose tissue as patients grow older.

According to the results presented, since the thermal conductivity of the breast has a great influence on the surface temperature of the breast, an empirical correlation has been proposed to determine this parameter according to the patient's age. The recalculated temperature results, using this correlation, were satisfactory.

REFERENCES

Acharya, U. R., Ng, E. Y. K., Tan, J. H., & Sree, S. V. (2012). Thermography based breast cancer detection using texture features and support vector machine. *Journal of Medical Systems*, *36*(3), 1503–1510. doi:10.100710916-010-9611-z PMID:20957511

Agnelli, J. P., Barrea, A. A., & Turner, C. V. (2011). Tumor location and parameter estimation by thermography. *Mathematical and Computer Modelling*, *53*(7-8), 1527–1534. doi:10.1016/j.mcm.2010.04.003

Araújo, M. C., Bezerra, L. A., Santos, L. C., Rolim, T. L., Santos, T. B., Lyra, P. R. M., & Lima, R. C. F. (2008). *Instrumentation and acquisition of the three-dimensional geometry of the breast of a phantom: comparison of temperatures calculated numerically and measured by thermographic imaging*. In *Annals of XXIX Iberian Latin-American Congress on Computational Methods in Engineering*, Maceió, Brazil.

Bezerra, L. A. (2013). *Estimativa de parâmetros termofísicos da mama utilizando método inverso* (Unpublished doctoral thesis). Universidade Federal de Pernambuco, Recife, Brazil.

Bezerra, L. A., Oliveira, M. M., Araújo, M. C., Viana, L. C., Santos, M. J. A., Santos, F. G. S., Rolim, T. L., Lyra, P. R. M., Lima, R. C. F., Borschartt, T. B., Resmini, R., & Conci, A. (2013b). Infrared Imaging for Breast Cancer Detection with Proper Selection of Properties: From Acquisition Protocol to Numerical Simulation. In *Multimodality Breast Imaging: Diagnosis and Treatment* (Vol. PM227). SPIE Press Book.

Bezerra, L. A., Oliveira, M. M., Rolim, T. L., Conci, A., Santos, F. G. S., Lyra, P. R. M., & Lima, R. C. F. (2013a). Estimation of breast tumor thermal properties using infrared images. *Signal Processing*, *93*(10), 2851–2863. doi:10.1016/j.sigpro.2012.06.002

Bezerra, L. A., Ribeiro, R. R., Lyra, P. R. M., & Lima, R. C. F. (2020). An empirical correlation to estimate thermal properties of the breast and of the breast nodule using thermographic images and optimization techniques. *International Journal of Heat and Mass Transfer*, *149*, 149. doi:10.1016/j.ijheatmasstransfer.2019.119215

Blackwell, B. F. (1989). Sensitivity analysis and uncertainty propagation of computational models. In W. J. Minkowywcz, E. M. Sparrow, & J. Y. Murthy (Eds.), *Handbook of numerical heat transfer* (2nd ed., pp. 53–71). J. Skilling.

Chang, C. L., & Chang, M. (2009). M. Inverse determination of thermal conductivity using semi-discretization method. *Applied Mathematical Modelling*, *33*(3), 1644–1655. doi:10.1016/j.apm.2008.03.001

Char, M. I., Chang, F. P., & Tai, B. C. (2008). Inverse determination of thermal conductivity by differential quadrature method. *International Communications in Heat and Mass Transfer*, *35*(2), 113–119. doi:10.1016/j.icheatmasstransfer.2007.06.006

Charny, C. (1992). Mathematical models of bioheat equation. In Y. I. Cho (Ed.), *Advances in Heat Transfer: Bioengineering Heat Transfer* (Vol. 22, pp. 19–155). Academic Press, Inc., Kluwer Academic. doi:10.1016/S0065-2717(08)70344-7

Diller, K. R. (1982). Modeling of bioheat transfer processes at high and low temperatures. In Y. I. Cho (Ed.), *Advances in Heat Transfer: Bioengineering Heat Transfer* (Vol. 22, pp. 157–357). Academic Press, Inc. doi:10.1016/S0065-2717(08)70345-9

El-Bastawissi, A. Y., White, E., Mandelson, M. T., & Taplin, S. (2001). Variation in mammographic breast density by race. *AEP*, *11*(4), 257–263. doi:10.1016/S1047-2797(00)00225-8 PMID:11306344

El-Bastawissi, A. Y., White, E., Mandelson, M. T., & Taplin, S. (2010). Can mammographic assessments lead to consider density as a risk factor for breast cancer. *European Journal of Radiology*. Advance online publication. doi:10.1016/j.ejrad.2010.01.001 PMID:20133095

Engl, H. W., Hanke, M., & Neubauer, A. (1996). *Regularization of inverse problems: Mathematics and its appplication*. Kluwer. doi:10.1007/978-94-009-1740-8

EtehadTavakol, M., Chandran, V., Ng, E. Y. K., & Kafieh, R. (2013). Breast cancer detection from thermal images using bispectral invariant features. *International Journal of Thermal Sciences*, 1–16.

Fluent. (2005). *Fluent 6.2 - User's Guide*. FLUENT Inc.

Fortuna, A. D. (2000). *O. Técnicas computacionais para dinâmica dos fluidos: conceitos básicos e aplicações*. Ed. Edusp.

Gautherie, M. (1980). Thermopathology of breast cancer: Measurements and analysis of in vivo temperature and blood flow. *Annals of the New York Academy of Sciences*, *335*(1 Thermal Chara), 383–415. doi:10.1111/j.1749-6632.1980.tb50764.x PMID:6931533

Gonzalez, F. (2007). Thermal simulation of breast tumors. *Revista Mexicana de Física*, *53*(4), 323–326.

Huang, C., & Huang, C. (2007). An inverse problem in estimating simultaneously the effective thermal conductivity and volumetric heat capacity of biological tissue. *Applied Mathematical Modelling*, *31*(9), 1785–1797. doi:10.1016/j.apm.2006.06.002

Jiang, L., Zhan, W., & Loew, M. H. (2011). Modeling static and dynamic thermography of the human breast under elastic deformation. *Physics in Medicine and Biology*, *56*(1), 187–202. doi:10.1088/0031-9155/56/1/012 PMID:21149948

Kim, S. K., Jung, B. S., Kim, H. J., & Lee, W. I. (2003). Inverse estimation of thermophysical properties for anisotropic composite. *Experimental Thermal and Fluid Science*, *24*(6), 697–704. doi:10.1016/S0894-1777(02)00309-6

Lahiri, B. B., Bagavathiappan S., Jayakumar T., & Philip, J. (2012) Medical applications of infrared thermography: A review. *International Journal Infrared Physics and Technology*, 222-232.

Liu, F. B., & Ozisik, M. N. (1995). Simultaneous estimation of fluid thermal conductivity and heat capacity in laminar duct flow. *Fluid Thermal Conductivity and Heat Capacity*, *333*(B), 583–591.

Maliska, C. R. (1995). *Transferência de calor e Mecânica dos fluidos computacional*. Ed. LTC.

Melo, J. R. F., Queiroz, J. R. A., Bezerra, L. A., & Lima, R. C. F. (2019). Development of a three-dimensional surrogate geometry of the breast and its use in estimating the thermal conductivities of breast tissue and breast lesions based on infrared images. *International Communications in Heat and Mass Transfer*, 108.

Mital, M. (2008). Breast tumor simulation and parameters estimation using evolucionary algorithms. *Modelling and Simulation in Engineering*, *10*(1), 7–14.

Mitra, S., & Balaji, C. (1992). A neural network based estimation of tumor parameters from a breast thermogram. *Modelling and Simulation in Engineering*, *10*(1), 7–14.

Ng, E. Y. K., & Sudarshan, N. M. (2001). Effect of blood flow, tumor and cold stress in a female breast: A novel time-accurate computer simulation. Proc. Instn Mech Enghs. *Part H*, *215*, 393–404. PMID:11521762

Ng, E. Y. K., & Sudarshan, N. M. (2001b). An improved three-dimensional direct numerical modelling and thermal analysis of a female breast with tumour. *Proceedings - Institution of Mechanical Engineers*, *215*(1), 25–36. doi:10.1243/0954411011533508 PMID:11323983

Ng, E. Y. K., & Sudarshan, N. M. (2004). Computer simulation in conjunction with medical thermography as an adjunct tool for early detection of breast cancer. *BMC Cancer*, *4*(17), 1–6. doi:10.1186/1471-2407-4-17 PMID:15113442

Nocedal, J., & Wright, S. J. (2006). Numerical Optimization. Springer.

Osman, M. M., & Afify, E. (1988). Thermal modeling of the malignant woman's breast. *Journal of Biomechanical Engineering*, *110*(4), 269–276. doi:10.1115/1.3108441 PMID:3205011

Partridge, P. W., & Wrobel, L. C. (2007). An inverse geometry problem for the localization of skin tumours by thermal analysis. *Engineering Analysis with Boundary Elements*, *31*(10), 803–811. doi:10.1016/j.enganabound.2007.02.002

Paruch, M., & Majchrzak, E. (2007). Identification of tumor region parameters using evolutionary algorithm and multiple reciprocity boundary element method. *Engineering Applications of Artificial Intelligence*, *20*(5), 647–655. doi:10.1016/j.engappai.2006.11.003

Pennes, H. H. (1948). Analysis of tissue and arterial blood temperature in the resting human forearm. *Journal of Applied Physiology*, *1*(2), 93–122. doi:10.1152/jappl.1948.1.2.93 PMID:18887578

Santos, L. C. (2009). *Desenvolvimento de ferramenta computacional para análise paramétrica da influência da posição e do tamanho de um tumor de mama em perfis de temperatura* (Master's thesis). Universidade Federal de Pernambuco, Recife, Brasil. Retrieved from https://repositorio.ufpe.br/handle/123456789/5021

Schaefer, G., Závišek, M., & Nakashima, T. (2009). Thermography based breast cancer analysis using statistical features and fuzzy classification. *Pattern Recognition*, *47*(6), 1133–1137. doi:10.1016/j.patcog.2008.08.007

Silva Neto, A. J., & Moura Neto, F. D. (2005). *Problemas Inversos - Conceitos fundamentais e aplicações*. Ed. UERJ.

Sundberg, J., & Hellstrom, G. (2009). Inverse modelling of thermal conductivity from temperature measurements at the prototype repository, aspo hrl. *International Journal of Rock Mechanics and Mining Sciences*, *46*(6), 1029–1041. doi:10.1016/j.ijrmms.2009.01.012

Tavakol, M. E., Lucas, C., Sadri, S., & Ng, E. Y. K. (2010). Analysis of Breast Thermography, an Objective Tool to Establish Possible Difference between Malignant or Benign Pattern Using Fractal Dimension. *Journal of Healthcare Engineering*, *1*(1), 27–43. doi:10.1260/2040-2295.1.1.27

Teles, M. L. & Gomes, H. M. (2010). Genetic algorithms and sequential quadratic programming comparisons for optimizing engineering problems. *Teoria e prática na Engenharia Civil, 15*, 29–39. (in Portuguese)

Udesc, U. (2007). *Câncer de mama*. Available in: https://www.joinville.udesc.br/processamentodeimagens/oCanc/oCanc.html

Viana, M. J. A. (2010). *Simulating the temperature profile in the breast using surrogate geometry obtained from an external breast prosthesis* (Master's thesis). Universidade Federal de Pernambuco, Recife, Brasil. Retrieved from https://repositorio.ufpe.br/handle/123456789/17939

Wissler, E. H. (1998). Pennes'1948 paper revisited. *Journal of Applied Physiology, 85*(1), 35–41. doi:10.1152/jappl.1998.85.1.35 PMID:9655751

Yang, L., Deng, Z. C., Yu, J. N., & Luo, G. W. (2009). Optimization method for the inverse problem of reconstructing the source term in a parabolic equation. *Mathematics and Computers in Simulation, 80*(2), 314–326. doi:10.1016/j.matcom.2009.06.031

Chapter 13
The Efforts of Deep Learning Approaches for Breast Cancer Detection Based on X-Ray Images

Aras Masood Ismael
Sulaimani Polytechnic University, Iraq

Juliana Carneiro Gomes
Universidade Federal de Pernambuco, Brazil

ABSTRACT

In this chapter, deep learning-based approaches, namely deep feature extraction, fine-tuning of pre-trained convolutional neural networks (CNN), and end-to-end training of a developed CNN model, are used to classify the malignant and normal breast X-ray images. For deep feature extraction, pre-trained deep CNN models such as ResNet18, ResNet50, ResNet101, VGG16, and VGG19 are used. For classification of the deep features, the support vector machines (SVM) classifier is used with various kernel functions namely linear, quadratic, cubic, and Gaussian, respectively. The aforementioned pre-trained deep CNN models are also used in fine-tuning procedure. A new CNN model is also proposed in end-to-end training fashion. The classification accuracy is used as performance measurements. The experimental works show that the deep learning has potential in detection of the breast cancer from the X-ray images. The deep features that are extracted from the ResNet50 model and SVM classifier with linear kernel function produced 94.7% accuracy score which the highest among all obtained.

DOI: 10.4018/978-1-7998-3456-4.ch013

INTRODUCTION

The Correct clarification of thyroid gland is very important for the diagnosis of breast infections. Breast is the most important part in the body for women's to be safe against any infections, and the diagnosis for treatment will help radiologist to decide faster. Working with the breast has an influence on most women's body organs.

Currently, malignant is a massive public health issue around the globe. According to the International Agency for Research on Cancer (IARC) Keller, et al (2012). Part of the World Health Organization (WHO), there is 8.2 million passing away caused by cancer in 2012 and 27 million of new cases of this disease are predicted to occur until 2030 [26]. The status of developing medicinal solution for the breast cancer classification allows medical specialists to obtain perfect datasets that guides their decision-making procedure. Analysis of the ANN Multi-Layer Perceptron depicts the neurons coordination within the breast nodules.

Cancer can be diagnosed by classifying lumps in two different types such as benign and malignant. Benign lumps represent an unusual outgrowth but rarely lead to a patient's passing away; yet, some types of benign tumors, too, can increase the probability of developing malignancy Kinzler et al.(1996). On the other hand, malignant lumps are more thoughtful and their timely diagnosis contributes to a successful action. As a result, diagnosis and predication of malignancy can boost the chances of treatment, decreasing the typically high costs of medical dealings for such patients Steyeberg et, al (2008)..

Breast cancer (BC) is the most commonly identified cancer and the principal cause of death for women in globe. Excluding cancer of skin, breast cancer is the second most common cancer in women Siegel et al (2011). in addition, the humanity of breast cancer is very high when associated to other types of cancer Miller et al (2016).Breast cancer, similar to other malignancies, starts with a rapid and uncontrolled outgrowth and multiplication of a fragment of the breast tissue, which depending on its potential damage, is divided into malignant and benign types.

Artificial Neural Network approaches helps medical doctors to diagnose diseases with a higher degree of proficiency, while minimizing inspection cost and time, as well as avoiding unnecessary excisional biopsy procedures. However, ANN systems not only allow a better imagining of mammograms, but also using different digital image processing (DIP), information discovery from data (KDD), artificial intelligence (AI) techniques such artificial neural networks (ANN) allow to preselect certain regions of interests (ROIs) for later analysis by the radiologists.

The contribution of this paper is as following;

A novel application of the deep learning on breast cancer detection is carried out based on the X-ray breast images. The remainder of this paper is as following. The next section gives the materials and methods that are used to in this work. CNN, and ELM, The methodology of the work is briefly introduced in this section too. Section 3 describes the experimental works and results. Section 4 gives the conclusions.

RELATED WORK

Artificial Neural Network (ANN) can be extensively used to analyze breast Infection and develop accurate diagnostics about the infections. Most researchers have been using ANN to develop solutions that enable medical practitioners too accurately and diagnose breast Infections. During developing optimal solutions, it's mandatory for computer scientists to determine the best log sigmoid activation functions, the series of layers (input and hidden layers) and Multi-Layer Perceptron's (MLP).

Umer et al (2019) In their study, they used several algorithms to diagnose Breast Disease Such as k nearest neighbors, Support vector machine, Decision tree and Naïve bayes, Among the algorithms used, the Sport Vector Machine obtained the best results from which all other approaches, the data used in the study were collected at a hospital in Kashmir, the highest test accuracy achieved in this study was 98.89% .

Li, x Zhan et al (2019 Proposed DCNN, multi-cohort, diagnostic find out about using ultrasound images sets from three hospitals in China. We developed and trained the DCNN model on the training set, 131 731 ultrasound pictures from 17627 patients with thyroid cancer and 180668 pictures from 25325 controls from the thyroid imaging database at Tianjin Cancer Hospital. Clinical diagnosis of the training set was once made through sixteen radiologists from Tianjin Cancer Hospital. Images from anatomical sites that had been judged as now not having most cancers have been excluded from the coaching set and solely individuals with suspected thyroid most cancers underwent pathological examination to verify diagnosis. The model's diagnostic performance was validated in an inner validation set from Tianjin Cancer Hospital (8606 pictures from 1118 patients) and two exterior datasets in China (the Integrated Traditional Chinese and Western Medicine Hospital, Jilin, 741 pictures from 154 patients; and the Weihai Municipal Hospital, Shandong, 11 039 images from 1420 patients). All persons with suspected thyroid most cancers after clinical examination in the validation sets had pathological examination. We also compared the specificity and sensitivity of the DCNN mannequin with the overall performance of six skilled thyroid ultrasound radiologists on the three validation sets. They obtained 0·889 test accuracy, 0·922 test Sensitivity and 0·856 Specificity using DCNN Li, X., Zhang et al (2019).

Rastogi et al(2014) proposed MLNN, they collected samples from hospital and worked in three different case for find out the impact of neural network against thyroid disease, the collected samples was T3, T4 and TSH, and applied to neural network in three different class types the experimental result showed that the MLNN can have advantage over such disease.

MATERIALS AND METHODS

The proposed method is illustrated in Fig. 1. As seen in Fig. 1, the X-ray chest images are used as input to the proposed breast cancer detection method. The input X-ray breast images are initially resized to 224×224 for being compatible with the CNN models. As mentioned earlier, three deep learning approaches namely deep feature extraction from pre-trained deep networks, fine-tuning of a pre-trained CNN model and end-to-end training of a CNN model are considered.

Figure 1. The illustration of the proposed methodology for Breast diagnosing

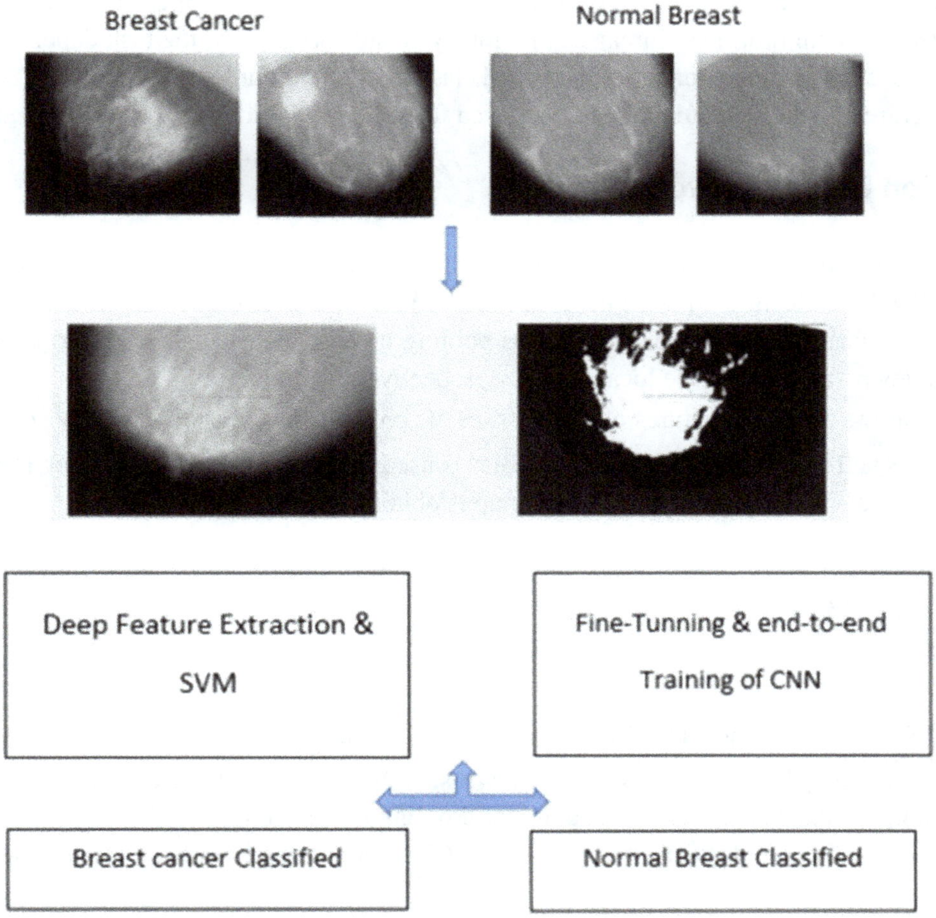

For both deep feature extraction and fine-tuning procedures, the ResNet18, ResNet50, ResNet101, VGG16 and VGG19 are used. For training of the deep features, the SVM classifier is used with various kernel functions namely linear, quadratic, cubic and Gaussian, respectively. A 21-layered new CNN model is also proposed and trained in the end-to-end training fashion. The proposed network model starts with input layer and there are five convolutions layers, five ReLu layers and five batch normalization layers, respectively. Two pooling layers are used after the first and second ReLu layers, respectively. A fully connected layer, softmax layer and classification layer are also used in the end of model.

Deep Transfer Learning

The procedure of deep feature extraction and fine-tuning of pre-trained CNN models is defined as deep transfer learning (DTL). While having a limited number of training images, DTL helps us to use deep learning in our own image classification task Pan et al (2009). DTL concept transfers a knowledge from the source domain where there are lots of training samples, to the target domain where there are considerably low samples when compared with the source domain. Thus, efficient image classification can be achieved with the support of the large dataset from the source domain. In deep learning prospective, especially in CNN aspect, the DTL is defined as transferring some layers of a pre-trained CNN model which was trained with millions of images, previously. More specifically, the task dependent layers of the CNN model such as fully connected layers and classification output layer are removed from the network architecture and the remaining layers are saved for the new classification task Deniz, et al (2018).

Convolution Neural Networks

A sequence of convolution, normalization and pooling layers are used to construct the main building blocks of a CNN architecture Qi, Z., Tian et al (2013). While the convolution layers are responsible to extract the local features, the normalization and pooling layers are responsible to normalize the local features and down-sampling of the local features, respectively.

Let X_i^{l-1} shows the local features obtained from the previous layers and k_{ij}^l and b_j^l denote the adjustable kernels and training bias, respectively. Bias is used to prevent over fitting during training of the CNN Başaran et al (2020). The output feature map is obtained in Eq. 1;

$$\mathrm{X}_j^l = \mathrm{f}\left(\sum_{i \in M_j} X_i^{l-1} * k_{ij}^l + b_j^l\right) \tag{1}$$

where, M_j and $f(.)$ denotes the input map selection and activation function, respectively. As mentioned earlier, pooling layer is employed for down-sampling of the feature maps. There are various pooling techniques namely average and maximum. Pooling layers are responsible to decrease the computational nodes and prevent the overfitting issue in CNN architecture Xu, et al (2017). The pooling is defined in Eq. 2;

$$\mathrm{X}_j^l = down\left(X_j^{l-1}\right) \tag{2}$$

where, the down-sampling is shown by the $down(.)$ function. It is worth noting that down-sampling provides an abstract of the local features for the next layer. The fully-connected (FC) layers have full connections to all of the activations in the previous layer. The FC layer provides discriminative features for the classification of the input image into its various classes.

Similar to the traditional machine learning techniques, the training of the CNN is carried out using an optimization process. Stochastic gradient descent with momentum (SGDM), and adaptive moment estimation (ADAM) are two well-known training methods for neural networks. The weights in the SGDM method are regularly updated for each training set to reach the goal Zeiler et al (2012). The optimization function is shown in Eq. 3;

$$V_t = \beta V_{t-1} + a\nabla_w L(W, X, y) \tag{3}$$

where, L, α and W indicates the loss function, learning rate, and the weights, respectively. During the training of the CNN, the new weights are calculated as follows;

$$W = W - aV_t \tag{4}$$

The ADAM optimizer, which also uses the average of the second moments of the slopes, updates the learning rate in each iteration and adopts the parameter learning rates based on the average first moment in the RMSProp method Shindjalova,et al (2014).

Support Vector Machines (SVM)

SVM, which was developed by Vapnik (Widodo & Yang, 2007), is a well-known classifier based on the structural risk reduction principle categorized in the supervised statistical learning theorem. The main idea of the SVM classifier is to determine an optimum hyper-plane between positive and negative samples (Qi, Tian & Shi, 2013). The linear separation of positive and negative samples can be handled by using the Eq. 5 (Adaminejad & Farjah, 2013);

$$f(x) = w^T x + b = 0 \tag{5}$$

where w indicates the weight vector and b is bias value that is used to determine the position of the hyper-plane. A kernel trick is employed to transfer the input data to another hyper-plane where the data is more convenient for linear separation. The best hyper-plane can be determined by using the following equation (Cheng & Bao, 2014);

$$\begin{cases} min\dfrac{w^2}{2} \\ y_i\left(w^T x_i + b\right) \geq 1 i = 1,2,\ldots,M \end{cases} \tag{6}$$

EXPERIMENTAL WORKS AND RESULTS

All coding were carried out with MATLAB software on a workstation equipped with the NVIDIA Quadro M4000 GPU with 8GB RAM. The X-ray breast images were collected from different sources (Outlier Detection DataSets, GitHub, & Kaggle). The labelling of the X-ray breast images was carried out by specialist doctors. The ODDS dataset contains 683 instances of 9 dimensionality, the matlignant class of this dataset is considered as outliers, while points in the benign class are considered inliers. And Github original dataset consisted of 162 whole mount slide images of Breast Cancer (BCa) specimens scanned at 40x. From that, 277,524 patches of size 224 x 224 were extracted (198,738 IDC negative and 78,786 IDC positive).

The X-ray breast images were re-sized to 224×224 for being compatible with the inputs of the CNN models. Some of the collected images were in gray scale and these images were converted to color image format by copying the gray scale image into all R, G and B channels, respectively. No other preprocessing methods were applied on the X-ray breast images. Five pre-trained CNN models namely, VGG16, VGG19, ResNet18, ResNet50 and ResNet101 were used in experiments. Moreover, SVM method with four kernel functions namely linear, quadratic, cubic, and Gaussian were considered in classification. The epsilon value of SVMs with the linear and quadratic kernel functions were set to 0.04 and 0.02, respectively. In cubic kernel SVM, the epsilon value was assigned to 0.01 and for Gaussian SVM, the epsilon parameters were set to 0.01. The classification accuracy score was used in performance evaluation. Table 1 shows the obtained accuracy scores. While the rows of the Table 1 show the SVM kernel types, the columns show the pre-trained CNN models. The last row and column show the average accuracy scores.

Table 1. The achievements of pre-trained deep CNN models and SVM classifiers on breast cancer detection

	Accuracy (%)					
Method: SVM	**ResNet18**	**ResNet50**	**ResNet101**	**VGG16**	**VGG19**	**Average**
Linear Kernel	86.3	94.7	88.4	89.5	88.4	89.5
Quadratic Kernel	87.4	91.6	89.5	89.5	87.4	89.1
Cubic Kernel	89.5	90.5	91.6	90.5	89.5	90.3
Gaussian Kernel	86.3	93.7	88.4	89.5	87.4	89.1
Average	87.4	92.6	89.5	89.8	88.1	

From Table 1, it was observed that ResNet50 model produced the highest average accuracy score, where the achievement was 92.6%. In addition, VGG16 model produced 89.8% average accuracy score, which the second best score. The ResNet101 model produced 89.5% average accuracy score. VGG19 and ResNet18 models produced 88.1% and 87.4% average accuracy scores, respectively. When the obtained results were observed from the view of kernel functions, it was seen that best average accuracy score 90.3% was produced by the Cubic kernel function. The second best average accuracy score 89.5% was produced by the linear kernel based SVM classifier. Quadratic and Gaussian kernels based SVM classifiers produced the identical 89.1% accuracy scores, respectively. From Table 1, it was also observed that the ResNet50 features and linear kernel SVM classifier produced the 94.7% accuracy score. This score was the highest among all achievements. The second best individual achievement 93.7% was also produced by the ResNet50 features and Gaussian kernel based SVM classifier. It is worth to mentioning that the worst accuracy score 86.3% were produced by the ResNet18 features and linear and Gaussian kernel functions. Confusion matrix is shown on Fig. 2.

Figure 2. The confusion matrix that was obtained for ResNet50 and linear SVM classifier

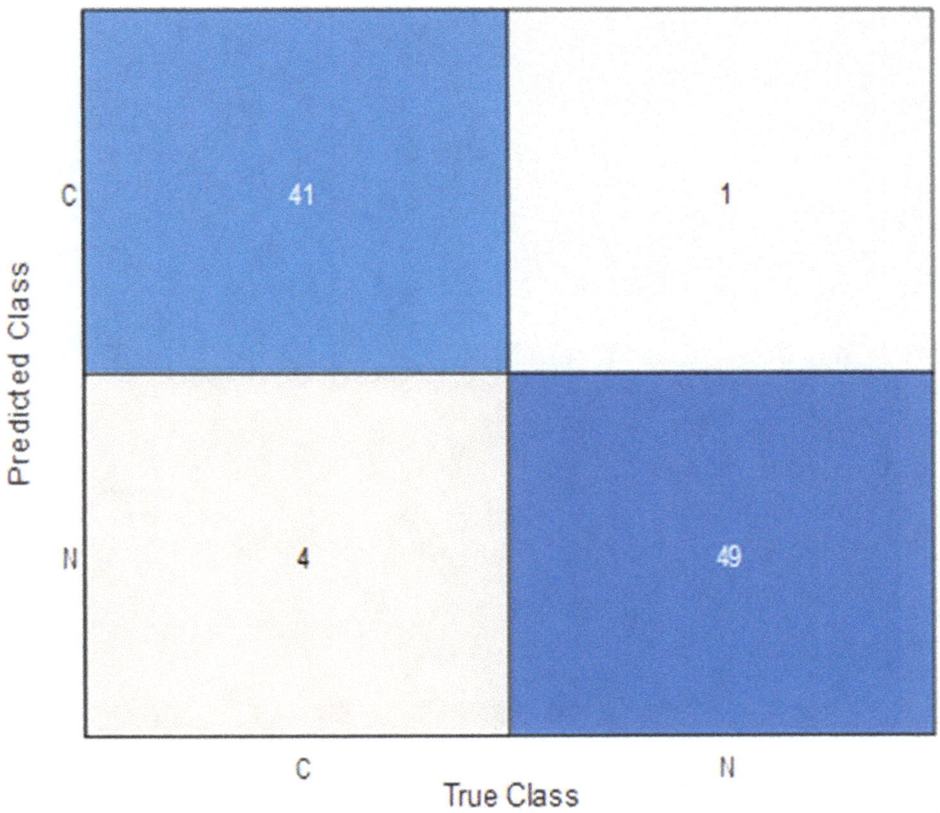

Fig. 2 shows the confusion matrix for ResNet50 features and Linear SVM classifier. The labels 'C' and 'N' show the breast cancer and normal breast cases, respectively. From Fig. 2, it is observed that while 41 breast cancer and 49 normal samples were classified correctly, 4 breast cancer and 1 normal samples were misclassified, respectively. The correct classification rate of the breast cancer samples was 91.11% and the correct classification rate of the normal cases was 98.0%.

Fig. 3 shows the training process of fine-tuning of the ResNet50 model. For fine-tuning and end-to-end training, the data augmentation was considered. The data augmentation was carried out by randomly rotating, shifting and flipping of the training images. The first row of Fig. 3 shows the training and average training accuracies (light-blue training (smoothed) and blue testing) and the second row of Fig. 3 shows the loss value for training samples (orange training (smoothed) and light-orange training). Table 2 gives the achievements of the fine-tuning of the pre-trained deep CNN models on breast classification.

Figure 3. The fine-tuning of ResNet50 model for Breast classification

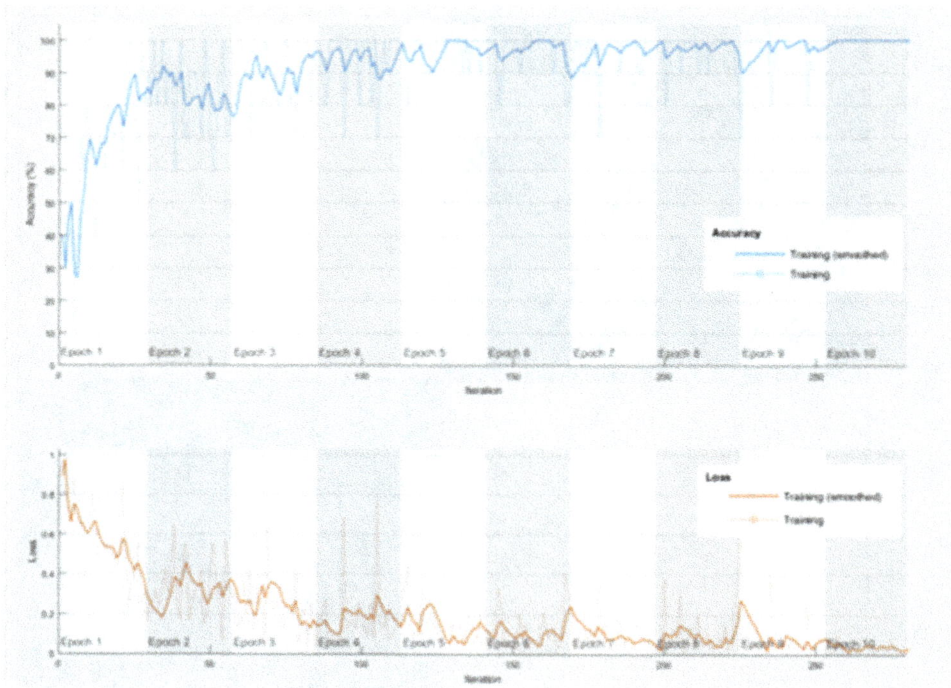

As seen in Table 2, all fine-tuned deep CNN models achieved classification accuracy scores above 85.00%. The highest accuracy score 92.63% was produced by the ResNet50 model. The second-best accuracy score 89.47% was obtained by the VGG19 model. Moreover, 88.42%, 87.37% and 85.26% accuracy scores were obtained by the ResNet18, ResNet101 and VGG16 models, respectively.

Table 2 The achievements of fine-tuning of pre-trained deep CNN models on Breast cancer classification

Fine-Tuning	Accuracy%
VGG16	85.26
ResNet18	88.42
ResNet50	92.63
ResNet101	87.37
VGG19	89.47

Fig. 4 shows the confusion matrix for fine-tuning of the ResNet50 model. From Fig. 4, it was observed that while 43 breast cancer and 45 normal samples were classified correctly.

Figure 4. The confusion matrix that was obtained by fine-tuning of ResNet50 model

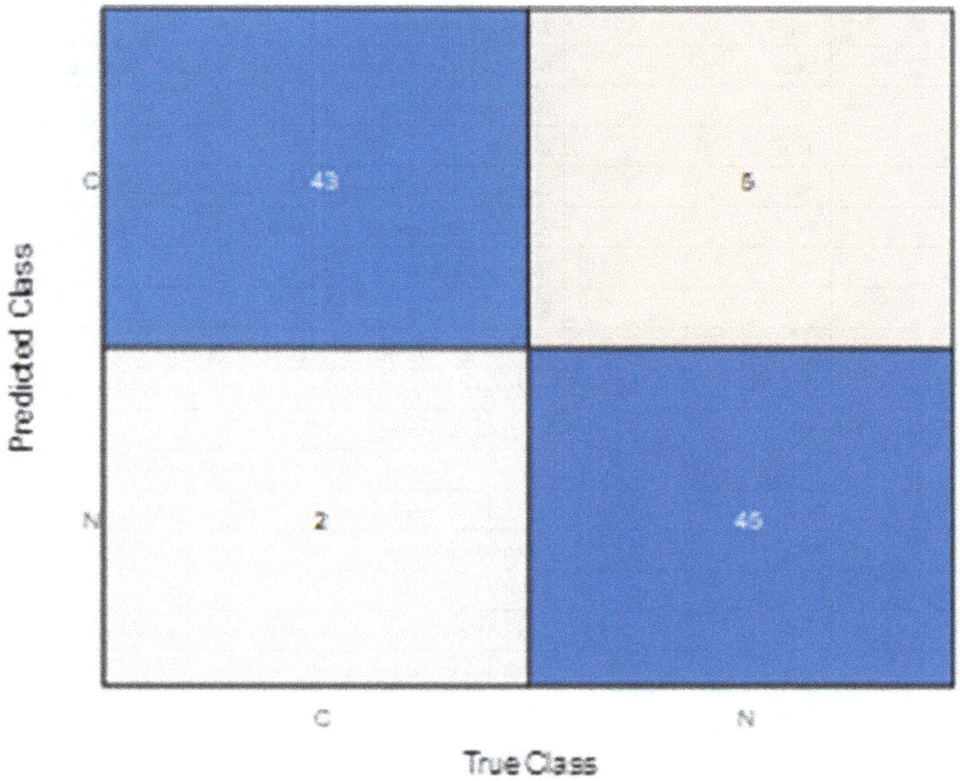

Figure 5. The developed CNN model for breast cancer detection.

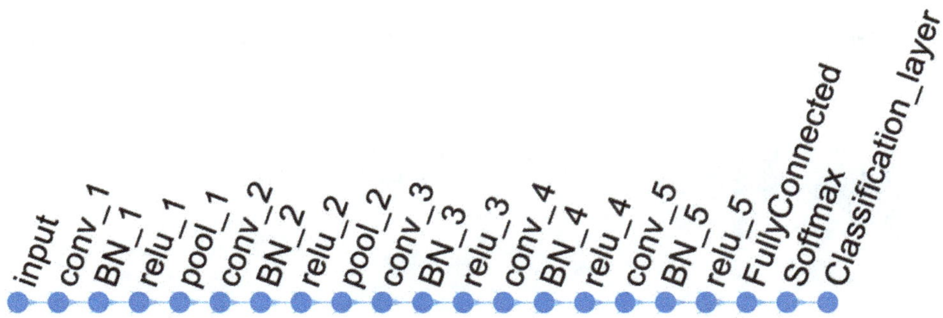

Table 3. Analysis of proposed CNN model for breast cancer detection

1	'input'	224x224x3 images
2	'conv_1'	64 3x3x3 convolutions with stride [1 1] and padding "same"
3	'BN_1'	Batch normalization
4	'relu_1'	ReLU
5	'pool_1'	2x2 max pooling with stride [2 2] and padding [0 0 0 0]
6	'conv_2'	32 3x3x8 convolutions with stride [1 1] and padding "same"
7	'BN_2'	Batch normalization
8	'relu_2'	ReLU
9	'pool_2'	2x2 max pooling with stride [2 2] and padding [0 0 0 0]
10	'conv_3'	16 3x3x16 convolutions with stride [1 1] and padding "same"
11	'BN_3'	Batch normalization
12	'relu_3'	ReLU
13	'conv_4'	8 3x3x16 convolutions with stride [1 1] and padding "same"
14	'BN_4'	Batch normalization
15	'relu_4'	ReLU
16	'conv_5'	4 3x3x16 convolutions with stride [1 1] and padding "same"
17	'BN_5'	Batch normalization
18	'relu_5'	ReLU
19	'fc'	5 fully connected layers
20	'softmax'	Softmax
21	'Classification'	crossentropyex with "0" and nine other classes

Figure 6. The end-to-end training of the developed CNN model for Breast cancer classification.

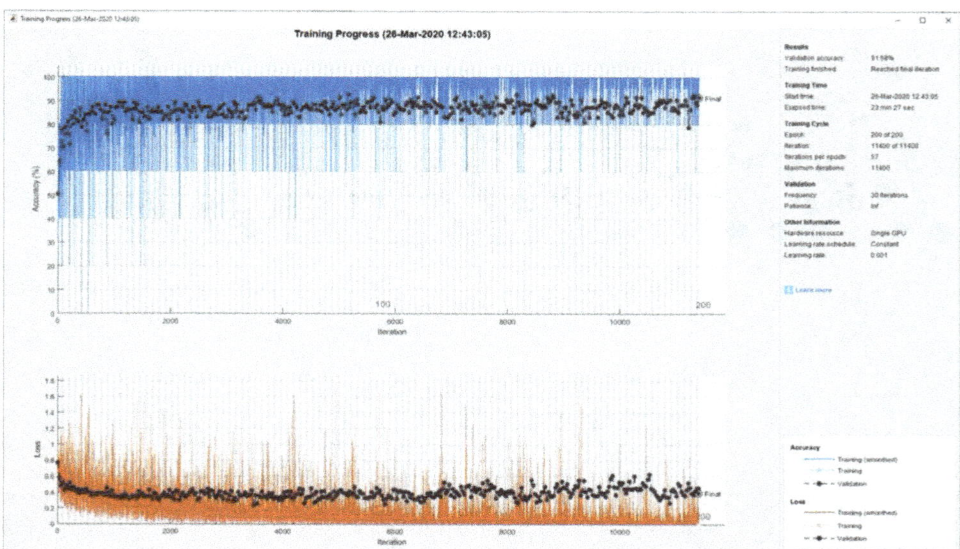

Figure 7. The confusion matrix that was obtained by end-to-end training of the developed CNN model

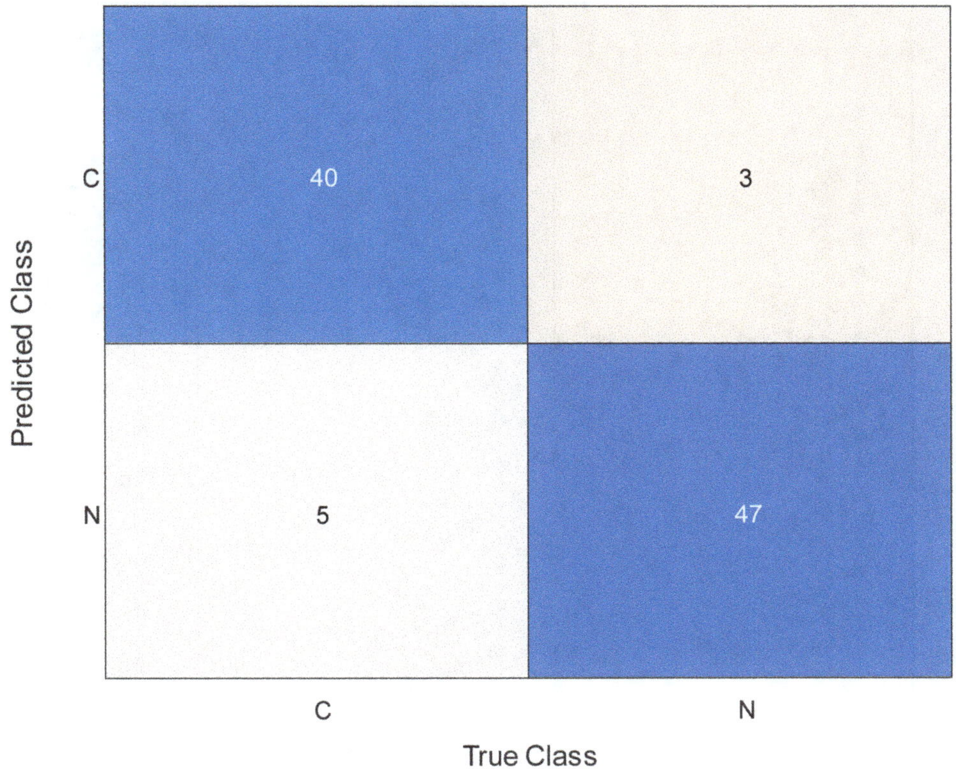

In the final experiments, a novel CNN model was constructed and trained in end-to-end fashion for breast cancer classification. The developed CNN model was depicted in Fig. 5. As seen in Fig. 5, the developed CNN model was composed of 21 layers. The network started with input layer and there were five convolutions layers namely conv_1, conv_2, conv_3, conv_4 and conv_5 in the model and batch normalization and ReLu layers followed each convolution layer. There were two pooling layers pool_1 and pool_2 which were come after ReLu_1 and ReLu_2 layers, respectively. A fully connected layer, softmax layer and classification layer were also used for classification. The conv_1, conv_2 and conv_3 layers contained 64, 32,16, 8 and 4 filters of size 3×3. The max operator was used in pooling layers.

Details of the end-to-end CNN architecture covering the description of layers, activations, and learnable weights are presented in Table 3. The training of the end-to-end CNN model was carried out with the "SGDM" optimizer with an initial learning rate of 0.001. The network trained for 300 iterations

The end-to-end training procedure of proposed CNN model was given in Fig. 6. The first row of Fig. 6 shows the training and testing accuracies (blue training and black testing) and the second row of Fig. 6 shows the loss values for both training and test samples (orange training and black testing). The obtained accuracy score was 91.58% and the training procedure was completed in 11400 iterations.

Fig. 7 presents the confusion matrix that was obtained with the end-to-end trained CNN model. While 40 breast cancer and 47 normal samples were classified correctly, 5 breast cancer and 3 normal samples were misclassified, respectively. The correct classification rate of the breast cancer samples was 88.89% and the correct classification rate of the normal cases was 94.0%.

Table 4. Shallow CNN models and their achievements

<table>
<tr><td>CNN Model</td><td>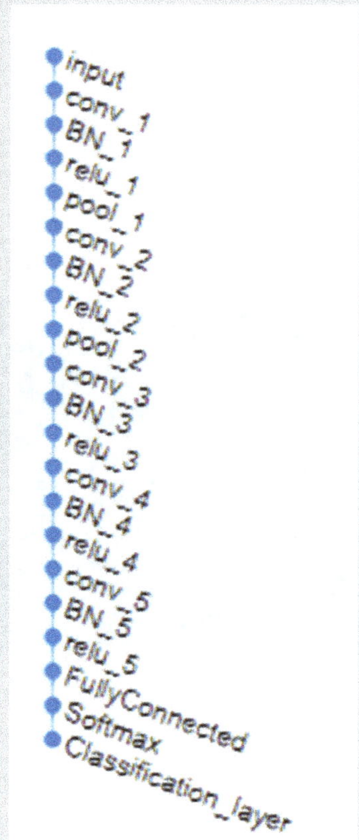
</td><td>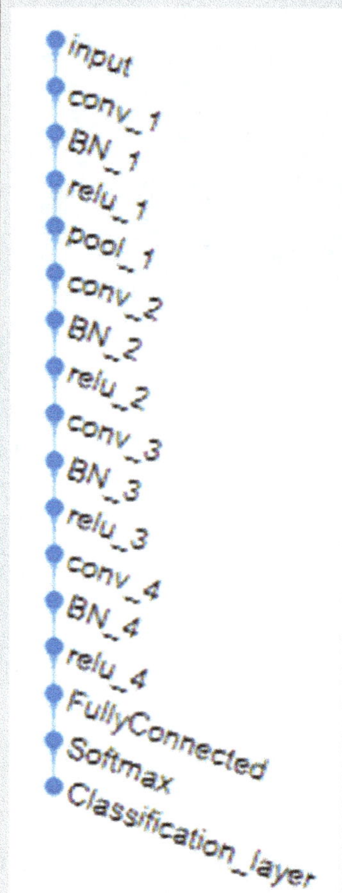
</td><td>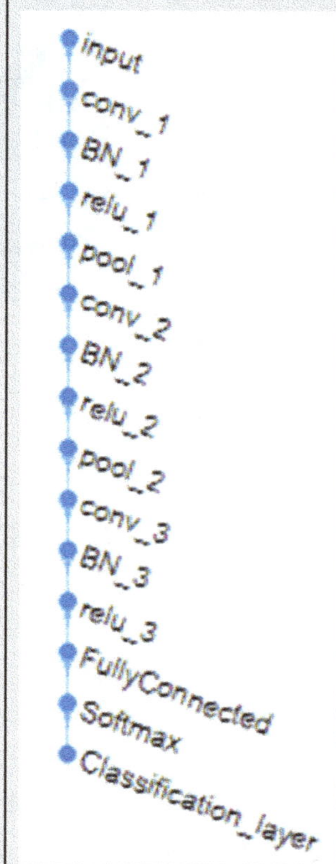
</td></tr>
<tr><td>Accuracy</td><td>91.58</td><td>88.42</td><td>86.32</td></tr>
</table>

Table 5. The obtained results for first experiment by using local feature descriptors and SVM classifiers

Local descriptors	**Accuracy scores (%)**				
	Linear SVM	**Quadratic SVM**	**Cubic SVM**	**Gaussian SVM**	**Average Accuracy (%)**
LBP	81.1	77.9	70.5	81.1	77.7
BGP	84.2	83.2	80.0	83.2	82.7
BSIF	90.5	90.5	90.5	88.4	90.0
CENTRIST	84.2	84.2	81.1	84.2	83.4
PHOG	85.3	83.2	83.2	84.2	84.0
LPQ	85.0	84.2	82.6	85.0	84.2
FDLBP	87.4	87.4	87.4	87.4	87.4
QLRBP	82.1	82.1	82.1	82.1	82.1
Average Accuracy (%)	85.0	84.1	82.2	84.5	

We further used more shallow CNN models to investigate their achievements on breast cancer classification. The shallow networks were also trained in end-to-end fashion and the obtained results were tabulated in Table 4.

As seen in Table 4, the first model contains 21 layers. These layers were input layer, 5 convolution layers, 5 batch normalization layers, 5 ReLu layers, 2 pooling layers and one fully connected layer, one softmax layer and one classification layer, respectively. The second model contains 17 layers. One input, four convolutions, four batch normalizations, four ReLu, one pooling, one fully connected layer, one softmax layer and one classification layer, respectively. Finally, the last model was composed of 15 layers. Three convolution layers, 3 batch normalization layers, 3 ReLu layers, 2 pooling layers and one fully connected layer, one Softmax layer and one classification layer, respectively. As mentioned earlier, the first model produced 91.58% accuracy score which is the best among all shallow CNN model's achievements. The second and third models produced 88.42% and 86.32% accuracy scores, respectively. From these results, it was observed that the deep CNN model produced the highest accuracy score.

Best of our knowledge, there has been no published works on breast cancer classification yet. Thus, for comparison purposes, various local descriptors were also used to extract features form the breast X-ray images for breast cancer detection. To this end, eight well-known local texture descriptors namely LBP (Ahonen, Hadid, & Pietikainen, 2006), FDLBP (Dubey, 2019), QLRBP (Lan, Zhou, & Tang, 2015), BGP (Zhang, Zhou & Li, 2012), LPQ (Ojansivu & Heikkilä, 2008), BSIF (Kannala & Rahtu, 2012), CENTRIST (Wu & Rehg, 2010) and PHOG (Bosch, Zisserman & Munoz, 2007) were considered. LBP summarizes local structures of images efficiently by comparing each pixel with its neighboring pixels. FDLBP improves the LBP by applying the decoder concept of multi-channel decoded local binary pattern over the multi-frequency patterns. QLRBP works on the quaternionic representation (QR) of the color image that encodes a color pixel using a quaternion. BGP was developed to integrate the advantages of both Gabor filters and LBP. LPQ was designed by quantizing the Fourier transform phase in local neighborhoods of a given pixel. Thus, a robust structure was obtained against to blur and low resolution. BSIF was produced by the binarization of the responses to linear filters that were learnt from natural images and independent component analysis. CENTRIST was designed similar to the LBP. After coding the pixel values, histogram was used as CENTRIST features. PHOG was developed for encoding an image utilizing its local shape at various scales with the help of distribution of direction of intensity and edges.

In the classification phase, the SVM classifier with linear, quadratic, cubic and Gaussian kernel functions were used. The obtained results with local descriptors and SVM classifier were given in Table 5.

The last column of Table 5 shows the average accuracy scores for the local descriptors and the last row of Table 5 shows the average achievements of the kernel functions of the SVM classifier. According to the represented results in Table 5, various observations can be extracted. For example, the BSIF local feature descriptor obtained the highest average classification accuracy score, where the calculated accuracy score was 90.0%. In other words, BSIF method outperformed other applied local feature descriptors. And, linear SVM technique outperformed other kernel functions where the obtained average accuracy score was 85.0%. LBP approach produced 77.7% average accuracy score, which was the worst accuracy score. Linear and Gaussian kernel functions produced the 81.1% accuracy scores with LBP features that was the highest among all other accuracy scores obtained with the LBP features. The BGP local descriptors produced 82.7% average accuracy score. And, the best BGP achievement 84.2% accuracy score was produced by the linear kernel function. 90.5% accuracy score, which was the best among all, was produced by BSIF and linear, quadratic and cubic kernel functions, respectively. CENTRIST technique produced accuracy scores 84.2% and 81.1%. while linear, quadratic and Gaussian kernel functions produced 84.2%

accuracy score, cubic kernel function produced 81.1% accuracy score. PHOG features produced the fourth best average accuracy score. The obtained score was 84.0% and LPQ technique produced 84.2% the third best average accuracy score. The FDLBP techniques' achievement was 87.4%, which was the second best average accuracy score. FDLBP technique produced the identical 87.4% accuracy scores for all kernel functions. QLRBP method produced the 82.1% average accuracy score and similar to the FDLBP technique, QLRBP also produced identical accuracy scores for all kernel functions too.

A final performance comparison of the used methods was given in Table 6. As seen in Table 6, the deep learning approached outperformed local descriptors.

Table 6 The performance comparison of the used methods

Method	Accuracy (%)
ResNet50 Features + SVM	94.7
Fine-tuning ResNet50	92.6
End-to-end training of CNN	91.6
BSIF + SVM	90.5

CONCLUSION

In this chapter, three deep CNN approaches are used to detect the breast cacner using X-Ray images. More specifically, two transfer learning approaches namely deep feature extraction and fine-tuning and an end-to end training of a new CNN model are considered. The deep features are classified with SVM classifier accompanied with different kernel functions. Eight well-known local descriptors are also considered. The obtained results revealed the following conclusions;

1) The deep learning approaches outperformed the local descriptors. Especially, deep features and SVM classifier performed better than the other approaches.
2) Fine-tuning and end-to-end training takes much time than deep feature extraction and local feature descriptor extraction.
3) Cubic kernel function generally outperformed other kernels in deep feature classification. ResNet50 model generally produced better results than the other pre-trained CNN models.
4) For the end-to-end training, the deep CNN models produced better results than shallow networks.

REFERENCES

Adaminejad, H., & Farjah, E. (2013). An Algorithm for Power Quality Events Core Vector Machine Based Classification. *The Modares Journal of Electrical Engineering*, *12*(4), 50–59.

Ahonen, T., Hadid, A., & Pietikainen, M. (2006). Face description with local binary patterns: Application to face recognition. *IEEE Transactions on Pattern Analysis and Machine Intelligence*, *28*(12), 2037–2041. doi:10.1109/TPAMI.2006.244 PMID:17108377

Alom, M. Z., Yakopcic, C., Nasrin, M. S., Taha, T. M., & Asari, V. K. (2019). Breast cancer classification from histopathological images with inception recurrent residual convolutional neural network. *Journal of Digital Imaging*, *32*(4), 605–617. doi:10.100710278-019-00182-7 PMID:30756265

Bal, P. R. (2018). Cross Project Software Defect Prediction using Extreme Learning Machine: An Ensemble based Study. *Proceedings of the 13th International Conference on Software Technologies*. 10.5220/0006886503540361

Başaran, E., Cömert, Z., & Çelik, Y. (2020). Convolutional neural network approach for automatic tympanic membrane detection and classification. *Biomedical Signal Processing and Control*, *56*, 101734. doi:10.1016/j.bspc.2019.101734

Bhandary, A., Prabhu, G. A., Rajinikanth, V., Thanaraj, K. P., Satapathy, S. C., Robbins, D. E., Shasky, C., Zhang, Y.-D., Tavares, J. M. R. S., & Raja, N. S. M. (2020). Deep-learning framework to detect lung abnormality–A study with chest X-Ray and lung CT scan images. *Pattern Recognition Letters*, *129*, 271–278. doi:10.1016/j.patrec.2019.11.013

Bosch, A., Zisserman, A., & Munoz, X. (2007). Representing shape with a spatial pyramid kernel. In *Proceedings of the 6th ACM international conference on Image and video retrieval* (pp. 401-408). 10.1145/1282280.1282340

Bray, F., Jemal, A., Grey, N., Ferlay, J., & Forman, D. (2012). Global cancer transitions according to the human development index (2008-2030): A population base study. *The Lancet. Oncology*, *13*(8), 790–801. doi:10.1016/S1470-2045(12)70211-5 PMID:22658655

Cheng, L., & Bao, W. (2014). Remote sensing image classification based on optimized support vector machine. *TELKOMNIKA Indonesian Journal of Electrical Engineering*, *12*(2), 1037–1045. doi:10.11591/telkomnika.v12i2.4325

Chouhan, V., Singh, S. K., Khamparia, A., Gupta, D., Tiwari, P., Moreira, C., Damaševičius, R., & de Albuquerque, V. H. C. (2020). A Novel Transfer Learning Based Approach for Pneumonia Detection in Chest X-ray Images. *Applied Sciences (Basel, Switzerland)*, *10*(2), 559. doi:10.3390/app10020559

Deniz, E., Şengür, A., Kadiroğlu, Z., Guo, Y., Bajaj, V., & Budak, Ü. (2018). Transfer learning based histopathologic image classification for breast cancer detection. *Health Information Science and Systems*, *6*(1), 18. doi:10.100713755-018-0057-x PMID:30279988

Ding, S., Zhao, H., Zhang, Y., Xu, X., & Nie, R. (2013). Extreme learning machine: Algorithm, theory and applications. *Artificial Intelligence Review*, *44*(1), 103–115. doi:10.100710462-013-9405-z

Dong, Y., Pan, Y., Zhang, J., & Xu, W. (2017, July). Learning to read chest X-ray images from 16000+ examples using CNN. In *2017 IEEE/ACM International Conference on Connected Health: Applications, Systems and Engineering Technologies*, (pp. 51-57). 10.1109/CHASE.2017.59

Dubey, S. R. (2019). Face retrieval using frequency decoded local descriptor. *Multimedia Tools and Applications*, *78*(12), 16411–16431. doi:10.100711042-018-7028-8

Elston, C. W., & Ellis, I. O. (1991). Pathological prognostic factors in breast cancer. I. The value of histological grade in breast cancer: Experience from a large study with long-term follow-up. *Histopathology*, *19*(5), 403–410. doi:10.1111/j.1365-2559.1991.tb00229.x PMID:1757079

Faust, O., Acharya, U. R., & Tamura, T. (2012). Formal design methods for reliable computer-aided diagnosis: A review. *IEEE Reviews in Biomedical Engineering*, *5*, 15–28. doi:10.1109/RBME.2012.2184750 PMID:23231986

Geng-he, L. (2013). Extension clustering-based extreme learning machine neural network. *Jisuanji Yingyong*, *33*(7), 1942–1945. doi:10.3724/SP.J.1087.2013.01942

Gupta, V., & Bhavsar, A. (2017). Breast cancer histopathological image classification: is magnification important? *Proceedings of the IEEE Conference on Computer Vision and Pattern Recognition Workshops*, 17–24. 10.1109/CVPRW.2017.107

Ho, T. K. K., & Gwak, J. (2019). Multiple feature integration for classification of thoracic disease in chest radiography. *Applied Sciences (Basel, Switzerland)*, *9*(19), 4130. doi:10.3390/app9194130

Huang, G.-B., Zhu, Q.-Y., & Siew, C.-K. (2004). Extreme learning machine: a new learning scheme of feedforward neural networks. *2004 IEEE International Joint Conference on Neural Networks* (IEEE Cat. No.04CH37541).

Huang, G. B., Zhu, Q. Y., & Siew, C. K. (2006). Extreme learning machine: Theory and applications. *Neurocomputing*, *70*(1-3), 489–501. doi:10.1016/j.neucom.2005.12.126

Kannala, J., & Rahtu, E. (2012). BSIF: Binarized statistical image features. In *Proceedings of the 21st international conference on pattern recognition (ICPR2012)* (pp. 1363-1366). Academic Press.

Keleş, A., & Keleş, A. (2008). ESTDD: Expert system for thyroid diseases diagnosis. *Expert Systems with Applications*, *34*(1), 242–246. doi:10.1016/j.eswa.2006.09.028

Keller, F., Muller, E., & Bohm, K. (2012). *HiCS: High-contrast subspaces for density-based outlier ranking*. ICDE.

Keller, F., Muller, E., & Bohm, K. (2012). *HiCS: High-contrast subspaces for density-based outlier ranking*. ICDE.

Kesim, E., Dokur, Z., & Olmez, T. (2019, April). X-Ray Chest Image Classification by A Small-Sized Convolutional Neural Network. In *2019 Scientific Meeting on Electrical-Electronics & Biomedical Engineering and Computer Science (EBBT)* (pp. 1-5). Academic Press.

Kinzler, K. W., & Vogelstein, B. (1996). Lessons from hereditary colorectal cancer. *Cell*, *87*(2), 159–170. doi:10.1016/S0092-8674(00)81333-1 PMID:8861899

Kowal, M., Filipczuk, P., Obuchowicz, A., Korbicz, J., & Monczak, R. (2013). Computer-aided diagnosis of breast cancer based on fine needle biopsy microscopic images. *Computers in Biology and Medicine, 43*(10), 1563–1572. doi:10.1016/j.compbiomed.2013.08.003 PMID:24034748

Lan, R., Zhou, Y., & Tang, Y. Y. (2015). Quaternionic local ranking binary pattern: A local descriptor of color images. *IEEE Transactions on Image Processing, 25*(2), 566–579. doi:10.1109/TIP.2015.2507404 PMID:26672041

Li, L.-N., Ouyang, J.-H., Chen, H.-L., & Liu, D.-Y. (2012). A Computer Aided Diagnosis System for Thyroid Disease Using Extreme Learning Machine. *Journal of Medical Systems, 36*(5), 3327–3337. doi:10.100710916-012-9825-3 PMID:22327384

Li, X., Shen, L., Xie, X., Huang, S., Xie, Z., Hong, X., & Yu, J. (2019). Multi-resolution convolutional networks for chest X-ray radiograph based lung nodule detection. *Artificial Intelligence in Medicine*, 101744. PMID:31732411

Li, X., Zhang, S., Zhang, Q., Wei, X., Pan, Y., Zhao, J., ... Yang, F. (2019). *Diagnosis of thyroid cancer using deep convolutional neural network models applied to sonographic images: a retrospective, multicohort, diagnostic study*. Academic Press.

Liu, C., Cao, Y., Alcantara, M., Liu, B., Brunette, M., Peinado, J., & Curioso, W. (2017). TX-CNN: Detecting tuberculosis in chest X-ray images using convolutional neural network. In *2017 IEEE International Conference on Image Processing (ICIP)* (pp. 2314-2318). 10.1109/ICIP.2017.8296695

Liu, F. T., Kai, M. T., & Zhou, Z.-H. (2008). Isolation forest. In *2008 Eighth IEEE International Conference on Data Mining*. IEEE. 10.1109/ICDM.2008.17

Loukas, C., Kostopoulos, S., Tanoglidi, A., Glotsos, D., Sfikas, C., & Cavouras, D. (2013). Breast cancer characterization based on image classification of tissue sections visualized under low magnification. *Computational and Mathematical Methods in Medicine, 2013*, 2013. doi:10.1155/2013/829461 PMID:24069067

Miller, K. D., Siegel, R. L., Lin, C. C., Mariotto, A. B., Kramer, J. L., Rowland, J. H., Stein, K. D., Alteri, R., & Jemal, A. (2016). Cancer treatment and survivorship statistics. *CA: a Cancer Journal for Clinicians, 66*(4), 271–289. doi:10.3322/caac.21349 PMID:27253694

Oh, S. H. (2011). Error back-propagation algorithm for classification of imbalanced data. *Neurocomputing, 74*(6), 1058–1061. doi:10.1016/j.neucom.2010.11.024

Ojansivu, V., & Heikkilä, J. (2008). Blur insensitive texture classification using local phase quantization. In *International conference on image and signal processing* (pp. 236-243). Springer. 10.1007/978-3-540-69905-7_27

Pan, S. J., & Yang, Q. (2009). A survey on transfer learning. *IEEE Transactions on Knowledge and Data Engineering, 22*(10), 1345–1359. doi:10.1109/TKDE.2009.191

Pedersen, M. E. H., & Chipperfield, A. J. (2008). *Tuning differential evolution for artificial neural networks*. HL0803 Hvass Laboratories.

Qi, Z., Tian, Y., & Shi, Y. (2013). Robust twin support vector machine for pattern classification. *Pattern Recognition*, *46*(1), 305–316. doi:10.1016/j.patcog.2012.06.019

Radiology assistant. (2020, March 23). *X-ray Chest images*. https://radiologyassistant.nl/chest/lk-jg-1

Rajpurkar, P., Irvin, J., Ball, R. L., Zhu, K., Yang, B., Mehta, H., ... Patel, B. N. (2018). Deep learning for chest radiograph diagnosis: A retrospective comparison of the CheXNeXt algorithm to practicing radiologists. *PLoS Medicine*, *15*(11), e1002686. doi:10.1371/journal.pmed.1002686 PMID:30457988

Rastogi, A. B., & Monika, A. (2014). *Study of neural network in diagnosis of thyroid. International Journal of Computer Technology and Electronics Engineering*, 4.

Shindjalova, R., Prodanova, K., & Svechtarov, V. (2014, November). Modeling data for tilted implants in grafted with bio-oss maxillary sinuses using logistic regression. In AIP Conference Proceedings (Vol. 1631, No. 1, pp. 58-62). American Institute of Physics. doi:10.1063/1.4902458

Shukla, A., Tiwari, R., Kaur, P., & Janghel, R. (2009). Diagnosis of Thyroid Disorders using Artificial Neural Networks. *2009 IEEE International Advance Computing Conference*. 10.1109/IADCC.2009.4809154

Siegel, R., Ward, E., Brawley, O., & Jemal, A. (2011). Jemal A. Cancer statistics. *CA: a Cancer Journal for Clinicians*, *61*(4), 212–236. doi:10.3322/caac.20121 PMID:21685461

Souza, J. C., Diniz, J. O. B., Ferreira, J. L., da Silva, G. L. F., Silva, A. C., & de Paiva, A. C. (2019). An automatic method for lung segmentation and reconstruction in chest X-ray using deep neural networks. *Computer Methods and Programs in Biomedicine*, *177*, 285–296. doi:10.1016/j.cmpb.2019.06.005 PMID:31319957

Spanhol, F. A., Oliveira, L. S., Cavalin, P. R., Petitjean, C., & Heutte, L. (2017). Deep features for breast cancer histopathological image classification. In *Systems, Man, and Cybernetics (SMC), 2017 IEEE International Conference on*, (pp. 1868–1873). IEEE. 10.1109/SMC.2017.8122889

Spanhol, F. A., Oliveira, L. S., Petitjean, C., & Heutte, L. (2016). A dataset for breast cancer histopathological image classification. *IEEE Transactions on Biomedical Engineering*, *63*(7), 1455–1462. doi:10.1109/TBME.2015.2496264 PMID:26540668

Steyeberg, E. (2008). *Clinical Prediction Models: A Practical Approach to Development, Validation and Updating*. Springer Science & Business Media.

Temurtas, F. (2009). A comparative study on thyroid disease diagnosis using neural networks. *Expert Systems with Applications*, *36*(1), 944–949. doi:10.1016/j.eswa.2007.10.010

Ting, K. M., Chuan, J. T. S., & Liu, F. T. (2009). Mass: A New Ranking Measure for Anomaly Detection. *IEEE Transactions on Knowledge and Data Engineering*.

Uçar, M., & Uçar, E. (2019). Computer-aided detection of lung nodules in chest X-rays using deep convolutional neural networks. *Sakarya University Journal of Computer and Information Sciences*, *2*(1), 41–52. doi:10.35377aucis.02.01.538249

Umar Sidiq, D., Aaqib, S. M., & Khan, R. A. (2019). Diagnosis of various Thyroid Ailments using Data Mining Classification Techniques. *Int J Sci Res Coput Sci Inf Technol*, *5*, 131–136.

Widodo, A., & Yang, B. S. (2007). Support vector machine in machine condition monitoring and fault diagnosis. *Mechanical Systems and Signal Processing*, *21*(6), 2560–2574. doi:10.1016/j.ymssp.2006.12.007

Wood-allum, C. A., & Shaw, P. J. (2014). Thyroid disease and the nervous system. *Handbook of Clinical Neurology*, *120*, 703–735. doi:10.1016/B978-0-7020-4087-0.00048-6 PMID:24365348

Woźniak, M., Połap, D., Capizzi, G., Sciuto, G. L., Kośmider, L., & Frankiewicz, K. (2018). Small lung nodules detection based on local variance analysis and probabilistic neural network. *Computer Methods and Programs in Biomedicine*, *161*, 173–180. doi:10.1016/j.cmpb.2018.04.025 PMID:29852959

Wu, J., & Rehg, J. M. (2010). Centrist: A visual descriptor for scene categorization. *IEEE Transactions on Pattern Analysis and Machine Intelligence*, *33*(8), 1489–1501. PMID:21173449

Xu, C., Yang, J., Lai, H., Gao, J., Shen, L., & Yan, S. (2019). UP-CNN: Un-pooling augmented convolutional neural network. *Pattern Recognition Letters*, *119*, 34–40. doi:10.1016/j.patrec.2017.08.007

Xu, S., Wu, H., & Bie, R. (2018). CXNet-m1: Anomaly detection on chest X-rays with image-based deep learning. *IEEE Access: Practical Innovations, Open Solutions*, *7*, 4466–4477. doi:10.1109/ACCESS.2018.2885997

Zeiler, M. D. (2012). *Adadelta: an adaptive learning rate method*. arXiv preprint arXiv:1212.5701

Zhang, L., Zhou, Z., & Li, H. (2012). Binary gabor pattern: An efficient and robust descriptor for texture classification. In 2012 19th IEEE international conference on image processing (pp. 81-84). IEEE.

Compilation of References

22Kopans, D. B. (1986). What is a useful adjunct to mammography? Radiology, 161(2), 560–561. doi:10.1148/radiology.161.2.3532197 PubMed doi:10.1148/radiology.161.2.3532197 PMID:3532197

Abdel-Dayem, A. R., & El-Sakka, M. R. (2005). Fuzzy entropy based detection of suspicious masses in digital mammogram images. *In Proceedings of 27th IEEE Engineering Annual Conference in Medicine and Biology* (pp. 4017-4022). Shanghai, China. 10.1109/IEMBS.2005.1615343

Acharya, U. R., Ng, E. Y. K., Tan, J.-H., & Sree, S. V. (2012). Thermography Based Breast Cancer Detection Using Texture Features and Support Vector Machine. *Journal of Medical Systems*, *36*(3), 1503–1510. doi:10.100710916-010-9611-z PMID:20957511

Adaminejad, H., & Farjah, E. (2013). An Algorithm for Power Quality Events Core Vector Machine Based Classification. *The Modares Journal of Electrical Engineering*, *12*(4), 50–59.

Adams, R., & Bischof, L. (1994). Seeded region growing. *IEEE Transactions on Pattern Analysis and Machine Intelligence*, *16*(6), 641–647. doi:10.1109/34.295913

Adler, A., Arnold, J. H., Bayford, R., Borsic, A., Brown, B., Dixon, P., ... Grychtol, B. (2009). GREIT: A unified approach to 2D linear EIT reconstruction of lung images. *Physiological Measurement*, *30*(6), S35–S55. doi:10.1088/0967-3334/30/6/S03 PMID:19491438

Adler, A., & Lionheart, W. R. B. (2006). Uses and abuses of EIDORS: An extensible software base for EIT. *Physiological Measurement*, *27*(5), S25–S42. doi:10.1088/0967-3334/27/5/S03 PMID:16636416

Agnelli, J. P., Barrea, A. A., & Turner, C. V. (2011). Tumor location and parameter estimation by thermography. *Mathematical and Computer Modelling*, *53*(7-8), 1527–1534. doi:10.1016/j.mcm.2010.04.003

Aguiar, P. S. Junior, Belfort, C. N. S., Silva, A. C., Diniz, P. H. B., Lima, R. C. F., Conci, A., & Paiva, A. C. (2013). Detecção de Regiões Suspeitas de Lesão na Mama em Imagens Térmicas Utilizando *Spatiogram* e Redes Neurais. *Cadernos de Pesquisa*, *20*(2), 56–63. doi:10.18764/2178-2229.v20n2p56-63

Ahonen, T., Hadid, A., & Pietikainen, M. (2006). Face description with local binary patterns: Application to face recognition. *IEEE Transactions on Pattern Analysis and Machine Intelligence*, *28*(12), 2037–2041. doi:10.1109/TPAMI.2006.244 PMID:17108377

Ai, L., & Yu, J., & He, Y., & Guan, T. (2013). High-dimensional indexing technologies for large scale content-based image retrieval: a review. *Journal of Zhejiang University SCIENCE C (Comput & Electron),* 14 (7), 505-520.

Alikhassi, A., Hamidpour, S. F., Firouzmand, M., Navid, M., & Eghbal, M. (2018). Prospective comparative study assessing role of ultrasound versus thermography in breast cancer detection. *Breast Disease*, *37*(4), 191–196. doi:10.3233/BD-180321 PMID:30124439

Ali, M. A. S., Sayed, G. I., Gaber, T., Hassanien, A. E., Snasel, V., & Silva, L. F. (2015). Detection of Breast Abnormalities of Thermograms based on a New Segmentation Method. *ACSIS*, *5*, 255–261. doi:10.15439/2015F318

Alom, M. Z., Yakopcic, C., Nasrin, M. S., Taha, T. M., & Asari, V. K. (2019). Breast cancer classification from histopathological images with inception recurrent residual convolutional neural network. *Journal of Digital Imaging*, *32*(4), 605–617. doi:10.100710278-019-00182-7 PMID:30756265

Alves, S. H., Amato, M. B., Terra, R. M., Vargas, F. S., & Caruso, P. (2014). Lung reaeration and reventilation after aspiration of pleural effusions. A study using electrical impedance tomography. *Annals of the American Thoracic Society*, *11*(2), 186–191. doi:10.1513/AnnalsATS.201306-142OC PMID:24308560

Amalu, W. C., Hobbins, W. B., Head, J. F., & Elliot, R. L. (2006). Infrared imaging of the breast - an overview. *The Biomedical Engineering Handbook*, *25*, 1–20.

Amalu, W. C., Hobbins, W. B., Head, J. F., & Elliott, R. L. (2006). Infrared imaging of the breast - an overview. In Biomedical Engineering Handbook. CRC Press.

American Cancer Society. (2019). Cancer Facts & Figures 2019. *CA: A Cancer Journal for Clinicians*, 1–71.

Ammer, K., & Ring, E. F. (2006). Standard Procedures for Infrared Imaging in Medicine. In Medical Devices and Systems, The Biomedical Engineering Handbook. CRC Press.

Ammer, K., & Ring, E. F. J. (2006). Standard procedures for infrared imaging in medicine. In Biomedical Engineering Handbook. CRC Press.

Amorim, A. M. A. M., Barbosa, J. da S., Freitas, A. P. L. de F., Viana, J. E. F., Vieira, L. E. M., Suassuna, F. C. M., Bento, P. M., & de Melo, D. P. (2019). Termografia Infravermelha na Odontologia. *HU Revista*, *44*(1), 15–22. doi:10.34019/1982-8047.2018.v44.13943

Amri, A., Pulko, S. H., & Wilkinson, A. J. (2016). Potentialities of steady-state and transient thermography in breast tumour depth detection: A numerical study. *Computer Methods and Programs in Biomedicine*, *123*, 68–80. doi:10.1016/j.cmpb.2015.09.014 PMID:26522612

Andrade, M. K. S., Santana, M. A., & Santos, W. P. (2018). Avaliação do Desempenho de Classificadores Inteligentes na Detecção da Doença de Alzheimer em Imagens de Ressonância Magnética Utilizando Extratores de Forma e Textura. In II Simpósio de Inovação em Engenharia Biomédica (SABIO 2018), Recife, Brazil.

Araújo, M. C. (2009). *Utilização de Câmera por Infravermelho para Avaliação de Diferentes Patologias em Clima Tropical e Uso Conjunto de Sistemas de Banco de Dados para Detecção do Câncer de Mama* [dissertation]. Recife: Universidade Federal de Pernambuco.

Araújo, M. C. (2014). *Uso de imagens termográficas para classificação de anormalidades de mama baseado em variáveis simbólicas intervalares* (Doctoral thesis). Universidade Federal de Pernambuco, Recife, Brazil.

Araújo, M. C. (2014). *Uso de imagens termográficas para classificação de anormalidades de mama baseado em variáveis simbólicas intervalares* [Use of thermographic images to classify breast abnormalities based on symbolic interval intervals] (Doctoral thesis). Universidade Federal de Pernambuco, Recife, Brazil.

Araújo, A. S., Conci, A., Moran, M. B., & Resmini, R. (2018, July). Comparing the Use of Sum and Difference Histograms and Gray Levels Occurrence Matrix for Texture Descriptors. In *2018 International Joint Conference on Neural Networks (IJCNN)* (pp. 1-8). 10.1109/IJCNN.2018.8489705

Araújo, M. C., Bezerra, L. A., Santos, L. C., Rolim, T. L., Santos, T. B., Lyra, P. R. M., & Lima, R. C. F. (2008). *Instrumentation and acquisition of the three-dimensional geometry of the breast of a phantom: comparison of temperatures calculated numerically and measured by thermographic imaging*. In *Annals of XXIX Iberian Latin-American Congress on Computational Methods in Engineering*, Maceió, Brazil.

Araújo, M. C., Lima, R. C. F., & Souza, R. M. C. R. (2014). Interval symbolic feature extraction for thermography breast cancer detection. *Expert Systems with Applications*, *41*(15), 6728–6737. doi:10.1016/j.eswa.2014.04.027

Araújo, M. C., Souza, R. M. C. R., Lima, R. C. F., & Filho, T. M. S. (2017). An interval prototype classifier based on a parameterized distance applied to breast thermographic images. *Medical & Biological Engineering & Computing*, *55*(6), 873–884. doi:10.100711517-016-1565-y PMID:27629552

Arridge. (2011). Methods in diffuse optical imaging. *Philos Trans A Math Phys Eng Sci.*, *369*(1955), 4558-76.

Asanuma, D., Sakabe, M., Kamiya, M., Yamamoto, K., Hiratake, J., Ogawa, M., Kosaka, N., Choyke, P. L., Nagano, T., Kobayashi, H., & Urano, Y. (2015). Sensitive beta-galactosidase-targeting fluorescence probe for visualizing small peritoneal metastatic tumours in vivo. Nature Communications, 6(1), 6463. doi:10.1038/ncomms7463 PubMed doi:10.1038/ncomms7463 PMID:25765713

Australian Government, Department of Health, Therapeutic Goods Administration. (2019). *Thermography should not be relied on for early detection of breast cancer*. Retrieved from https://www.tga.gov.au/media-release/thermography-should-not-be-relied-early-detection-breast-cancer

Avila-Castro, I. A., Hernández-Martínez, A. R., Estevez, M., Cruz, M., Esparza, R., Pérez, R., & Rodríguez, A. L. (2017). Thorax thermographic simulator for breast pathologies. *Journal of Applied Research and Technology*, *15*(2), 143–151. doi:10.1016/j.jart.2017.01.008

Azevedo, W. W., Lima, S. M. L., Fernandes, I. M. M., Rocha, A. D. D., Cordeiro, F. R., Silva-Filho, A. G., & Santos, W. P. (2015). *Morphological extreme learning machines applied to detect and classify masses in mammograms*. In *2015 International Joint Conference of Neural Networks (IJCNN)*, Killarney, Ireland. 10.1109/IJCNN.2015.7280774

Azevedo, W. W., Lima, S. M., Fernandes, I. M., Rocha, A. D., Cordeiro, F. R., da Silva-Filho, A. G., & dos Santos, W. P. (2015, August). *Fuzzy morphological extreme learning machines to detect and classify masses in mammograms. In 2015 IEEE international conference on fuzzy systems (fuzz-IEEE)*. IEEE.

Baâzaoui, A., Barhoumi, W., Ahmed, A., & Zagrouba, E. (2018). Modeling clinician medical-knowledge in terms of med-level features for semantic content-based mammogram retrieval. *Expert Systems with Applications*, *94*(1), 11–20. doi:10.1016/j.eswa.2017.10.034

Baeza-Yates, R., & Ribeiro-Neto, B. (Eds.). (1999). *Modern Information Retrieval*. ACM Press/Addison-Wesley.

Baines, C. J., & Miller, A. B. (1997). Mammography versus clinical examination of the breasts. Journal of the National Cancer Institute. Monographs, 1997(22), 125–129. doi:10.1093/jncimono/1997.22.125 PubMed doi:10.1093/jncimono/1997.22.125 PMID:9709288

Bal, P. R. (2018). Cross Project Software Defect Prediction using Extreme Learning Machine: An Ensemble based Study. *Proceedings of the 13th International Conference on Software Technologies*. 10.5220/0006886503540361

Bankman, I. N. (2009). *Handbook of medical imaging: Processing and analysis* (3rd ed.). Academic Press.

Baraldi, A., & Parmiggiani, F. (1995). An Investigation of the Textural Characteristics Associated with Gray Level Cooccurrence Matrix Statistical Parameters. *IEEE Transactions on Geoscience and Remote Sensing*, *33*(2), 293–304. doi:10.1109/TGRS.1995.8746010

Barbosa, V. A. F., Ribeiro, R. R., Feitosa, A. R. S., Freitas, R. C., Melo, M. F. B., da Silva, V. L. B. A., de Souza, R. E., & dos Santos, W. P. (2016). Reconstrução de imagens de TIE usando busca por cardume de peixes e density based on fish school search. *XXV Congresso Brasileiro de Engenharia Biomédica.*

Barbosa, V. A., dos Santos, W. P., de Souza, R. E., Ribeiro, R. R., Feitosa, A. R. S., da Silva, V. L. B. A., & Valença, R. B. (2018). Image Reconstruction of Electrical Impedance Tomography Using Fish School Search and Differential Evolution. In *Critical Developments and Applications of Swarm Intelligence* (pp. 301–338). IGI Global. doi:10.4018/978-1-5225-5134-8.ch012

Barbosa, V. A., Ribeiro, R. R., Feitosa, A. R., da Silva, V. L., Rocha, A. D., Freitas, R. C., Melo, M. F. B., da Silva, V. L. B. A., de Souza, R. E., & dos Santos, W. P. (2015). Reconstrução de imagens de tomografia por impedância elétrica usando cardume de peixes, busca não-cega e algoritmo genético. In *Anais do 12 Congresso Brasileiro de Inteligência Computacional* (pp. 1–6). ABRICOM. doi:10.21528/CBIC2015-043

Barbosa, V. A., Ribeiro, R. R., Feitosa, A. R., Silva, V. L., Rocha, A. D., Freitas, R. C., Souza, R. E., & Santos, W. P. (2017). Reconstruction of Electrical Impedance Tomography Using Fish School Search, Non-Blind Search, and Genetic Algorithm. *International Journal of Swarm Intelligence Research, 8*(2), 17–33. doi:10.4018/IJSIR.2017040102

Barhoumi, W., & Baâzaoui, A. (2014). Pigment network detection in dermatoscopic images for melanoma diagnosis. *Innovation and Research in BioMedical Engineering, 35*(3), 128-138.

Barnes, R. B. (1963). Thermography of the Human body. *Science, 140*(3569), 870–877. doi:10.1126cience.140.3569.870 PMID:13969373

Barros, A. C. S. D., Pompei, L. M., & Silveira, J. B. M. (2010). *Manual de Orientação Mastologia.* Federação Brasileira das Associações de Ginecologia e Obstetrícia.

Barton, M. B., Harris, R., & Fletcher, S. W. (1999). The rational clinical examination. Does this patient have breast cancer? The screening clinical breast examination: Should it be done? How? Journal of the American Medical Association, 282(13), 1270–1280. doi:10.1001/jama.282.13.1270 PubMed doi:10.1001/jama.282.13.1270 PMID:10517431

Başaran, E., Cömert, Z., & Çelik, Y. (2020). Convolutional neural network approach for automatic tympanic membrane detection and classification. *Biomedical Signal Processing and Control, 56*, 101734. doi:10.1016/j.bspc.2019.101734

Basilion, J. P. (2001). Current and future technologies for breast cancer imaging. Breast Cancer Research, 3(1), 14–16. doi:10.1186/bcr264 PubMed doi:10.1186/bcr264 PMID:11300100

Bayford, R. H. (2006). Bioimpedance tomography (electrical impedance tomography). *Annual Review of Biomedical Engineering, 8*(1), 63–91. doi:10.1146/annurev.bioeng.8.061505.095716 PMID:16834552

Belfort, C. N. S., Silva, A. C., & Paiva, A. C. (2015). *Detecção de lesões em imagens termográficas de mama utilizando Índice de Similaridade de Jaccard e Artificial Crawlers.* In *XV Workshop de Informática Médica*, Recife, Brazil.

Belfort, C. N., Silva, A. C., & de Paiva, A. C. (2015). *Detecção de lesões em imagens termograficas da mama utilizando Índice de Similaridade de Jaccard e Artificial Crawlers.* XXXV CONGRESSO DA SOCIEDADE BRASILEIRA DE COMPUTAÇÃO.

Belkacémi, Y., Boussen, H., Hamdi-Cherif, M., Benider, A., Errihani, H., Mrabti, H., Bouzid, K., Bensalem, A., Fettouki, S., Ben Abdalah, M., Abid, L., & Gligorov, J. (2010). Young women breast cancer epidemiology in North Africa. In Proceedings of thirty two SFSPM days (pp. 56-68), Strasbourg: Academic Press.

Bellman, R. (1961). *Adaptive control processes: A guided tour.* Princeton University Press. doi:10.1515/9781400874668

Ben Abdallah, M., Zehani, S., Maalej, M., Hsairi, M., Hechiche, M., Ben Romdhane, K., Boussen, H., Saadi, A., Achour, N., & Ben Ayed, F. (2009). Cancer du sein en Tunisie: Caractéristiques épidémiologiques et tendance évolutive de l'incidence. *La Tunisie Medicale*, *87*(7), 417–425. PMID:20063673

Bera, T. K., Biswas, S. K., Rajan, K., & Nagaraju, J. (2019). Improving image quality in electrical impedance tomography (EIT) using projection error propagation-based regularization (PEPR) technique: A simulation study. *Journal of Electrical Bioimpedance*, *2*(1), 2–12. doi:10.5617/jeb.158

Bezerra, L. A. (2007). *Uso de imagens termográficas em tumores mamários para validação de simulação computacional* (Master's thesis). Universidade Federal de Pernambuco, Recife, PE, Brazil. Retrieved from https://repositorio.ufpe.br/handle/123456789/5486

Bezerra, L. A. (2013). Estimativa de parâmetros termofísicos da mama e de distúrbios mamários a partir de termografia por infravermelho utilizando técnicas de otimização [Estimation of thermophysical parameters of the breast and maternal disturbances from infrared thermography using otimization techniques] (Doctoral thesis). Universidade Federal de Pernambuco, Recife, Brazil.

Bezerra, L. A. (2013). *Estimativa de parâmetros termofísicos da mama utilizando método inverso* (Unpublished doctoral thesis). Universidade Federal de Pernambuco, Recife, Brazil.

Bezerra, L. A., Oliveira, M. M., Araújo, M. C., Viana, L. C., Santos, M. J. A., Santos, F. G. S., Rolim, T. L., Lyra, P. R. M., Lima, R. C. F., Borschartt, T. B., Resmini, R., & Conci, A. (2013b). Infrared Imaging for Breast Cancer Detection with Proper Selection of Properties: From Acquisition Protocol to Numerical Simulation. In *Multimodality Breast Imaging: Diagnosis and Treatment* (Vol. PM227). SPIE Press Book.

Bezerra, L. A., Oliveira, M. M., Rolim, T. L., Conci, A., Santos, F. G. S., Lyra, P. R. M., & Lima, R. C. F. (2013). Estimation of breast tumor thermal properties using infrared images. *Signal Processing*, *93*(10), 2851–2863. doi:10.1016/j.sigpro.2012.06.002

Bezerra, L. A., Ribeiro, R. R., Lyra, P. R. M., & Lima, R. C. F. (2020). An empirical correlation to estimate thermal properties of the breast and of the breast nodule using thermographic images and optimization techniques. *International Journal of Heat and Mass Transfer*, *149*, 149. doi:10.1016/j.ijheatmasstransfer.2019.119215

Bhandary, A., Prabhu, G. A., Rajinikanth, V., Thanaraj, K. P., Satapathy, S. C., Robbins, D. E., Shasky, C., Zhang, Y.-D., Tavares, J. M. R. S., & Raja, N. S. M. (2020). Deep-learning framework to detect lung abnormality–A study with chest X-Ray and lung CT scan images. *Pattern Recognition Letters*, *129*, 271–278. doi:10.1016/j.patrec.2019.11.013

Bhowmik, M. K., Gogoi, U. R., Das, K., Ghosh, A. K., Bhattacharjee, D., & Majumdar, G. (2016). Standardization of Infrared Breast Thermogram Acquisition Protocols and Abnormality Analysis of Breast Thermograms. *Thermosense: Thermal Infrared Applications XXXVIII. SPIE, 9861.*

Bhowmik, M. K., Gogoi, U. R., Majumdar, G., Bhattacharjee, D., Datta, D., & Ghosh, A. K. (2017). Designing of Ground-Truth-Annotated DBT-TU-JU Breast Thermogram Database Toward Early Abnormality Prediction. *IEEE Journal of Biomedical and Health Informatics*, *22*(4), 1238–1249. doi:10.1109/JBHI.2017.2740500 PMID:28829321

Billard, L., & Diday, E. (2006). *Symbolic Data Analysis: Conceptual Statistics and Data Mining*. John Wiley and Sons. doi:10.1002/9780470090183

Birnbaum, S. J., & Kliot, D. (1964). Thermography-obstetrical applications. *Annals of the New York Academy of Sciences*, *121*(1), 209–222. doi:10.1111/j.1749-6632.1964.tb13697.x PMID:14237513

Blackwell, B. F. (1989). Sensitivity analysis and uncertainty propagation of computational models. In W. J. Minkowywcz, E. M. Sparrow, & J. Y. Murthy (Eds.), *Handbook of numerical heat transfer* (2nd ed., pp. 53–71). J. Skilling.

Bohren, C. F., & Huffman, D. R. (1998). *Absorption and scattering of light by small particles*. John Wiley & Sons. doi:10.1002/9783527618156

Borcea, L. (2002). Electrical impedance tomography. *Inverse Problems*, *18*(6), R99–R136. doi:10.1088/0266-5611/18/6/201

Borchartt, T. B. (2013). *Análise De Imagens Termográficas Para a Classificação De Alterações Na Mama* (Doctoral thesis). Universidade Federal Fluminense, Rio de Janeiro, RJ, Brasil.

Borchartt, T. B. (2013). *Análise de imagens termográficas para a classificação de alterações na mama* (M Sc. Dissertation). Computer Institute, Universidade Federal Fluminense, Niterói, RJ, Brazil.

Borchartt, T. B., Conci, A., Lima, R. C. F., Resmini, R., & Sanchez, A. (2013). Breast thermography from an image processing viewpoint: A survey. *Signal Processing*, *93*(10), 2785–2803. doi:10.1016/j.sigpro.2012.08.012

Bosch, A., Zisserman, A., & Munoz, X. (2007). Representing shape with a spatial pyramid kernel. In *Proceedings of the 6th ACM international conference on Image and video retrieval* (pp. 401-408). 10.1145/1282280.1282340

Bouchette, G., Church, P., Mcfee, J. E., & Adler, A. (2013). Imaging of compact objects buried in underwater sediments using electrical impedance tomography. *IEEE Transactions on Geoscience and Remote Sensing*, *52*(2), 1407–1417. doi:10.1109/TGRS.2013.2250982

Brasileiro Filho, G. (2011). *Bogliolo Patologia* (8th ed.). Guanabara Koogan.

Bray, F., Ferlay, J., Soerjomataram, I., Siegel, R. L., Torre, L. A., & Jemal, A. (2019, April 15). (in press). Global Cancer Statistics 2018: GLOBOCAN estimates of incidence and mortality worldwide for 36 cancers in 185 countries. CA: a Cancer Journal for Clinicians, 144(8), 1941–1953. 10.1002/ijc.31937 PubMed PMID:30207593

Bray, F., Ferlay, J., Soerjomataram, I., Siegel, R. L., Torre, L. A., & Jemal, A. (2018). Global cancer statistics 2018: GLOBOCAN estimates of incidence and mortality worldwide for 36 cancers in 185 countries. *CA: a Cancer Journal for Clinicians*, *68*(6), 394–424. doi:10.3322/caac.21492 PMID:30207593

Bray, F., Jemal, A., Grey, N., Ferlay, J., & Forman, D. (2012). Global cancer transitions according to the human development index (2008-2030): A population base study. *The Lancet. Oncology*, *13*(8), 790–801. doi:10.1016/S1470-2045(12)70211-5 PMID:22658655

Breiman, L. (2001). Article. *Machine Learning*, *45*(1), 5–32. doi:10.1023/A:1010933404324

Brem, R. F., Floerke, A. C., Rapelyea, J. A., Teal, C., Kelly, T., & Mathur, V. (2008). Breast-specific gamma imaging as an adjunct imaging modality for the diagnosis of breast cancer. Radiology, 247(3), 651–657. doi:10.1148/radiol.2473061678 PubMed doi:10.1148/radiol.2473061678 PMID:18487533

Brem, R. F., Rapelyea, J. A., Zisman, G., Mohtashemi, K., Raub, J., Teal, C. B., Majewski, S., & Welch, B. L. (2005). Occult breast cancer: Scintimammography with high-resolution breast-specific gamma camera in women at high risk for breast cancer. Radiology, 237(1), 274–280. doi:10.1148/radiol.2371040758 PubMed doi:10.1148/radiol.2371040758 PMID:16126919

Brioschi, M., Teixeira, M. J., Silva, F., & Colman, D. (2010). *Medical thermography textbook: principles and applications*. Andreoli.

Brown, B. H., Barber, D. C., & Seagar, A. D. (1985). Applied potential tomography: Possible clinical applications. *Clinical Physics and Physiological Measurement*, *6*(2), 109–121. doi:10.1088/0143-0815/6/2/002 PMID:4017442

Burges, C. J. C. (1998). A Tutorial on Support Vector Machines for Pattern Recognition. *Data Mining and Knowledge Discovery*, *2*(2), 121–167. doi:10.1023/A:1009715923555

BUS. (n.d.). *Breast ultrasound.* Retrieved from https://densebreast-info.org/breast-ultrasound.aspx

Campbell, H. S., Fletcher, S. W., Pilgrim, C. A., Morgan, T. M., & Lin, S. (1991). Improving physicians' and nurses' clinical breast examination: A randomized controlled trial. American Journal of Preventive Medicine, 7(1), 1–8. doi:10.1016/S0749-3797(18)30957-7 PubMed doi:10.1016/S0749-3797(18)30957-7 PMID:1867894

Cancer Institute Hospital of JFCR. (2019). Retrieved from https://www.jfcr.or.jp/hospital-en/

Catmul, E. A. (1974). Subdivision algorithm for computer display of curved surfaces. Univ. Utah Computer Sci Dept, 74–133.

Chandy, D. A., Christinal, A. H., Theodore, A. J., & Selvan, S. E. (2017). Neighbourhood search feature selection method for content-based mammogram retrieval. *Medical & Biological Engineering & Computing, 55*(3), 493–505. doi:10.100711517-016-1513-x PMID:27262458

Chang, C. L., & Chang, M. (2009). M. Inverse determination of thermal conductivity using semi-discretization method. *Applied Mathematical Modelling, 33*(3), 1644–1655. doi:10.1016/j.apm.2008.03.001

Char, M. I., Chang, F. P., & Tai, B. C. (2008). Inverse determination of thermal conductivity by differential quadrature method. *International Communications in Heat and Mass Transfer, 35*(2), 113–119. doi:10.1016/j.icheatmasstransfer.2007.06.006

Charny, C. (1992). Mathematical models of bioheat equation. In Y. I. Cho (Ed.), *Advances in Heat Transfer: Bioengineering Heat Transfer* (Vol. 22, pp. 19–155). Academic Press, Inc., Kluwer Academic. doi:10.1016/S0065-2717(08)70344-7

Cheney, M., Isaacson, D., & Newell, J. C. (1999). Electrical impedance tomography. *SIAM Review, 41*(1), 85–101. doi:10.1137/S0036144598333613

Cheng, H. D., Shi, X. J., Min, R., Hu, L. M., Cai, X. P., & Du, H. N. (2005). Approaches for automated detection and classification of masses in mammograms. *Pattern Recognition, 39*(2006), 646-668.

Cheng, H., Shi, X., Min, R., Hu, L., Cai, X., & Du, H. (2006). Approaches for automated detection and classification of masses in mammograms. *Pattern Recognition, 39*(4), 646–668. doi:10.1016/j.patcog.2005.07.006

Cheng, J., & Greiner, R. (2001). *Learning Bayesian Belief Network Classifiers: Algorithms and System.* Advances in Artificial Intelligence - Springer Berlin Heidelberg. doi:10.1007/3-540-45153-6_14

Cheng, L., & Bao, W. (2014). Remote sensing image classification based on optimized support vector machine. *TELKOMNIKA Indonesian Journal of Electrical Engineering, 12*(2), 1037–1045. doi:10.11591/telkomnika.v12i2.4325

Cherepenin, V. A., Karpov, A. Y., Korjenevsky, A. V., Kornienko, V. N., Kultiasov, Y. S., Ochapkin, M. B., Trochanova, O. V., & Meister, J. D. (2002). Three-dimensional EIT imaging of breast tissues: System design and clinical testing. *IEEE Transactions on Medical Imaging, 21*(6), 662–667. doi:10.1109/TMI.2002.800602 PMID:12166863

Cherepenin, V., Karpov, A., Korjenevsky, A., Kornienko, V., Mazaletskaya, A., Mazourov, D., & Meister, D. (2001). A 3D electrical impedance tomography (EIT) system for breast cancer detection. *Physiological Measurement, 22*(1), 9–18. doi:10.1088/0967-3334/22/1/302 PMID:11236894

Chica-Olmo, M., & Abarca-Hernandez, F. (2000). Computing geostatistical image texture for remotely sensed data classification. *Computers & Geosciences, 26*(4), 373–383. doi:10.1016/S0098-3004(99)00118-1

Choi, M. H., Kao, T. J., Isaacson, D., Saulnier, G. J., & Newell, J. C. (2007). A reconstruction algorithm for breast cancer imaging with electrical impedance tomography in mammography geometry. *IEEE Transactions on Biomedical Engineering, 54*(4), 700–710. doi:10.1109/TBME.2006.890139 PMID:17405377

Chouhan, V., Singh, S. K., Khamparia, A., Gupta, D., Tiwari, P., Moreira, C., Damaševičius, R., & de Albuquerque, V. H. C. (2020). A Novel Transfer Learning Based Approach for Pneumonia Detection in Chest X-ray Images. *Applied Sciences (Basel, Switzerland)*, *10*(2), 559. doi:10.3390/app10020559

Chung, S. H., Mehta, R., Tromberg, B. J., & Yodh, A. G. (2011). Non-invasive measurement of deep tissue temperature changes caused by apoptosis during breast cancer neoadjuvant chemotherapy: A case study. *Journal of Innovative Optical Health Sciences*, *4*(04), 361–372. doi:10.1142/S1793545811001708 PMID:22408653

Church, P., McFee, J. E., Gagnon, S., & Wort, P. (2006). Electrical impedance tomographic imaging of buried landmines. *IEEE Transactions on Geoscience and Remote Sensing*, *44*(9), 2407–2420. doi:10.1109/TGRS.2006.873208

Cockburn, W. (2018). *The Truth About Breast Thermography*. Retrieved from https://www.healingwell.com/articles/post/the-truth-about-breast-thermography

Coelho, A. S., Santos, M. A. S., Caetano, R. I., Piovesan, C. F., Fiuza, L. A., Machado, R. L. D., & Furini, A. A. C. (2018). Predisposição hereditária ao câncer de mama e sua relação com os genes BRCA1 e BRCA2: Revisão da literatura. *Revista Brasileira de Análises Clínicas*, *50*(1), 17–21.

Coleman, G. B., & Andrews, H. C. (1979). Image segmentation by clustering. *Proceedings of the IEEE*, *67*(5), 773–785. doi:10.1109/PROC.1979.11327

Collins, A. J., Ring, E. F., Cosh, J. A., & Bacon, P. A. (1974). Quantitation of thermography in arthritis using multi-isothermal analysis. I. The thermographic index. *Annals of the Rheumatic Diseases*, *33*(2), 113–115. doi:10.1136/ard.33.2.113 PMID:4821383

Colombo, P. E., Milanezi, F., Weigelt, B., & Reis-Filho, J. S. (2011). Microarrays in the 2010s: The contribution of microarray-based gene expression profiling to breast cancer classification, prognostication and prediction. Breast Cancer Research, 13(3), 212. doi:10.1186/bcr2890 PubMed doi:10.1186/bcr2890 PMID:21787441

Conci, A., Azevedo, E., & Leta, F. R. (2008). *Computação Gráfica (in portuguese)*. Campus/Elsevier.

Cordeiro, F. R., Bezerra, K. F. P., & dos Santos, W. P. (2017, June). Random Walker with Fuzzy Initialization Applied to Segment Masses in Mammography Images. In *2017 IEEE 30th International Symposium on Computer-Based Medical Systems (CBMS)* (pp. 156-161). IEEE. 10.1109/CBMS.2017.40

Cordeiro, F. R., Lima, S. M., Silva-Filho, A. G., & Santos, W. P. (2012, August). Segmentation of mammography by applying extreme learning machine in tumor detection. In *International Conference on Intelligent Data Engineering and Automated Learning* (pp. 92-100). Springer.

Cordeiro, F. R., Santos, W. P., & Silva-Filho, A. G. (2013). Segmentation of mammography by applying GrowCut for mass detection. *Studies in Health Technology and Informatics*, *192*, 87–91. PMID:23920521

Cordeiro, F. R., Santos, W. P., & Silva-Filho, A. G. (2016). A semi-supervised fuzzy GrowCut algorithm to segment and classify regions of interest of mammographic images. *Expert Systems with Applications*, *65*, 116–126. doi:10.1016/j.eswa.2016.08.016

Cordeiro, F. R., Santos, W. P., & Silva-Filho, A. G. (2016). An adaptive semi-supervised Fuzzy GrowCut algorithm to segment masses of regions of interest of mammographic images. *Applied Soft Computing*, *46*, 613–628. doi:10.1016/j.asoc.2015.11.040

Cortazar, P., Zhang, L., Untch, M., Mehta, K., Costantino, J. P., Wolmark, N., Bonnefoi, H., Cameron, D., Gianni, L., Valagussa, P., Swain, S. M., Prowell, T., Loibl, S., Wickerham, D. L., Bogaerts, J., Baselga, J., Perou, C., Blumenthal, G., Blohmer, J., ... von Minckwitz, G. (2014). Pathological complete response and long-term clinical benefit in breast cancer: The CTNeoBC pooled analysis. *Lancet*, *384*(9938), 164–172. doi:10.1016/S0140-6736(13)62422-8 PMID:24529560

Cotrim, D. S., Silva, A. M., & Bezerra, E. A. (2007). Infra-estrutura de informática para sistemas de apoio ao diagnóstico aplicada a servidores pacs [Infrastructure of computing for support systems or diagnosis applied to servers pacs]. *III-SIIM*, 1-4.

Cover, T., & Hart, P. (1967). Nearest neighbor pattern classification. *IEEE Transactions on Information Theory*, *13*(1), 21–27. doi:10.1109/TIT.1967.1053964

da Silva, A. L., de Santana, M. A., Azevedo, W. W., Bezerra, R. S., dos Santos, W. P., & de Lima, R. C. (2018). *Seleção de Atributos para Apoio ao Diagnóstico do Câncer de Mama Usando Imagens Termográficas, Algoritmos Genéticos e Otimização por Enxame de Partículas.* II Simpósio de Inovação em Engenharia Biomédica - SABIO.

da Silva, A. S. (2015). *Classificação e segmentação de termogramas de mama para triagem de pacientes residentes em regiões de poucos recursos médicos.* Federal University of Pernambuco.

Daily, W., & Ramirez, A. (1995). Electrical resistance tomography during in-situ trichloroethylene remediation at the Savannah River Site. *Journal of Applied Geophysics*, *33*(4), 239–249. doi:10.1016/0926-9851(95)90044-6

Dai, M., Li, B., Hu, S., Xu, C., Yang, B., Li, J., Fu, F., Fei, Z., & Dong, X. (2013). In vivo imaging of twist drill drainage for subdural hematoma: A clinical feasibility study on electrical impedance tomography for measuring intracranial bleeding in humans. *PLoS One*, *8*(1), e55020. doi:10.1371/journal.pone.0055020 PMID:23372808

Dalvi-Garcia, F., Souza, M. N. D., & Pino, A. V. (2013). Algoritmo de reconstrução de imagens para um sistema de Tomografia por Impedância Elétrica (TIE) baseado em configuração multiterminais. *Rev. Bras. Eng. Biomed., Rio de Janeiro, 29*(2), 133-143.

Davidson, N. (1997). Diseases of the Breast. *Journal of the National Cancer Institute*, *89*(1), 85–85. doi:10.1093/jnci/89.1.85

de Jesus Guirro, R. R., & Vaz, M. M. O. L. L. (2017). Accuracy and Reliability of Infrared Thermography in Assessment of the Breasts of Women Affected by Cancer. *Journal of Medical Systems*, *41*(5), 87. doi:10.100710916-017-0730-7 PMID:28405947

de Lima, S. M., da Silva-Filho, A. G., & dos Santos, W. P. (2016). Detection and classification of masses in mammographic images in a multi-kernel approach. *Computer Methods and Programs in Biomedicine*, *134*, 11–29. doi:10.1016/j.cmpb.2016.04.029 PMID:27480729

de Oliveira, P. M., Silva, G. S., de Souza, G. M., Azevedo, W. W., de Santana, M. A., & dos Santos, W. P. (2019). Uso de classificadores na predição de lesões de mama a partir de imagens termográficas. *Anais do III Simpósio de Inovação em Engenharia Biomédica - SABIO 2019*, 69.

de Souza, T. K. S., de Santana, M. A., de Andrade, J. F. S., dos Santos, W. P., & de Almeida, M. B. J. (2019). Métodos Computacionais Aplicados ao Diagnóstico de Câncer de Mama por Termografia: uma revisão de literatura. *Anais do III Simpósio de Inovação em Engenharia Biomédica - SABIO 2019.*

Dean, J. C., & Ilvento, C. C. (2006). Improved cancer detection using computer-aided detection with diagnostic and screening mammography: Prospective study of 104 cancers. *AJR. American Journal of Roentgenology*, *187*(1), 20–28. doi:10.2214/AJR.05.0111 PMID:16794150

Dehghani, H., Pogue, P. W., Poplack, S. P., & Paulsen, K. D. (2003). Multiwavelength three-dimensional near-infrared tomography of the breast: Initial simulation, phantom, and clinical results. Applied Optics, 42(1), 135–145. doi:10.1364/AO.42.000135 PubMed doi:10.1364/AO.42.000135 PMID:12518832

Dehghani, Srinivasan, Pogue, & Gibson. (2009). Numerical modelling and image reconstruction in diffuse optical tomography. *Philos Trans A Math Phys Eng Sci, 367*(1900), 3073-93.

Deniz, E., Şengür, A., Kadiroğlu, Z., Guo, Y., Bajaj, V., & Budak, Ü. (2018). Transfer learning based histopathologic image classification for breast cancer detection. *Health Information Science and Systems*, *6*(1), 18. doi:10.100713755-018-0057-x PMID:30279988

Dhahbi, S., Barhoumi, W., & Zagrouba, E. (2015). Multi-view score fusion for content-based mammogram retrieval. In *Proceedings of Eighth International Conference on Machine Vision* (*vol. 9875*). Barcelona, Spain: Academic Press.

Dhahbi, S., Barhoumi, W., & Zagrouba, E. (2016). Multi-scale Kernel PCA and Its Application to Curvelet-Based Feature Extraction for Mammographic Mass Characterization. In H. Boström, A. Knobbe, C. Soares, & P. Papapetrou (Eds.), *Advances in Intelligent Data Analysis XV* (pp. 183–191). Lecture Notes in Computer Science. Springer. doi:10.1007/978-3-319-46349-0_16

Diaby, V., Tawk, R., Sanogo, V., Xiao, H., & Montero, A. J. (2015). A review of systematic reviews of the cost-effectiveness of hormone therapy, chemotherapy, and targeted therapy for breast cancer. Breast Cancer Research and Treatment, 151(1), 27–40. doi:10.1007/s10549-015-3383-6 PubMed doi:10.100710549-015-3383-6 PMID:25893588

Diakides, N., Diakides, M., Lupo, J., Paul, J., & Balcerak, R. (2006). Advances in Medical Infrared Imaging. In J. D. Bronzino (Ed.), Medical Devices and Systems, The Biomedical Engineering Handbook (3rd ed.). CRC Press. doi:10.1201/9781420003864.sec3

Díaz-Cortés, M., Ortega-Sánchez, N., Hinojosa, S., Oliva, D., Cuevas, E., Rojas, R., & Demin, A. (2018). A multi-level thresholding method for breast thermograms analysis using Dragonfly algorithm. *Infrared Physics & Technology*, *93*, 346–361. doi:10.1016/j.infrared.2018.08.007

Dibai-Filho, A. V., Costa, A. C., Packer, A. C., de Castro, E. M., & Rodrigues-Bigaton, D. (2015). Women with more severe degrees of temporomandibular disorder exhibit an increase in temperature over the temporomandibular joint. *The Saudi Dental Journal*, *27*(1), 44–49. doi:10.1016/j.sdentj.2014.10.002 PMID:25544814

Dickhaut, M., Schreer, I., & Frischbier, H. J. (1996). The value of BBE in the assessment of breast lesions. In Electropotentials in the Clinical Assessment of Breast Neoplasia. New York, NY: Springer-Verlag.

Diday, E., & Noirhomme-Fraiture, M. (2008). *Symbolic Data Analysis and the SODAS Software*. John Wiley and Sons.

Diller, K. R. (1982). Modeling of bioheat transfer processes at high and low temperatures. In Y. I. Cho (Ed.), *Advances in Heat Transfer: Bioengineering Heat Transfer* (Vol. 22, pp. 157–357). Academic Press, Inc. doi:10.1016/S0065-2717(08)70345-9

Ding, S., Zhao, H., Zhang, Y., Xu, X., & Nie, R. (2013). Extreme learning machine: Algorithm, theory and applications. *Artificial Intelligence Review*, *44*(1), 103–115. doi:10.100710462-013-9405-z

DMR, Database For Mastology Research. (2020). Retrieved from http://visual.ic.uff.br/dmi/

Dong, F., Xu, Y., Hua, L., & Wang, H. (2006). Two methods for measurement of gas-liquid flows in vertical upward pipe using dual-plane ERT system. *IEEE Transactions on Instrumentation and Measurement*, *55*(5), 1576–1586. doi:10.1109/TIM.2006.881564

Dong, Y., Pan, Y., Zhang, J., & Xu, W. (2017, July). Learning to read chest X-ray images from 16000+ examples using CNN. In *2017 IEEE/ACM International Conference on Connected Health: Applications, Systems and Engineering Technologies*, (pp. 51-57). 10.1109/CHASE.2017.59

dos Santos, W. P., de Souza, R. E., Ribeiro, R. R., Feitosa, A. R. S., de Freitas Barbosa, V. A., da Silva, V. L. B. A., . . . de Freitas, R. C. (2018). Electrical Impedance Tomography Using Evolutionary Computing: A Review. In Bio-Inspired Computing for Image and Video Processing (pp. 93-128). Chapman and Hall/CRC.

dos Santos, W. P., de Souza, R. E., Ribeiro, R. R., Feitosa, A. R. S., de Freitas Barbosa, V. A., da Silva, V. L. B. A., Ribeiro, D. E., & de Freitas, R. C. (2018). Electrical Impedance Tomography Using Evolutionary Computing: A Review. In Bio-Inspired Computing for Image and Video Processing (pp. 93-128). Chapman and Hall/CRC.

Dougherty, G. (2009). *Digital Image Processing for Medical Applications*. Cambridge University Press. doi:10.1017/CBO9780511609657

Dourado Neto, H. (2014). Egmentação e análise automática de termogramas: um método auxiliar na detecção do câncer de mama. *Dissertation Respomse to the Graduate Program in Mechanical Engineering*. Federal University of Pernambuco.

Dourado Neto, H. M. (2014). *Segmentação e análise automática de termogramas: um método auxiliar na detecção do câncer de mama* [dissertation]. Recife: Universidade Federal de Pernambuco.

Dourado Neto, H. M. (2014). *Segmentação e análise automáticas de termogramas : um método auxiliar na detecção do câncer de mama um método auxiliar na detecção do câncer de mama* (Master's thesis). Universidade Federal de Pernambuco, Recife, PE, Brazil.

Dourado Neto, H. M. (2014). *Segmentação e análise automáticas de termogramas: um método auxiliar na detecção do câncer de mama um método auxiliar na detecção do câncer de mama* [Automatic segmentation and analysis of thermograms: an auxiliary method for detecting breast cancer, an auxiliary method for detecting breast cancer] (Dissertação de mestrado). Universidade Federal de Pernambuco, Recife, PE, Brasil.

Dubey, S. R. (2019). Face retrieval using frequency decoded local descriptor. *Multimedia Tools and Applications*, *78*(12), 16411–16431. doi:10.100711042-018-7028-8

Dumansky, Y., Lyakh, Y., Gorshkov, O., Gurianov, V., & Prihodchenko, V. (2012). Fractal dimensionality analysis of normal and cancerous mammary gland thermograms. *Chaos, Solitons, and Fractals*, *45*(12), 1494–1500. doi:10.1016/j.chaos.2012.07.006

Dyakowski, T., York, T., Mikos, M., Vlaev, D., Mann, R., Follows, G., Boxman, A., & Wilson, M. (2000). Imaging nylon polymerisation processes by applying electrical tomography. *Chemical Engineering Journal*, *77*(1-2), 105–109. doi:10.1016/S1385-8947(99)00132-1

Ebert, D. S., & Musgrave, F. K. (2003). *Texturing & modeling: a procedural approach*. Morgan Kaufmann.

EBME & Clinical Engineering Articles. (2019, October 4). Retrieved from https://www.ebme.co.uk/articles/clinical-engineering/medical-thermography

El-Bastawissi, A. Y., White, E., Mandelson, M. T., & Taplin, S. (2001). Variation in mammographic breast density by race. *AEP*, *11*(4), 257–263. doi:10.1016/S1047-2797(00)00225-8 PMID:11306344

El-Bastawissi, A. Y., White, E., Mandelson, M. T., & Taplin, S. (2010). Can mammographic assessments lead to consider density as a risk factor for breast cancer. *European Journal of Radiology*. Advance online publication. doi:10.1016/j.ejrad.2010.01.001 PMID:20133095

Elston, C. W., & Ellis, I. O. (1991). Pathological prognostic factors in breast cancer. I. The value of histological grade in breast cancer: Experience from a large study with long-term follow-up. *Histopathology*, *19*(5), 403–410. doi:10.1111/j.1365-2559.1991.tb00229.x PMID:1757079

Engl, H. W., Hanke, M., & Neubauer, A. (1996). *Regularization of inverse problems: Mathematics and its appplication.* Kluwer. doi:10.1007/978-94-009-1740-8

Espíndola, N. A., Bezerra, L. A., Santos, L. C., & Lima, R. C. F. (2018). Estimating Breast Thermophysical Parameters by the Use of Mapping Surface Temperatures Measured by Infrared Images. *IEEE Latin America Transactions, 16*(10).

Espíndola, N. A., Bezerra, L. A., Santos, L. C., & Lima. R. C. F. (2018). Estimating Breast Thermophysical Parameters by the Use of Mapping Surface Temperatures Measured by Infrared Images. *IEEE Latin America Transactions, 16*(10).

EtehadTavakol, M., Chandran, V., Ng, E. Y. K., & Kafieh, R. (2013). Breast cancer detection from thermal images using bispectral invariant features. *International Journal of Thermal Sciences*, 1–16.

Etehadtavakol, M., & Ng, E. Y. (2017). Potential of thermography in pain diagnosing and treatment monitoring. In *Application of infrared to biomedical sciences* (pp. 19–32). Springer. doi:10.1007/978-981-10-3147-2_2

Etehadtavakol, M., & Ng, E. Y. K. (2013). Breast Thermography As a Potential Non-Contact Method in the Early Detection of Cancer: A Review. *Journal of Mechanics in Medicine and Biology*, *13*(02), 1330001. doi:10.1142/S0219519413300019

EurekAlert. (2019). Retrieved from https://www.eurekalert.org/pub_ releases/2019-06/riot-iit062619.php

Eyuboglu, B. M., Brown, B. H., Barber, D. C., & Seager, A. D. (1987). Localisation of cardiac related impedance changes in the thorax. *Clinical Physics and Physiological Measurement*, *8*(4A), 167–173. doi:10.1088/0143-0815/8/4A/021 PMID:3568566

Farewell, V. T., Bulbrook, R. D., & Hayward, J. L. (1978). Risk factors in breast cancer: A prospective study in the island of Gnernsy, in early diagnosis of Breast cancer. New York: E. Grandmann and L. Beck Gustav Fisher Verlag Stuttgart, 1978, 43–51.

Fass, L. (2008). Imaging and cancer: A review. Molecular Oncology, 2(2), 115–152. doi:10.1016/j.molonc.2008.04.001 PubMed doi:10.1016/j.molonc.2008.04.001 PMID:19383333

Faust, O., Acharya, U. R., & Tamura, T. (2012). Formal design methods for reliable computer-aided diagnosis: A review. *IEEE Reviews in Biomedical Engineering*, *5*, 15–28. doi:10.1109/RBME.2012.2184750 PMID:23231986

Feitosa, A. R., Ribeiro, R. R., Barbosa, V. A., de Souza, R. E., & dos Santos, W. P. (2014, May). Reconstruction of electrical impedance tomography images using particle swarm optimization, genetic algorithms and non-blind search. In *5th ISSNIP-IEEE Biosignals and Biorobotics Conference (2014): Biosignals and Robotics for Better and Safer Living (BRC)* (pp. 1-6). IEEE.

Feitosa, A. S. (2015). Reconstrução de imagens de tomografia por impedância elétrica utilizando o método Dialético de otimização. *Dissertation Response to the Graduate Program in biomedical engineering*. Federal University of Pernambuco.

Feitosa, A. R., Ribeiro, R. R., Barbosa, V. A., de Souza, R. E., & dos Santos, W. P. (2014, October). Reconstruction of electrical impedance tomography images using chaotic ring-topology particle swarm optimization and non-blind search. In *2014 IEEE International Conference on Systems, Man, and Cybernetics (SMC)* (pp. 2618-2623). IEEE. 10.1109/SMC.2014.6974322

Figueiredo, A. A. A., do Nascimento, J. G., Malheiros, F. C., da Silva Ignacio, L. H., Fernandes, H. C., & Guimaraes, G. (2019). Breast tumor localization using skin surface temperatures from a 2D anatomic model without knowledge of the thermophysical properties. *Computer Methods and Programs in Biomedicine*, *172*, 65–77. doi:10.1016/j.cmpb.2019.02.004 PMID:30902128

FLIR Systems. (2004). *ThermaCAM S45: Manual do operador*. Author.

Fluent. (2005). *Fluent 6.2 - User's Guide*. FLUENT Inc.

Folkman, J. (1971). Tumor angiogenesis: Therapeutic implications. *The New England Journal of Medicine*, *285*(21), 1182–1186. doi:10.1056/NEJM197111182852108 PMID:4938153

Fornage, B. D. (2000). Recent advances in breast sonography. JBR-BTR; Organe de la Societe Royale Belge de Radiologie (SRBR), 83(2), 75–80. PubMed PMID:10859903

Fornell, D. (2017). *New Technology and Clinical Data in Breast Imaging, ITN, "Breast Imaging" website channel.* https://www.itnonline.com/article/new-technology-and-clinical-data-breast-imaging

Fortuna, A. D. (2000). *O. Técnicas computacionais para dinâmica dos fluidos: conceitos básicos e aplicações*. Ed. Edusp.

Furuichi, M., Makie, T., Honma, Y., Isoda, T., & Miyake, S. (2015). Laboratory-Confirmed Dengue Fever and Chikungunya Fever Cases at the Narita Airport Quarantine Station in 2013. *Japanese Journal of Infectious Diseases*, *68*(2), 142–144. doi:10.7883/yoken.JJID.2014.242 PMID:25420667

Furuie, S., Gutierrez, M., Bertozzo, N., Figueriedo, J. C. B., & Yamaguti, M. (1999). Archiving and Retrieving Long-Term Cineangiographic Images in a PACS. *Computers in Cardiology*, 142–144. doi:10.1109/CIC.1999.826001

Gallas, A., & Barhoumi, W. (2015). Locality-sensitive hashing for region-based large-scale image indexing. *IET Image Processing*, *9*(9), 804–810. doi:10.1049/iet-ipr.2014.0910

Galvão, S. D. S. L. (2015). *Registro de imagens térmicas da mama adquiridas dinamicamente. Doctoral dissertation* (PhD thesis). Computer Institute, Universidade Federal Fluminense, Niterói, RJ, Brazil.

Galvão, S. D., & Júnior Hruschka, E. R. (2004). Ponderação do knn utilizando-se de métodos. *da Vinci, Curitiba, 1*(1), 115-125.

Gan, G., Ma, C., & Wu, J. (2007). Data clustering: Theory, algorithms, and applications. *International Statistical Review*, *76*(1), 141–141.

Garduño-Ramón, M. A., Vega-Mancilla, S. G., Morales-Henández, L. A., & Osornio-Rios, R. A. (2017). Supportive Noninvasive Tool for the Diagnosis of Breast Cancer Using a Thermographic Camera as Sensor. *Sensors (Basel)*, *17*(3), 497. doi:10.339017030497 PMID:28273793

Gasiorowicz, S. (1979). Física Quântica (G. Dois, Ed.). Academic Press.

Gautherie, M. (1980). Thermopathology of breast cancer: Measurements and analysis of in vivo temperature and blood flow. *Annals of the New York Academy of Sciences*, *335*(1), 383–415. doi:10.1111/j.1749-6632.1980.tb50764.x PMID:6931533

Gautherie, M. (1983). Thermobiological assessment of benign and malignant breast diseases. *American Journal of Obstetrics and Gynecology*, *147*(8), 861–869. doi:10.1016/0002-9378(83)90236-3 PMID:6650622

Geng-he, L. (2013). Extension clustering-based extreme learning machine neural network. *Jisuanji Yingyong*, *33*(7), 1942–1945. doi:10.3724/SP.J.1087.2013.01942

Gershen-Cohen, J., Haberman, J., & Brueschke, E. (1965). Medical thermography: A summary of current status. *Radiologic Clinics of North America*, 3. PMID:5846852

Geurts, P., Ernst, D., & Wehenkel, L. (2006). Extremely randomized trees. *Machine Learning*, *63*(1), 3–42. doi:10.100710994-006-6226-1

Ghafir, M. F. M., Batcha, M. F. M., & Raghavan, V. R. (2009). Prediction of the thermal conductivity of metal hydrides - the inverse problem. *International Journal of Hydrogen Energy*, *34*(16), 7125–7130. doi:10.1016/j.ijhydene.2008.06.033

Giger, M., Inciardi, M., Edwards, A., Papaioannou, J., Drukker, K., Jiang, Y., Brem, R., & Brown, J. (2016). Automated Breast Ultrasound in Breast Cancer Screening of Women with Dense Breasts: Reader Study of Mammography-Negative and Mammography-Positive Cancers. AJR. American Journal of Roentgenology, 206(6), 1–10. doi:10.2214/AJR.15.15367 PubMed doi:10.2214/AJR.15.15367 PMID:27043979

Glickman, Y.A., Filo, O., & Nachaliel, U. (2002). Novel EIS postprocessing algorithm for breast cancer diagnosis. *IEEE Trans Med Imag, 21*(710).

Global Cancer Control. (2019, October 4). Retrieved from https://www.uicc.org/membership/national-cancer-research-center-japan

Godavarty, A., Thompson, A. B., Roy, R., Gurfinkel, M., Eppstein, M. J., Zhang, C., & Sevick-Muraca, E. M. (2004, May-June). Diagnostic imaging of breast cancer using fluorescence-enhanced optical tomography: Phantom studies. Journal of Biomedical Optics, 9(3), 488–496. doi:10.1117/1.1691027 PubMed doi:10.1117/1.1691027 PMID:15189086

Gogoi, U. R., Bhowmik, M. K., Bhattacharjee, D., & Ghosh, A. K. (2018). Singular value based characterization and analysis of thermal patches for early breast abnormality detection. *Australasian Physical & Engineering Sciences in Medicine*, *41*(4), 861–879. doi:10.100713246-018-0681-4 PMID:30171500

Gogoi, U. R., Majumdar, M., Bhowmik, M. K., & Ghosh, A. K. (2019). Evaluating the efficiency of infrared breast thermography for early breast cancer risk prediction in asymptomatic population. *Infrared Physics & Technology*, *99*, 201–211. doi:10.1016/j.infrared.2019.01.004

Goldschmidt, R. R. (2010). *Uma Introdução à Inteligência Computacional: fundamentos, ferramentas e aplicações.* IST-Rio.

Gonzalez, F. (2007). Thermal simulation of breast tumors. *Revista Mexicana de Física*, *53*(4), 323–326.

Gonzalez-Hernandez, J., Recinella, A. N., Kandlikar, S. G., Dabydeen, D., Medeiros, L., & Phatak, P. (2019). Technology, application and potential of dynamic breast thermography for the detection of breast cancer. *International Journal of Heat and Mass Transfer*, *131*, 558–573. doi:10.1016/j.ijheatmasstransfer.2018.11.089

Gonzalez, R. C., & Woods, R. E. (2002). *Digital image processing.* Pearson.

Gonzalez, R. C., Woods, R. E., & Eddins, E. L. (2004). *Digital Image Processing Using Matlab.* Pearson Prentice Hall.

Gourd, E. (2017). Breast thermography alone no substitute for mammography. *The Lancet. Oncology*, *18*(12), e713. doi:10.1016/S1470-2045(17)30833-1 PMID:29103872

Gowda, K., & Diday, E. (1992). Symbolic clustering using a new similarity measure. *IEEE Transactions on Systems, Man, and Cybernetics*, *22*(2), 368–378. doi:10.1109/21.148412

Gu, X., Zhang, Q., Bartlett, M., Schutz, L., Fajardo, L. L., & Jiang, H. (2004). Differentiation of cysts from solid tumors in the breast with diffuse optical tomography. Academic Radiology, 11(1), 2094–2107. doi:10.1016/S1076-6332(03)00562-2 PubMed doi:10.1016/S1076-6332(03)00562-2 PMID:14746402

Guardo, R., Boulay, C., Murray, B., & Bertrand, M. (1991). An experimental study in electrical impedance tomography using backprojection reconstruction. *IEEE Transactions on Biomedical Engineering*, *38*(7), 617–627. doi:10.1109/10.83560 PMID:1879853

Gupta, V., & Bhavsar, A. (2017). Breast cancer histopathological image classification: is magnification important? *Proceedings of the IEEE Conference on Computer Vision and Pattern Recognition Workshops*, 17–24. 10.1109/CVPRW.2017.107

Guyon, I., Gunn, S., Nikravesh, M., & Zadeh, L. A. (2008). *Feature extraction: foundations and applications*. Springer.

Guyton, A. C., & Hall, J. E. (2011). *Tratado de fisiologia médica* (12th ed.). Elsevier Brasil.

Haddad, D. S., Brioschi, M. L., & Arita, E. S. (2012). Thermographic and clinical correlation of myofascial trigger points in the masticatory muscles. *Dento Maxillo Facial Radiology*, *41*(8), 621–629. doi:10.1259/dmfr/98504520 PMID:23166359

Haddad, D. S., Brioschi, M. L., Vardasca, R., Weber, M., Crosato, E. M., & Arita, E. S. (2014). Thermographic characterization of masticatory muscle regions in volunteers with and without myogenous temporomandibular disorder: Preliminary results. *Dento Maxillo Facial Radiology*, *43*(8), 20130440. doi:10.1259/dmfr.20130440 PMID:25144605

Halliday, D., Resnick, R., & Walker, J. (2009). *Fundamentos de Física* (8th ed.). LTC.

Halter, R. J., Hartov, A., & Paulsen, K. D. (2008). A broadband high-frequency electrical impedance tomography system for breast imaging. *IEEE Transactions on Biomedical Engineering*, *55*(2), 650–659. doi:10.1109/TBME.2007.903516 PMID:18270001

Hamilton, S. J., & Hauptmann, A. (2018). Deep D-Bar: Real-time electrical impedance tomography imaging with deep neural networks. *IEEE Transactions on Medical Imaging*, *37*(10), 2367–2377. doi:10.1109/TMI.2018.2828303 PMID:29994023

Han, F., Shi, G., Liang, C., Wang, L., & Li, K. (2015). A simple and efficient method for breast cancer diagnosis based on infrared thermal imaging. *Cell Biochemistry and Biophysics*, *71*(1), 491–498. doi:10.100712013-014-0229-5 PMID:25194831

Han, S., Kang, H. K., Jeong, J. Y., Park, M. H., Kim, W., Bang, W. C., & Seong, Y. K. (2017). A deep learning framework for supporting the classification of breast lesions in ultrasound images. *Physics in Medicine and Biology*, *62*(19), 7714–7728. doi:10.1088/1361-6560/aa82ec PMID:28753132

Haralick, R. M. (1979). Statistical and structural approaches to texture. *Proceedings of the IEEE*, *67*(5), 786–804. doi:10.1109/PROC.1979.11328

Haralick, R. M., Shanmugam, K., & Dinstein, I. (1973). Textural Features for Image Classification. *IEEE Transactions on Systems, Man, and Cybernetics*, *3*(6), 610–621. doi:10.1109/TSMC.1973.4309314

Haralick, R. M., Sternberg, S. R., & Zhuang, X. (1987). Image analysis using mathematical morphology. *IEEE Transactions on Pattern Analysis and Machine Intelligence*, *PAMI-9*(4), 532–550. doi:10.1109/TPAMI.1987.4767941 PMID:21869411

Hardy, J. D., & Muschenheim, C. (1936). The radiation of heat from the human body. V. *The Journal of Clinical Investigation*, *15*(1), 1–8. doi:10.1172/JCI100746 PMID:16694368

Harris, D. L., Greeining, W. P., & Aichroth, P. M. (1966). Infra-red in the diagnosis of a lump in the breast. *British Journal of Cancer*, *20*(4), 710–721. doi:10.1038/bjc.1966.82 PMID:5964605

Hastie, T., Tibshirani, R., & Friedman, J. (2009). *The Elements of Statistical Learning* (2nd ed.). Springer. doi:10.1007/978-0-387-84858-7

Hatwar, R., & Herman, C. (2017). Inverse method for quantitative characterisation of breast tumours from surface temperature data. *International Journal of Hyperthermia, 33*(7), 741–757. doi:10.1080/02656736.2017.1306758 PMID:28540793

Haykin, S. (2003). Redes neurais, Princípios e Prática. *The Bookman.*

Haykin, S. (2007). *Redes neurais: princípios e prática.* Bookman Editora.

Heckbert, P. (1986). Survey of texture mapping. *IEEE Computer Graphics and Applications, 6*(11), 56–67. doi:10.1109/MCG.1986.276672

He, D. C., & Wang, L. (1990). Texture unit, texture spectrum, and texture analysis. *IEEE Transactions on Geoscience and Remote Sensing, 28*(4), 509–512. doi:10.1109/TGRS.1990.572934

Herborn, C. U., Marincek, B., Erfmann, D., Meuli-Simmen, C., Wedler, V., Bode-Lesniewska, B., & Kubik-Huch, R. A. (2002). Breast augmentation and reconstructive surgery: MR imaging of implant rupture and malignancy. European Radiology, 12(9), 2198–2206. doi:10.1007/s00330-002-1362-x PubMed doi:10.100700330-002-1362-x PMID:12195470

Hildebrandt, C., Raschner, C., & Ammer, K. (2010). An overview of recent application of medical infrared thermography in sports medicine in Austria. *Sensors (Basel), 10*(5), 4700–4715. doi:10.3390100504700 PMID:22399901

Holder, D. (2004). *Electrical impedance tomography: methods, history and applications.* CRC Press. doi:10.1201/9781420034462

Hong, S., Lee, K., Ha, U., Kim, H., Lee, Y., Kim, Y., & Yoo, H. J. (2014). A 4.9 mΩ-sensitivity mobile electrical impedance tomography IC for early breast-cancer detection system. *IEEE Journal of Solid-State Circuits, 50*(1), 245–257. doi:10.1109/JSSC.2014.2355835

Hosaki, Y., Mitsunobu, F., Ashida, K., Tsugeno, H., Okamoto, M., Nishida, N., Takata, S., Yokoi, T., Tanizaki, Y., Ochi, K., & Tsuji, T. (2002). Non-invasive study for peripheral circulation in patients with diabetes mellitus. *Annual Reports of Misasa Medical Branch, 72*, 31–37.

Hossain, S., Abdelaal, M., & Mohammadi, F. A. (2016). Thermogram Assessment for Tumor Parameter Estimation Considering Body Geometry. *Canadian Journal of Electrical and Computer Engineering, 39*(3), 219–234. doi:10.1109/CJECE.2016.2541661

Hossain, S., & Mohammadi, F. A. (2016). Tumor parameter estimation considering the body geometry by thermography. *Computers in Biology and Medicine, 76*, 80–93. doi:10.1016/j.compbiomed.2016.06.023 PMID:27416548

Ho, T. K. K., & Gwak, J. (2019). Multiple feature integration for classification of thoracic disease in chest radiography. *Applied Sciences (Basel, Switzerland), 9*(19), 4130. doi:10.3390/app9194130

Houdas, Y., & Ring, E. F. J. (1982). *Human Body Temperature.* Plenum Press. doi:10.1007/978-1-4899-0345-7

Hrung, J. M., Sonnad, S. S., Schwartz, J. S., & Langlotz, C. P. (1999). Accuracy of MR imaging in the work-up of suspicious breast lesions: A diagnostic meta-analysis. Academic Radiology, 6(7), 387–397. doi:10.1016/S1076-6332(99)80189-5 PubMed doi:10.1016/S1076-6332(99)80189-5 PMID:10410164

Hsieh, J. (2009, November). *Computed tomography: principles, design, artifacts, and recent advances.* Bellingham, WA: SPIE.

Huang, G.-B., Zhu, Q.-Y., & Siew, C.-K. (2004). Extreme learning machine: a new learning scheme of feedforward neural networks. *2004 IEEE International Joint Conference on Neural Networks* (IEEE Cat. No.04CH37541).

Huang, C., & Huang, C. (2007). An inverse problem in estimating simultaneously the effective thermal conductivity and volumetric heat capacity of biological tissue. *Applied Mathematical Modelling*, *31*(9), 1785–1797. doi:10.1016/j.apm.2006.06.002

Huang, G. B., Zhou, H., Ding, X., & Zhang, R. (2011). Extreme learning machine for regression and multiclass classification. *IEEE Transactions on Systems, Man, and Cybernetics. Part B, Cybernetics*, *42*(2), 513–529. doi:10.1109/TSMCB.2011.2168604 PMID:21984515

Huang, G. B., Zhu, Q. Y., & Siew, C. K. (2006). Extreme learning machine: Theory and applications. *Neurocomputing*, *70*(1-3), 489–501. doi:10.1016/j.neucom.2005.12.126

Huang, Z., Wang, B., & Li, H. (2003). Application of electrical capacitance tomography to the void fraction measurement of two-phase flow. *IEEE Transactions on Instrumentation and Measurement*, *52*(1), 7–12. doi:10.1109/TIM.2003.809087

Hua, P., Woo, E. J., Webster, J. G., & Tompkins, W. J. (1993). Finite element modeling of electrode-skin contact impedance in electrical impedance tomography. *IEEE Transactions on Biomedical Engineering*, *40*(4), 335–343. doi:10.1109/10.222326 PMID:8375870

Huber, N., Béqo, N., Adams, C., Sze, G., Tunstall, B., Qiao, G., & Wang, W. (2010). Further investigation of a contactless patient-electrode interface of an Electrical Impedance Mammography system. *Journal of Physics: Conference Series*, *224*(1), 012166. doi:10.1088/1742-6596/224/1/012166

Hudson, R. D. Jr. (1969). *Infrared System Engineering*. John Wiley and Sons Inc.

Hu, L., Gupta, A., Gore, J. P., & Xu, L. X. (2004). Effect of forced convection on the skin thermal expression of breast cancer. *Journal of Biomechanical Engineering*, *126*(2), 204–211. doi:10.1115/1.1688779 PMID:15179850

HyperPhysics. (2019). *The Interaction of Radiation with the Matter*. Department of Physics and Astronomy, Georgia State University. Retrieved from http://hyperphysics.phy-astr.gsu.edu/hbase/mod3.html

Iljaž, J., Wrobel, L. C., Hriberšek, M., & Marn, J. (2019). Numerical modelling of skin tumour tissue with temperature-dependent properties for dynamic thermography. *Computers in Biology and Medicine*, *112*, 112. doi:10.1016/j.compbiomed.2019.103367 PMID:31386971

Incropera, F. P., & Witt, D. P. (1996). Introduction to heat transfer (3rd ed.). Wiley Ed.

Instituto Nacional de Câncer. (2002). *Falando sobre câncer de mama*. INCA.

Iorio, M. V., Casalini, P., Piovan, C., Braccioli, L., & Tagliabue, E. (2011). Breast cancer and microRNAs: Therapeutic impact. The Breast, 20, S63–S70. doi:10.1016/S0960-9776(11)70297-1 PubMed doi:10.1016/S0960-9776(11)70297-1 PMID:22015296

Isard, H. J., Becker, W., Shilo, R., & Ostrum, B. J. (1972). Breast thermography after four years and 10,000 studies. *AJR. American Journal of Roentgenology*, *115*(4), 811–821. doi:10.2214/ajr.115.4.811 PMID:5054275

Jia, M., Zheng, R., Zhang, S., Zeng, H., Zou, X., & Chen, W. (2015). Female breast cancer incidence and mortality in 2011, China. Journal of Thoracic Disease, 7, 1221–1226. PubMed PMID:26380738

Jiang, L., Zhan, W., & Loew, M. H. (2011). Modeling static and dynamic thermography of the human breast under elastic deformation. *Physics in Medicine and Biology*, *56*(1), 187–202. doi:10.1088/0031-9155/56/1/012 PMID:21149948

Jiang, M., Zhang, S., Li, H., & Metaxas, D. (2015). Computer-aided diagnosis of mammographic masses using scalable image retrieval. *IEEE Transactions on Biomedical Engineering*, *62*(2), 783–792. doi:10.1109/TBME.2014.2365494 PMID:25361497

Jiang, M., Zhang, S., & Metaxas, D. N. (2018). Detecting Mammographic Masses via Image Retrieval and Discriminative Learning. In K. Suzuki & Y. Chen (Eds.), *Artificial Intelligence in Decision Support Systems for Diagnosis in Medical Imaging*. Springer. doi:10.1007/978-3-319-68843-5_5

Joensuu, H., Asola, R., Holli, K., Kumpulainen, E., Nikkanen, V., & Parvinen, L. M. (1994). Delayed diagnosis and large size of breast cancer after a flase negative mammogram. European Journal of Cancer (Oxford, England), 30(9), 1299–1302. doi:10.1016/0959-8049(94)90177-5 doi:10.1016/0959-8049(94)90177-5

Jordana, J., Gasulla, M., & Pallás-Areny, R. (1999, April). Leakage detection in buried pipes by electrical resistance imaging. In *Proc. 1st World Congress on Industrial Process Tomography (Buxton)* (pp. 28-34). Academic Press.

Jordan, M. I., & Mitchell, T. M. (2015). Machine learning: Trends, perspectives, and prospects. *Science, 349*(6245), 255–260. doi:10.1126cience.aaa8415 PMID:26185243

Jorgensen, B., & Wewn, G. (2010). *The benefits and harms of screening for cancer with a focus on breast screening*. Academic Press.

Jouirou, A., Baâzaoui, A., & Barhoumi, W. (2019). Multi-view information fusion in mammograms: A comprehensive overview. *Information Fusion, 52*, 308–321. doi:10.1016/j.inffus.2019.05.001

Jouirou, A., Baâzaoui, A., Barhoumi, W., & Zagrouba, E. (2015). Curvelet-based locality sensitive hashing for mammogram retrieval in large-scale datasets. In *Proceedings of 12th IEEE/ACS International Conference of Computer Systems and Applications* (pp. 1-8). IEEE. 10.1109/AICCSA.2015.7507106

Jumuga, C., Macota, G., & Stoian, I. (2009). The role of sonoelastography for the diagnosis of breast cancer. *Gineco. ro, 5*, 258-262.

Kan, C., & Srinath, M. D. (2001). Combined Features of Cubic B-Spline Wavelet Moments and Zernike Moments for Invariant Character Recognition. In *IEEE International Conference on Information Technology: Coding and Computing (ITCC'01)*. IEEE.

Kandlikar, S. G., Perez-Raya, I., Raghupathi, P. A., Gonzalez-Hernandez, J., Dabydeen, D., Medeiros, L., & Phatak, P. (2017). Infrared imaging technology for breast cancer detection – Current status, protocols and new directions. *International Journal of Heat and Mass Transfer, 108*(Part B), 2303 – 2320.

Kannala, J., & Rahtu, E. (2012). BSIF: Binarized statistical image features. In *Proceedings of the 21st international conference on pattern recognition (ICPR2012)* (pp. 1363-1366). Academic Press.

Kapoor, P., Prasad, S. V., & Patni, S. (2012). Image Segmentation and Asymmetry Analysis of Breast Thermograms for Tumor Detection. *International Journal of Computers and Applications, 50*(9), 40–45. doi:10.5120/7803-0932

Keleş, A., & Keleş, A. (2008). ESTDD: Expert system for thyroid diseases diagnosis. *Expert Systems with Applications, 34*(1), 242–246. doi:10.1016/j.eswa.2006.09.028

Keller, F., Muller, E., & Bohm, K. (2012). *HiCS: High-contrast subspaces for density-based outlier ranking*. ICDE.

Kelly, K. M., Dean, J., Comulada, W. S., & Lee, S. J. (2010). Breast cancer detection using automated whole breast ultrasound and mammography in radiographically dense breasts. European Radiology, 20(3), 734–742. doi:10.1007/s00330-009-1588-y PubMed doi:10.100700330-009-1588-y PMID:19727744

Kerlikowske, K., Grady, D., Rubin, S. M., Sandrock, C., & Ernster, V. L. (1995). Efficacy of screening mammography. A meta-analysis. Journal of the American Medical Association, 273(2), 149–154. doi:10.1001/jama.1995.03520260071035 PubMed doi:10.1001/jama.1995.03520260071035 PMID:7799496

Kermani, S., Samadzadehaghdam, N., & EtehadTavakol, M. (2015). Automatic color segmentation of breast infrared images using a Gaussian mixture model. *Optik (Stuttgart)*, *126*(21), 3288–3294. doi:10.1016/j.ijleo.2015.08.007

Kesim, E., Dokur, Z., & Olmez, T. (2019, April). X-Ray Chest Image Classification by A Small-Sized Convolutional Neural Network. In *2019 Scientific Meeting on Electrical-Electronics & Biomedical Engineering and Computer Science (EBBT)* (pp. 1-5). Academic Press.

Key, T. J., Appleby, P. N., Reeves, G. K., Roddam, A., Dorgan, J. F., Longcope, C., ... (2003). Body mass index, serum sex hormones, and breast cancer risk in postmenopausal women. Journal of the National Cancer Institute, 95(16), 1218–1226. doi:10.1093/jnci/djg022 PubMed doi:10.1093/jnci/djg022 PMID:12928347

Keyserlingk, J. R., Ahlgren, P. D., Yu, E., & Belliveau, N. (1998). Infrared Imaging of the Breast: Initial Reappraisal Using High-Resolution Digital Technology in 100 Successive Cases of Stage I and II Breast Cancer. *The Breast Journal*, *4*(4), 245–251. doi:10.1046/j.1524-4741.1998.440245.x PMID:21223443

Kim, S. K., Jung, B. S., Kim, H. J., & Lee, W. I. (2003). Inverse estimation of thermophysical properties for anisotropic composite. *Experimental Thermal and Fluid Science*, *24*(6), 697–704. doi:10.1016/S0894-1777(02)00309-6

Kinzler, K. W., & Vogelstein, B. (1996). Lessons from hereditary colorectal cancer. *Cell*, *87*(2), 159–170. doi:10.1016/S0092-8674(00)81333-1 PMID:8861899

Kirubha, A. S. P., Anburajan, M., Venkataraman, B., & Menaka, M. (2015). Comparison of PET–CT and thermography with breast biopsy in evaluation of breast cancer: A case study. *Infrared Physics & Technology*, *73*, 115–125. doi:10.1016/j.infrared.2015.09.008

Kirubha, A. S. P., Anburajan, M., Venkataraman, B., & Menaka, M. (2018). A case study on asymmetrical texture features comparison of breast thermogram and mammogram in normal and breast cancer subject. *Biocatalysis and Agricultural Biotechnology*, *15*, 390–401. doi:10.1016/j.bcab.2018.07.001

Koga, S., Nakano, S., Honma, Y., & Ogasawara, N. (2007, June 28). FDG-PET (positron emission tomography) in the detection of primary breast cancer and lymph nodes involvement [Japanese]. Japanese Journal of Clinical Medicine, 65(Suppl 6), 379–384. PubMed PMID:17682181

Kohavi, R., & John, G. (1997). Wrappers for feature subset selection. *Artificial Intelligence*, *97*(1-2), 273–324. doi:10.1016/S0004-3702(97)00043-X

Kong, X., Moran, M. S., Zhang, N., Haffty, B., & Yang, Q. (2011). Meta-analysis confirms achieving pathological complete response after neoadjuvant chemotherapy predicts favourable prognosis for breast cancer patients. *European Journal of Cancer*, *47*(14), 2084–2090. doi:10.1016/j.ejca.2011.06.014 PMID:21737257

Kowal, M., Filipczuk, P., Obuchowicz, A., Korbicz, J., & Monczak, R. (2013). Computer-aided diagnosis of breast cancer based on fine needle biopsy microscopic images. *Computers in Biology and Medicine*, *43*(10), 1563–1572. doi:10.1016/j.compbiomed.2013.08.003 PMID:24034748

Krawczyk, B., Schaefer, G., & Woźniak, M. (2015). A hybrid cost-sensitive ensemble for imbalanced breast thermogram classification. *Artificial Intelligence in Medicine*, *65*(3), 219–227. doi:10.1016/j.artmed.2015.07.005 PMID:26319694

Kulshreshtha, D., Singh, V. P., Shrivastava, A., Chaudhary, A., & Srivastava, R. (2017). Content-based mammogram retrieval using k-means clustering and local binary pattern. In *Proceedings of 2nd International Conference on Image, Vision and Computing* (pp. 634-638). Academic Press. 10.1109/ICIVC.2017.7984633

Kumar, S. P., Sriraam, N., Benakop, P. G., & Jinaga, B. C. (2010, July). Reconstruction of brain electrical impedance tomography images using particle swarm optimization. In *2010 5th International Conference on Industrial and Information Systems* (pp. 339-342). IEEE.

Kumar, I., Bhadauria, H. S., Virmani, J., & Thakur, S. (2017). A classification framework for prediction of breast density using an ensemble of neural network classifiers. *Biocybernetics and Biomedical Engineering*, *37*(1), 217–228. doi:10.1016/j.bbe.2017.01.001

Kumar, V., Abbas, A. K., Fausto, N., & Aster, J. C. (2010). *Robbins & Cotran Patologia Bases Patológicas das Doenças* (8th ed.). Elsevier.

Kuncheva, L. I. (2014). *Combining pattern classifiers: methods and algorithms*. John Wiley & Sons.

Ladis, R. J., & Koch, G. G. (1977). The Measurement of Observer Agreement for Categorical Data. *Biometrics*, *33*(1), 159–174. doi:10.2307/2529310 PMID:843571

Lahiri, B. B., Bagavathiappan S., Jayakumar T., & Philip, J. (2012) Medical applications of infrared thermography: A review. *International Journal Infrared Physics and Technology*, 222-232.

Lahiri, B. B., Bagavathiappan S., Jayakumar T., & Philip, J. (2012). Medical applications of infrared thermography: A review. *International Journal Infrared Physics and Technology*, 222-232.

Lahiri, B. B., Bagavathiappan, S., Soumya, C., Jayakumar, T., & Philip, J. (2015). Infrared thermography based studies on mobile phone induced heating. *Infrared Physics & Technology*, *71*, 242–251. doi:10.1016/j.infrared.2015.04.010

Lan, R., Zhou, Y., & Tang, Y. Y. (2015). Quaternionic local ranking binary pattern: A local descriptor of color images. *IEEE Transactions on Image Processing*, *25*(2), 566–579. doi:10.1109/TIP.2015.2507404 PMID:26672041

Lawson, R. (1957). Thermography: A new tool in the investigation of breast lesions. *Canadian Services Medical Journal*, *8*(8), 517–524. PMID:13460932

Lawson, R. N. (1956). Implications of surface temperatures in the diagnosis of breast cancer. *Canadian Medical Association Journal*, *75*(5), 309–310. PMID:13343098

Lawson, R. N. (1957). Thermography – a new tool in the investigation of breast lesions. *Canadian Services Medical Journal*, *13*, 517–524. PMID:13460932

Leach, M. O. (2001). Application of magnetic resonance imaging to angiogenesis in breast cancer. Breast Cancer Research, 3(1), 22–27. doi:10.1186/bcr266 PubMed doi:10.1186/bcr266 PMID:11300102

Leão, M. P. V., & Macedo, V. G. (2014). Comparação entre os métodos analítico e iterativo na reconstrução de imagens tomográficas. In *XXIV Congresso Brasileiro de Engenharia Biomédica. Uberlândia: Canal* (*Vol. 6*). Academic Press.

Leichter, I., Buchbinder, S., Bamberger, P., Novak, B., Fields, S., & Lederman, R. (2000). Quantitative characterization of mass lesions on digitized mammograms for computer-assisted diagnosis. Investigative Radiology, 35(6), 366–372. doi:10.1097/00004424-200006000-00005 PubMed doi:10.1097/00004424-200006000-00005 PMID:10853611

Lei, J., Mu, H. P., Liu, Q. B., Wang, X. Y., & Liu, S. (2018). Data-driven reconstruction method for electrical capacitance tomography. *Neurocomputing*, *273*, 333–345. doi:10.1016/j.neucom.2017.08.006

Lemaître, G., & Yong, E. W. (n.d.). Evaluation measures for segmentation. *Matrix, 1.*

Li, X., Zhang, S., Zhang, Q., Wei, X., Pan, Y., Zhao, J., ... Yang, F. (2019). *Diagnosis of thyroid cancer using deep convolutional neural network models applied to sonographic images: a retrospective, multicohort, diagnostic study.* Academic Press.

Liberman, M., Sampalis, F., Mulder, D. S., & Sampalis, J. S. (2003). Breast Cancer Diagnosis by Scintimammography: A Meta-analysis and Review of the Literature. *Breast Cancer Research and Treatment, 80*(1), 115–126. doi:10.1023/A:1024417331304

Librelotto, S. R., & Mozzaquatro, P. (2014). Análise dos algoritmos de mineração j48 e apriori aplicados na detecção de indicadores da qualidade de vida e saúde. *Revista Interdisciplinar de Ensino, Pesquisa e Extensão - RevInt.*

Li, L.-N., Ouyang, J.-H., Chen, H.-L., & Liu, D.-Y. (2012). A Computer Aided Diagnosis System for Thyroid Disease Using Extreme Learning Machine. *Journal of Medical Systems*, *36*(5), 3327–3337. doi:10.100710916-012-9825-3 PMID:22327384

Li, Q., Zhao, T., Zhang, L., Sun, W., & Zhao, X. (2017). Ferrography wear particles image recognition based on extreme learning machine. *Journal of Electrical and Computer Engineering*, *2017*, 2017. doi:10.1155/2017/3451358

Liu, F. B., & Ozisik, M. N. (1995). Simultaneous estimation of fluid thermal conductivity and heat capacity in laminar duct flow. *Fluid Thermal Conductivity and Heat Capacity, 333*(B), 583–591.

Liu, C., Cao, Y., Alcantara, M., Liu, B., Brunette, M., Peinado, J., & Curioso, W. (2017). TX-CNN: Detecting tuberculosis in chest X-ray images using convolutional neural network. In *2017 IEEE International Conference on Image Processing (ICIP)* (pp. 2314-2318). 10.1109/ICIP.2017.8296695

Liu, C., Heijden, F., Klein, M. E., Baal, J. G., Bus, S. A., & Netten, J. J. (2013). Infrared dermal thermography on diabetic feet soles to predict ulcerations: A case study. *Advanced Biomedical and Clinical Systems*, *11*, 8572. doi:10.1117/12.2001807

Liu, F. T., Kai, M. T., & Zhou, Z.-H. (2008). Isolation forest. In *2008 Eighth IEEE International Conference on Data Mining*. IEEE. 10.1109/ICDM.2008.17

Liu, J. G., & Mason, P. J. (2016). *Image Processing and GIS for Remote Sensing: Techniques and Applications* (2nd ed.). Wiley-Blackwell. doi:10.1002/9781118724194

Liu, J., Zhang, S., Liu, W., Deng, C., Zheng, Y., & Metaxas, D. N. (2017). Scalable Mammogram Retrieval Using Composite Anchor Graph Hashing With Iterative Quantization. *IEEE Transactions on Circuits and Systems for Video Technology*, *27*(11), 2450–2460. doi:10.1109/TCSVT.2016.2592329

Liu, Y., & Sun, F. (2011). A fast differential evolution algorithm using k-Nearest Neighbour predictor. *Expert Systems with Applications*, *38*(4), 4254–4258. doi:10.1016/j.eswa.2010.09.092

Li, X., Shen, L., Xie, X., Huang, S., Xie, Z., Hong, X., & Yu, J. (2019). Multi-resolution convolutional networks for chest X-ray radiograph based lung nodule detection. *Artificial Intelligence in Medicine*, 101744. PMID:31732411

Loukas, C., Kostopoulos, S., Tanoglidi, A., Glotsos, D., Sfikas, C., & Cavouras, D. (2013). Breast cancer characterization based on image classification of tissue sections visualized under low magnification. *Computational and Mathematical Methods in Medicine*, *2013*, 2013. doi:10.1155/2013/829461 PMID:24069067

Lozano, A. III, & Hassanipour, F. (2019). Infrared imaging for breast cancer detection: An objective review of foundational studies and its proper role in breast cancer screening. *Infrared Physics & Technology*, *97*, 244–257. doi:10.1016/j.infrared.2018.12.017

Luz, L. M. S. (2007). *Segmentação em ultra-sonografia de mama com operadores morfológicos associados à função gaussiana* (Master's thesis). Universidade Federal do Rio de Janeiro, Rio de Janeiro, RJ, Brazil.

Lv, X., & Wang, Y. (2016). Multiple-Feature Kernel Hashing for Mass Detection. In *Proceedings of the International Conference on Internet Multimedia Computing and Service* (pp. 99-104). Xi'an, China: Academic Press.

Madhu, H., Kakileti, S. T., Venkataramani, K., & Jabbireddy, S. (2016). *Extraction of medically interpretable features for classification of malignancy in breast thermography*. 38th Annual International Conference of the IEEE Engineering in Medicine and Biology, Orlando, FL.

Mahmoudzadeh, E., Montazeri, M. A., Zekri, M., & Sadri, S. (2015). Extended hidden Markov model for optimized segmentation of breast thermography images. *Infrared Physics & Technology*, *72*, 19–28. doi:10.1016/j.infrared.2015.06.012

Mahmoudzadeh, E., Zekri, M., Montazeri, M. A., Sadri, S., & Dabbagh, S. T. (2016). Directional SUSAN image boundary detection of breast thermogram. *IET Image Processing*, *10*(7), 552–560. doi:10.1049/iet-ipr.2015.0347

Makes D Department of Radiology. (2005). Faculty of Medicine, University of Indonesia Ciptomangunkusumo General Hospital. Jakarta Biomed Imaging Interv J, 1(1), e6–e1.

Maliska, C. R. (1995). *Transferência de calor e Mecânica dos fluidos computacional*. Ed. LTC.

Mambou. (2018). *Breast Cancer Detection Using Infrared Thermal Imaging and a Deep Learning Model*. Academic Press.

Mambou, S. J., Maresova, P., Krejcar, O., Selamat, A., & Kuca, K. (2018). Breast Cancer Detection Using Infrared Thermal Imaging and a Deep Learning Model. *Sensors (Basel)*, *18*(9), 2799. doi:10.339018092799 PMID:30149621

Mamounas, E. P. (2015). Impact of neoadjuvant chemotherapy on locoregional surgical treatment of breast cancer. *Annals of Surgical Oncology*, *22*(5), 1425–1433. doi:10.124510434-015-4406-6 PMID:25727558

Manginas, A., Andreanides, E., Leontiadis, E., Sfyrakis, P., Maounis, T., Degiannis, D., Alivizatos, P., & Cokkinos, D. (2010). Right ventricular endocardial thermography in transplanted and coronary artery disease patients: First human application. *The Journal of Invasive Cardiology*, *22*, 400–404. PMID:20814045

Marchena-Menéndez, J., Ramírez-Torres, A., Penta, R., Rodríguez-Ramos, R., & Merodio, J. (2019). Macroscopic thermal profile of heterogeneous cancerous breasts. A three-dimensional multiscale analysis. *International Journal of Engineering Science*, *144*, 144. doi:10.1016/j.ijengsci.2019.103135

Marques, R. S. (2012). *Segmentação automática das mamas em imagens térmicas* (M Sc. Dissertation). Computer Institute, Universidade Federal Fluminense, Niterói, RJ, Brazil.

Marques, R. S., Conci, A., Perez, M. G., Andaluz, V. H., & Mejia, T. M. (2016). An approach for automatic segmentation of thermal imaging in Computer Aided Diagnosis. *IEEE Latin America Transactions*, *14*(4), 1856–1865. doi:10.1109/TLA.2016.7483526

Martins, J. G., Costa, Y. M. G., Gonçalves, D. B., & Oliveira, L. E. S. (2011). Uso de descritores de textura extraídos de GLCM para o reconhecimento de padrões em diferentes domínios de aplicação. In *XXXVII Conferencia Latinoamericana de Informática*. Elsevier.

Massardo, T., Alonso, O., Llamas-Ollier, A., Kabasakal, L., Ravishankar, U., Morales, R., Delgado, L., & Padhy, A. K. (2005). Planar Tc99m—sestamibi scintimammography should be considered cautiously in the axillary evaluation of breast cancer protocols: Results of an international multicenter trial. BMC Nuclear Medicine, 5(1), 4. doi:10.1186/1471-2385-5-4 PubMed doi:10.1186/1471-2385-5-4 PMID:16048648

Materka, A., & Strzelecki, M. (1998). Texture analysis methods–a review. Technical university of lodz, institute of electronics, COST B11 report.

McKinlay, J. B., Burns, R. B., Feldman, H. A., Freund, K. M., Irish, J. T., Kasten, L. E., Moskowitz, M. A., Potter, D. A., & Woodman, K. (1998). Physician Variability and Uncertainty in the Management of Breast Cancer: Results from a Factorial Experiment. *Medical Care*, *36*(3), 385–396. doi:10.1097/00005650-199803000-00014 PMID:9520962

Medical Xpress. (2019). *Infrared imaging technology being developed to better detect breast cancer*. Retrieved from https://medicalxpress.com/ news/2019-06-infrared-imaging-technology-breast-cancer.html?utm_sour ce=TrendMD&utm_medium=cpc&utm_campaign=MedicalXpress_TrendMD_1

Melo, J. F. R. (2019). *Metodologia para desenvolvimento de geometria tridimensional de mama e seu uso na estimativa de parâmetros usando imagens termográficas* [Methodology for the development of three-dimensional geometry of the breast and its use in estimating parameters using thermographic images] (Master's thesis). Universidade Federal de Pernambuco, Recife, PE, Brazil.

Melo, J. R. F., Queiroz, J. R. A., Bezerra, L. A., & Lima, R. C. F. (2019). Development of a three-dimensional surrogate geometry of the breast and its use in estimating the thermal conductivities of breast tissue and breast lesions based on infrared images. *International Communications in Heat and Mass Transfer*, 108.

Menczer, J., & Eskin, B. A. (1969). Evaluation of postpartum breast engorgement by thermography. *Magazine Obstetrics and Gynecology*, *33*(2), 260–263. PMID:4886952

Menin, O. H. (2009). *Método dos elementos de contorno para tomografia de impedância elétrica* (Doctoral dissertation). Universidade de São Paulo.

Menke, C. H. (2000). *Rotinas em Mastologia* (2nd ed.). ArtMed Editora.

Migowski, A., Silva, G. A. E., Dias, M. B. K., Diz, M. D. P. E., Sant'Ana, D. R., & Nadanovsky, P. (2018). Guidelines for early detection of breast cancer in Brazil. II - New national recommendations, main evidence, and controversies. *Cadernos de Saude Publica*, *34*(6). PMID:29947654

Miles, D. W., Thomsen, L. L., Happerfield, L., Bobrow, L. G., Knowles, R. G., & Moncada, S. (1995). Nitric oxide synthase activity in human breast cancer. *Journal of Cancer*, *72*(1), 41–44. doi:10.1038/bjc.1995.274 PMID:7541238

Miller, K. D., Siegel, R. L., Lin, C. C., Mariotto, A. B., Kramer, J. L., Rowland, J. H., Stein, K. D., Alteri, R., & Jemal, A. (2016). Cancer treatment and survivorship statistics. *CA: a Cancer Journal for Clinicians*, *66*(4), 271–289. doi:10.3322/caac.21349 PMID:27253694

Milosevic, M., Jankovic, D., Milenkovic, A., & Stojanov, D. (2018). Early diagnosis and detection of breast cancer. *Technology and Health Care*, *26*(4), 729–759. doi:10.3233/THC-181277 PMID:30124455

Milosevic, M., Jankovic, D., & Peulic, A. (2015). Comparative analysis of breast cancer detection in mammograms and thermograms. *Biomedizinische Technik. Biomedical Engineering*, *60*(1), 49–56. doi:10.1515/bmt-2014-0047 PMID:25720034

Ministério da Saúde. (2017). *Instituto Nacional de Câncer José Alencar Gomes da Silva*. Estimativa 2018: Incidência de Câncer no Brasil, Rio de Janeiro.

Mital, M., & Scott, E. P. (2007, February). Thermal detection of embedded tumors using infrared imaging. Journal of Biomechanical Engineering, 129(1), 33–39. doi:10.1115/1.2401181 PubMed doi:10.1115/1.2401181 PMID:17227096

Mital, M. (2008). Breast tumor simulation and parameters estimation using evolucionary algorithms. *Modelling and Simulation in Engineering*, *10*(1), 7–14.

Mitra, S., & Balaji, C. (1992). A neural network based estimation of tumor parameters from a breast thermogram. *Modelling and Simulation in Engineering*, *10*(1), 7–14.

Modest, M. F. (2013). *Radiative heat transfer* (3rd ed.). Academic Press. doi:10.1016/B978-0-12-386944-9.50023-6

Mohanty, F., Rup, S., Dash, B., Majhi, B., & Swamy, M. N. S. (2019). Digital mammogram classification using 2D-BDWT and GLCM features with FOA-based feature selection approach. *Neural Computing & Applications*, 1–15. doi:10.100700521-019-04186-w

Montoya Vallejo, M. F. (n.d.). *Algoritmo de tomografia por impedância elétrica utilizando programação linear como método de busca da imagem* (Doctoral dissertation). Universidade de São Paulo.

Montreal Breast Center. (2019, October 8). Retrieved from http://www.vmmed.com

Moore, K. L., Dalley, A. F., & Agur, A. M. R. (2001). *Anatomia orientada para a clínica* (6th ed.). Guanabara Koogan.

Moran, M. B., Apostolo, G. H., Araujo, A., Andrade, E., Viterbo, J. V., & Conci, A. (2019). A novel approach for the segmentation of breast thermal images combining image processing and collective intelligence. In *IEEE 19th International Conference on Bioinformatics and Bioengineering (BIBE)*. 10.1109/BIBE.2019.00099

Moran, M. B., Conci, A., & Araujo, A. S. (2019). Evaluation of quantitative features and convolutional neural networks for nodule identification in thyroid thermographies. In *IEEE 19th International Conference on Bioinformatics and Bioengineering (BIBE)*. 10.1109/BIBE.2019.00140

Moran, M. B., Conci, A., Gonzalez, J. R., Araujo, A. S., Fiirst, W., Damiao, C., Lima, G., & Filho, R. (2018). Identification of thyroid nodules in infrared images by convolutional neural networks. In *31st International Joint Conference on Neural Networks (IJCNN)*. 10.1109/IJCNN.2018.8489032

Morasiewicz, L., Dudek, K., Orzechowski, W., Kulej, M., & Stepniewski, M. (2008). Use of thermography to monitor the bone regenerate during limb lengthening - preliminary communication. *Ortop Traumatol Rehabil 2, 10*(3), 279-85.

Moskowitz, M., Fox, S. H., del Re, R. B., Milbrath, J. R., Bassett, L. W., Gold, R. H., & Shaffer, K. A. (1981). The potential value of liquid-crystal thermography in detecting significant mastopathy. *Radiology*, *140*(3), 659–662. doi:10.1148/radiology.140.3.7280232 PMID:7280232

Moskowitz, M., Milbrath, J., Gartside, P., Ermeno, A., & Mandel, D. (1976). Lack of efficiency of thermography as a screening tool for minimal and Stage I breast cancer. *Journal of Medicine*, *295*(5), 249–252. PMID:934189

Motta, L. S. (2010). *Obtenção automática da região de interesse em termogramas frontais da mama para o auxílio à detecção precoce de doenças* (M Sc. Dissertation). Computer Institute. UFF, Niteroi, Brazil.

MS & INCA. (2002). *Falando sobre câncer de mama.* Rio de Janeiro: Instituto Nacional de Câncer. Coordenação de Prevenção e Vigilância – (Conprev).

Mudigonda, N. R., Rangayyan, R. M., & Desautels, J. L. (2001). Detection of breast masses in mammograms by density slicing and texture flow-field analysis. *IEEE Transactions on Medical Imaging*, *20*(12), 1215–1227. doi:10.1109/42.974917 PMID:11811822

Müller-Schimpfle, M., Ohmenhäuser, K., Sand, J., Stoll, P., & Claussen, C. D. (1997). Dynamic 3D – MR mammography: Is there a benefit of sophisticated evaluation of enhancement curves for clinical routine? Journal of Magnetic Resonance Imaging, 7(1), 236–240. doi:10.1002/jmri.1880070137 PubMed doi:10.1002/jmri.1880070137 PMID:9039622

Muramatsu, C., Higuchi, S., Morita, T., Oiwa, M., Kawasaki, T., & Fujita, H. (2018). Retrieval of reference images of breast masses on mammograms by similarity space modeling. In *Proceedings of Fourteenth International Workshop on Breast Imaging* (Vol. 1071809). Atlanta, GA: Academic Press.

Murtaza, G., Shuib, L., Wahab, A. W., Mujtaba, A. G., Mujtaba, G., Nweke, H. F., Al-garadi, M. A., Zulfiqar, F., Raza, G., & Azmi, N. A. (2019). Deep learning-based breast cancer classification through medical imaging modalities: State of the art and research challenges. *Artificial Intelligence Review*, 1–66.

Narvaez, F., Diaz, G., & Romero, E. (2011). Multi-view information fusion for automatic BI-RADS description of mammographic masses. In Proceedings of SPIE 7963, Medical Imaging 2011: Computer-Aided Diagnosis (pp. 84–89). Academic Press.

Nascimento, F. B., Pitta, M. G., & Rêgo, M. J. (2015). Análise dos principais métodos de diagnóstico de câncer de mama como propulsores no processo inovativo. *Arquivos de Medicina*, *29*(6).

Nathan, B. E., Burn, J. I., & MacErlean, D. P. (1972). Value of mammary thermography in differential diagnosis. *British Medical Journal*, *2*(5809), 316–317. doi:10.1136/bmj.2.5809.316 PMID:5022040

National Cancer Institute. (n.d.). *Breast Cancer Screening (PDQ®)–Health Professional Version*. Retrieved from https://www.cancer.gov/types/breast/hp/breast-screening-pdq#_543

Neal, C. H., Flynt, K. A., Jeffries, D. O., & Helvie, M. A. (2018). Breast Imaging Outcomes following Abnormal Thermography. *Academic Radiology*, *25*(3), 273–278. doi:10.1016/j.acra.2017.10.015 PMID:29275941

Newcomb, P. A., Titus-Ernstoff, L., Egan, K. M., Trentham-Dietz, A., Baron, J. A., Storer, B. E., ... (2002). Postmenopausal estrogen and progestin use in relation to breast cancer risk. Cancer Epidemiology, Biomarkers & Prevention, 11, 593–600. PubMed PMID:12101105

Ng, E. K. (2009). A review of thermography as promising non-invasive detection modality for breast tumor. *International Journal of Thermal Sciences*, *48*(5), 849–859. doi:10.1016/j.ijthermalsci.2008.06.015

Ng, E. K., & Sudharsan, N. M. (2001). Numerical computation as a tool to aid thermographic interpretation. *Journal of Medical Engineering & Technology*, 53–60. doi:10.1080/03091900110043621 PMID:11452633

Ng, E. Y. (2005). Is thermal scanner losing its bite in mass screening of fever due to SARS? *Medical Physics*, *32*(1), 93–97. doi:10.1118/1.1819532 PMID:15719959

Ng, E. Y. K., & Kee, E. C. (2008). Advanced integrated technique in breast cancer thermography. *Journal of Medical Engineering & Technology*, *32*(2), 103–114. doi:10.1080/03091900600562040 PMID:17852648

Ng, E. Y. K., & Sudarshan, N. M. (2001). Effect of blood flow, tumor and cold stress in a female breast: A novel time-accurate computer simulation. *Proc. Instn Mech Enghs. Part H*, *215*, 393–404. PMID:11521762

Ng, E. Y. K., & Sudarshan, N. M. (2001b). An improved three-dimensional direct numerical modelling and thermal analysis of a female breast with tumour. *Proceedings - Institution of Mechanical Engineers*, *215*(1), 25–36. doi:10.1243/0954411011533508 PMID:11323983

Ng, E. Y. K., & Sudarshan, N. M. (2004). Computer simulation in conjunction with medical thermography as an adjunct tool for early detection of breast cancer. *BMC Cancer*, *4*(17), 1–6. doi:10.1186/1471-2407-4-17 PMID:15113442

Nguyen, A. V., Cohen, N. J., Lipman, H., Brown, C. M., Molinari, N. A., Jackson, W. L., Kirking, H. P., Szymanowski, T. W., Wilson, B. A., Salhi, R. R., Roberts, D. W., & Strykar, D. B. (2010). Comparison of 3 infrared thermal detection systems and self-report for mass fever screening. *Emerging Infectious Diseases*, *16*(11), 1710–1717. doi:10.3201/eid1611.100703 PMID:21029528

Nishiura, H., & Kamiya, K. (2011). Fever screening during the influenza (H1N1-2009) pandemic at Narita International Airport, Japan. *BMC Infectious Diseases*, *11*(1), 11–121. doi:10.1186/1471-2334-11-111 PMID:21539735

Nocedal, J., & Wright, S. J. (2006). Numerical Optimization. Springer.

Nogueira, C. H. F. V., Nogueira, C. F., & Ely, J. B. (2015). Termografia por Infravermelho em Cirurgia Plástica – Novos Horizontes. *Pan American Journal Medical Thermology*, *2*(1), 81–87.

Norton, P. R., Horn, S. B., Pelleggrino, J. G., & Perconti, P. (2008). Infrared detector and detectors arrays. In N. A. Diakides, & J. D. Bronzino (Eds.), Medical Infrared Imaging. CRC Press.

Norvig, P., & Russell, S. (2014). *Inteligência Artificial* (3rd ed.). Elsevier.

Nyirjesy, I., & Ayme, Y. (1986). *Clinical evaluation, mammography, and thermography in the diagnosis of breast carcinoma* (Vol. 1). Thermology.

Nyström, L., Andersson, I., Bjurstam, N., Frisell, J., Nordenskjöld, B., & Rutqvist, L. E. (2002). Long-term effects of mammography screening: Updated overview of the Swedish randomised trials. Lancet, 359(9310), 909–919. doi:10.1016/S0140-6736(02)08020-0 PubMed doi:10.1016/S0140-6736(02)08020-0 PMID:11918907

O'Connor, M., Rhodes, D., & Hruska, C. (2009). Molecular breast imaging. *Expert Review of Anticancer Therapy*, *9*(8), 1073–1080. doi:10.1586/era.09.75 PMID:19671027

Ogava, R. L. T., Soares, N. S., Gomes, J. C., Barbosa, V. A. F., Ribeiro, R. R., Ribeiro, D. E., de Souza, R. E., & dos Santos, W. P. (2017). Algoritmo de Evolução Diferencial hibridizado e Simulated Annealing aplicados a Tomografia por Impedância Elétrica. *Anais do I Simpósio de Inovação em Engenharia Biomédica - SABIO 2017*, 65.

Oh, S. H. (2011). Error back-propagation algorithm for classification of imbalanced data. *Neurocomputing*, *74*(6), 1058–1061. doi:10.1016/j.neucom.2010.11.024

Ojala, T., Pietikäinen, M., & Harwood, D. (1996). A comparative study of texture measures with classification based on featured distributions. *Pattern Recognition*, *29*(1), 51–59. doi:10.1016/0031-3203(95)00067-4

Ojansivu, V., & Heikkilä, J. (2008). Blur insensitive texture classification using local phase quantization. In *International conference on image and signal processing* (pp. 236-243). Springer. 10.1007/978-3-540-69905-7_27

Oliveira, M. M. (2012). *Desenvolvimento de protocolo e construção de um aparato mecânico para padronização da aquisição de imagens termográficas de mama* (Unpublished Master's dissertation). Universidade Federal de Pernambuco, Recife, Brazil.

Oliveira, M. M. (2012). *Desenvolvimento de protocolo e construção de um aparato mecânico para padronização da aquisição de imagens termográficas de mama* [dissertation]. Recife: Universidade Federal de Pernambuco.

Oliveira, M. M. (2012). *Desenvolvimento de protocolo e construção de um aparato mecânico para padronização da aquisição de imagens termográficas de mama*. Federal University of Pernambuco.

Oliver, A., Freixenet, J., Marti, J., Perez, E., Pont, J., Denton, E. R., & Zwiggelaar, R. (2010). A review of automatic mass detection and segmentation in mammographic images. *Medical Image Analysis*, *14*(2), 87–110. doi:10.1016/j.media.2009.12.005 PMID:20071209

Osman, M. M., & Afify, E. (1984). Thermal modeling of the normal woman's breast. *Journal of Biomechanical Engineering*, *106*(2), 123–130. doi:10.1115/1.3138468 PMID:6738016

Osman, M. M., & Afify, E. (1988). Thermal modeling of the malignant woman's breast. *Journal of Biomechanical Engineering*, *110*(4), 269–276. doi:10.1115/1.3108441 PMID:3205011

Pak, D. D., Rozhkova, N. I., Kireeva, M. N., Ermoshchenkova, M. V., Nazarov, A. A., Fomin, D. K., & Rubtsova, N. A. (2012). Diagnosis of breast cancer using electrical impedance tomography. *Biomedical Engineering*, *46*(4), 154–157. doi:10.100710527-012-9292-7 PMID:23035354

Pan, S. J., & Yang, Q. (2009). A survey on transfer learning. *IEEE Transactions on Knowledge and Data Engineering*, *22*(10), 1345–1359. doi:10.1109/TKDE.2009.191

Pappa, G. L., Freitas, A. A., & Kaestner, C. A. (2002). Attribute Selection with a Multi-objective Genetic Algorithm. *Advances in Artificial Intelligence: 16th Brazilian Symposium on Artificial Intelligence, SBIA*, 280-290. doi:10.1007/3-540-36127-8_27

Parker, J. R. (1997). *Algorithms for image processing and computer vision*. John Wiley & Sons.

Partridge, P. W., & Wrobel, L. C. (2007). An inverse geometry problem for the localization of skin tumours by thermal analysis. *Engineering Analysis with Boundary Elements*, *31*(10), 803–811. doi:10.1016/j.enganabound.2007.02.002

Paruch, M., & Majchrzak, E. (2007). Identification of tumor region parameters using evolutionary algorithm and multiple reciprocity boundary element method. *Engineering Applications of Artificial Intelligence*, *20*(5), 647–655. doi:10.1016/j.engappai.2006.11.003

Pedersen, M. E. H., & Chipperfield, A. J. (2008). *Tuning differential evolution for artificial neural networks*. HL0803 Hvass Laboratories.

Pedrini, H., & Schwartz, W. (2008). *Análise de Imagens Digitais: Princípio, Algoritmos e aplicações*. Cengage Learning.

Pedrini, H., & Schwartz, W. R. (2008). *Análise de imagens digitais: princípios, algoritmos e aplicações*. Thomson Learning.

Pellegrino, J. G., Zeibel, J., Driggers, R. G., & Perconti, P. (2008). Infrared Camera Characterization. In N. A. Diakides & J. D. Bronzino (Eds.), Medical Infrared Imaging. CRC Press.

Pennes, H. H. (1948). Analysis of tissue and arterial blood temperature in the resting human forearm. *Journal of Applied Physiology*, *1*(2), 93–122. doi:10.1152/jappl.1948.1.2.93 PMID:18887578

Pereira, J. M. S., Santana, M. A., Lima, N. M., Sousa, F. N., de Lima, R. C. F., & dos Santos, W. P. (2017) *Método para Classificação do Tipo da Lesão na Mama Presentes nas Imagens Termográficas utilizando Classificador ELM*. Paper presented at the I Simpósio de Inovação em Engenharia Biomédica (SABIO 2017), Recife, PE, Brazil.

Piperno, G., & Lenington, S. (2002). Breast electrical impedance and estrogen use in postmenopausal women. *Maturitas, 41*(17).

Piperno, G., Frei, E.H., & Moshitzky, M. (1990). Breast cancer screening by impedance measurements. *Front Med Biol Eng, 2*(111).

Polidori, G., Renard, Y., Lorimier, S., Pron, H., Derruau, S., & Taiar, R. (2017). Medical Infrared Thermography assistance in the surgical treatment of axillary Hidradenitis Suppurativa: A case report. *International Journal of Surgery Case Reports*, *34*, 56–59. doi:10.1016/j.ijscr.2017.03.015 PMID:28359047

Pontes, R. (2011). *Inteligência Artificial nos Investimentos*. Joinville: Clube dos Autores Publicações.

Prabha, S., Suganthi, S. S., & Sujatha, C. M. (2015). An approach to analyze the breast tissues in infrared images using nonlinear adaptive level sets and Riesz transform features. *Technology and Health Care*, *23*(4), 429–442. doi:10.3233/THC-150915 PMID:26409908

Prabha, S., & Sujatha, C. M. (2018). Proposal of index to estimate breast similarities in thermograms using fuzzy C means and anisotropic diffusion filter based fuzzy C means clustering. *Infrared Physics & Technology*, *93*, 316–325. doi:10.1016/j.infrared.2018.08.018

Pracella, D., Bonin, S., Barbazza, R., Sapino, A., Castellano, I., Sulfaro, S., & Stanta, G. (2013). Are breast cancer molecular classes predictive of survival in patients with long follow-up? Disease Markers, 35, 595–605. doi:10.1155/2013/347073 PubMed doi:10.1155/2013/347073 PMID:24288429

Prasad, S. N., & Houserkova, D. (2007). The Role of Various Modalities in Breast Imaging. Biomed Pap Med., 151(2), 209–218. doi:10.5507/bp.2007.036 doi:10.5507/bp.2007.036

Prasad, S. S., Ramachandra, L., Kumar, V., Dave, A., Mestha, L. K., & Venkatarmani, K. (2016). Evaluation of efficacy of thermographic breast imaging in breast cancer: A pilot study. *Breast Disease*, *36*(4), 143–147. doi:10.3233/BD-160236 PMID:27767959

Prats, E., Aisa, F., Abós, M. D., Villavieja, L., García-López, F., Asenjo, M. J., Razola, P., & Banzo, J. (1999). Mammography and 99mTc-MIBI scintimammography in suspected breast cancer. Journal of Nuclear Medicine, 40, 296–301. PubMed PMID:10025838

Price, K., Storn, R. M., & Lampinen, J. A. (2006). *Differential evolution: a practical approach to global optimization.* Springer Science & Business Media.

Qi, H., Kuruganti, P. T., & Snyder, W. E. (2006). Detecting breast cancer from thermal infrared images by asymmetry analysis. In Biomedical Engineering Handbook. CRC Press.

Qi, Z., Tian, Y., & Shi, Y. (2013). Robust twin support vector machine for pattern classification. *Pattern Recognition*, *46*(1), 305–316. doi:10.1016/j.patcog.2012.06.019

Quaresma, V., Matcher, S. J., & Ferrari, M. (1998, January). Identification and quantification of intrinsic optical contrast for near-infrared mammography. Photochemistry and Photobiology, 67(1), 4–14. doi:10.1111/j.1751-1097.1998.tb05159.x PubMed doi:10.1111/j.1751-1097.1998.tb05159.x PMID:9477760

Queiroz, K. F. F. C. (2014). *Análise da repetitividade e melhoria de segmentação semiautomática de ROIs em imagens termográficas de mama* (Unpublished bachelor's degree dissertation). Universidade Federal de Pernambuco, Recife, Brazil.

Radiology assistant. (2020, March 23). *X-ray Chest images*. https://radiologyassistant.nl/chest/lk-jg-1

Raghavendra, U., Gudigar, A., Rao, T. N., Ciaccio, E. J., Ng, E. Y. K., & Acharya, U. R. (2019). Computer-aided diagnosis for the identification of breast cancer using thermogram images: A comprehensive review. *Infrared Physics & Technology*, *102*, 102. doi:10.1016/j.infrared.2019.103041

Rahmatinia, S., & Fahimi, B. (2017). Magneto-Thermal Modeling of Biological Tissues: A Step Toward Breast Cancer Detection. *IEEE Transactions on Magnetics*, *53*(6), 1–4. doi:10.1109/TMAG.2017.2671780

Rajmanova, P., Nudzikova, P., & Vala, D. (2015). Application and technology of thermal imaging camera in medicine. *IFAC-PapersOnLine*, *48*(4), 492–497. doi:10.1016/j.ifacol.2015.07.083

Rajpurkar, P., Irvin, J., Ball, R. L., Zhu, K., Yang, B., Mehta, H., ... Patel, B. N. (2018). Deep learning for chest radiograph diagnosis: A retrospective comparison of the CheXNeXt algorithm to practicing radiologists. *PLoS Medicine*, *15*(11), e1002686. doi:10.1371/journal.pmed.1002686 PMID:30457988

Ramírez-Torres, A., Rodríguez-Ramos, R., Sabina, F. J., García-Reimbert, C., Penta, R., Merodio, J., Guinovart-Díaz, R., Bravo-Castillero, J., Conci, A., & Preziosi, L. (2017). The role of malignant tissue on the thermal distribution of cancerous breast. *Journal of Theoretical Biology*, *426*, 152–161. doi:10.1016/j.jtbi.2017.05.031 PMID:28552555

Rastgar-Jazi, M., & Mohammadi, F. (2017). Parameters sensitivity assessment and heat source localization using infrared imaging techniques. *Biomedical Engineering Online*, *16*(1), 113. doi:10.118612938-017-0403-2 PMID:28934956

Rastghalam, R., & Pourghassem, H. (2016). Breast cancer detection using MRF-based probable texture feature and decision-level fusion-based classification using HMM on thermography images. *Pattern Recognition*, *51*, 176–186. doi:10.1016/j.patcog.2015.09.009

Rastogi, A. B., & Monika, A. (2014). *Study of neural network in diagnosis of thyroid. International Journal of Computer Technology and Electronics Engineering*, 4.

Resmini, R. (2011). *Análise de imagens térmicas da mama usando descritores de textura* (M Sc. Dissertation). Computer Institute, Universidade Federal Fluminense, Niterói, RJ, Brazil.

Resmini, R. (2016). *Classificação De Doenças Da Mama Usando Imagens Por Infravermelho* (Doctoral dissertation). Instituto de Computação, Universidade Federal Fluminense, Brazil.

Resmini, R., Araujo, A., Conci, A., Silva, L., & Moran, M. (2018). Number of Texture Unit as Feature to Breast's Disease Classification from Thermal Images. In *2018 IEEE/ACS 15th International Conference on Computer Systems and Applications (AICCSA)* (pp. 1-6). IEEE. 10.1109/AICCSA.2018.8612826

Resmini, R., Conci, A., Borchartt, T. B., de Lima, R. d., Montenegro, A. A., & Pantaleão, C. A. (2012). Diagnóstico precoce de doenças mamárias usando imagens térmicas e aprendizado de máquina. *Revista Eletrônica do Vale do Itajaí*, 55-67.

Resmini, R., Conci, A., Borchartt, T. B., Lima, R. C. F., Montenegro, A. A., & Pantaleão, C. A. (2012). Diagnóstico Precoce de Doenças Mamárias Usando Imagens Térmicas e Aprendizado de Máquina. *Revista Eletrônica do Alto Vale de Itajaí*, *1*(1), 55–67.

Ribeiro, P. B., Schiabel, H., Patrocinio, A. C., & Romero, R. A. F. (2008). Análise da Variação de Textura em Imagens Mamográficas para Classificação de Massas Suspeitas. In 4o Workshop de Visão Computacional, 2008, São Paulo, Brazil.

Ribeiro, R. R., Feitosa, A. R., de Souza, R. E., & dos Santos, W. P. (2014, April). Reconstruction of electrical impedance tomography images using genetic algorithms and non-blind search. In *2014 IEEE 11th International Symposium on Biomedical Imaging (ISBI)* (pp. 153-156). IEEE. 10.1109/ISBI.2014.6867832

Ribeiro, R. R., Feitosa, A. R., de Souza, R. E., & dos Santos, W. P. (2014, May). A modified differential evolution algorithm for the reconstruction of electrical impedance tomography images. In *5th ISSNIP-IEEE Biosignals and Biorobotics Conference (2014): Biosignals and Robotics for Better and Safer Living (BRC)* (pp. 1-6). IEEE.

Ribeiro, R. R., Feitosa, A. R., Barbosa, V. A., da Silva, V. L., Rocha, A. D., Freitas, R. C., ... dos Santos, W. P. (2015). Reconstrução de Imagens de TIE usando Simulated Annealing, Evolução Diferencial e Algoritmos Genéticos. *XII Congresso Brasileiro de Inteligência Computacional*. 10.21528/CBIC2015-063

Ribeiro, R. R., Feitosa, A. R., de Souza, R. E., & dos Santos, W. P. (2014, October). Reconstruction of electrical impedance tomography images using chaotic self-adaptive ring-topology differential evolution and genetic algorithms. In *2014 IEEE International Conference on Systems, Man, and Cybernetics (SMC)* (pp. 2605-2610). IEEE. 10.1109/SMC.2014.6974320

Riis, C., Lernevall, A., Sorensen, F. B., & Nygaard, H. (2005). 3D Ultrasound-Based Evaluation of Lesions in the Uncompressed Breast. In E. Ueno, T. Shiina, M. Kubota, & K. Sawai (Eds.), Research and Development in Breast Ultrasound. Springer. doi:10.1007/4-431-27008-6_22 doi:10.1007/4-431-27008-6_22

Rimpiläinen, V., Kuosmanen, M., Ketolainen, J., Järvinen, K., Vauhkonen, M., & Heikkinen, L. M. (2010). Electrical impedance tomography for three-dimensional drug release monitoring. *European Journal of Pharmaceutical Sciences*, *41*(2), 407–413. doi:10.1016/j.ejps.2010.07.008 PMID:20654713

Ring, E. F. J., & Ammer, K. (2000). The technique of infrared imaging in medicine. Thermology Int., 10, 7–14.

Ring, E. F., & Ammer, K. (2012). Infrared thermal imaging in medicine. *Physiological Measurement*, *33*(3), 33–46. doi:10.1088/0967-3334/33/3/R33 PMID:22370242

Ring, F. (2010). Thermal imaging today and its relevance to diabetes. *Journal of Diabetes Science and Technology*, *4*(4), 857–862. doi:10.1177/193229681000400414 PMID:20663449

Ring, F., Jung, A., & Zuber, J. (2015). *A Case Book of Infrared Imaging in Clinical Medicine*. IOP Publishing.

Robinson, G. P., Tagare, H. D., Duncan, J. S., & Jaffe, C. C. (1996). Medical image collection indexing: Shape-based retrieval using KD-trees. *Computerized Medical Imaging and Graphics*, *20*(4), 209–217. doi:10.1016/S0895-6111(96)00014-6 PMID:8954229

Rocha, A. D. (2006). Detecção e classificação de lesões em imagens de mamografia usando classificadores SVM. *Dissertation Response to the Graduate Program in Biomedical Engineering*. Federal University of Pernambuco.

Rochester Institute of Technology. (2019). Retrieved from https:// www.rit.edu/news/rit-rrh-working-improve-cancer-screening

Rodrigues, A. L., Bezerra, R. S., de Santana, M. A., dos Santos, W. P., Azevedo, W. W., & de Lima, R. C. (2018). Seleção de Atributos para Apoio ao Diagnóstico do Câncer de Mama Usando Imagens Termográficas, Algoritmos Genéticos e Otimização por Enxame de Partículas. *Anais do II Simpósio de Inovação em Engenharia Biomédica - SABIO 2018*.

Rodrigues, A. L., Santana, M. A., Azevedo, W. W., Bezerra, R. S., Santos, W. P., & Lima, R. C. F. (2018). *Seleção de Atributos para Apoio ao Diagnóstico do Câncer de Mama Usando Imagens Termográficas, Algoritmos Genéticos e Otimização por Enxame de Partículas*. Paper presented at the II Simpósio de Inovação em Engenharia Biomédica (SABIO), Recife, Brazil.

Rodrigues, C. I. H. (2008). *Sistemas CAD em Patologia Mamária* [dissertation]. Porto: Universidade do Porto.

Rolnik, V. P., & Seleghim, P. Jr. (2006). A specialized genetic algorithm for the electrical impedance tomography of two-phase flows. *Journal of the Brazilian Society of Mechanical Sciences and Engineering*, *28*(4), 378–389. doi:10.1590/S1678-58782006000400002

Sadoughi. (2018). *Artificial intelligence methods for the diagnosis of breast cancer by image processing: a review*. Academic Press.

Saladin, K. S., & Porth, C. (2010). *Anatomy & physiology: the unity of form and function* (Vol. 5). McGraw-Hill.

Saniei, E., Setayeshi, S., Akbari, M. E., & Navid, M. (2016). Parameter estimation of breast tumour using dynamic neural network from thermal pattern. *Journal of Advanced Research*, *7*(6), 1045–1055. doi:10.1016/j.jare.2016.05.005 PMID:27857851

Santana, M. A. D., Pereira, J. M. S., Silva, F. L. D., Lima, N. M. D., Sousa, F. N. D., Arruda, G. M. S. D., de Lima, R. C. F., da Silva, W. W. A., & Santos, W. P. D. (2018). Breast cancer diagnosis based on mammary thermography and extreme learning machines. *Research on Biomedical Engineering*, *34*(1), 45–53. doi:10.1590/2446-4740.05217

Santana, M. A., da Silva, W. W., da Silva, A. L., Pereira, J. M., Barbosa, V. A., Diniz, C. A., ... dos Santos, W. P. (2018). Desempenho de máquinas de aprendizado extremo com operadores morfológicos para identificação e classificação de lesões em imagens frontais de termografia de mama. *XXII Congresso Brasileiro de Automática. SBA Sociedade Brasileira de Automática*. doi:10.20906/CPS/CBA2018-0202

Santos dos, W. P., de Souza, R. E., Santos Filho, P. B., Lima Neto, F. B., & de Assis, F. M. (2008). A dialectical approach for classification of DW-MR Alzheimer. *IEEE Congress on Evolutionary Computation (IEEE World Congress on Computational Intelligence)*. doi:10.1109/CEC.2008.4631023

Santos, L. C. (2009). *Desenvolvimento de ferramenta computacional para análise paramétrica da influência da posição e do tamanho de um tumor de mama em perfis de temperatura* (Master's thesis). Universidade Federal de Pernambuco, Recife, Brasil. Retrieved from https://repositorio.ufpe.br/handle/123456789/5021

Santos, L. C. (2009). *Desenvolvimento de ferramenta computacional para análise paramétrica da influência da posição e do tamanho do tumor da mama e perfis de temperatura* [Development of computational hardware for parametric analysis of the influence of the position and size of the breast and temperature profiles] (Master's thesis). Universidade Federal de Pernambuco, Recife, PE, Brazil.

Santos, W. P. (2009). Método Dialético de Busca e Otimização para Análise de Imagens de Ressonância Magnética. *Master Thesis Response to the Graduate Program in Electrical engineering*. Federal University of Pernambuco.

Santos, W. P., & de Assis, F. M. (2009). Método Dialético de Otimização usando o Princípio da Máxima Entropia. *Learning and Nonlinear Models – Revista da Sociedade Brasileira de Redes Neurais (SBRN), 7*(2), 54-64. doi:10.21528/CBRN2009-010

Santos, W. P., Souza, R., Santos filho, P., Lima neto, F., & Assis, F. (2008). A Dialectical Approach for Classification of DW-MR Alzheimer's. *IEEE Congress on Evolutionary Computation*, 1728-1735.

Santos, E. B., Bianco, H. T., & Brioschi, M. L. (2015). Thermography in Assessing Cardiovascular Risk. *Pan American Journal Medical Thermology*, *2*(1), 23–25. doi:10.18073/2358-4696/pajmt.v2n1p23-25

Santos, W. P., & Assis, F. (2009). Optimization based on Dialectics. *International Joint Conference on Neural Networks*, 2804-2811.

Santos, W. P., & De Assis, F. M. (2013). *Algoritmos dialéticos para inteligência computacional*. Universitária da UFPE.

Santos, W., Assis, F., Souza, R., Mendes, P., Monteiro, H., & Alves, H. (2009). Dialectical Non-Supervised Image Classification. *IEEE Congress on Evolutionary Computation*, 2480-2487.

Santos, W., Assis, F., Souza, R., Santos Filho, P. B., & Lima Neto, F. B. (2009). Dialectical multispectral classification of diffusion-weighted magnetic. *Computerized Medical Imaging and Graphics*, *33*(6), 442–460. doi:10.1016/j.compmedimag.2009.04.004 PMID:19446434

Sarigoz, T., Ertan, T., Topuz, O., Sevim, Y., & Cihan, Y. (2018). Role of digital infrared thermal imaging in the diagnosis of breast mass: A pilot study: Diagnosis of breast mass by thermography. *Infrared Physics & Technology*, *91*, 214–219. doi:10.1016/j.infrared.2018.04.019

Saxena, A., Ng, E. Y. K., & Lim, T. S. (2019). Infrared (IR) thermography as a potential screening modality for carotid artery stenosis. *Computers in Biology and Medicine*, *113*, 113. doi:10.1016/j.compbiomed.2019.103419 PMID:31493579

Scaperrotta, G., Ferranti, C., Costa, C., Mariani, L., Marchesini, M., Suman, L., Folini, C., & Bergonzi, S. (2008). Role of sonoelastography in non-palpable breast lesions. European Radiology, 18(11), 2381–2389. doi:10.1007/s00330-008-1032-8 PubMed doi:10.100700330-008-1032-8 PMID:18523780

Schaefer, G., Závišek, M., & Nakashima, T. (2009). Thermography based breast cancer analysis using statistical features and fuzzy classification. *Pattern Recognition*, *42*(6), 1133–1137. doi:10.1016/j.patcog.2008.08.007

Schilling, K., Narayanan, D., & Kalinyak, J.E. (2008). Effect of breast density, menopausal status, and hormone use in high resolution positron emission mammography. *Radiol Soc North Am.*, VB31–04.

Schnall, M. D. (2001). Application of magnetic resonance imaging to early detection of breast cancer. Breast Cancer Research, 3(1), 17–21. doi:10.1186/bcr265 PubMed doi:10.1186/bcr265 PMID:11300101

Schnepper, C. A., & Stadtherr, M. A. (1996). Robust process simulation using interval methods. *Computers & Chemical Engineering*, *20*(2), 187–199. doi:10.1016/0098-1354(95)00014-S

Scholz, B., & Anderson, R. (2000). On electrical impedance scanning: Principles and simulations. *Electromedica, 68*(35).

Serrano, R. C., Lima, R. C. F., Melo, R. H. C., & Conci, A. (2010). Using fractal geometry to extract features of thermal images for early breast diseases. *ICGG - Proceedings of the 14th International Conference on Geometry and Graphics.*

Sessler, D. I. (1994). Consequences and treatment of perioperative hypothermia. *Anesthesiology Clinics of North America, 12*, 425–456.

Shanthi, S., & Bhaskaran, V. (2013). A Novel Approach for Detecting and Classifying Breast Cancer in Mammogram Images. *International Journal of Intelligent Information Technologies, 9*(1), 21–39. doi:10.4018/jiit.2013010102

Sheikhbahaei, S., Trahan, T. J., Xiao, J., Taghipour, M., Mena, E., Connolly, R. M., & Subramaniam, R. M. (2016). FDG-PET/CT and MRI for evaluation of pathologic response to neoadjuvant chemotherapy in patients with breast cancer: A meta-analysis of diagnostic accuracy studies. *The Oncologist, 21*(8), 931–939. doi:10.1634/theoncologist.2015-0353 PMID:27401897

Shindjalova, R., Prodanova, K., & Svechtarov, V. (2014, November). Modeling data for tilted implants in grafted with bio-oss maxillary sinuses using logistic regression. In AIP Conference Proceedings (Vol. 1631, No. 1, pp. 58-62). American Institute of Physics. doi:10.1063/1.4902458

Shukla, A., Tiwari, R., Kaur, P., & Janghel, R. (2009). Diagnosis of Thyroid Disorders using Artificial Neural Networks. *2009 IEEE International Advance Computing Conference.* 10.1109/IADCC.2009.4809154

Siegel, R., Naishadham, D., & Jemal, A. (2012). Cancer statistics, 2012. CA: a Cancer Journal for Clinicians, 62(1), 10–29. doi:10.3322/caac.20138 PubMed doi:10.3322/caac.20138 PMID:22237781

Siegel, R., Ward, E., Brawley, O., & Jemal, A. (2011). Jemal A. Cancer statistics. *CA: a Cancer Journal for Clinicians, 61*(4), 212–236. doi:10.3322/caac.20121 PMID:21685461

Silva Neto, A. J., & Moura Neto, F. D. (2005). *Problemas Inversos - Conceitos fundamentais e aplicações*. Ed. UERJ.

Silva, A. P. D., & Brito, P. (2006). Linear discriminant analysis for interval data. *Computational Statistics, 21*(2), 289–308. doi:10.100700180-006-0264-9

Silva, L. F., Saade, D. C. M., Sequeiros, G. O., Silva, A. C., Paiva, A. C., Bravo, R. S., & Conci, A. (2014). A new database for breast research with infrared image. *Journal of Medical Imaging and Health Informatics, 4*(1), 92–100. doi:10.1166/jmihi.2014.1226

Silva, L. F., Santos, A. A. S. M. D., Bravo, R. S., Silva, A. C., Muchaluat-Saade, D. C., & Conci, A. (2016). Hybrid analysis for indicating patients with breast cancer using temperature time series. *Computer Methods and Programs in Biomedicine, 130*, 142–153. doi:10.1016/j.cmpb.2016.03.002 PMID:27208529

Silva, L. F., Sequeiros, G. O., Santos, M. L., Fontes, C. A., Muchaluat-Saade, D. C., & Conci, A. (2015). Thermal Signal Analysis for Breast Cancer Risk Verification. *Studies in Health Technology and Informatics, 216*, 746–750. PMID:26262151

Simard, P., Le Cun, Y., & Denker, J. (1992). Efficient Pattern Recognition Using a New Transformation Distance. *Proceedings of the 5th International Conference on Neural Information Processing Systems*, 50-58.

Singh, G., Anand, S., Lall, B., Srivastava, A., & Singh, V. (2015, May). Development of a microcontroller based electrical impedance tomography system. In 2015 Long Island Systems, Applications and Technology (pp. 1-4). IEEE. doi:10.1109/LISAT.2015.7160174

Singh, D., & Singh, A. K. (2019). Role of image thermography in early breast cancer detection- Past, present and future. *Computer Methods and Programs in Biomedicine*, 183. PMID:31525547

Singh, V. P., & Srivastava, R. (2017). Content-based mammogram retrieval using wavelet based complete-LBP and K-means clustering for the diagnosis of breast cancer. *International Journal of Hybrid Intelligent Systems, 14*(1-2), 31–39. doi:10.3233/HIS-170240

Sivic, J., & Zisserman, A. (2003). Video google: a text retrieval approach to object matching in video. In *Proceedings of Ninth IEEE International Conference on Computer Vision* (Vol. 2, pp. 1470-1477). 10.1109/ICCV.2003.1238663

Soni, N. K., Hartov, A., Kogel, C., Poplack, S. P., & Paulsen, K. D. (2004). Multi-frequency electrical impedance tomography of the breast: New clinical results. *Physiological Measurement, 25*(1), 301–314. doi:10.1088/0967-3334/25/1/034 PMID:15005324

Soomro, M. H. (2017). Haralick's texture analysis applied to colorectal T2-weighted MRI: A preliminary study of significance for cancer evolution. In *2017 13th IASTED International Conference on Biomedical Engineering (BioMed)* (pp. 16-19). IEEE. 10.2316/P.2017.852-019

Souza, R. M. C. R., Carvalho, F. A. T., & Tenorio, C. P. (2004). Dynamic cluster methods for interval data based on Mahalanobis distances. *Proceedings of the meeting of the international federation of classification societies (ifcs). Classification, Clustering, and Data Mining Applications*, 351–360. 10.1007/978-3-642-17103-1_34

Souza, T. K., Andrade, J. F. S., Almeida, M. B. J., Santana, M. A., & Santos, W. P. (2019). *Métodos Computacionais Aplicados ao Diagnóstico de Câncer de Mama por Termografia: uma revisão de literatura.* Paper presented at the III Simpósio de Inovação em Engenharia Biomédica (SABIO 2019), Recife, Brazil.

Souza, G. A., Brioschi, M. L., Vargas, J. V., Morais, K. C., Dalmaso Neto, C., & Neves, E. B. (2015). Reference breast temperature: Proposal of an equation. *Einstein (Sao Paulo, Brazil), 13*(4), 518–524. doi:10.1590/S1679-45082015AO3392 PMID:26761549

Souza, J. C., Diniz, J. O. B., Ferreira, J. L., da Silva, G. L. F., Silva, A. C., & de Paiva, A. C. (2019). An automatic method for lung segmentation and reconstruction in chest X-ray using deep neural networks. *Computer Methods and Programs in Biomedicine, 177*, 285–296. doi:10.1016/j.cmpb.2019.06.005 PMID:31319957

Spanhol, F. A., Oliveira, L. S., Cavalin, P. R., Petitjean, C., & Heutte, L. (2017). Deep features for breast cancer histopathological image classification. In *Systems, Man, and Cybernetics (SMC), 2017 IEEE International Conference on,* (pp. 1868–1873). IEEE. 10.1109/SMC.2017.8122889

Spanhol, F. A., Oliveira, L. S., Petitjean, C., & Heutte, L. (2016). A dataset for breast cancer histopathological image classification. *IEEE Transactions on Biomedical Engineering, 63*(7), 1455–1462. doi:10.1109/TBME.2015.2496264 PMID:26540668

Spitalier, H., & Giraud, D. (1982). *Does infrared thermography truly have a role in present-day breastcancer management?Biomedical Thermology.* Alan R. Liss.

Spritzer, P. (2003). TRHM e proliferação do tecido mamário normal: O debate continua. *Brasileiros de Endocrinologia & Metabologia, 5-6*(1), 5–6. Advance online publication. doi:10.1590/S0004-27302003000100003

Sree, S. V., Ng, E. Y., Acharya, R. U., & Faust, O. (2011). Breast imaging: A survey. *World Journal of Clinical Oncology, 2*(4), 171–178. doi:10.5306/wjco. v2.i4.171

Staffa, E., Bernard, V., Kubicek, L., Vlachovsky, R., Vlk, D., Mornstein, V., Bourek, A., & Staffa, R. (2017). Infrared thermography as option for evaluating the treatment effect of percutaneous transluminal angioplasty by patients with peripheral arterial disease. *Vascular, 25*(1), 42–49. doi:10.1177/1708538116640444 PMID:26993145

Stark, A. M., & Way, S. (1974). The screening of well women for the early detection of breast cancer using clinical examination with thermography and mammography. *Cancer, 33*(6), 1671–1679. doi:10.1002/1097-0142(197406)33:6<1671::AID-CNCR2820330630>3.0.CO;2-4 PMID:4834162

Stark, A. M., & Way, S. (1974). The use of thermovision in the detection of early breast cancer. *Cancer, 33*(6), 1664–1670. doi:10.1002/1097-0142(197406)33:6<1664::AID-CNCR2820330629>3.0.CO;2-7 PMID:4834161

Steyeberg, E. (2008). *Clinical Prediction Models: A Practical Approach to Development, Validation and Updating*. Springer Science & Business Media.

Sundberg, J., & Hellstrom, G. (2009). Inverse modelling of thermal conductivity from temperature measurements at the prototype repository, aspo hrl. *International Journal of Rock Mechanics and Mining Sciences, 46*(6), 1029–1041. doi:10.1016/j.ijrmms.2009.01.012

Tan, T. Z., & Queck, C. (2007). A novel cognitive interpretation of breast cancer thermography with complementary learning fuzzy neural memory structure. *International Journal of Thermal Sciences, 33*, 652–666. PMID:32288331

Tan, X., & Triggs, B. (2007). Enhanced local texture feature sets for face recognition under difficult lighting conditions. In *International workshop on analysis and modeling of faces and gestures* (pp. 168-182). Springer. 10.1007/978-3-540-75690-3_13

Tavakol, M. E., Lucas, C., Sadri, S., & Ng, E. Y. K. (2010). Analysis of Breast Thermography, an Objective Tool to Establish Possible Difference between Malignant or Benign Pattern Using Fractal Dimension. *Journal of Healthcare Engineering, 1*(1), 27–43. doi:10.1260/2040-2295.1.1.27

Tehrani, J. N., Jin, C., McEwan, A., & van Schaik, A. (2010, August). A comparison between compressed sensing algorithms in electrical impedance tomography. In *2010 Annual International Conference of the IEEE Engineering in Medicine and Biology* (pp. 3109-3112). IEEE. 10.1109/IEMBS.2010.5627165

Teles, M. L. & Gomes, H. M. (2010). Genetic algorithms and sequential quadratic programming comparisons for optimizing engineering problems. *Teoria e prática na Engenharia Civil, 15*, 29–39. (in Portuguese)

Temurtas, F. (2009). A comparative study on thyroid disease diagnosis using neural networks. *Expert Systems with Applications, 36*(1), 944–949. doi:10.1016/j.eswa.2007.10.010

Thermography Clinic Inc. (2019). Retrieved from http:// www.thermography-mw.com

Thomassin, L. (1984). *Proceedings of the third international congress of thermology*. New York: Plenum Press.

Ting, K. M., Chuan, J. T. S., & Liu, F. T. (2009). Mass: A New Ranking Measure for Anomaly Detection. *IEEE Transactions on Knowledge and Data Engineering*.

Tofts, P. S., Berkowitz, B., & Schnall, M. D. (1995). Quantitative analysis of dynamic Gd – DTPA enhancement in breast tumours using a permeability model. Magnetic Resonance Imaging, 33, 564–568. PubMed PMID:7776889

Tofts, P. S., Berkowitz, B., & Schnall, M. D. (1995). Quantitative analysis of dynamic Gd – DTPA enhancement in breast tumours using a perme-ability model. Magnetic Resonance Imaging, 33, 564–568. PubMed PMID:7776889

Torre, L., Siegel, R., & Jemal, A. (2015). *Global cancer facts & figures*. American Cancer Society.

Trafarski, A., Róanski, L., Straburzynska-Lupa, A., & Korman, P. (2008). The Quality of Diagnosis by IR Thermography as a Function of Thermal Stimulation in Chosen Medical Applications. *9th International Conference on Quantitative InfraRed Thermography*, Krakow, Poland. 10.21611/qirt.2008.03_13_17

Traldi, M., Galvão, P., de Morais, S., & Fonseca, M. (2016). Demora no diagnóstico de câncer de mama de mulheres atendidas no Sistema Público de Saúde. *Cadernos Saúde Coletiva*, *24*(2), 185–191. doi:10.1590/1414-462X201600020026

Trokhanova, O. V., Okhapkin, M. B., & Korjenevsky, A. V. (2008). Dual-frequency electrical impedance mammography for the diagnosis of non-malignant breast disease. *Physiological Measurement*, *29*(6), S331.

Tyson, J. (2001). *How Night Vision Works*. Retrieved from https://electronics.howstuffworks.com/gadgets/high-tech-gadgets/nightvision.htm

Uçar, M., & Uçar, E. (2019). Computer-aided detection of lung nodules in chest X-rays using deep convolutional neural networks. *Sakarya University Journal of Computer and Information Sciences*, *2*(1), 41–52. doi:10.35377aucis.02.01.538249

Udesc, U. (2007). *Câncer de mama*. Available in: https://www.joinville.udesc.br/processamentodeimagens/oCanc/oCanc.html

Umar Sidiq, D., Aaqib, S. M., & Khan, R. A. (2019). Diagnosis of various Thyroid Ailments using Data Mining Classification Techniques. *Int J Sci Res Coput Sci Inf Technol*, *5*, 131–136.

United Breast Cancer Foundation. (2019). Retrieved from https://www.ubcf.org/your-health/breast-thermography/

Unser, M. (1986). Sum and difference histograms for texture classification. *IEEE Transactions on Pattern Analysis and Machine Intelligence*, *PAMI-8*(1), 118–125. doi:10.1109/TPAMI.1986.4767760 PMID:21869331

Van Ongeval, Ch. (2007, May-June). Department of Radiology, KULeuven, UZ Gasthuisberg, Leuven, Belgium. Digital mammography for screen-ing and diagnosis of breast cancer: An overview. JBR-BTR; Organe de la Societe Royale Belge de Radiologie (SRBR), 90(3), 163–166.

Varela, C., Tahoces, P. G., Mendez, A. J., Souto, M., & Vidal, J. J. (2007). Computerized detection of breast masses in digitized mammograms. *Computers in Biology and Medicine*, *37*(2), 214–226. doi:10.1016/j.compbiomed.2005.12.006 PMID:16620805

Vasconcelos, J., Santos, W., & de Lima, R. (2018). *Analysis of Methods of Classification of Breast*. IEEE Latin America Transactions. doi:10.1109/TLA.2018.8444159

Vauhkonen, M., Lionheart, W. R., Heikkinen, L. M., Vauhkonen, P. J., & Kaipio, J. P. (2001). A MATLAB package for the EIDORS project to reconstruct two-dimensional EIT images. *Physiological Measurement*, *22*(1), 107–111. doi:10.1088/0967-3334/22/1/314 PMID:11236871

Vázquez, A. (2007). *Filosofia da práxis*. Expressão Popular.

Venkataramani, K., Mestha, L. K., Ramachandra, L., Prasad, S. S., Kumar, V., & Raja, P. J. (2015). Semi-automated breast cancer tumor detection with thermographic video imaging. *Conference Proceedings; ... Annual International Conference of the IEEE Engineering in Medicine and Biology Society. IEEE Engineering in Medicine and Biology Society. Conference*, 2022–2025. doi:10.1109/EMBC.2015.7318783 PMID:26736683

Viana, M. J. A. (2010). *Simulating the temperature profile in the breast using surrogate geometry obtained from an external breast prosthesis* (Master's thesis). Universidade Federal de Pernambuco, Recife, Brasil. Retrieved from https://repositorio.ufpe.br/handle/123456789/17939

Wahab, A. A., Salim, M. I., Ahamat, M. A., Manaf, N. A., Yunus, J., & Lai, K. W. (2016). Thermal distribution analysis of three-dimensional tumor-embedded breast models with different breast density compositions. *Medical & Biological Engineering & Computing*, *54*(9), 1363–1373. doi:10.100711517-015-1403-7 PMID:26463520

Walker, D., & Kaczor, T. (2012). Breast thermography: history, theory, and use. Is this screening tool adequate for standalone use. *Nat Med J, 4*(7).

Wang, H., Xu, G., Zhang, S., & Yan, W. (2015). An implementation of generalized back projection algorithm for the 2-D anisotropic EIT problem. *IEEE Transactions on Magnetics, 51*(3), 1–4. doi:10.1109/TMAG.2014.2356648

Wang, J., Chang, K., Chen, C., Chien, K., Tsai, Y., Wu, Y., Teng, Y., & Shih, T. T. (2010). Evaluation of the diagnostic performance of infrared imaging of the breast: A preliminary study. *Biomedical Engineering Online, 9*(3), 1–14. doi:10.1186/1475-925X-9-3 PMID:20055999

Wan, Y., Borsic, A., Heaney, J., Seigne, J., Schned, A., Baker, M., Wason, S., Hartov, A., & Halter, R. (2013). Transrectal electrical impedance tomography of the prostate: Spatially coregistered pathological findings for prostate cancer detection. *Medical Physics, 40*(6Part1), 063102. doi:10.1118/1.4803498 PMID:23718610

Warner, E., Plewes, D. B., Shumak, R. S., Catzavelos, G. C., Di Prospero, L. S., Yaffe, M. J., Goel, V., Ramsay, E., Chart, P. L., Cole, D. E. C., Taylor, G. A., Cutrara, M., Samuels, T. H., Murphy, J. P., Murphy, J. M., & Narod, S. A. (2001). Comparison of Breast Magnetic Resonance Imaging, Mammography, and Ultrasound for Surveillance of Women at High Risk for Hereditary Breast Cancer. *Journal of Clinical Oncology, 19*(15), 3524–3531. doi:10.1200/JCO.2001.19.15.3524 PMID:11481359

Watt, A., & Policarpo, F. (1998). *The computer image*. Academic Press.

Weinberg, R. A. (2008). *A biologia do câncer*. Artmed.

Weiss, L. K., Burkman, R. T., Cushing-Haugen, K. L., Voigt, L. F., Simon, M. S., Daling, J. R., ... (2002). Hormone replacement therapy regimens and breast cancer risk (1). Obstetrics and Gynecology, 100, 1148–1158. PubMed PMID:12468157

Weum, S., Mercer, J. B., & de Weerd, L. (2016). Evaluation of dynamic infrared thermography as an alternative to CT angiography for perforator mapping in breast reconstruction: A clinical study. *BMC Medical Imaging, 16*(1), 43. doi:10.118612880-016-0144-x PMID:27421763

WHO. (2019). *Global Health Observatory*. Geneva: World Health organization. Retrieved from who.int/gho/database/en/

Wibmer, A., Hricak, H., Gondo, T., Matsumoto, K., Veeraraghavan, H., Fehr, D., Zheng, J., Goldman, D., Moskowitz, C., Fine, S. W., Reuter, V. E., Eastham, J., Sala, E., & Vargas, H. A. (2015). Haralick texture analysis of prostate MRI: Utility for differentiating non-cancerous prostate from prostate cancer and differentiating prostate cancers with different Gleason scores. *European Radiology, 25*(10), 2840–2850. doi:10.100700330-015-3701-8 PMID:25991476

Widodo, A., & Yang, B. S. (2007). Support vector machine in machine condition monitoring and fault diagnosis. *Mechanical Systems and Signal Processing, 21*(6), 2560–2574. doi:10.1016/j.ymssp.2006.12.007

Wiecek, B., Wiecek, M., Strakowski, R., Jakubowska, T., & Ng, E. Y. K. (2010). Wavelet-based thermal image classification for breast screening and other medical applications. In E. Y. K. Ng, R. U. Acharya, & J. S. Suri (Eds.), Performance Evaluation Techniques in Multi-modality Breast Cancer Screening, Diagnosis and Treatment. American Scientific Publishers.

Wilcox, R. H. (1961). Adaptive control processes - A guided tour. *Naval Research Logistics Quarterly, 8*(3), 315–316. doi:10.1002/nav.3800080314

Williams, K. L., Phillips, B. H., Jones, P. A., Beaman, S. A., & Fleming, P. J. (1990). Thermography in screening for breast cancer. *Journal of Epidemiology and Community Health, 44*(2), 112–113. doi:10.1136/jech.44.2.112 PMID:2370497

Wissler, E. H. (1998). Pennes' 1948 paper revisited. *Journal of Applied Physiology, 85*(1), 35–41. doi:10.1152/jappl.1998.85.1.35 PMID:9655751

Witten, I. H., Frank, E., Hall, M. A., & Pal, C. J. (2016). *Data Mining: Practical machine learning tools and techniques*. Morgan Kaufmann.

Wood-allum, C. A., & Shaw, P. J. (2014). Thyroid disease and the nervous system. *Handbook of Clinical Neurology, 120*, 703–735. doi:10.1016/B978-0-7020-4087-0.00048-6 PMID:24365348

World Health Organization. (2014). *WHO position paper on mammography screening*. WHO.

World Health Organization. (2018). Early Detection. In Cancer control: knowledge into action: WHO guide for effective programmes. Geneva: WHO.

Woźniak, M., Połap, D., Capizzi, G., Sciuto, G. L., Kośmider, L., & Frankiewicz, K. (2018). Small lung nodules detection based on local variance analysis and probabilistic neural network. *Computer Methods and Programs in Biomedicine, 161*, 173–180. doi:10.1016/j.cmpb.2018.04.025 PMID:29852959

Wu, T., Stewart, A., Stanton, M., McCauley, T., Phillips, W., Kopans, D. B., Moore, R. H., Eberhard, J. W., Opsahl-Ong, B., Niklason, L., & Williams, M. B. (2003). Tomographic mammography using a limited number of low-dose cone-beam projection images. Medical Physics, 30(3), 365–380. doi:10.1118/1.1543934 PubMed doi:10.1118/1.1543934 PMID:12674237

Wu, J., & Rehg, J. M. (2010). Centrist: A visual descriptor for scene categorization. *IEEE Transactions on Pattern Analysis and Machine Intelligence, 33*(8), 1489–1501. PMID:21173449

Wu, L. A., Kuo, W. H., Chen, C. Y., Tsai, Y. S., & Wang, J. (2016). The association of infrared imaging findings of the breast with prognosis in breast cancer patients: An observational cohort study. *BMC Cancer, 16*(1), 541. doi:10.118612885-016-2602-9 PMID:27464553

Xie, F., & Bovik, A. C. (2013). Automatic segmentation of dermoscopy images using. *Pattern Recognition, 46*(3), 1012–1019. doi:10.1016/j.patcog.2012.08.012

Xu, C., Yang, J., Lai, H., Gao, J., Shen, L., & Yan, S. (2019). UP-CNN: Un-pooling augmented convolutional neural network. *Pattern Recognition Letters, 119*, 34–40. doi:10.1016/j.patrec.2017.08.007

Xu, S., Wu, H., & Bie, R. (2018). CXNet-m1: Anomaly detection on chest X-rays with image-based deep learning. *IEEE Access: Practical Innovations, Open Solutions, 7*, 4466–4477. doi:10.1109/ACCESS.2018.2885997

Yamamoto, A., Fukushima, H., Okamura, R., Nakamura, Y., Morimoto, T., Urata, Y., Mukaihara, S., & Hayakawa, K. (2006). Dynamic helical CT mam-mography of breast cancer. Radiation Medicine, 24(1), 35–40. doi:10.1007/BF02489987 PubMed doi:10.1007/BF02489987 PMID:16715660

Yang, L., Deng, Z. C., Yu, J. N., & Luo, G. W. (2009). Optimization method for the inverse problem of reconstructing the source term in a parabolic equation. *Mathematics and Computers in Simulation, 80*(2), 314–326. doi:10.1016/j.matcom.2009.06.031

Yassin, N. R., Omran, S., El Houby, E. M. F., & Allam, H. (2018). Machine learning techniques for breast cancer computer aided diagnosis using different image modalities: A systematic review. *Computer Methods and Programs in Biomedicine, 156*, 25–45. doi:10.1016/j.cmpb.2017.12.012 PMID:29428074

Yorkey, T. J., Webster, J. G., & Tompkins, W. J. (1987). Comparing reconstruction algorithms for electrical impedance tomography. *IEEE Transactions on Biomedical Engineering, BME-34*(11), 843–852. doi:10.1109/TBME.1987.326032 PMID:3692503

Zadeh, H. G., Haddadnia, J., Ahmadinejad, N., & Baghdadi, M. R. (2015). Assessing the Potential of Thermal Imaging in Recognition of Breast Cancer. *Asian Pacific Journal of Cancer Prevention, 16*(18), 8619–8623. doi:10.7314/APJCP.2015.16.18.8619 PMID:26745126

Zeiler, M. D. (2012). *Adadelta: an adaptive learning rate method.* arXiv preprint arXiv:1212.5701

Zhang, L., Zhou, Z., & Li, H. (2012). Binary gabor pattern: An efficient and robust descriptor for texture classification. In 2012 19th IEEE international conference on image processing (pp. 81-84). IEEE.

Zhang, H., He, L., & Zhu, L. (2009). Critical conditions for the thermal diagnosis of the breast cancer. *3rd International Conference on Bioinformatics and Biomedical Engineering.* 10.1109/ICBBE.2009.5162563

Zhang, L. F., & Zhang, L. (2008). Study of index for mammogram database. *Journal of Shanghai Jiaotong University, 28*(5), 548–551. doi:10.100711741-008-0615-2

Zhang, X., Wang, W., Sze, G., Barber, D., & Chatwin, C. (2014). An image reconstruction algorithm for 3-D electrical impedance mammography. *IEEE Transactions on Medical Imaging, 33*(12), 2223–2241. doi:10.1109/TMI.2014.2334475 PMID:25014954

Zhiqiong, W., Junchang, X., Yukun, H., Chen, L., Ling, X., & Yang, L. (2018). A similarity measure method combining location feature for mammogram retrieval. *Journal of X-Ray Science and Technology, 26*(4), 553–571. doi:10.3233/XST-18374 PMID:29865106

Zhou, Y., & Herman, C. (2018). Optimization of skin cooling by computational modeling for early thermographic detection of breast cancer. *International Journal of Heat and Mass Transfer, 126*(Part B), 864 – 876.

Zhu, Q., Cronin, E. B., Currier, A. A., Vine, H. S., Huang, M., Chen, N., & Xu, C. (2005, October). Benign versus malignant breast masses: Optical differentiation with US-guided optical imaging reconstruction. Radiology, 237(1), 57–66. doi:10.1148/radiol.2371041236 PubMed doi:10.1148/radiol.2371041236 PMID:16183924

Zore, Z., Filipović-Zore, I., Stanec, M., Batinjan, B., & Matejčić, A. (2015). Association of clinical, histopathological and immunohistochemical prognostic factors of invasive breast tumors and thermographic findings. *Infrared Physics & Technology, 68,* 101–205. doi:10.1016/j.infrared.2014.12.009

Zou, Y., & Guo, Z. (2003). A review of electrical impedance techniques for breast cancer detection. *Medical Engineering & Physics, 25*(2), 79–90. doi:10.1016/S1350-4533(02)00194-7 PMID:12538062

Zuluaga-Gomez, J., Zerhouni, N., Al Masry, Z., Devalland, C., & Varnier, C. (2019). A survey of breast cancer screening techniques: Thermography and electrical impedance tomography. *Journal of Medical Engineering & Technology, 43*(5), 305–322. doi:10.1080/03091902.2019.1664672 PMID:31545114

About the Contributors

Wellington Pinheiro dos Santos received a bachelor's degree in Electrical Electronics Engineering (2001) and MSc in Electrical Engineering (2003) from the Federal University of Pernambuco, and Ph.D. in Electrical Engineering from the Federal University of Campina Grande (2009). He is currently a Professor of the Department of Biomedical Engineering at the Federal University of Pernambuco, acting in Undergraduate and Graduate Programs in Biomedical Engineering. He is a member of the Graduate Program in Computer Engineering from the Polytechnic School of Pernambuco, University of Pernambuco, since 2009. He has experience in the area of Computer Science, acting on the following themes: digital image processing, pattern recognition, computer vision, evolutionary computation, numerical methods of optimization, computational intelligence, computer graphics, virtual reality, game design and applications of Computing and Engineering in Medicine and Biology. He is a member of the Brazilian Society of Biomedical Engineering (SBEB), the Brazilian Society of Computational Intelligence, and the International Federation of Medical and Biological Engineering (IFMBE).

Washington Wagner Azevedo da Silva holds a PhD in Computer Science from the Federal University of Pernambuco - UFPE (2017) and a master in Computer Science from the Federal University of Pernambuco - UFPE (2011). He graduated in Systems Analysis at Universidade Salgado de Oliveira - UNIVERSO (2004). He did a post-doctorate at the Department of Biomedical Engineering at the Federal University of Pernambuco - UFPE (10/2017 to 10/2019) with Prof. Dr. Wellington Pinheiro dos Santos. He was a Test Engineer for the CIn / Motorola project (in the period from 10/05/2006 to 10/31/2007). He has experience in Computer Science, acting on the following subjects: Software Test Engineering, Artificial Intelligence, Artificial Neural Networks, Hybrid Intelligent Systems, Handwriting Recognition, pattern recognition and Biomedical Engineering.

Maira Araujo de Santana has a Master's degree in Biomedical Engineering at the Federal University of Pernambuco (UFPE) and member of the Biomedical Computing Research Group. She holds a degree in Biomedical Engineering from the Federal University of Pernambuco (2017). She has fluency in Portuguese (native language) and English, as well as basic knowledge of Spanish and German. She completed an internship in Clinical Engineering at Hospital das Clínicas de Pernambuco (09/2016 - 01/2017). She was a Scholarship for Science for Borders Program of the Federal Government / CAPES in the United States for one year (edict 180: 08/2015 - 08/2016), of which nine months (08/2015 - 05/2016) were dedicated to She has a BA in Biomedical Engineering at the University of Alabama at Birmingham (UAB), AL (USA) and in the last three months (05/2016 - 08/2016) she worked as a researcher at the Carl E Ravin Advanced Imaging Laboratories (RAILabs) - Duke University, NC, USA - deepening specific knowledge of the area of image processing (sub-area of Biomedical Engineering) and acquiring experience in laboratory stage, scientific production, programming in MATLAB language and Office package.

* * *

Adriel dos Santos Araújo holds a master's degree in Computer Science at the Fluminense Federal University (2018) and a bachelor's degree in Information Systems at the Federal University of Mato Grosso (2015). His experiences involve acting mainly in projects in the fields of Computer Vision, Artificial Intelligence, Data Science, and Human-Computer Interaction. In recent years, he has been involved in research related to biomedical imaging for scientific applications. These studies support the medical diagnosis of diseases through infrared examinations. Currently, Adriel is a Ph.D. Student at the Fluminense Federal University.

Marcus C. Araújo is a professor and researcher at the Department of Mechanical Engineering from the Federal University of Pernambuco - Brazil. His current research interests include Bioengineering, Thermography and Heat Transfer in Medical Procedures.

Abir Baâzaoui is a PhD Student of Informatics at Université de Tunis El Manar, Institut Supérieur d'Informatique El Manar.

Valter Augusto de Freitas Barbosa received his Master's (2017) and Bachelor's (2014) in Biomedical Engineering from the Federal University of Pernambuco, Recife, Brazil. Actually his an Assistant Professor at the Department of Physics and is engaged in a Doctorate's in Mechanical Engineering at the Federal University of Pernambuco, Brazil, since 2017. His main research interests are biomedical instrumentation, image Diagnosis, breast cancer early diagnosis, thermography applications, intelligent systems for health, and evolutionary algorithms for optimizations.

Walid Barhoumi holds a Pre-PhD diploma (DEA) from the National Polytechnic Institute of Toulouse, a Ph.D. from the National School of Computer Science (Tunisia), and a Habilitation (HU) from the University of Carthage. From 2009 to 2010, he served as the ICT National Contact Point (ICT-NCP) of Tunisia in the context of the FP7 Program and since 2015 he is the ICT-NCP of Tunisia in the context of the Horizon 2020 Program. In 2006, he joined the National Engineering School of Carthage, where he is currently an Associate Professor.

Luciete Alves Bezerra holds a degree in Chemical Engineering from the Federal University of Pernambuco (UFPE) (2005), a master's degree in mechanical engineering from the Federal University of Pernambuco (2007) and a PhD in Mechanical Engineering from the Federal University of Pernambuco (2013). She is currently an Adjunct Professor in the Department of Mechanical Engineering at UFPE and her research areas are: Biomechanics, Heat Transfer, Computer Simulation, Dynamic Computational Fluids, Inverse Heat Transfer Problems and Thermography.

Aura Conci graduated in civil engineering with M.Sc. and Ph. D. in the same area. Professor of PUC-RJ from 1988 to 1994 and since 1994 at Universidade Federal Fluminense (UFF), where she works in computer science. Her main research areas are computer modeling, computer vision, image analysis and processing, bioinformatics and pattern recognition. She has oriented more than 100 students in all academic levels. Member of the International Society for Geometry and Graphics – ISGG (since 1998 and North America / South America vice-president from 2013 to 2020). Member of Brazilian Society of

Mechanical Science - ABCM (since 1989). She acts in the editorial office of a number of international journals and has cooperated on research with many scholars in various countries (e.g. Bosnia-Herzegovina, Canada, China, Cuba, Croatia, Ecuador, France, Romania, Spain, UAE and UK). She has a number of high quality publications, according to https://scholar.google.com.br/citations?user=lojRGVgAAAAJ &hl=en-BR: her total score has more than 2500 citations in general, where more than 1500 is related to citations of the last 5 years. She has grants from Brazilian government (she was has elaborated a number of works with a various remote regions in Brazil).and acts as coordinator or participant over 20 research projects under public resources from international agencies as well.

Amanda Lays Rodrigues da Silva graduated in Nursing (2014) and has a Master in Biomedical Engineering (2019) from the Federal University of Pernambuco. His research interests are digital medical image analysis, attribute selection, genetic algorithms and development of tools to support early diagnosis of breast cancer.

Maria Beatriz de Almeida is a Biomedical Engineering student at the Federal University of Pernambuco, Recife, Brazil.

José Filipe de Andrade is a Biomedical Engineering student at the Federal University of Pernambuco, Recife, Brazil.

Sidney Marlon de Lima holds a PhD in Computer Science from UFPE (Federal University of Pernambuco) and a Post-Doctorate in Computer Engineering from UPE (University of Pernambuco). In 2018, Sidney Lima was approved in 1st place in the public contest for Assistant Professor of the Department of Electronics and Systems of UFPE. Sidney Lima is currently an author and reviewer for Science Elsevier and also coordinates research lines at UPE's Stricto Sensu Masters in Computer Engineering. As for the laurels, Sidney Lima was the first engineer in the history of the UPE Computing Department to graduate before the conventional period. Sidney Lima became an engineer in 9 (nine) periods in a course of 10 (ten) periods. Similarly, Sidney Lima was the first master in all history of the UPE Computing Department to graduate early. Sidney Lima became a Master of Computer Engineering in three (3) semesters in a four (4) term program. At only 23 years old, Sidney Lima began his career as a university professor. The teacher has teaching experience at the undergraduate and postgraduate level, both in private colleges and in a public university.

Thifany Ketuli de Souza is a Biomedical Engineering student at the Federal University of Pernambuco, Recife, Brazil.

Nadja Espíndola is a PhD student in Mechanical Engineering at Federal University of Pernambuco (PPGEM - UFPE). Graduated in Mechanical Engineering from the University of Pernambuco (UPE / 1998), Master in Production Engineering (UFPE / 2011) and Mechanical Engineering (UFPE / 2017). Has professional experience in the area of production engineering, with emphasis on production management and quality management.

Juliana Gomes is a Biomedical Engineer (Federal University of Pernambuco, UFPE - 2016) with an international experience through the program Science without Borders (CAPES) in the United States, which provided know how in the Imaging Processing field. Master Degree in Biomedical Engineering program (UFPE), with scholarship by CAPES, and research in the Electrical Impedance Tomography field. PhD student in Computer Engineering (Polytechnic School of Pernambuco, UPE), with scholarship by FACEPE, and research in Neuroengineering field.

Abhimanyu Kumar Jha is presently working as Dean, Faculty of Life Sciences and Head, Department of Biotechnology at Institute of Applied Medicines and Research, Ghaziabad, Uttar Pradesh, India. Previously, he worked as Head in Department of Biotechnology, IMS Engineering College, Ghaziabad (U.P.), India. He did Ph.D. from Department of Biotechnology, Punjab University, Chandigarh (India). He has published 32 papers in international journals and 3 papers in national journals of repute, having good impact factors. He got 3 awards for best oral and poster presentation. He got the Young Scientist Travel Award from the Organizing Committee for presenting his research in International Congress on Cell Biology (ICCB) held at Seoul, South Korea in 2008. He has also published 9 book chapters in books published by Elsevier and Springer. He has delivered three keynote lectures, several invited talks and chaired the scientific sessions in several international as well as national conferences. He is presently working on the epidemiology and epigenetics of Oral Squamous Cell Carcinoma (OSCC) and Liver cancer. He is also working on Alzheimer's disease as well as the correlation of contaminants present in ground water with epigenetic changes in cancer.

Darko Kolarić, PhD, senior research fellow at the Ruđer Bošković Institute is a member of the Division of Electronics. During his career, he was the leader of several dozen national science and technology projects. He was a participant in a European Community projects. He is currently a participant in the project of the Croatian Science Foundation. He has led numerous development projects in the field of optoelectronics and computing. These projects resulted in a prototype model and series in the industry. The scientific and professional work to date includes 69 papers.

Clarisse Lins de Lima obtained her Bachelor's Degree in Biomedical Engineering in 2017, from the Federal University of Pernambuco, Brazil. Currently, she is working toward a Master's Degree in Biomedical Engineering from the Federal University of Pernambuco. Her main research interests are digital epidemiology, epidemics forecasting, serious games and applied artificial intelligence for health systems.

Rita de Cássia Fernandes de Lima holds a bachelor's degree in Physics, and a Master's and Doctorate degrees in Nuclear Engineering (sub-area: thermalhydraulics). Since 2005, her research interests are biomedical engineering, focusing on biological phenomena modeling, acting on the following topics: biomechanics, heat transfer in medical procedures, thermography, breast cancer detection and numerical simulations using the finite volume method. Nowadays, she is Full Professor at the Federal University of Pernambuco/Brazil.

Paulo Roberto Maciel Lyra is Full Professor in the Department of Mechanical Engi-neering at Federal University of Pernambuco (UFPE), where he is the Leader of the High Performance Computing on Computational Mechanics (PADMEC) group and Responsible for the Implantation and Head of the Research Institute on Petroleum and Energy LITPEG – UFPE, being also the head of the Scientific

Computation and Visualization Laboratory. He has been a Research Fellow from the Brazilian National Scientific Research Council (CNPq), and a Permanent Member of the Graduate Programs on Mechanical and on Civil Engineering. Lyra is a member of the Brazilian Association on Computational Methods in Engineering (ABMEC) General Council and a Brazilian representative in the International Association for Computational Mechanics (IACM) General Council, IACM Fellows Award 2020. Lyra holds the following degrees in Civil Engineer: BS from UFPE (1984), an MS (1988) from Federal University of Rio de Janeiro (COPPE-UFRJ) and a PhD (1994) from University of Wales at Swansea (UWS), with a postdoctoral assignment (Research Assistant) at UWS (1994-1995) and at Massachusetts Institute of Technology (MIT) (Visiting Associate Professor) (2002–2003). He has coauthored more than 350 research publications in referred journals and in conference proceedings on different subjects. His main research areas of interest are computational fluid dynamics, high performance computation, reservoir simulation and bioheatransfer.

João Roberto Ferreira de Melo was graduated in Mechanical Engineering at the Federal University of Pernambuco (UFPE) with one year of academic exchange at Institut National des Sciences Appliquées in Bourges-FR. He has received his M.Sc. degree in 2019 in the area of thermal processes and systems at UFPE. His work is focused on the development of a methodology based on thermographic images for the development of a more reliable three-dimensional model of patient's breast with abnormalities. Currently, he is working at the Federal Police Department of Brazil.

Maira Beatriz Moran graduated in Computer Science by the Universidade Estadual do Norte Fluminense Darcy Ribeiro (2015) and technician in Industrial Informatics by the Instituto Federal Fluminense (2010). Master in Computing by the Universidade Federal Fluminense (2018) and currently a PhD student in the same institution. Her research works cover mainly the following subjects: image processing and analysis, artificial intelligence and health information systems.

Iskra Alexandra Nola currently works as Associate Professor at Department of Environmental and Occupational Health and Sports Medicine. The area of scientific work and interests include public health emergencies; environmental factors and related health effects; sociological aspects of environmental health; health/medical tourism; air pollutants and related health effects; and harmful environmental/variable factors and related effects in cardiovascular and breast cancer patients. She teaches at several different subjects in the area of environmental health; health and public health risks in disaster risk management; genes and environment; crisis situations management etc. at graduate, postgraduate and doctoral levels, including study in English – graduate and postgraduate as well. She is a course leader of one subject at the postgraduate (doctoral) study of Biomedicine at the School of Medicine, University of Zagreb, and one at the postgraduate specialist interdisciplinary study on Crisis Management at the University of Zagreb. She has participated actively at seven research projects and currently she participates at two, at one of them she is a leader and principal investigator. She has held several invited lectures in health tourism domain. She is a mentor of about twenty graduate and postgraduate theses. She is a mentor of Student section of Public Health at Andrija Stampar School of Public Health, School of Medicine, University of Zagreb.

Jessiane Monica Pereira is a Master in Computer Engineering at UPE with emphasis in Artificial Intelligence, Renewable Energy Specialist at UNINTER, Graduate in Electrical Engineering at UNINASSAU (2017) and member of research group Development of Intelligent Systems to Support Complementary Diagnosis of Breast Cancer using Thermography from the Department of Biomedical Engineering of UFPE under the guidance of Professor Dr. Wellington Pinheiro dos Santos. With professional experience in Electrical Project Development in (Low Voltage), (Medium Voltage) and Network Connected Photovoltaic Systems. I also have a technical degree in electrotechnics from SENAI-PE (2011) and a Renewable Energy Systems technician from IFPE (2016). He is interested in the areas of Biomedical Computing, Neural Networks, Machine Learning and Pattern Recognition.

Kamila Queiroz is a PhD student in Mechanical Engineering at the Federal University of Pernambuco, in the area of Energy. Master in Mechanical Engineering, Federal University of Pernambuco, in the area of concentration in Thermal Processes and Systems (2016) .Graduation in Biomedical Engineering, Federal University of Pernambuco (2014). Currently, I am a professor at the Federal Institute of Education, Science and Technology of Rio Grande do Norte (IFRN), acting on the following subjects: bioengineering, thermography, and heat transmission.

Roger Resmini is a Computer Science from UNIR (Rondonópolis, Mato Grosso, Brazil) in 2008. Holds a Master's degree (2010) and a Doctor's degree in Computer Science at Federal Fluminense University (UFF, Niterói, Rio de Janeiro, Brazil) in 2016. Nowadays is Professor at Universidade Federal de Rondonópolis (UFR). Main interest are image analysis, smart cities, artificial intelligence, entrepreneurship and software development.

David Edson Ribeiro is a Computer Engineer from the University of Pernambuco (UPE-2010), holds a Master's degree in Biomedical Engineering in the field of Biomedical Computing from the Federal University of Pernambuco (UFPE-2018), and is an Electronic Technician with an emphasis on industrial automation from the Institute. Federal of Pernambuco (IFPE-2009). He is currently a laboratory technician in the area of computer science and information systems at the Federal University of Pernambuco acting by the Department of Nuclear Energy in support of teaching, research and extension. Has experience in Computer Engineering and Electronics, working in Embedded Systems, Computer Architecture, Industrial Electronics, Electronic Systems and Controls, Free Hardware, Electrical Impedance Tomography and technical, vocational and higher education.

Reiga Ramalho Ribeiro has a degree in Biomedical Engineering (2013) and a Master in Biomedical Engineering (2016) both from the Federal University of Pernambuco. He is currently a Clinical Engineer at the Cobrape-LEME-L + M-ANENGE Consortium providing consulting services to the Bahia State Department of Health. He has experience in the areas of Clinical Engineering, Medical Instrumentation and Computer Science, the latter acting on the following subjects: development of electronic circuits from an Arduino-based free hardware platform, digital image processing, digital signal processing, recognition of patterns, evolutionary computation and numerical methods. He is a member of the Biomedical Computing Research Group of the Department of Biomedical Engineering of the Federal University of Pernambuco.

Debasray Saha obtained his graduation in biotechnology major from Vidyasagar University, West Bengal, India (2015-2018). He is currently in his second year of post-graduation in biotechnology at Institute of Applied Medicines & Research, Ghaziabad, U.P., India. His undergraduate thesis focused on Multidrug –Resistant Bacteria with Activated and Diversified MDR in Kolkata Water: Ganga Action Plan and Heterogeneous Phyto-Antibiotics Tacking Superbug Spread in India. He is also worked on Profile of bacteria isolated from blood culture samples from a tertiary care center & the correlation with C-reactive protein (CRP) and Serum Procalcitonin from Apollo Gleneagles Hospitals, Kolkata, India. His research focus on Cancer Biology, Drug Development & Discovery. He has two publication in an International journal publish and three book chapter in Springer Nature.

Francisco George de Siqueira Santos received his M.D. from the Federal University of Pernambuco (UFPE). He works in Mastology at the Hospital das Clínicas da UFPE and is also the coordinator of the Mastology Department at the Gynecologic Clinical of the same hospital. He is an expert in evidence-based medicine, teaching undergraduates and interns at the Gynecology Department. He is also a member of the research group on breast cancer.

Ladjane Coelho dos Santos is an electronic engineer from the University of Pernambuco (1998). He received a master's degree in mechanical engineering from the Federal University of Pernambuco (2008) and a PhD in mechanical engineering from the Federal University of Pernambuco (2014). Now she is an effective professor at the Federal Institute of Sergipe. She has experience in the field of Electrical Engineering, and is interested in research on thermography, breast cancer, parametric analysis, computer simulation and coordinate measuring machine and weather station.

Renata Maria Cardoso Rodrigues de Souza is Associate Professor at Centro de Informática of the Universidade Federal de Pernambuco (UFPE). She has been fellowship researcher of the CNPq (Brazilian Agency) since 2010. She has published 97 articles in scientific journals and conferences. Her current research includes methods in Data Science such as supervised (regression) and unsupervised (clustering) learning and applied statistics.

Ricardo Emmanuel de Souza holds a degree in Electrical Engineering (Electronic modality) from the Federal University of Pernambuco - UFPE (1983), a master's degree in Physics from UFPE (1986) and a doctorate in Physics from UFPE (1991). He worked as a researcher in the area of industrial engineering at the Technological Institute of Pernambuco (ITEP) (1991-1995). He held a postdoctoral internship at the Department of Chemistry at the University of California (Berkeley) (1998-1999). He is a full professor at the UFPE Department of Biomedical Engineering. Research in physics has an emphasis on Nuclear Magnetic Resonance (NMR), acting mainly in the area of NMR imaging of biological materials and systems. In Physics and Biomedical Engineering, research involves the reconstruction and processing of NMR images, optical coherence tomography (OCT), electrical impedance tomography (TIE) and X-ray tomography. In Biomedical Engineering we develop research in the field. of biomedical electronic instrumentation for patient assessment, monitoring and therapy. In h-Museometry, research focuses on the study of photochemical degradation of paper collections and the development of methods for performing virtual unwinding and unfolding of paper, parchment or tissue documents through X-ray based techniques. In these areas of research, the researcher has also carried out scientific museology projects. He is a member of the Brazilian Society of Biomedical Engineering (SBEB). From September 2018 until August 2019, he was a visiting professor at the University of Évora, Portugal.

Neeraj Vaishnav obtained his graduation in Bio-science (Zoology, Botany, and Chemistry) major from University of Kota, Rajasthan, India (2015-2017). He is currently pursuing his second year of post-graduation in biotechnology at University of Rajasthan, Jaipur, Rajasthan, India. Presently he is working on "The Status of Promoter Hypermethylation of RASSF1A, Lats1 and Lats2 Genes in Liver Cancer among North Indian Population" from Institute of Applied Medicines and Research (IAMR), Ghaziabad, Uttar Pradesh, India. His research focus on Cancer Biology, Genetics or Epigenetics alterations, and Molecular biology.

Index

G

H

I

K

M

N

O

P

S

T

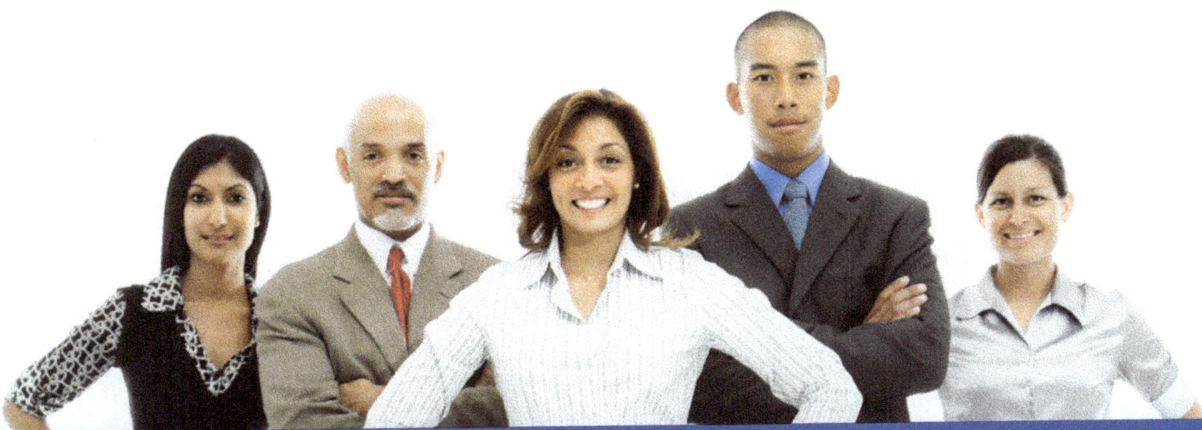

www.ingramcontent.com/pod-product-compliance
Lightning Source LLC
LaVergne TN
LVHW060302011026
849161LV00011B/2762